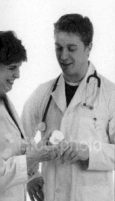

PHARMACY MANAGEMENT

ESSENTIALS FOR

ALL PRACTICE SETTINGS

Notice

Medicine is an ever-changing science. As new research and clinical experience broaden our knowledge, changes in treatment and drug therapy are required. The authors and the publisher of this work have checked with sources believed to be reliable in their efforts to provide information that is complete and generally in accord with the standards accepted at the time of publication. However, in view of the possibility of human error or changes in medical sciences, neither the authors nor the publisher nor any other party who has been involved in the preparation or publication of this work warrants that the information contained herein is in every respect accurate or complete, and they disclaim all responsibility for any errors or omissions or for the results obtained from use of the information contained in this work. Readers are encouraged to confirm the information contained herein with other sources. For example and in particular, readers are advised to check the product information sheet included in the package of each drug they plan to administer to be certain that the information contained in this work is accurate and that changes have not been made in the recommended dose or in the contraindications for administration. This recommendation is of particular importance in connection with new or infrequently used drugs.

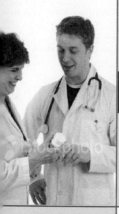

PHARMACY MANAGEMENT

ESSENTIALS FOR

ALL PRACTICE SETTINGS

FIFTH EDITION

David P. Zgarrick, PhD, FAPhA
Professor
School of Pharmacy
Bouvé College of Health Sciences
Northeastern University
Boston, Massachusetts

Greg L. Alston, PharmD
Professor and Associate Dean
South University Savannah Campus
Savannah, Georgia

Leticia R. Moczygemba, PharmD, PhD
Associate Professor
Health Outcomes Division
The University of Texas College of Pharmacy
Associate Director
Texas Center for Health Outcomes Research
    and Education
Austin, Texas

Shane P. Desselle, RPh, PhD, FAPhA
Professor, College of Pharmacy
Touro University California
Vallejo, California

McGraw Hill

New York   Chicago   San Francisco   Athens   London   Madrid   Mexico City
Milan   New Delhi   Singapore   Sydney   Toronto

Pharmacy Management: Essentials for All Practice Settings, Fifth Edition

Copyright © 2020 by McGraw Hill Education. All rights reserved. Printed in the United States of America. Except as permitted under the United States Copyright Act of 1976, no part of this publication may be reproduced or distributed in any form or by any means, or stored in a data base or retrieval system, without the prior written permission of the publisher.

1 2 3 4 5 6 7 8 9   LCR   24 23 22 21 20 19

ISBN 978-1-260-45638-7
MHID 1-260-45638-2

This book was set in Adobe Garamond Pro by Cenveo® Publisher Services.
The editors were Michael Weitz and Kim J. Davis.
The production supervisor was Richard Ruzycka.
Project management was provided by Sarika Gupta, Cenveo Publisher Services.
The cover designer was W2 Design.
Cover image credits: Getty Images and iStockphoto.

This book is printed on acid-free paper.

Library of Congress Cataloging-in-Publication Data

Names: Zgarrick, David P., editor. | Moczygemba, Leticia R., editor. | Alston, Greg L., editor. | Desselle,
    Shane P., editor.
Title: Pharmacy management : essentials for all practice settings / [edited by] David P. Zgarrick, Leticia R. Moczygemba,
    Greg L. Alston, Shane P. Desselle.
Description: Fifth edition. | New York : McGraw Hill, [2020] | Includes bibliographical references and index. | Summary:
    "The editors believed that there would be value in a comprehensive pharmacy management textbook that covered
    many content areas and gathered a variety of resources into one text. They also aimed to develop a text that uses
    "evidence-based management"; that is, material derived from the best and most contemporary primary literature,
    but that which at the same time focuses on the application of knowledge into skills that pharmacists will use every
    day"— Provided by publisher.
Identifiers: LCCN 2019022917 (print) | LCCN 2019022918 (ebook) | ISBN 9781260456387 (paperback) alk.
    paper | ISBN 9781260456394 (ebook)
Subjects: MESH: Pharmacy Administration | Pharmacies—organization & administration
Classification: LCC RS100 (print) | LCC RS100 (ebook) | NLM QV 737.1 | DDC 615/.1068—dc23
LC record available at https://lccn.loc.gov/2019022917
LC ebook record available at https://lccn.loc.gov/2019022918

McGraw Hill books are available at special quantity discounts to use as premiums and sales promotions, or for use in corporate training programs. To contact a representative, please visit the Contact Us page at www.mhprofessional.com.

CONTENTS

Contributors | ix

Preface | xiii

Acknowledgments | xvii

I. WHY STUDY MANAGEMENT IN PHARMACY SCHOOL?   1

Chapter 1   The "Management" in Medication Therapy Management   3
Chapter 2   Management Functions   21
Chapter 3   Leadership in Pharmacy Practice   35
Chapter 4   Ethical Decision-Making, Problem-Solving, and Delegating Authority   55
Chapter 5   Creating and Managing Value   75

II. MANAGING OPERATIONS   89

Chapter 6   Strategic Planning in Pharmacy Operations   91
Chapter 7   Business Planning for Pharmacy Programs   109
Chapter 8   Operations Management   127
Chapter 9   Managing Technology that Supports the Medication Use Process   141
Chapter 10   Ensuring Quality in Pharmacy Operations   161
Chapter 11   Risk Management in Contemporary Pharmacy Practice   187
Chapter 12   Preventing and Managing Medication Errors: The Pharmacist's Role   205
Chapter 13   Compliance with Regulations and Regulatory Bodies   233

III. MANAGING PEOPLE   253

Chapter 14   Managing Yourself for Success   255
Chapter 15   Negotiation Skills   275
Chapter 16   Organizational Structure and Behavior   293
Chapter 17   Human Resources Management Functions   325
Chapter 18   The Basics of Employment Law and Workplace Safety   347
Chapter 19   Pharmacy Technicians   367
Chapter 20   Performance Appraisal Systems   391

IV. MANAGING MONEY   415

Chapter 21   Financial Reports   417
Chapter 22   Budgeting   437
Chapter 23   Third-Party Payer Considerations   455

V. MANAGING TRADITIONAL GOODS AND SERVICES   481

Chapter 24   Marketing Fundamentals   483
Chapter 25   Marketing Applications   513
Chapter 26   Customer Service   535
Chapter 27   Supply Chain Management   557
Chapter 28   Merchandising   585

VI. MANAGING VALUE-ADDED SERVICES   607

Chapter 29   Value-Added Services as a Component of Enhancing Pharmacists' Roles in Public Health   609
Chapter 30   Implementing Value-Added Pharmacist Services   625

VII. MANAGEMENT APPLICATIONS IN SPECIFIC PHARMACY PRACTICE SETTINGS   655

Chapter 31   Entrepreneurship and Innovation   657
Chapter 32   Applications in Independent Community Pharmacy   671

Index | 695

CONTRIBUTORS

Jennifer L. Adams, PharmD, EdD
Clinical Associate Professor and Associate Dean for Academic Affairs, College of Pharmacy, Idaho State University, Sam and Aline Skaggs Health Science Center, Meridian, Idaho

Greg L. Alston, PharmD
Professor and Associate Dean, South University Savannah Campus, Savannah, Georgia
Chief Value Officer, Pharmacist Success Academy

Mitch Barnett, PharmD, MS
Associate Professor, Touro University California, Vallejo, California

John P. Bentley, PhD
Professor and Chair, Department of Pharmacy Administration, School of Pharmacy, University of Mississippi, University, Mississippi

Steve Boone
Pharmacy Insurance Practice Leader, Heffernan Insurance Brokers, Chesterfield, Missouri

Peter T. Bulatao, PharmD, MS, MMAS, BCPS, BCACP
Associate Professor, Pharmacy Practice, South University Savannah Campus, Savannah, Georgia

Leigh Ann Bynum, PhD
Associate Professor, Pharmaceutical Sciences, Belmont University College of Pharmacy, Nashville, Tennessee

Lauren M. Caldas, PharmD, BCACP
Assistant Professor, School of Pharmacy, Virginia Commonwealth University, Richmond, Virginia

Patrick J. Campbell, PharmD
Director of Measurement Outcomes Research, Pharmacy Quality Alliance, Alexandria, Virginia

Antoinette B. Coe, PharmD, PhD
Assistant Professor, University of Michigan College of Pharmacy, Ann Arbor, Michigan

Edward Cohen, PharmD
Executive Vice President, Pharmacy Advocacy, Michael J Hennessy Associates, Inc., Plainsboro, New Jersey

Michael R. Cohen, RPh, MS, ScD
Founder and President, Institute for Safe Medication Practices, Huntington Valley, Pennsylvania

Shane P. Desselle, RPh, PhD, FAPhA
Professor, College of Pharmacy, Touro University California, and President, Applied Pharmacy Solutions, Vallejo, California

Andrew J. Donnelly, PharmD, MBA
Director, Pharmacy Services, University of Illinois Hospital and Health Sciences System, Clinical Professor of Pharmacy Practice and Associate Dean for Clinical Affairs, University of Illinois at Chicago, College of Pharmacy, Chicago, Illinois

Brent I. Fox, PhD, PharmD
Associate Professor, Department of Health Outcomes Research and Policy, Harrison School of Pharmacy, Auburn University, Auburn, Alabama

Perry L. Fri
Executive Vice President of Industry Relations, Membership and Education, Healthcare Distribution Alliance (HDA) and Chief Operating Officer, HDA Research Foundation, Alexandria, Virginia

Eric Fromhart, PharmD
Co-founder and President, Secure340B.com, Philadelphia, Pennsylvania

Caroline M. Gaither, PhD
Professor, Department of Pharmaceutical Care and Health Systems, Senior Associate Dean, Professional Education Division, College of Pharmacy, University of Minnesota, Minneapolis, Minnesota

David Gettman, MBA, PhD
Professor, D'Youville College School of Pharmacy, Buffalo, New York

Matthew Grissinger, RPh, FISMP, FASCP
Director, Error Reporting Programs, Institute for Safe Medication Practices, Huntington Valley, Pennsylvania

Dana P. Hammer, RPh, PhD
Faculty Lead for Student Professional Development, Skaggs School of Pharmacy and Pharmaceutical Sciences, University of Colorado, Denver, Colorado

Karl M. Hess, PharmD, APh, CTH, FCPhA, AFTM RCPS (Glasg)
Associate Professor of Pharmacy Practice, Director, Community Pharmacy Practice Innovations, Department of Pharmacy Practice, Chapman University School of Pharmacy, Harry and Diane Rinker Health Science Campus, Irvine, California

Susan E. Higgins, MBA
Independent Management and Strategy Consulting Serving the Health Care Industry

Kenneth C. Hohmeier, PharmD
Associate Professor of Clinical Pharmacy and Translational Science, Director of Community Affairs, University of Tennessee Health Science Center College of Pharmacy, Memphis, Tennessee

Erin R. Holmes, PhD, PharmD
Associate Professor, University of Mississippi School of Pharmacy, Oxford, Mississippi

Jan M. Keresztes, PharmD, FASHP
Senior Educator, Pharmacy, Talent First PBC, Orland Park, Illinois

Michael L. Manolakis, PhD
Vice President, National Pharmacy Practice Group, Aon Consulting, Charlotte, North Carolina

Erna Mesic, MPH
Manager, Retail and Pharmacy Projects, Walgreens, Deerfield, Illinois

Leticia R. Moczygemba, PharmD, PhD
Associate Professor and Associate Director, Texas Center for Health Outcomes Research and Education, Health Outcomes Division, The University of Texas College of Pharmacy, Austin, Texas

Rashid Mosavin, PhD
Dean and Professor, College of Pharmacy and Health Sciences, Texas Southern University

Mel L. Nelson, PharmD
Director of Research and Academic Affairs, Pharmacy Quality Alliance, Alexandria, Virginia

Jacob T. Painter, PharmD, MBA, PhD
Associate Professor, Division of Pharmaceutical Evaluation and Policy, University of Arkansas for Medical Sciences, Little Rock, Arkansas

Evan T. Robinson, PhD
Dean and Professor, College of Pharmacy and Health Sciences, Creighton University, Omaha, Nebraska

Meagan Rosenthal, PhD
Assistant Professor, Department of Pharmacy Administration, University of Mississippi School of Pharmacy, Oxford, Mississippi

Thad Schumacher, PharmD
Pharmacist and Owner, Fitchburg Family Pharmacy, Fitchburg, Wisconsin

Glen T. Schumock, PharmD, MBA, PhD
Dean and Professor, University of Illinois at Chicago College of Pharmacy, Chicago, Illinois

Mark H. Siska, BS Pharm, MBA/TM
Chief Pharmacy Informatics Officer, Mayo Clinic, Rochester, Minnesota

Todd D. Sorenson, PharmD, FAPhA, FCCP
Professor and Associate Head, Department of Pharmaceutical Care and Health Systems, College of Pharmacy, University of Minnesota, Minneapolis, Minnesota

Rachel Sullivan
Project Manager, HDA Research Foundation, Alexandria, Virginia

Benjamin S. Teeter, PhD
Assistant Professor, University of Arkansas for Medical Sciences, Little Rock, Arkansas

Kyle M. Turner, PharmD, BCACP
Assistant Clinical Professor, University of Utah College of Pharmacy, Salt Lake City, Utah

Benjamin Y. Urick, PharmD, PhD
Research Assistant Professor, Center for Medication Optimization, Eshelman School of Pharmacy, University of North Carolina, Chapel Hill, North Carolina

Julie M. Urmie, PhD
Associate Professor, University of Iowa College of Pharmacy, Iowa City, Iowa

Terri L. Warholak, PhD, RPh
Professor and Assistant Dean of Academic Affairs and Assessment, University of Arizona College of Pharmacy, Tucson, Arizona

William Wynn, PharmD
Assistant Professor, Experiential Education Coordinator, and Director of Interprofessional Education, South University Columbia Campus, Columbia, South Carolina

David P. Zgarrick, PhD, FAPhA
Professor, School of Pharmacy, Bouvé College of Health Sciences, Northeastern University, Boston, Massachusetts

PREFACE

■ WHY DID WE CREATE THIS TEXTBOOK?

Pharmacy remains a very exciting profession; in fact, more opportunities are available for pharmacists, pharmacy students, and educators than ever before. The roles of pharmacists in interprofessional health care teams continue to evolve, as does their recognition by payers and policy makers. Pharmacists continue to transform the delivery of their services to accentuate the critical nature of public health and proactive health care. But with new opportunities also come challenges, including the challenge of how to manage the personal and professional resources necessary to succeed in today's ever-changing environment.

Educators must not only keep up with changes in pharmacy practice, but also anticipate and prepare our students for opportunities and contingencies that will arise throughout their professional careers. In our efforts to best prepare students, pharmacy management educators have increasingly had to gather teaching materials from a variety of textbooks, journals, and other educational resources. This is due to the fact that many resources only focus on a specific management function (marketing, personnel, accounting, and finance) or a specific practice setting (independent pharmacies, hospital pharmacies). We believed that there would be value in a comprehensive pharmacy management textbook that covered many content areas and gathered a variety of resources into one text. We also aimed to develop a text that uses "evidence-based management"; that is, material derived from the best and most contemporary primary literature, but that which at the same time focuses on the application of knowledge into skills that pharmacists will use every day.

■ NEW CONTENT IN THIS EDITION!

In planning for a fifth edition of this text, we sought input from faculty who teach pharmacy management, as well as from pharmacy students and pharmacists who apply management principles in their daily practice. We listened carefully to users also while scanning the latest advances in teaching strategies to produce the fifth edition. Of course, we also considered the many changes in pharmacy practice, management, and health systems reform that have occurred during the past few years.

- Every chapter has been updated to reflect the fluid nature of its respective management topic.
- New trends in the management literature are reflected in each of the chapters, including management trends within and beyond pharmacy.
- Some chapters have been revised substantially and with new authors to provide users of the text with the most relevant information. Examples include the following:
  - Sustaining medication therapy management services through implementation science as well as other models of care delivery, such as continuous medication monitoring (CoMM).
  - Leveraging leadership skills into practice by guiding change management, establishing a culture of employee self-motivation, extracting the most from your resources and infrastructure, all while advocating for your profession and the patients you serve.
  - Broadening our views of how pharmacists manage the supply chain, particularly to ensure that they can access safe and effective medications and other resources that are needed by their patients.

- Maintaining compliance with laws, rules, and regulations which impact a pharmacy manager's ability to care for patients and manage their practice.
- Developing new ways of organizing and managing our time for our own success and the success of others, particularly given the challenges and opportunities provided by social media and other forms of technology.

We have also added new chapters commensurate with contemporary pharmacy practice in anticipation of continually evolving models of care. These include:

- Ethical Decision Making, Problem Solving, and Delegating Authority, where pharmacists utilize appropriate judgment processes when faced with decisions of how to optimize care in the face of budgetary constraints and preferences of various stakeholders in the medication use process.
- Negotiation Skills, a skill needed through various components of practice, ranging from encouraging treatment adherence from patients, to requesting a change from the prescriber in a patient's medication regimen, to adjudicating a fair contract with a third-party payer for the services renders to covered enrolees.
- Pharmacy Technicians, the persons to whom pharmacists are increasingly delegating more responsibility and greater numbers of tasks that pharmacists used to perform so that they can now spend more time in direct patient care activities.

■ NEW FEATURES IN THIS EDITION!

Management education encompasses a broad constellation of knowledge, skills, abilities, and attitudes required to become an effective leader. It is difficult for instructors to possess the breadth of experience across all aspects of pharmacy management to intuitively design structured lesson plans to effectively educate their students. With that in mind, the editors of the fifth edition have developed tools to assist instructors with teaching the concepts covered in this book. Instructors who adopt the textbook will have full access to these resources which include: (1) PowerPoint™ slides that cover the core content of each chapter; (2) lesson plans built on the *Understanding by Design* model developed by Jay McTighe and Grant Wiggins. These plans guide the course leader through the three stages of lesson design: (1) focusing on the big ideas within the content; (2) crafting fair, valid, and reliable assessments of the desired results; and (3) creating an effective and engaging learning unit.

■ WHAT WILL THE READER FIND IN THIS TEXTBOOK?

This textbook is organized to reflect all of the major management functions performed by pharmacists in any practice setting. The book is divided into sections representing each function, and is further divided into chapters that detail the various components of each function.

Our experience as educators has taught us that students are the most effective learners when they are "ready" to learn. Many students selected pharmacy as a major in part from the desire to help people, but also due to their fascination and intrigue with how such small amounts of various medicinal substances have such profound effects on the body. Many of these students also believe that they only need to learn about management after they graduate, and then only if they take on a managerial or administrative position at their pharmacy. The first section of this book makes the case that management skills are important for all people and pharmacists, regardless of their position or practice setting. In an environment of increasingly scarce resources and higher accountability, we also help the reader to understand and create the value proposition for themselves, their services, and their organization. After establishing the need for management in both our personal and professional lives, the next four sections describe the management functions and resources that are common to all pharmacy practice settings (operations, people, money, traditional pharmacy goods and services). Chapters within each section focus on important aspects of each function or resource.

As pharmacy practice moves from a product orientation to a patient orientation, there are unique challenges that arise in managing the value-added services that pharmacists are developing to meet patient needs in medication therapy management. A section of this book is dedicated to the planning, implementation, and reimbursement of these new patient care services offered by pharmacists.

Several chapters are dedicated to describing the risks inherent in pharmacy practice and the impact that laws, regulations, and medication errors have on pharmacy management. The final section describes how management functions are applied by entrepreneurs and intrapreneurs in settings ranging from independently owned community pharmacies to those developing new goods, services, and ideas in any setting to meet needs related to medications and their use.

■ HOW EACH CHAPTER IS ORGANIZED?

Each chapter is divided into several sections to facilitate the reader's understanding and application of the material. Chapters begin with a list of learning objectives that outline the major topics to be addressed. A brief scenario is used to describe how a pharmacy student or pharmacist may need or apply the information described in this book in their daily lives or practice. Questions at the start of each chapter provide direction and assist the reader in understanding what they can expect to learn.

The text of each chapter provides comprehensive coverage of the content and theory underlying the major concepts. References to the management and pharmacy literature are commonly used to provide readers with links to additional background information. Explanations and applications are also used to help readers better understand the need to master and apply each concept. Questions at the end of each chapter encourage readers to think about what they have just learned and apply these concepts in new ways.

■ WHAT WE HOPE YOU WILL GAIN FROM THIS BOOK?

If you are a pharmacy student, we hope that using this book will help you gain an appreciation for the roles of management in pharmacy practice, regardless of your future position or practice setting. This book will also provide you with a variety of management theories and tools that you can apply in your daily life.

We realize that many pharmacists have not had much management coursework in their formal education or professional training. We hope that this book serves as a valuable guide to pharmacists who may require some assistance in dealing with matters they did not anticipate when embarking on their careers. For those pharmacists with formal management education and experience, we hope that this book serves as a valuable reference or as a source of new ideas that can be applied in daily practice.

For educators, this book has been designed as a comprehensive pharmacy management textbook. As a whole, it is meant to be used in survey courses that cover many areas of pharmacy management. The section format also allows the book to be used in courses that focus on specific pharmacy management functions or topics. The sections and content of each chapter are meant not only to provide valuable information that is easy for students to understand but also to stimulate further discussion and motivate students to learn more on their own.

■ WE WOULD LIKE TO HEAR FROM YOU!

The creators of each chapter have put a great deal of time and effort into getting their final outputs ready for consumers, but it rarely can be considered a "finished product." Textbooks are "works in progress" that can always be improved. The best way to improve these products is to seek input from our users. As you use this book, we would like to learn what you like about it, what could be improved, and what topics or features you would like to see included in the future. Please feel free to share your thoughts at any time by contacting us through *pharmacy@mcgraw-hill.com*. We plan to improve this book over future editions by listening to your feedback and continuing to reflect changes in the management sciences and pharmacy practice.

For Ancillaries, please go to the Pharmacy tab at:
https://www.mhprofessional.com/desselle5e

ACKNOWLEDGMENTS

We would like to thank the colleagues who have played an important role in our development throughout our undergraduate, professional, and graduate studies, as well as at our institutions. In addition, as our careers have advanced, we also have come to know many great academicians in other disciplines and other leaders in pharmacy who have greatly influenced our careers and provided keen guidance. We have learned so much from all these people and feel fortunate that they have been willing to share their knowledge and experience with us.

Thanks must also go to all the faculty, staff, and administrators at Northeastern University, University of Texas College of Pharmacy, South University Savannah Campus, and Touro University who have provided an environment that makes this type of endeavor possible. We would also like to thank all of the students we have taught who have inspired us to continue to strive to become better educators.

We would like to thank everyone at McGraw-Hill Education and, in particular, our editor, Michael Weitz, for working with us to improve this comprehensive pharmacy management textbook.

Finally, we would like to acknowledge the efforts of each of our chapter authors. We chose our authors not only because of their expertise but also because of their dedication to teaching and the professional development of pharmacy students and pharmacists. There is no way in which we could have completed this textbook without their efforts.

SECTION I

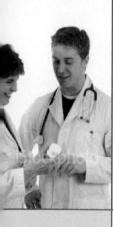

WHY STUDY MANAGEMENT IN PHARMACY SCHOOL?

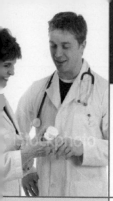

1

THE "MANAGEMENT" IN MEDICATION THERAPY MANAGEMENT

Shane P. Desselle, Leticia R. Moczygemba, David P. Zgarrick, and Greg L. Alston

About the Authors: Dr. Desselle is a professor of Social, Behavioral, and Administrative Pharmacy at Touro University California College of Pharmacy. His research program focuses on optimizing roles for pharmacy technicians, development of mentorship programs, and in promoting healthy organizational cultures and citizenship behaviors in professional settings. He is a Fulbright Specialist Scholar having completed a project to develop a Center of Assessment for the University of Pristina in Kosovo. Dr. Desselle is a Founding Editor-in-Chief of the international peer-reviewed journal, Research in Social and Administrative Pharmacy with graduate students and collaborations worldwide on various projects such as medication safety and medication adherence issues with informal caregivers. Dr. Desselle also is a primary author for the Pharmacy Management Tips of the Week on AccessPharmacy that accompany this textbook.

Dr. Moczygemba is an associate professor and associate director of the Texas Center for Health Outcomes Research and Education at The University of Texas College of Pharmacy. Her research program focuses on working with communities and health systems to mitigate health disparities by developing patient-centered interventions to optimize medication-related health outcomes. She has worked to advance the health care of homeless individuals, older adults, and those living in rural areas through the development, implementation, and evaluation of care models that integrate pharmacists with health care teams. She teaches in the health care systems course in the Doctor of Pharmacy (PharmD) program and is engaged in interprofessional education initiatives with a focus on quality improvement and patient safety.

Dr. Zgarrick is a professor in the School of Pharmacy at Northeastern University's Bouvé College of Health Sciences. He received a BS degree in pharmacy from the University of Wisconsin and a MS and PhD in pharmaceutical administration from the Ohio State University. He has practice experience in both independent and chain community pharmacy settings. He has taught courses in pharmacy management, business planning for professional services, and drug literature evaluation. His scholarly interests include pharmacist workforce research, pharmacy management and operations, pharmacy education, and the development of postgraduate programs.

Dr. Alston is Associate Dean and professor, Savannah Campus, South University School of Pharmacy. He has over 30 years of experience in community pharmacy management, both

3

as a chain pharmacy administrator and an independent pharmacy owner. He earned a Doctor of Pharmacy degree from the University of the Pacific and has published three best-selling management books, *The Bosshole Effect—Managing People Simplified* and *The Ten Things A New Manager Must Get Right From the Start,* and *Own Your Value- The Real Future of Pharmacy Practice.* His passion lies in teaching the next generation of pharmacists how to create value for the stakeholders they serve.

■ LEARNING OBJECTIVES

After completing this chapter, readers should be able to

1. Identify changes in the roles of pharmacists since the early 1900s.
2. Describe how pharmacy practitioners and educators viewed the need for management skills as the roles of pharmacists evolved.
3. Identify principal domains of pharmacy care.
4. Describe how management skills and functions fit within the context of providing medication therapy management services.
5. Identify myths surrounding the practice of pharmacy and health care as a business.
6. Evaluate the need for a management perspective to better serve patients and improve outcomes to drug therapy.
7. List the managerial sciences and describe their use as tools to assist pharmacists in practice.

■ SCENARIO

Stephanie Chen has just completed the first 2 years of a PharmD curriculum. Despite many long hours of hard work and a few anxious moments preparing for examinations, she has been pleased with her educational experience. She perceives that as she continues progressing through the curriculum, the upcoming courses will be more integrated and directly applicable to pharmacy practice. She is especially excited about taking courses in pharmacology and therapeutics so that she can "really learn about how to be a pharmacist." As she glances down at her schedule and sees that she is enrolled in a required course in pharmacy management, her enthusiasm becomes somewhat tempered. She immediately consults with fellow students on what they have heard about the course, and they tell her that the course is about "finance, accounting, personnel management, and marketing." Despite some positive comments provided by students having already completed the course, she is concerned. "What do I have to take this course for? I did not come to pharmacy school for this. I'm very good at science. If I liked this kind of stuff, I would have majored in business. How is this going to help me to become a better pharmacist?" she asks herself.

After some thought, she comes to realize that, at worst, taking this course will not be the end of the world, and even better, it simply might be a moderate intrusion in her Monday–Wednesday–Friday routine. She begins to focus on other issues, such as her part-time job at Middletown South Pharmacy. Lately, she has been dreading each day she goes to work there. The staff consistently seems rushed and impatient. There always seems to be conflict among the employees, and as soon as one fire has been put out, another larger one begins to burn. She regrets her decision to quit her job at Middletown North Pharmacy 3 months ago, even though it took 20 minutes longer to get there. Things always seemed to run smoothly at Middletown North. Mary even noticed that the patients at Middletown North seemed happier and healthier than those at Middletown South.

■ CHAPTER QUESTIONS

1. How have pharmacists' roles in delivering goods and services evolved over the past few decades? What roles and functions do pharmacists perform today?
2. What is the significance of management within the context of the profession's movement toward the provision of direct patient-care services such as medication therapy management? Why has its significance typically been overlooked by pharmacists and pharmacy students?
3. What are some of the myths surrounding the confluence of business practices and the provision of patient care by pharmacists?
4. What evidence exists that a business perspective is critical to provide effective pharmacy services to patients?
5. What are the managerial sciences, and how can pharmacists use them effectively?

■ INTRODUCTION

The preceding scenario, though perhaps overly simplistic, captures the feelings of many students who select pharmacy as a major. They generally are interested in science, have a desire to help people in need, and prefer a career offering long-term financial security. Given that the pharmacy curriculum consists of courses that apply knowledge from physics, chemistry, anatomy, physiology, and therapeutics, most pharmacy students achieved success in science and math courses throughout their pre-pharmacy studies (Keshishian et al., 2010). Second, students selecting pharmacy as a major typically are attracted to health care fields and may have contemplated nursing, medicine, or other health professions. Research has demonstrated that people in health care are caring

and empathic and seek personal reward and self-actualization through the helping of others (Meyer-Juncol., 2015, Pohontsch et al., 2018; Warshawski et al., 2018). Finally, many pharmacy students also consider the relatively high salaries of their chosen profession prior to choosing a college major and a career pathway. While few fields guarantee graduates a job, and certainly not one with entry-level salaries in the six figures, pharmacy students take comfort in knowing that employment in their profession will provide them with a generous and steady stream of income. It comes as no surprise that pharmacists and pharmacy students have been shown to be risk-averse individuals who do not deal with uncertainties particularly well (Latif, 2000; Leung et al., 2018). This further explains their gravitation toward science-oriented courses that offer straightforward solutions to problems.

Unbeknown to many pharmacy students is that the actual practice of pharmacy does not present a succession of problems that can be resolved in such a linear manner. While the sequential processes involved in community pharmacy practice have remained the same—patients present with prescriptions, pharmacy personnel fill them, and the necessary counseling is offered or provided by the pharmacist—a careful introspection reveals that the profession has undergone a rapid, head-turning transformation over just the past few decades. Pharmacists now are increasingly involved with providing direct patient-care services in addition to dispensing medications, and are taking greater responsibility for patients' outcomes arising from drug therapy. Pharmacists have become more integrated into health care delivery teams that coordinate patient care through the implementation of evidence-based guidelines and treatment algorithms. This has been even further accelerated by recent changes in states' pharmacist scope of practice regulations, collaborative practice agreements, reimbursement incentives from payers, and the reorganization of health care delivery into medical home models and accountable care organizations (George et al., 2018; Isasi & Krofah, 2015; McConaha et al., 2015).

For students to better understand the way that pharmacy is practiced today, time should be devoted to understanding the major forces that have shaped the profession. This chapter begins with a brief history of the evolution of pharmacy practice in the 20th century. This history, coupled with a snapshot of contemporary pharmacy practice, will make it clear that the past and current pharmacy practice models are as much about management as they are about clinical pharmacy practice. The chapter proceeds by pointing out myths about the exclusivity of the pharmacy business and patient outcomes and by providing evidence that what is best for the operation of a pharmacy business is often also best for the patients and other stakeholders that it serves. The chapter concludes with a brief discussion of the managerial sciences—tools that every practitioner will find useful at one point or another regardless of the practice setting. This chapter and all other succeeding chapters use an *evidence-based approach* to discuss pharmacy management, relying on recent literature and research findings to describe and explain what is happening in practice today. Students are encouraged to explore readings of interest among the references cited throughout the text.

■ A BRIEF HISTORICAL OVERVIEW OF PHARMACY PRACTICE

There have been several noteworthy efforts to describe the evolution of pharmacy practice. Some have described the process within the context of "waves," or shifts, in educational and industrial forces (Hepler, 1987), another through identifying stages of professional identity (Hepler & Strand, 1990), and still another through describing activation of pharmacists' services as stewards of public health in a medical care system increasingly challenging for patients to navigate (Blanchard et al., 2017). While these approaches appear quite different, their descriptions of the principal drivers of change closely mirror one another.

Pharmacy in the Early Twentieth Century
Pharmacy in the United States began in the 20th century much like it existed in the latter 1800s.

Pharmacy was, at best, a "marginal" profession. Most practitioners entered the occupation through apprenticeships rather than formal education. The pharmacist's principal job function was described as the "daily handling and preparing of remedies in common use" (Sonnedecker, 1963, p. 204). Pharmacists, or "apothecaries," were often engaged in the wholesale manufacture and distribution of medicinal products. Pharmacists' roles during this time were considerably different than they are today. In the early 20th century, pharmacists' primary roles were to procure raw ingredients and extemporaneously compound them into drug products for consumer use. While pharmacists had yet to achieve recognition as health care professionals, they often had considerable autonomy in their practice. There was no clear distinction between "prescription" and "nonprescription" drugs. Although physicians were engaged in the process of writing prescriptions, pharmacists were not precluded from dispensing preparations without a physician's order. Consumers commonly relied on their pharmacists' advice on minor ailments, and often entrusted the nickname of "doc" to their neighborhood pharmacist (Hepler, 1987).

Pharmacists had little choice but to have sharp business acumen to survive. Since few of the products they dispensed were prefabricated by manufacturers, pharmacists had to be adept at managing inventories of bulk chemicals and supplies used in compounding the preparations they dispensed. They also had to have a keen sense of how to manage time and people to accomplish a series of complex tasks throughout the workday.

A series of studies commissioned by the US government in the early 1900s produced what became known as the "Flexner reports" in 1915. These reports were critical for health care professionals and their education, including pharmacists. The reports questioned the validity and necessity of pharmacists as health care professionals. Shortly thereafter, the American Association of Colleges of Pharmacy (AACP) commissioned a study directed by W. W. Charters that ultimately served as the basis for requiring a 4-year baccalaureate degree program for all colleges of pharmacy (Hepler, 1987). These and other forces led to dramatic changes in pharmacy in the coming years.

Pharmacy in the Middle of the Twentieth Century

The 1940s through the 1960s often have been referred to as the "era of expansion" in health care (Smyrl, 2014). The Flexner reports paved the way for a more scientifically sound, empirically based allopathic branch of medicine to become the basis by which health care was practiced and organized. The federal government invested significant funds to expand the quantity and quality of health care services. The Hospital Survey and Construction (Hill-Burton) Act of 1946 provided considerable funding for the renovation and expansion of existing hospitals and the construction of new ones, primarily in underserved inner city and rural areas (Torrens, 1993).

Ironically, pharmacists began to see their roles diminish during this era of expansion in health care. Among the factors responsible for this decline were advances in technology and in the pharmaceutical sciences, coupled with societal demands that drug products become uniform in their composition. These brought about the mass production of prefabricated drug products in tablet, capsule, syrup, and elixir dosage forms, thus significantly reducing the need for pharmacists to compound prescription orders. The passage of the Durham–Humphrey amendment to the Food, Drug, and Cosmetic Act in 1951 created a prescription, or "legend," category of drugs. Pharmacists did not have the ability to dispense these drugs without an order from a licensed prescriber. Finally, pharmacy's own "Code of Ethics" promulgated by the American Pharmaceutical Association (APhA) stated that pharmacists were not to discuss the therapeutic effects or composition of a prescription with a patient (Buerki & Vottero, 1994, p. 93). This combination of forces relegated the role of the pharmacist largely to a dispenser of pre-prepared drug products.

The response of schools and colleges of pharmacy to these diminishing professional roles was the creation of curricula that were more technical, scientific, and content driven. A fifth year of education was added to the 4-year baccalaureate degree by colleges and schools of pharmacy during the late 1940s and early 1950s following the AACP Committee on Curriculum report entitled, "The Pharmaceutical Curriculum" (Hepler, 1987). It was during this time that pharmacology, pharmaceutics, and medicinal chemistry matured as disciplines and became the core of pharmacy education. Pharmacy students were required to memorize an abundance of information about the physical and chemical nature of drug products and dosage forms. Courses in the business aspects of pharmacy took a secondary role, whereas education in patient care (e.g., communications, therapeutics) was for all intents and purposes nonexistent.

With the APhA Code of Ethics suggesting that pharmacists not discuss drug therapies with patients, the profession lost sight of the need for pharmacists to communicate effectively with patients and other health care professionals. As the number of hospital and chain pharmacies expanded, resulting in pharmacists being more likely to be an employee than a business owner, the importance of practice management skills was not stressed in schools of pharmacy. Ironically, studies such as the "Dichter report" commissioned by the APhA revealed that consumers regarded pharmacists more as merchants than as health care professionals (Maine & Penna, 1996).

Pharmacy in the Latter Part of the Twentieth Century

The era of expansion slowed in the 1970s when society began to question the value obtained from the larger amount of resources being allocated toward health care. Congress passed the Health Maintenance Act of 1973, which helped to pave the way for health maintenance organizations (HMOs) to become an integral player in the delivery of health care services. Governments, rather than the private sector, took the lead in attempting to curb costs when they implemented a prospective payment system of reimbursement for Medicare hospitalizations based on categories of diagnosis-related groups (Pink, 1991).

In 1975 the Millis Commission's report, *Pharmacists for the Future: The Report of the Study Commission on Pharmacy* (Millis, 1975), suggested that pharmacists were inadequately prepared in systems analysis and management skills and had particular deficiencies in communicating with patients, physicians, and other health care professionals. A subsequent report suggested incorporating more of the behavioral and social sciences into pharmacy curricula and encouraged faculty participation and research into real problems inherent in pharmacy practice (Millis, 1976).

Prior to these reports, the American Society of Hospital Pharmacists had published *Mirror to Hospital Pharmacy* stating that pharmacy had lost its purpose, falling short of producing health care professionals capable of engendering change and noting that frustration and dissatisfaction among practitioners were beginning to affect students (Hepler, 1987, p. 371). The clinical pharmacy movement evolved in the 1970s to capture the essence of the drug use control concept forwarded by Brodie (1967) and promoted the pharmacist's role as therapeutic advisor. The clinical pharmacy movement brought about changes in pharmacy education and practice. After being introduced in 1948, the 6-year PharmD degree became the only entry-level degree offered by a small number of colleges of pharmacy as early as the late 1960s and early 1970s. The additional year of study was devoted mostly to therapeutics or "disease-oriented courses" and experiential education. The PharmD degree became the entry-level degree into the profession in the early 2000s, with colleges of pharmacy phasing out their baccalaureate programs.

These trends toward a more clinical practice approach may at first glance appear to be an ill-conceived response given recent changes in health care delivery. These changes placed a heightened concern over spiraling costs and have resulted in the deinstitutionalization of patients and the standardization of care using tools such as protocols, treatment algorithms, and disease-based therapeutic guidelines. Adoption of a clinical practice approach may also appear to fly in the face of changes in the organization of the pharmacy workforce and current market for pharmaceuticals. Studies have suggested that pharmacists willing and knowledgeable enough to provide patient-oriented clinical services face significant barriers when practicing in a community pharmacy environment (Blalock et al., 2013; Kennelty et al., 2015; Schommer & Gaither, 2014). In addition, the growth of mail order services in the outpatient pharmacy setting virtually excludes face-to-face consultation with patients. Mail order pharmacy has become a significant channel for the distribution of pharmaceuticals and is used by the Veterans Administration system and many pharmacy benefits managers. Many brick-and-mortar pharmacy operations now have a significant mail order component to their business as well. While providing consumers with a convenient way to obtain drug products, this form of commerce has the potential to further remove the pharmacist from patients and others who could benefit from their clinical services. Moreover, this trend has continued; at the time of writing this chapter, the massive e-retailer Amazon had begun its foray into the prescription drug market initially through the purchase of a company (PillPack) that delivers medication to patients through the mail in packaging aimed to improve patient adherence (LaVito & Hirsch, 2018). With Amazon's advantages in supply chain and operational cost-savings (see Chapter 27), this could provide for a momentous disruption in the prescription drug market. However, as described further in this chapter and in many places throughout the text, sometimes challenges such as this can end up being a boon to practice and with the proper management and leadership can be among a number of phenomena that could result in a greater opportunity for pharmacists to become more highly involved in direct patient-care activities.

■ PHARMACEUTICAL CARE AND MEDICATION THERAPY MANAGEMENT AS MANAGEMENT MOVEMENTS

With these changes in mind, adopting pharmaceutical care as a practice philosophy in the 1990s would have appeared "a day late and a dollar short" for both the profession and the patients it serves. And indeed, that might have been the case had the concept of *pharmaceutical care* been entirely clinical in nature. The originators of the concept fervently stressed that pharmaceutical care was not simply a list of clinically oriented activities to perform for each and every patient but was, in fact, a new mission and way of thinking that takes advantage of pharmacists' accessibility and the frequency to which they are engaged by patients—a way of thinking that engenders the pharmacist to take responsibility for managing a patient's drug therapy to resolve current problems and prevent future problems related to their medications.

It has been argued that the focus on preventing and resolving medication-related problems is simply an extension of *risk management* (Heringa et al., 2016 see also Chapter 11). Risks are an inherent part of any business activity, including the provision of pharmacy services. Common risks to a business include fire, natural disasters, theft, economic downturns, and employee turnover, as well as the fact that there is no guarantee that consumers will accept or adopt any good or service that the business offers. The practice of pharmacy involves additional risks, specifically the risk that patients will suffer untoward events as a result of their drug therapy or from errors in the medication dispensing process. These events are significant because they may result in significant harm and even death to a patient. They can also harm pharmacists and their businesses. Risk management suggests that risk cannot be avoided entirely, but rather it should be assessed, measured, and reduced to some feasible extent (Flyvbjerg, 2006).

The idea that pharmaceutical care should be viewed strictly as a clinical movement was called into question (Wilkin, 1999). Evidence that pharmaceutical care existed in part as a management movement was provided in a study that sought to identify standards of practice for providing pharmaceutical care (Desselle, 1997). A nationwide panel of experts identified 52 standards of pharmacy practice, only to have a statewide sample of pharmacists judge many of them as unfeasible to implement in everyday practice. Of the practice standards that were judged to be feasible, the researchers constructed a system of "factors" or

"domains" in which these standards could be classified (Desselle & Rappaport, 1995). These practice domains can be found in Table 1-1. Figuring prominently into this classification was the "risk management" domain, which included activities related to documentation, drug review, triage, and dosage calculations. However, the contributions of the managerial sciences do not stop there. The remaining four domains connote significant involvement by pharmacists into managerial processes. Two of the domains ("services marketing" and "business management") are named specifically after managerial functions.

From Pharmaceutical Care to Medication Therapy Management and Other Paradigms

While the pharmaceutical care movement made an indelible mark on the profession, its use in the modern lexicon describing pharmacists' services is fading. It has been replaced with terminology that more accurately reflects pharmacists' growing roles in the provision of public health services and reorganization of care into medical homes. In recognizing the morbidity and mortality resulting from medication errors as a public health problem, the profession embraced the concept of medication therapy management (MTM). MTM represents a comprehensive and proactive approach to help patients maximize the benefits from drug therapy and includes services aimed to facilitate or improve patient adherence to drug therapy, educate entire populations of persons, conduct wellness programs, and become more intimately involved in disease management and monitoring. The MTM movement has been strengthened by language in the Medicare Prescription Drug, Improvement and Modernization Act (MMA) of 2003 (Public Law Number 108–173, 2010), which mandates payment for MTM services and proffers pharmacists as viable health professionals that may offer such services. The place of MTM in health care delivery was advanced even further in the Patient Protection and Affordable Care Act, which established pilots for integrated care delivery, comprehensive medication review for Medicare beneficiaries, and grants specifically for MTM programs (Public Law Number 111–148, 2010). As

Table 1-1.   Pharmacy Care Practice Domains

I. *Risk management*
Devise system of data collection
Perform prospective drug utilization review
Document therapeutic interventions and activities
Obtain over-the-counter medication history
Calculate dosages for drugs with a narrow therapeutic index and special populations, such as children and older adults
Report adverse drug events to FDA
Triage patients' needs for proper referral
Remain abreast of newly uncovered adverse effects and drug–drug interactions

II. *Patient-centered care delivery*
Serve as patient advocate with respect to social, economic, and psychological barriers to drug therapy
Attempt to change patients' medication orders when barriers to adherence exist
Counsel patients on new and refill medications as necessary
Promote patient wellness
Maintain caring, friendly relationship with patients
Telephone patients to obtain medication orders called in and not picked up

III. *Disease and medication therapy management*
Provide information to patients on how to manage their disease state/conditions and medication regimens
Monitor patients' progress resulting from pharmacotherapy
Carry inventory of products necessary for patients to execute and monitor a therapeutic plan (e.g., -inhalers, nebulizers, glucose monitors)
Supply patients with information on support and educational groups (e.g., American Diabetes Association, Multiple Sclerosis Society)

IV. *Pharmacy care services marketing*
Meet prominent prescribers in the local area of practice
Be an active member of professional associations that support the concept of pharmaceutical care
Make available an area for private consultation services for patients as necessary
Identify software that facilitates pharmacists' patient care–related activities

V. *Business management*
Utilize technicians and other staff to free up the pharmacist's time
Identify opportunities for billing and reimbursement of pharmacist services

such, MTM is now considered a key component in the provision of pharmacy care services.

Pharmacy has seldom come short in developing new acronyms and proposed models of practice. Moving beyond MTM, the concept of comprehensive medication management (CMM) is designed to optimize medication-related medication outcomes

in collaborative practice environments (American College of Clinical Pharmacy, 2015). This is light of emphasis on patient-centered, team-based care and increasingly linked to reimbursement through pay-for-performance, even while those reimbursement systems do not always recognize clinical pharmacy services as uniquely billable. It focuses attention on high-risk medications and/or high-risk patients. Another model, Continuous Medication Monitoring (CoMM), on the other hand, occurs in community pharmacy settings and is proposed to monitor all medications for drug therapy problems for all patients and seeks to take advantage of and seize efficiencies from bundling clinical services with the process of dispensing (Goedken et al., 2018).

The Commonality of Management and Leadership

A cynic could potentially be critical of the need for this many practice paradigms and acronyms; however, each has their place and speaks to subtleties that might be more or less in the vernacular preferred or used by the audience for which they are intended. Regardless of the paradigm being described, management concepts and leadership are paramount for their optimal execution. This is reflected in the revised Standards 2016 from the American Council for Pharmacy Education (ACPE), which places requirements for curricular and other types of outcomes among US colleges/schools of pharmacy (American Council for Pharmacy Education, 2015). Standard 1 on foundational knowledge for curriculums refers to administrative sciences; standard 2 on essentials for practice and care refers to key elements in medication use systems management along with designing strategies for wellness and population-based care; standard 3 on approach to practice and care refers to problem-solving, patient advocacy, and communication; standard 4 on personal and professional development refers to leadership and innovation, and professionalism; and other standards refer to the leadership and management of the institution, itself, including its organizational culture, innovation, strategic plan, mission, vision, governance, and change planning. These factors have all been shown to be indispensable in promoting advanced pharmacy care services (Rosenthal et al., 2016) and in promoting a culture of safety (Sawan et al., 2017). As such, professional pharmacy organizations and education regulators recognize the momentous contribution of management and leadership in MTM and other practice paradigms.

■ MYTHS CONCERNING THE CONFLUENCE OF BUSINESS PRACTICE AND PHARMACY

Despite evidence that would suggest otherwise, the need for a management perspective in pharmacy is often overlooked by some pharmacy students and practitioners. Common misconceptions about the need for a management perspective have been documented (Tootelian & Gaedeke, 1993, p. 23):

- *The practice of pharmacy is ethically inconsistent with good business.* The origin of this myth probably evolved from the unethical business practices of some organizations. Scandals involving abuses by corporate executives at large international firms in the early 2000s have done little to mitigate these perceptions. Physicians, pharmacists, and other professionals who commit insurance fraud or knowingly bill for goods and services they did not provide demonstrate that health care professions are not without unscrupulous members (Agar, 2015). Furthermore, some people believe that companies involved in the sale of health care goods and services should be philanthropic in nature and are upset that companies profit from consumers' medical needs. Despite occasional examples of misconduct, most companies and persons involved in business operations conduct themselves in an appropriate manner.
- *Business is not a profession guided by ethical standards.* Pharmacists and pharmacy students are generally cognizant of the vast number of rules and regulations that govern pharmacy, but are less aware of the standards governing practice in advertising, accounting, and interstate commerce. Many of the rules and regulations governing pharmacy practice were borrowed from legislation existing in sectors other than health care.
- *In business, quality of care is secondary to generating profits.* This misconception likely results from the efforts by payers of health care and by managers to control costs. In light of the fact that in 2015 health care accounted for 17.2%

of the United States' gross national product and cost $9,892 per person (Organisation for Economic Co-operation and Development [OECD], 2017), health care consumers have little choice but to become more discerning shoppers of health care goods and services. Because resources are limited, the number of goods and services provided to consumers cannot be boundless. Conscientiousness in the allocation of resources helps to ensure that more of the right people receive the right goods and services at the right time and place. Many people do not stop to think that if a company in the health care business is not able to pay its own workforce and cover its other costs of doing business, it will have little choice but to close its doors, leaving a void in the array of goods and services previously afforded to consumers. Even not-for-profit entities have to pay the bills, because if they cannot break even, they too have to shut down operations. Students may be surprised to learn that most not-for-profit companies in health care both depend on and compete with companies that are structured on a for-profit basis.

- *The good pharmacist is one who is a "clinical purist."* This is perhaps a manifestation of the other misconceptions, in addition to a false pretense that the complexities of modern drug therapy do not allow time for concern with other matters. On the contrary, a lack of knowledge on how to manage resources and a lack of understanding on how to work within the current system of health care delivery only impede pharmacists' ability to provide MTM and other patient-care services. Pharmacists who "don't want to be bothered with management" face the same logistical constraints, such as formularies, generic substitution, prior authorizations, limited networks, employee conflict and lack of productivity, breakdowns in computer hardware and software, budgetary limitations, and changes in policy, that all other pharmacists face. The problem with the "don't want to be bothered with management" pharmacists is that they will be less likely to operate efficiently within the system, becoming frustrated and ultimately less clinically effective

than the pharmacists who accept these challenges as part of their practice.

The profession has come under more intense pressure to reduce the incidence of medication errors in both institutional and ambulatory settings (Institute of Medicine, 2006). This is placing a burden on pharmacists to be especially productive, efficient, and error-free. Productivity is a function of a pharmacist's ability to manage workflow, technology, the quality and efficiency of support personnel, phone calls, and other problems that arise in day-to-day practice.

Moreover, pharmacy administrators reward pharmacists who can manage a pharmacy practice. New PharmD graduates may obtain entry-level administrative positions (e.g., pharmacy department manager, area manager, clinical coordinator) within their first few years of practice. It is not uncommon to see pharmacy graduates move up into even higher-level administrative positions (e.g., district or regional manager of a chain, associate director or director of a hospital pharmacy department) within 5 to 10 years of graduation. Pharmacists who can manage a practice successfully (i.e., reduce errors, engender patient satisfaction, improve profitability, reduce employee turnover) are in the best position for promotions.

A final point to consider is that even if a pharmacist does not ascend to an administrative position, that person inherently "manages" a practice the instant he or she takes a position as a pharmacist. Staff pharmacists in every practice setting manage technicians, clerks, and other personnel every hour of every day. They also manage the flow of work through their sites and the use of medications by patients. Closely tied to this issue is the issue of personal job satisfaction. The pressures on the modern pharmacist are unmistakable. Satisfaction with one's job and career are important because they are closely related to one's satisfaction with life (Gubbins et al., 2015). Pharmacists' ability to manage their work environment can have a significant impact on their ability to cope with the daily stressors of practice, increasing job satisfaction, and diminishing the likelihood of career burnout or impairment through the abuse of alcohol and drugs.

■ GOOD MANAGEMENT PRACTICE AND MEDICATION THERAPY MANAGEMENT—A WINNING COMBINATION

Evidence of the success of a management perspective in pharmacy practice abounds. A series of studies examined the use of strategic planning by pharmacists in both community and hospital settings (Harrison & Bootman, 1994; Harrison & Ortmeier, 1995, 1996). These studies showed that among community pharmacy owners, those who fully incorporated strategic planning saw higher sales volume and profitability than did those who did not. Pharmacies owned by "strategic planners" were also significantly more likely to offer clinical or value-added services than pharmacies run by owners who were not. Likewise, better administrative, distributive, and clinical performance among hospital pharmacies was also associated with their respective directors' involvement in the strategic planning process. Since that time, professional organizations in recognizing the importance of strategic planning have published environmental forecasts to encourage and facilitate strategic planning and organizational structuring (Killingsworth & Eschenbacher, 2018; Vermeulen et al., 2019).

Another study pointed out that support from supervisors and colleagues had a positive impact on the commitment that pharmacists display toward their respective organizations, thus enhancing the likelihood that these pharmacists would not quit their jobs (Gaither, 1998). It has also been reported that pharmacists' effectiveness in managing personnel, particularly the provision of timely feedback, was associated with the quality of care provided to patients (Patterson et al., 2017), and pharmacists designating themselves as "managers" were less satisfied with their own jobs, likely as a result of their lack of managerial training (Ferguson et al., 2011).

Surveys of pharmacists commonly indicate that, looking at their practices today, they wish they had more training in management during their professional education. It has been reported that inadequate staffing, lack of time, reimbursement challenges, and poor communication with patients and providers are obstacles to delivering pharmacy care services (Blake et al., 2009; Law et al., 2009; Moczygemba et al., 2012; Robinson et al., 2016; Shah & Chawla, 2011). Studies have concluded that it would benefit practicing pharmacists to seek continuing education in management, business plan development, health care systems and policy, and pharmacotherapeutics (Blake et al., 2009; Shah & Chawla, 2011). It has been argued that to achieve excellence in the implementation of MTM services, pharmacists must obtain and properly allocate resources, design efficient distribution systems, select and train adequate support staff, develop systems for disseminating knowledge on new drugs and technology, and document and evaluate the cost-effectiveness of the services provided—all of which are tasks that require management skills (Brummel et al., 2014).

Table 1-2 summarizes many of the principal factors that affect the delivery of pharmacy goods and services and is used to further illustrate the existing synergy between patient care and good business practice. First, the demographic composition of the patient population has changed dramatically. The mean age of Americans continues to increase, as does their life expectancy. This results in a greater proportion of patients presenting with multiple disease states and complex therapeutic regimens. Although many of our nation's seniors lead normal, productive lives, their visual acuity, sense of hearing, mobility, and ability to use and/or obtain viable transportation may be compromised. Pharmacists must take on additional responsibilities in managing these patients' care and coordinating their services. Also, the population of patients that pharmacists serve is becoming more diverse in age/generational beliefs, race/ethnicity, socioeconomic status, and in other ways. Good pharmacy managers will benefit from a heightened sensitivity toward the needs of all patients and efforts to provide goods and services that appeal to specific populations.

The shift in the demographic composition of patients also brings to bear the varying beliefs people

Table 1-2.	Factors Affecting the Delivery of Pharmacy Goods and Services

Patient demographics
  Aging population
  Females as decision makers
  Ethnic composition of patients
Attitudes and belief systems
  Beliefs about disease, sick role, and medication taking
  Trust in the health care delivery system
  Direct-to-consumer advertising of prescription drugs
Third-party payers and coverage issues
  Complexity/differences among payers' policies
  Formularies
  Limited networks
  Limited access for some patients
  Lack of knowledge by patients
Competitive markets
  Diminished margins
  Diversity in the types of providers offering products and services
Technology
  Software
  Automated dispensing technology

have about treating their disease states, taking medications, and their trust in the health care delivery system. All the clinical and scientific knowledge in the world is rendered useless if pharmacists lack basic knowledge about the patients whom they serve. Even the most carefully devised and therapeutically correct medication care plan will not work if the patient does not put faith in the pharmacist's recommendations. Good pharmacists are able to relate to patients of all persuasions and convince them to put faith in the consultation they provide. This requires cultural competence by pharmacists and other pharmacy personnel. An additional consideration is the increased marketing of health care products directly to consumers. This has resulted inevitably in an increase in the frequency of medication-specific queries from patients. Good

pharmacists do not bias their answers but are able to triage the patient's request with appropriate information and recommendations.

A management perspective is essential when it comes to issues dealing with third-party payers (e.g., private insurers, government-sponsored programs—see Chapter 23). Unlike other countries, whose health care systems are founded on single-payer reimbursement structures, practitioners in the United States face a mix of payers, including individual patients, private insurers, employers, and government health plans. Each payer differs in its formularies (list of approved drugs), rules for reimbursement, quality indicators, and the network of pharmacists qualified to accept its coverage. Pharmacists must identify payers that compensate their practices to provide high-quality patient care, while at the same time managing their own resources to maintain an appropriate level of profit. Pharmacists must provide information about insurance coverage to patients, particularly those with low health literacy, who often do not know about the intricacies of their plans and the health care system (Loignon et al., 2018). In addition, pharmacists must coordinate therapeutic plans for patients whose financial situation may preclude them from receiving certain therapies and services.

An additional challenge facing pharmacies and pharmacists is that of shrinking profit margins. A pharmacy's net profit margin is the excess of revenues after covering expenses that it secures as a percentage of its total revenues. As the percentage of prescriptions paid for by sources other than patients has increased, pharmacy profit margins have decreased. In addition to selecting the right mix of plans in which to participate, pharmacists must seek other opportunities to bring in additional revenues and decrease expenses, such as implementing patient-care services, selling ancillary products, effectively purchasing and maintaining proper levels of inventory, effective marketing, and having the appropriate amount and type of personnel needed to do the job. This is especially important in light of the fact that consumers have more choices than ever in seeking health care solutions, ranging from nontraditional sources (complementary and alternative medicine) to more traditional sources (grocery stores, convenience stores, gift shops, the Internet).

Pharmacists must also maintain technologies that enhance the dispensing and drug distribution processes, enable the provision of clinical services, and manage information used to make business and patient care decisions (see Chapter 9). Effectively managing technology gives pharmacists more time to provide patient care and perform other practice and management functions.

Changes in the legal and regulatory environments (see Chapter 13), which have impacted both the types of goods and services pharmacists may provide as well as their levels of reimbursement, further underscore the need for practice management skills among pharmacists. In addition to knowledge required to help patients navigate the health care system, pharmacists must be able to maximize efficiency in human, capital, and technological resources to serve patients, provide services, and take advantage of the unique opportunities arising to gain reimbursement for their goods and services.

■ THE MANAGERIAL SCIENCES

Although mentioned throughout this chapter, a more formal examination of the managerial sciences should put into perspective their use as tools to implement pharmacy services effectively. The managerial sciences are summarized in Table 1-3. The reason they are referred to as *sciences* is that their proper application stems from the scientific process of inquiry, much the same as with other pharmaceutical sciences. The science of *accounting* (see Chapter 21) involves "keeping the books," or adequately keeping track of the business' transactions, such as sales revenues, wages paid to employees, prescription product purchases from suppliers, rent, and utility bills. This must be done to ensure that the company is meeting its debts and achieving its financial goals. Accounting is also used to determine the amount of taxes owed, make reports to external agencies and/or auditors, and identify

areas where the company's assets could be managed more efficiently. While accounting is used to evaluate a company's financial position, *finance* is more concerned with the sources and uses of funds (e.g., Where will the money come from to pay for new and existing goods and services? Which goods and services are most likely to enhance profitability for a pharmacy?).

The other managerial science commonly associated with managing money is *economics*. Economics is a tool to evaluate the inputs and outcomes of any number of processes, including and even transcending financial considerations. It can be used to determine the right mix of personnel and automated dispensing technologies, the optimal number of prescriptions dispensed given current staffing levels, whether or not a pharmacy should remain open for additional hours of business, and how much to invest in theft deterrence. It is also used to determine the most appropriate drugs to place on a formulary or to include in a critical pathway.

Human resources management (HRM, see Chapter 17) is used to optimize the productivity of any pharmacy's most critical asset—its people. It involves determining the jobs that need to be done, recruiting people for those jobs, hiring the right persons for those jobs, training them appropriately, appraising their performance, motivating them, and seeing that they are justly rewarded for their efforts. Pharmacy managers are beginning to realize the value in support personnel, particularly technicians, if they are going to transform their practice to include more direct patient-care services (see Chapter 19). HRM also involves issues such as determining the right mix of fringe benefits and retirement, setting vacation and absentee policies, assistance with career planning, ensuring employees' on-the-job safety, and complying with laws and rules established by regulatory bodies. Melding HRM with other aspects of management requires excellent leadership skills (see Chapter 3).

It may be easy to assume that *marketing* is simply another word for *advertising* (see Chapters 24 and 25). While promotional activities are a significant component of marketing, its activities include identifying the company's strengths over

Table 1-3.   The Managerial Sciences

Accounting
  Keep the books
  Record financial transactions
  Prepare financial statements
  Manage cash flows
  Analysis of profitability
  Determine business strengths and weaknesses
  Compute taxes owed to federal, state, and
    local governments
Finance
  Determine financial needs
  Identify sources of capital
  Develop operating budgets
  Invest profits
  Manage assets
Economics
  Determine optimal mix of labor and capital
  Determine optimal output
  Determine optimal hours of business operation
  Determine levels of investment into risk
    management
Human resources management
  Conduct job analyses
  Hire personnel
  Orient and train personnel
  Motivate personnel for performance
  Appraise personnel performance
  Allocate organizational rewards
  Terminate employment

Marketing
  Identify competitive advantages
  Implement competitive advantages
  Identify target markets
  Evaluate promotional strategies
  Implement promotional strategies
  Evaluate promotional strategies
  Select proper mix of merchandise
  Properly arrange and merchandise products
  Price goods and services
Operations management
  Design workflow
  Control purchasing and inventory
  Perform continuous quality improvement
    initiatives
Value creation
  Sell yourself and/or your ideas to stakeholders
  Leverage knowledge and skill sets to enhance
    success
  Develop or enhance a process or good that
    enhances a stakeholder's position
  Leverage existing knowledge, skills, and
    abilities to develop a product or service
    offering for stakeholders:
  At the correct price
  With the proper amount of additional service
  To be freely chosen as a viable alternative
    in the marketplace

its competitors, properly identifying consumers to which marketing strategies will be directed, carrying the right mix of goods and services, arranging these products for optimal "visual selling," and establishing the right prices for goods and services. Price setting is critical not only for goods but also especially important for services, particularly MTM and other patient-care services that are increasingly becoming part of pharmacy practice.

Operations management (see Chapter 8) involves establishing policies delineating the activities of each employee on a day-to-day basis, what tools they will use to accomplish the tasks, and where those tasks will be performed (i.e., workflow design). It also entails maintaining the proper inventory of prescription and nonprescription products so that, on the one hand, the pharmacy is not consistently running out of drug products that patients need, and on the other hand, there are not excess amounts of products reaching their expiration date prior to sale or otherwise taking up valuable space that could be used for other purposes (see Chapter 27).

Knowledge and skill sets in each of these areas assist and inform yet another very important component of management, which is *value creation*, which can be defined as the art of utilizing foundational assets (e.g., knowledge, skills, and experiences) to generate the ability to create value for other stakeholders in the health care marketplace. This not only employs some aspect of personal selling but also requires a firm grasp of internal and external environments to help individual and organizations gain the most from current resources, and/or acquire needed resources to improve a business or create a new niche. In that way, it is an application of all the other managerial sciences and will be elaborated upon in Chapter 5.

■ SMOOTH OPERATIONS— REVISITING THE SCENARIO

The preceding discussion of the managerial sciences, especially the issue of workflow design in operations management, brings us back to the scenario involving Stephanie Chen. Pharmacy students questioning the significance of management and the importance of having a management perspective need not look much further than this case. Stephanie is faced with a dilemma all too common to pharmacy students and practitioners. Students and pharmacists can likely recall that at some practice sites things just seemed to be "going well." Both the customers and the employers were happy, and it was pleasant to come to work. At other practice sites there always appears to be a crisis. While this may be an oversimplification, the latter sites are not being managed well, whereas the former ones probably are. The tremendous variability that exists from one workplace to another is indicative of how critical management is for both the employees working there and the patients they serve. Now ask yourself: Where do you think that you would rather work, and where do you think that patients are receiving the best care, Middletown North Pharmacy or Middletown South Pharmacy?

■ CONCLUSION

Contrary to popular belief, good business practice and good patient care are not mutually exclusive. In fact, they are almost entirely mutually dependent. Superior

1. Would you be willing to extend your commute or make other similar sacrifices to work at a place where you enjoyed your job? Why or why not?
2. How do you feel about the role that management plays in the practice of pharmacy?
3. Can you identify someone in a managerial position who is very good at what he or she does? What is it that makes him or her effective?
4. Do you believe that you are going to be an effective pharmacist? What makes you think so?
5. Do you think that you are going to ascend eventually to a managerial position? Why or why not?

patient care and the implementation of clinical services are made possible by pharmacists who are skilled in management. Pharmacists must be attuned to the internal and external forces that shape the practice of pharmacy. The managerial sciences of accounting, finance, economics, HRM, marketing, and operations management are indispensable tools for today's practitioner.

REFERENCES

Accreditation Council for Pharmacy Education (ACPE). *Accreditation Standards and Key Elements for the Professional Program in Pharmacy Leading to the Doctor of Pharmacy Degree ("Standards 2016")*. Available at https://www.acpe-accredit.org/pharmd-program-accreditation/. Accessed November 6, 2018.

Agar J. 2015. Pharmacy CEO gets maximum sentence in drug repackaging scheme. Available at http://www.mlive.com/news/grand-rapids/index.ssf/2015/08/kentwood_pharmacy_ceo_kim_muld_1.html#incart_river. Accessed September 2, 2015.

American College of Clinical Pharmacy. 2015. Collaborative drug therapy management and comprehensive medication management—2015. *Pharmaotherapy* 35:e39–e50.

Blake KB, Madhavan SS, Scott VG, Elswick BL. 2009. Medication therapy management in West Virginia: Pharmacists' perceptions of educational and training needs. *Res Social Adm Pharm* 5:182–188.

Blalock SJ, Roberts AW, Lauffenburger JC, Thompson T, O'Connor SK. 2013. The effect of community pharmacy-based interventions on patient health outcomes: A systematic review. *Med Care Res Rev* 70:235–266.

Blanchard C, Livet M, Ward C, et al. 2017. The active implementation frameworks: A roadmap for implementation of comprehensive medication management in primary care. *Res Social Adm Pharm* 13:922–929.

Brodie DC. 1967. Drug use control: Keystone to pharmaceutical service. *Drug Intell Clin Pharm* 1:63–65.

Brummel A, Lustiq A, Westrich K, et al. 2014. Best practices: Improving patient outcomes and costs in an ACO through comprehensive medication therapy management. *J Manag Care Spec Pharm* 20:1152–1158.

Buerki RA, Vottero LD. 1994. *Ethical Responsibility in Pharmacy Practice*. Madison, WI: American Institute of the History of Pharmacy.

Desselle SP. 1997. Pharmacists' perceptions of pharmaceutical care practice standards. *J Am Pharm Assoc (Wash)* NS37:529–534.

Desselle SP, Rappaport HM. 1995. Feasibility and relevance of identified pharmaceutical care practice standards for community pharmacists. Paper presented at the American Association of Pharmaceutical Scientists Annual Meeting, Miami, FL, November 7.

Ferguson J, Ashcroft D, Hassell K. 2011. Qualitative insight into job satisfaction and dissatisfaction with management among community and hospital pharmacists. *Res Social Adm Pharm* 7:306–316.

Flyvbjerg B. 2006. From Nobel Prize to project management: Getting risks right. *Proj Manage J* 37:5–15.

Gaither CA. 1998. Predictive validity of work/career-related attitudes and intentions on pharmacists' turnover behavior. *J Pharm Market Manage* 12:3–25.

George DL, Smith MJ, Draugalis JR, et al. 2018. The use of think-aloud protocols to identify a decision-making process of community pharmacists aimed at improving CMS Star Ratings scores. *Res Social Adm Pharm* 14:262–268.

Goedken AM, Butler CM, McDonough RP, Deninger MJ, Doucette WR. 2018. Continuous Medication Monitoring (CoMM): A foundational model to support the clinical work of community pharmacists. *Res Social Adm Pharm* 14:106–111.

Gubbins PO, Ragland D, Castleberry AN, Payakachat N. 2015. Family commitment and work satisfaction among pharmacists. *Pharmacy (Basel)* 17:386–398.

Harrison DL, Bootman JL. 1994. Strategic planning by institutional pharmacy administrators. *J Pharm Market Manage* 8:73–96.

Harrison DL, Ortmeier BG. 1995. Levels of independent community pharmacy strategic planning. *J Pharm Market Manage* 10:38–52.

Harrison DL, Ortmeier BG. 1996. Predictors of community pharmacy strategic planning. *J Pharm Market Manage* 11:1–14.

Hepler CD. 1987. The third wave in pharmaceutical education: The clinical movement. *Am J Pharm Educ* 51:369–385.

Hepler CD, Strand LM. 1990. Opportunities and responsibilities in pharmaceutical care. *Am J Hosp Pharm* 47:533–543.

Heringa M, Floor-Schreudering A, Tromp BC, et al. 2016. Nature and frequency of drug therapy alerts generated by clinical decision support in community pharmacy. *Pharmacoepidemiol Drug Saf* 25:82–89.

Institute of Medicine. 2006. *Preventing Medication Errors: Quality Chasm Series*. Washington, DC: National Academy of Sciences.

Isasi F, Krofah E. 2015. *The Expanding Role of Pharmacists in a Transformed Health Care System*. Washington, DC: National Governors Association Center for Best Practices.

Kennelty KA, Chewning B, Wise M, Kind A, Roberts T, Kreling D. 2015. Barriers and facilitators of medication reconciliation processes for recently discharged patients from community pharmacists' perspectives. *Res Social Adm Pharm* 11:517–530.

Keshishian F. 2010. Factors influencing pharmacy students' choice of major and its relationship to anticipatory socialization. *Am J Pharm Educ* 74:75.

Killingsworth P, Eschenbacher L. 2018. Designing organizational structures: Key thoughts for development. *Am J Health Syst Pharm* 75:482–492.

Latif DA. 2000. Relationship between pharmacy students' locus of control, Machiavellianism, and moral reasoning. *Am J Pharm Educ* 64:33–37.

LaVito A, Hirsch A. Amazon shakes up drugstore business with deal to buy PillPack. Available at https://www.cnbc.com/2018/06/28/amazon-to-acquire-online-pharmacy-pillpack.html. Accessed November 5, 2018.

Law AV, Okamoto MP, Brock K. 2009. Ready, willing, and able to provide MTM services? A survey of community pharmacists in the USA. *Res Social Adm Pharm* 5:376–381.

Leung HY, Saini B, Ritchie HE. 2018. Medications and pregnancy: The role of community pharmacists—A descriptive study. *PLoS One* 13: doi: 10.1371/journal.pone.0195101

Loignon C, Dupere S, Fortin M, Ramden VR, Truchon K. 2018. Health literacy—Engaging in the co-creation of meaningful health navigation services: A study protocol. *BMC Health Serv Res* 18: Article 505.

Maine LL, Penna RP. 1996. Pharmaceutical care: An overview. In Knowlton C, Penna R (eds.) *Pharmaceutical Care*. New York, NY: Chapman & Hall, p. 133.

McConaha JL, Tedesco GW, Civitarese L, Hebda MF. 2015. A pharmacist's contribution within a patient-centered medical home. *J Am Pharm Assoc* 55:302–306.

Meyer-Junco L. 2015. Empathy and the new practitioner. *Am J Health Syst Pharm* 72:2042–2058.

Millis JS. 1975. *Pharmacists for the Future: The Report of the Study Commission on Pharmacy*. Ann Arbor, MI: Health Administration Press.

Millis JS. 1976. Looking ahead: The Report of the Study Commission on Pharmacy. *Am J Hosp Pharm* 33:134–138.

Moczygemba LR, Goode JV, Silvester JA, Matzke GR. 2012. Pharmacy practice in Virginia in 2011. *Ann Pharmacother* 46:S13–S26.

Organisation for Economic Co-operation and Development (OECD). Health at a glance 2017: OECD indicators. 2017. Available at https://www.oecd.org/unitedstates/Health-at-a-Glance-2017-Key-Findings-UNITED-STATES.pdf. Accessed January 2, 2019.

Patterson PJ, Bakken BK, Doucette WR, Urmie JM, McDonough RP. 2017. Informal learning processes in support of clinical service delivery in service-oriented community pharmacy. *Res Social Adm Pharm* 13:224–232.

Pink LA. 1991. *Hospitals*. In Fincham JE, Wertheimer AI (eds.) *Pharmacists and the U.S. Healthcare System*. Binghamton, NY: Pharmaceutical Products Press, p. 158.

Pohontsch NJ, Stark A, Ehrhardt M, Kotter T, Scherer M. 2018. Influences on students' empathy in medical education: An exploratory interview with medical students in their third and last year. *BMC Med Educ* 18:231.

Public Law 108–173. 2010. Available at http://www.medicare.gov/medicarereform/108s1013.htm. Accessed December 6, 2010.

Public Law 111–148. 2010. Available at http://www.gpo.gov/fdsys/pkg/PLAW-111publ148/pdf/PLAW-111publ148.pdf. Accessed December 6, 2010.

Robinson E, Shcherbakova N, Backer L. 2016. Assessment of pharmacy manpower and services in New England. *J Pharm Pract* 29:549–555.

Rosenthal M, Tsao NW, Tsyuki RT, Marra CA. 2016. Identifying relationships between the professional culture of pharmacy, pharmacists' personality traits, and the provision of advanced pharmacy services. *Res Social Adm Pharm* 12:56–67.

Sawan M, Jeon YH, Fois RA, Chen TF. 2017. Exploring the link between organizational climate and the use of psychotropic medicines in nursing homes: A qualitative study. *Res Social Adm Pharm* 13:513–523.

Schommer JC, Gaither CA. 2014. A segmentation analysis for pharmacists' and patients' views of pharmacists' roles. *Res Soc Admin Pharm* 10:508–528.

Shah B, Chawla S. 2011. A needs assessment for development and provision of medication therapy management services in New York City. *J Pharm Pract* 24:339–344.

Smyrl ME. 2014. Beyond interests and institutions: US health policy reform and the surprising silence of big business. *J Health Polit Policy Law* 39:5–34.

Sonnedecker G. 1963. *Kremers and Urdang's History of Pharmacy*. Philadelphia, PA: Lippincott.

Tootelian DH, Gaedeke RM. 1993. *Essentials of Pharmacy Management*. St. Louis, MO: Mosby.

Torrens PR. 1993. Historical evolution and overview of health service in the United States. In Williams JS, Torrens PR (eds.) *Introduction to Health Services*, 4th ed. Albany, NY: Delmar, p. 3.

Vermeulen LC, Eddington ND, Gourdine MA, et al. 2019. ASHP Foundation Forecast 2019; Strategic planning advice for pharmacy departments in hospital and health systems. *Am J Health Syst Pharm* 76:71–100.

Warshawski S, Itzhaki M, Barnoy S. 2018. The associations between peer caring behaviours and social support to nurse students' caring perceptions. *Nurse Pract Educ* 31:88–94.

Wilkin NE. 1999. Pharmaceutical care: A clinical movement? *Mississippi Pharm* 26:13.

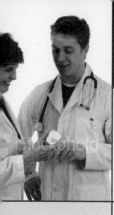

2

MANAGEMENT FUNCTIONS

David P. Zgarrick

About the Author: Dr. Zgarrick is a professor in the School of Pharmacy at Northeastern University's Bouvé College of Health Sciences. He received a BS degree in pharmacy from the University of Wisconsin and MS and PhD in pharmaceutical administration from the Ohio State University. He has practice experience in both independent and chain community pharmacy settings. He has taught courses in pharmacy management, business planning for professional services, and drug literature evaluation. His scholarly interests include pharmacist workforce research, pharmacy management and operations, pharmacy education, and the development of postgraduate programs.

■ LEARNING OBJECTIVES

After completing this chapter, readers should be able to

1. Define the terms *management* and *manager*. Describe how concepts in management figure into our everyday lives.
2. Compare and contrast *management* and *leadership*.
3. Compare and contrast classical views of management with modern views.
4. Describe the management process within the contexts of what managers do, resources they manage, and levels at which managers perform their roles.
5. Integrate modern views of management with the management process.
6. Apply the management process to a variety of activities, ranging from performing professional roles to accomplishing one's tasks of daily living.

■ SCENARIO

Krista Connelly is a second-year pharmacy student. Like most second-year students, she describes her life as "incredibly stressed out." A typical day consists of getting up at 6 AM, getting dressed and running out the door by 7 AM, and driving to school to get to her first class by 8 AM (making sure to avoid the accident on the expressway that she heard about on her way out the door). While at school, she finds time to squeeze in cups of coffee and snack bars between the lectures, labs, and workshops that usually last until at least 4 PM. She also makes a point to go to the library to prepare upcoming assignments, as well as to meet with her professors to review how she did on her examinations.

After class today, Krista has an Academy of Students of Pharmacy (ASP) meeting. Krista is the president of her chapter and works with committee chairs to accomplish the goals of the organization. In the past few weeks, she has helped the new professional service chairperson develop a diabetes screening program, talked her fundraising chairperson out of quitting, and wrote a report on each committee's activities for the chapter website. While Krista enjoys her leadership role in ASP, she finds some of the people she works with to be frustrating and wonders how she can motivate them to do a better job.

After her meeting, Krista drives to a fast-food restaurant to grab a quick dinner on her way to her part-time pharmacy intern job. When she is not working, she will usually head to a friend's house to study for an upcoming examination. She typically gets back to her apartment between 10 and 11 PM and mentally prepares for what she needs to do in the next few days. She might stream a new show or spend some time on social media before heading to bed at around midnight.

On weekends, Krista catches up on what one might call "activities of daily living." She does her laundry, pays her bills, calls her parents and friends back home, and gets together with her friends on Saturday nights. When Krista and her friends (most of whom are also pharmacy students) go out, they often talk about their plans after they graduate from pharmacy school. They talk about how exciting it will be to treat patients, work with other health care professionals, and finally start making a pharmacist's salary to begin paying down their student loans. None of them says that they want to be pharmacy managers. "The pharmacy manager at my store is always on my case about coming in late or having to arrange my hours around my examination schedule," said Krista.

"I don't see how being a manager can help me do the things I want to as a pharmacist."

■ CHAPTER QUESTIONS

1. Why is it that all pharmacists should be considered managers regardless of their titles or positions?
2. Why should pharmacy students study management?
3. What is the difference between management and leadership?
4. How does management affect every aspect of our daily lives?
5. Will the same approach to management be effective for all types of situations encountered by pharmacists?

■ WHAT IS MANAGEMENT?

For many people, a distinct set of images comes to mind when they hear the word *management*. First and foremost, they think of a person (or possibly a group of people) who is "the boss" to whom they report at work. While some people view their relationships with management as positive, many of us have had experiences where this has not been the case. This is why when you ask people what they think of management, they often provide negative views and experiences. Ask pharmacy students what they think about entering careers in pharmacy management, and you likely will get answers similar to those provided by Krista Connelly and her friends in the scenario.

Perhaps it may be better to start by looking a bit more closely at the term *management*. The stem of the word is *manage,* which according to the *Merriam-Webster Dictionary* is a verb meaning "to handle or direct with a degree of skill, to work upon or try to alter for a purpose, or to succeed in accomplishing" (Merriam-Webster, 2019). Think about how this definition applies to your daily life. Have you ever handled or directed something with a degree of skill (even if it was just yourself)? Have you worked upon or altered something for a purpose (your appearance, perhaps)? Have you ever succeeded in accomplishing a task (even if it was just getting to an examination on time)?

Management educators focus on processes, the "how" tasks are accomplished and goals are achieved. Daft (2018) defines management as "attainment of organizational goals in an efficient and effective manner through planning, organizing, leading, and controlling organizational resources." Tootelian and Gaedeke (1993) describe management as "a process which brings together resources and unites them in such a way that, collectively, they achieve goals or objectives in the most efficient manner possible." A *process* which is simply a method of doing something. Processes are used to perform simple everyday tasks (e.g., checking your phone or driving to school) as well as more complex activities (e.g., hiring a pharmacy technician or monitoring the outcomes of a patient's drug therapy). People perform processes because they want to achieve a goal or objective. Goals and objectives can be personal (e.g., keeping track of your friends or getting to school on time) or professional (e.g., a smoothly operating pharmacy or high-quality patient care). Because processes require resources, and because resources are scarce (they are not present in unlimited supply), it is important that resources be used in such a way as to achieve goals and objectives in the most efficient manner possible. While one could achieve one's goal of getting to school on time by driving 90 miles an hour, one also could argue that this would not be the most efficient use of the driver's resources, especially if there is a sharp turn ahead or a police officer waiting around the corner.

Managers are simply people who perform management activities. While people whom we think of as "the boss" and those with administrative titles within an organization certainly are managers, the fact is that anyone who has a task to accomplish or a goal to achieve is also a manager (see Chapter 14). Pharmacy students and pharmacists who say that they do not want to be managers may not desire the authority and responsibilities of having an administrative position, but there is no getting around their need to use resources efficiently to perform the tasks related to their jobs. All pharmacists, regardless of their job responsibilities or position, should view themselves as managers.

Another term that is often used in concert with management is *leadership*. While some people use the terms interchangeably to describe characteristics that are expected of people who are "in charge" of organizations, leadership is a distinctly different skill from *management*. Leadership involves the ability to guide, inspire, and direct others. While it certainly is desirable that managers have leadership skills, the two do not necessarily go hand in hand. You can learn more about leadership and its role in effective pharmacy management in Chapter 3. Because managers use resources, including resources that may or may not belong to them, managers must also apply ethical principles when making decisions and solving problems. Chapter 4 provides an overview of ethical principles that are applied by pharmacists in the context of managing their operations and caring for patients, in addition to reminding us that both managerial and leadership skills are important.

■ CLASSICAL AND MODERN VIEWS OF MANAGEMENT

While management activities have been part of human existence since there have been tasks to perform and goals to accomplish (e.g., gathering food or finding shelter), the study of management as a scientific and academic curriculum is relatively new. Before the industrial revolution of the 18th and 19th centuries, most people lived and worked alone or in small groups. While people at that time still had goals and objectives that needed to be accomplished efficiently, there was little formal study of the best ways to do so. The advent of the industrial revolution brought together groups of hundreds and thousands of people who shared a common objective. To get large groups of people to work together effectively, industrialists and academics established hierarchies and systems that allowed large industrial organizations to accomplish their goals, especially goals related to growth and profitability.

Around the turn of the 20th century, an American industrialist and a French engineer began to publish observations in what would become known as the *classical,* or *administrative,* school of management thought. F.W. Taylor, an executive with Bethlehem Steel, published *The Principles of Scientific Management* in 1911. He was among the first to espouse applying scientific principles to management of the workplace. Henri Fayol, a French mining engineer and corporate executive, published *Administration Industrielle et Generale* in 1916. Both Taylor and Fayol argued that all organizations, regardless of size or objective, had to perform a standard set of functions to operate efficiently. Fayol's five management functions (i.e., forecasting and planning, organizing, commanding, coordinating, and controlling) became widely accepted throughout the industrialized world. Both Fayol's five management functions and 14 principles for organizational design (Table 2-1) are still used by managers today. For example, while in the scenario Krista Connelly has the responsibility for working with her ASP chapter's committee chairs,

Table 2-1.   Classical Management Theory (Fayol)

Fayol's five management functions
1. Forecast and plan
2. Organize
3. Command
4. Coordinate
5. Control

Fayol's 14 principles for organizational design and effective administration
- *Specialization/division of labor.* People should perform tasks specific to their skills. No one should be expected to perform all the skills needed to run an organization.
- *Authority with corresponding responsibility.* People with responsibility also have sufficient authority within an organization to ensure that a task is performed.
- *Discipline.* People should follow rules, with consequences for not following rules.
- *Unity of command.* The organization has an administrator who is recognized as having the ultimate authority (e.g., CEO or president).
- *Unity of direction.* The organization has a sense of direction or vision that is recognized by all members (e.g., mission statement).
- *Subordination of individual interest to general interest.* The goals of the organization supersede the goals of any individuals within the organization.
- *Remuneration of staff.* Employees should be paid appropriately given the market for their skills and their level of responsibility.
- *Centralization.* Performing similar tasks at a single location is more effective than performing these tasks at multiple locations.
- *Scalar chain/line of authority.* Each employee has one, and only one, direct supervisor.
- *Order.* Tasks should be performed in a systematic fashion.
- *Equity.* Supervisors should treat employees with a sense of fairness.
- *Stability of tenure.* Benefits should go to employees who have stayed with an organization longer.
- *Initiative.* Organizations and employees are more effective when they are proactive, not reactive.
- *Esprit de corps.* Teamwork, harmony.

she cannot be effective in her ability to carry out her responsibilities unless her position provides her with authority that is recognized by the committee chairs.

Much of Taylor's and Fayol's work was developed based on the workplace conditions of the 19th and early 20th centuries. The great industries of those times focused primarily on the mass production of tangible goods. Very few people were educated beyond high school. The few people with higher levels of education (almost always men) generally were given administrative positions. They were expected to supervise large numbers of less educated production-line employees. In this hierarchy, the role of administrators generally was to command and control their employees, and the role of workers was to carry out the tasks at hand without question.

On the other hand, the workforce and workplace of the early 21st century have evolved into something quite different. According to the U.S. Bureau of Labor Statistics (2019), more than three times the number of people are employed in positions which provide services than are employed in jobs which produce tangible goods. Today's workforce is better educated and more highly skilled than workers have been in the past. In many cases, today's administrators have less formal education and fewer technical skills than the people they are supervising.

These trends have led many to question the relevance of classical management theories in today's rapidly changing world. Browse the "Business" section of practically any bookstore or online bookseller and you'll find literally hundreds of works written by management "gurus" such as Covey, Drucker, Peters, and many others espousing modern management techniques and offering "hands on" advice about how to deal with day-to-day workplace issues. This text recognizes the value of classical management theories by using them as the foundation from which each chapter is built. Classical theories also serve as the foundation upon which well-renowned management researchers, educators, and practitioners perform their work. Researchers apply scientific methods to the study of management and publish their results in scholarly journals, similar to what we see in pharmacy

and medicine. These books and research studies make important contributions to management science, given the continued need to use scarce resources to achieve goals and objectives in an ever-changing business climate. Readers will also see many quotes from management practitioners throughout the text, describing how they have applied management theories, evidence, and experience in the real world. As such, we have leveraged all of these aspects into a text that provides practical advice and strategies for readers to translate into everyday practice, both in a pharmacy and in our personal lives.

■ THE MANAGEMENT PROCESS

Figure 2-1 describes one way in which Fayol's management functions can be adapted to describe what managers do in today's world. There are three dimensions of management: (1) activities that managers perform, (2) resources that managers need, and (3) levels at which managers make decisions. Every action taken by a manager involves at least one aspect of each of the three dimensions.

Management Activities

Fayol's five management functions have been adapted to describe four activities that all managers perform. While managers who hold administrative positions in their organizations may have formal ways of performing these activities (and are evaluated on their ability to get them done), all managers (which means all of us!) perform each of these activities every day, whether we are thinking of them or not.

The first of these four activities is planning. *Planning* is predetermining a course of action based on one's goals and objectives. Managers must consider many factors when planning, including their internal and external environments. The pharmacy manager at a community pharmacy or the chief pharmacy officer of a hospital will develop plans to predetermine which drug products she wishes to carry or what professional services she might offer. Some pharmacists will even

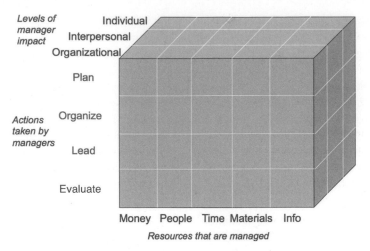

Figure 2-1. The management process.

go so far as to develop formal strategic and business plans for their pharmacies (see Chapters 6, 7, 29, and 30). On the other hand, planning can also be very informal. Anyone who goes to work or school in the morning develops a plan for how he will get there (i.e., What time do I need to leave? What form of transportation should I take? What route should I follow? With whom am I going to ride/carpool?).

The next management activity is organizing. *Organizing* is the arrangement and relationship of activities and resources necessary for the effective accomplishment of a goal or objective. Once a pharmacist has decided which drug products or services they should offer, they need to ask themselves *what* resources they need to provide them, *how* they will go about obtaining these resources, and then determine *when* they will need to obtain them. Once the person going to work or school has a plan, they need to think about what else they may need to do to accomplish their goal (e.g., check the weather and traffic reports, get gas in the car, drop kids off with a child care provider).

The third step is the leading or directing step. This step combines Fayol's command and coordinate steps to provide a better description of what managers actually do in today's world. *Leading* or *directing* involves bringing about purposeful action toward

some desired outcome. It can take the form of actually doing something yourself (the person going to work or school just needs to get up and go) or working with others to lead them to where you want your organization to be. A pharmacist eventually may offer the goods and services described in their plans, but almost certainly will need to work with a number of other people within her organization to accomplish this task. In the scenario, Krista Connelly, in her role as president of her ASP chapter, is responsible for seeing that the chapter's committees work effectively to accomplish their objectives. Working with others often requires leadership skills, which will be discussed in Chapter 3.

The fourth step is the control or evaluation step. *Control* or *evaluation* involves reviewing the progress that has been made toward the objectives that were set out in the plan. This step involves not only determining *what* actually happened but also *why* it happened. Performing quality control checks to help ensure that patients are receiving the desired medication in the appropriate manner is a very important function of a pharmacy practice. Pharmacists can also ask themselves if the goods and services they offered met their goals. These goals can be from the perspective of their patients (e.g., Did the goods and services result in high-quality patient care or improved clinical outcomes?) as well as from other perspectives (e.g., Did the service improve the pharmacist's job satisfaction? Did it improve the profitability of the pharmacy or organization?). The person going to work or school not only should ask himself if he arrived on time but also should know why he did or did not (e.g., the traffic accident on the expressway, hitting the snooze button that third time before getting up). Chapters 8 through 12 review methods that pharmacists use to ensure the quality of their operations, manage the risks inherent in medication use and pharmacy practice, and reduce the occurrence of medication errors.

Management activities should be performed in order, starting with the planning step. They are also meant to be cyclic, meaning that what a manager learns in the control/evaluation step should be incorporated back into the planning step the next time she needs to accomplish that objective (Figure 2-2). For example, if a pharmacy student receives a score on an examination that did not meet his goal, he should use what he learned in the evaluation step (e.g., what questions he got wrong, time spent studying) to help him plan for the next examination.

Resources that are Managed

Regardless of their level or position within an organization, managers must use resources to achieve their goals and objectives. Keep in mind that resources are scarce, meaning that they are not available in unlimited supply. Both organizations and individuals must use resources efficiently to achieve their goals and objectives.

The first resource that many managers think of is money. Customers generally provide money to pharmacies and pharmacists in exchange for goods and services. Employers generally pay their employees money in exchange for the services they provide to the organization. Managing money is important to any organization or individual, and several chapters of this book are dedicated to explaining how pharmacies and pharmacists manage money and use economic information to make decisions (see Chapters 21 to 23). Money in and of itself can be an important yardstick for measuring the success of an organization or an individual. However, most managers value money for its ability to allow them to obtain additional resources that are necessary to achieve other goals and objectives.

Another resource that is very important to managers is people. In pharmacy practice, there is very little that any one person can accomplish on his or her own, regardless of the practice setting. Pharmacists must work with other employees in their pharmacies, other health care professionals, and especially the patients and customers they serve. Given the importance of this topic, an entire section of this book (Chapters 14 to 20) is dedicated to the management of people.

How many times have you heard someone say, "I'd have gotten that done if I'd have had more time"? Of all the resources managers have at their disposal, time can be the most limiting. After all, there are only 24 hours in a day! Time management is essential for today's busy pharmacist, as well as for most other people. In the scenario, Krista Connelly is a great example of a pharmacy student who could benefit from time and stress management. Chapter 14 is dedicated to managing one's self; that is, time management, stress management, and organizational skills that can help you to get the most out of this precious resource. It is aligned with other chapters on the management of people because one has to be able to manage themselves and their time effectively in order to manage those of other people.

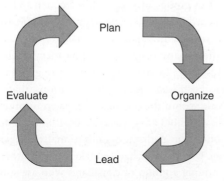

Figure 2-2. Management activities cycle.

When many people think of a pharmacy, they still think of a pharmacist standing behind a counter compounding drug products and dispensing prescriptions. While pharmacy practice continues to evolve from a product to a patient orientation, managing material resource is still an important function in any pharmacy. Community pharmacies filled over 4 billion prescriptions in 2017, an increase of more than 15% over the past decade (Kaiser Family Foundation, 2019). The costs of these drug products, as well as the costs of the equipment and supplies necessary to dispense them safely and efficiently to patients, continue to rise in all practice settings. Just as people need to assess their needs and supplies of material goods (e.g., food, clothing, household supplies) before going on a shopping trip, pharmacies need to make the same assessments before purchasing drug products, equipment, and supplies. Chapters 8, 27, and 28 are all designed to help readers learn more about managing material resources.

While the 18th and 19th centuries were known as the time of the industrial revolution, the 21st century certainly will be known as the information age. The advent of the computer and the Internet in the late 20th century has resulted in an explosion of information that is literally at most people's fingertips. This already has had a tremendous impact on pharmacy practice, providing pharmacists with information about drugs and patients that they did not have only a few years ago. While it is not certain what implications this will have for pharmacy practice in the future, it is certain that information management is becoming an important job for pharmacists. Chapter 9 provides an overview of technologies that pharmacists use to manage information, as well as insights into what role information management may have on the future of pharmacy practice.

Levels of Management

When managers perform management activities, they can do so at a number of levels within an organization, and with a variety of different purposes in mind. While some people think of management activities occurring only in corporations and other complex organizations, management activities take place in all types of organizations, involving all levels of interactions among their members.

There is not a person reading this chapter who has not performed self-management activities. Just the fact that you are a pharmacy student or pharmacist attests to the fact that you have performed a number of activities on your own just to get to this point. Self-management is the most frequently occurring level of management, if for no other reason than that practically every decision we make every day (both professional and personal) requires self-management. For example, pharmacists must prioritize and manage their time efficiently so that they can accomplish a wide variety of tasks, from ensuring that every prescription is dispensed accurately to making sure that they have time to consult with other health care professionals and counsel their patients.

Next to self-management, the most frequent level on which managers find themselves performing is the interpersonal level. Interpersonal management occurs between the manager and one other person. In a pharmacy, this might involve a pharmacist counseling a patient about a medication, training a technician on how to submit a claim for a medication therapy management service with a third-party payer, or consulting with a prescriber regarding a patient's drug therapy. Our personal lives are full of interpersonal relationships, including those with our parents, siblings, spouse, children, friends, and significant others.

The level of management that occurs least often is organizational management. This involves actions that affect groups of people. We frequently think of this occurring at work, especially when a pharmacist needs to develop a policy or make a decision that may affect many people at the pharmacy. High-level administrators in large organizations (e.g., pharmacy chains, hospitals) often make decisions that affect everyone within the organization. Keep in mind that people who hold administrative positions are not the only ones who perform organizational management. Anyone who has ever had to make an "executive decision" among a group of classmates who are studying for an examination or deciding where to go for lunch can relate to the kinds of organizational-level decisions that business leaders make every day.

■ INTEGRATING MODERN AND CLASSICAL VIEWS OF MANAGEMENT

Much of what was first described by Taylor and Fayol at the beginning of the 20th century is still applied today by managers at all levels of administration in all types of organizations. However, much has changed in both pharmacy practice and the workplace over that time, and management science has grown to keep up with those changes.

In the past, the relationship between an administrator and a worker was often hierarchical. The authority of the administrator generally went unquestioned, and workers simply did what they were told. In today's workplace, there is often more of a partnership between administrators and workers. While administrators are still responsible for achieving organizational goals and objectives, workers generally expect to have input as to how goals and objectives will be developed and expect to share in the rewards when those goals are accomplished.

Health care organizations such as hospitals and pharmacies present a number of managerial challenges to administrators. Unlike the workers of Taylor's and Fayol's day, most health care workers are highly educated and skilled professionals. Trends toward specialization among health care professionals often create situations where even entry-level health care workers have more knowledge and expertise of their particular area than their administrators. As you can imagine, administrators of health care professionals who attempt to use their authority to command and control these employees may find this not to be an effective way to achieve organizational goals and objectives. According to Drucker, "knowledge workers" in today's information age need to ask "what *should*" they be doing in light of their own values, in accordance with the objectives and values of the organization (Drucker, 1999).

Modern views of management suggest that managers must adapt their management activities to their workers. These functions generally occur in addition to the classical management functions. According to Nelson and Economy (2010), today's manager also needs to

- *Energize.* Today's managers need to have a vision of what they want to create and the energy to make it happen. When you think of good managers with whom you have worked with, they are probably not the kind of people who just want to maintain the status quo for the rest of their lives. They have ideas about what they would like to see their organizations become in the future, and the energy and enthusiasm to attract others to want to join them in achieving their goals. They are always trying to make the best of stressful situations, especially when the level of resources available may be less than they desire. In pharmacy today, good managers are often pharmacists who want to see the profession move forward by developing new goods and services, especially those that improve patient care. Their energy and enthusiasm attract motivated pharmacists and other personnel who share their vision and want to work with them. These managers also are able to advocate to obtain new resources they need to carry out their vision, or make the most of resources that they already have. Not only does the power of energy and enthusiasm work for pharmacists, but it also benefits pharmacy students. Do you think that Krista Connelly would be an effective chapter president if she did not have a high level of energy and enthusiasm for ASP's goals and objectives?
- *Empower.* If you are a highly educated and skilled health professional, the last thing you want is to have an administrator questioning your decisions and telling you how you should do your job. In today's environment, managers should empower their employees to do what needs to be done. In many ways, today's manager is very much like the coach of a team. Coaches develop a game plan; select players; provide them with training, resources, and advice; and then step back and let the players execute the game plan. Good coaches

empower their players to carry out the game plan. Managers who empower their employees provide them with training, resources, and advice and then let the employees get the job done. Krista Connelly can empower her ASP committee chairpersons by providing them with goals, resources, and advice and then letting them get to work.

This is not to say that managers do not need to supervise their employees. Managers are still responsible for seeing that organizational goals are met, which may mean having to intervene with workers. Just as coaches need to provide resources and advice to their players during a game, and occasionally replace a player who is not executing the game plan, managers need to provide resources, advice, and occasionally discipline to see that organizational goals are met.

- *Support.* After a manager has empowered her employees to do their jobs, she should not just leave them on their own, especially when things start to go wrong. Today, good managers need to be coaches, collaborators, and sometimes even cheerleaders for their employees. Providing support for employees does not mean that managers should be willing to do their employees' work or always agree with the decisions employees make on the job. It does mean that managers need to provide employees with the training, resources, and authority needed to do their jobs. Managers also need to be good coaches, letting employees know when they have done a good job, as well as helping them learn when things are not going so well. Even pharmacy students like Krista Connelly know that a few kind words to her committee chairpersons will help the ASP chapter in the long run.

In providing support, managers must also be mindful to balance the needs and resources of their organizations with what employees need. As much as a manager may wish to give a valued employee a big raise, the manager must also consider how much money is available for a raise among other potential uses of his organization's financial resources.

- *Communicate.* In today's information-laden environment, communication between managers and

employees is more important than ever. While managers can energize, empower, and support their employees, if they cannot communicate their messages, they will not be effective and their organizations will suffer. The cornerstone of communications in any environment is trust. If employees feel that they can bring up any question or concern to a manager, they will likely be more receptive to what the manager has to say.

One major challenge for managers and employees today is the vast number of ways in which they can communicate. Communication that once took place between managers and employees in person now can take place over the telephone, via voice mail or e-mail, in a text message, or even through a social network, such as Facebook, Twitter, or Instagram. While these additional methods can make it easier for managers and employees to communicate with each other, care must be taken in using these methods. As you can imagine, not every method of communication is appropriate for every type of message (e.g., disciplining or firing an employee in a text message is generally *not* a good idea).

■ WHY SHOULD I STUDY MANAGEMENT?

After reading the first two chapters of this book, you still may be asking yourself, "Why should I study management?" You may think that being a good manager just involves using your common sense and applying the Golden Rule (act toward others as you would have others act toward you). After all, you probably have done a good job managing yourself up to this point without taking a management course or reading a management textbook. Can managing a pharmacy practice be that much different?

While there is certainly a role for applying self-management skills, most pharmacy managers agree that managing a pharmacy practice successfully requires a unique set of skills. Some of these skills can be quite technical (e.g., financial management [see Chapters 21 to 23] and marketing [see Chapters 24 and 25]), requiring a knowledge base that goes beyond what many pharmacists bring to their practices. These skills should be learned just as one would learn medicinal chemistry, pharmacology, or pharmacotherapeutics. And just pharmacists and other health professionals who seek evidence based on validated research to answer questions regarding patient care, managers can use a similar approach to addressing their management questions. Learning to search, read, and critically evaluate the management literature will help you make more informed management decisions.

Something else to keep in mind is that in today's workplace, what might be common sense to you may not make sense at all to the other people you encounter. Pharmacists today work with employees, other health professionals, and especially patients who come from a wide variety of backgrounds. People from diverse backgrounds bring with them an incredible amount of insight and experience. Pharmacists who do not take this diversity into account when working with people may find themselves frustrated and not able to achieve their goals and objectives effectively, as well as at risk of harming the very employees, professionals, and patients which they serve. Working with others who have diverse backgrounds and expectations, while at the same time achieving your own personal goals, as well as the goals of your employer or organization, can be especially challenging. To aid pharmacy managers in working with others who may hold views and have expectations different than their own, we have added a chapter on negotiation (Chapter 15). You will come to learn that pharmacists use negotiation skills every day to care for their patients, supervise their employees, work with other health care professionals, and to advocate for themselves and their profession.

This book presents material that is relevant to both pharmacy students and pharmacists. Pharmacy students who use this book will find that many of the scenarios that start each chapter are directed toward experiences to which they can relate. There may be some of you right now who think that your life has a lot in common with Krista Connelly's. The information provided in each chapter not only will help students to better deal with management issues they are currently experiencing but will also help to prepare them for what to expect in the future as pharmacists. Pharmacists will find the information provided in each chapter applicable to almost everything that they do, from dispensing a prescription to implementing a new clinical service. Figure 2-3 provides just one example of how a pharmacist could use information from throughout this book to guide them through the planning, organization, implementation, and evaluation of a new service.

Pharmacists who use this book often have a good idea of why they need to have management skills. After all, they are living pharmacy practice management on a daily basis! The information provided in this book should help provide pharmacists with the skills they will need to better meet the challenges they face every day.

■ QUESTIONS FOR FURTHER DISCUSSION

Listed below are three scenarios that represent how pharmacists use the management process on a daily basis. For each scenario, please describe (1) the level of management being performed, (2) the type of management activity being performed, and (3) the resources that the pharmacist needs to perform this activity.

Scenario 1: Sabin Patel, PharmD, is trying to decide what form of education (graduate degree, certificate program, continuing education) would best allow her to advance through a career ladder in her organization.

Scenario 2: Doug Danforth, PharmD, is training a technician regarding information that needs to be collected during an initial patient interview.

Scenario 3: Casey Kulpinski, PharmD, is reviewing her pharmacy's financial statements to determine if her diabetes care center has met the financial goals set by the parent corporation.

Step 1—Justify their idea within the broader goals and objectives of their organization, of other organizations, and for themselves
• Organization Structure and Behavior—Chapter 16
• Strategic Planning—Chapter 6

Step 2—Advocate for the service with others who may have competing priorities and limited resources, as well as with those who may see this service as a threat
• Leadership—Chapter 3
• Negotiation—Chapter 15

Step 3—Develop plans, set goals, and describe the potential implications of the service for all relevant parties (patients, other providers, payors, the pharmacists providing the service, the organization's profitability)
• Business Planning—Chapter 7

Step 4—Actually implement the service, which may entail:
• Obtaining financial resources
  Financial Reports—Chapter 21
• Hiring & training personnel to provide the service
  Human Resource Management Functions—Chapter 17
• Purchasing equipment, supplies, and other services needed to provide the service
  Supply Chain Management—Chapter 27
• Obtaining and remodeling physical space to provide the service
  Merchandising—Chapter 28
• Obtaining regulatory approval
  Compliance with Regulations and Regulatory Bodies—Chapter 13
• Insuring against risks that may arise from the service
  Risk Management in Contemporary Pharmacy Practice—Chapter 11

Figure 2-3. Steps needed to add a pharmacist to an outpatient primary clinic.

Step 5—Manage the day-to-day operation of the service itself, which may entail:

• Applying operations management principles to assure that the service is provided in an appropriate manner
  Operations Management—Chapter 8
  Employment Law and Workplace Safety—Chapter 18
• Utilizing technology to manage needed information and document services and their outcomes
  Informatics—Chapter 9
• Ensure the quality of the service
  Ensuring Quality in Pharmacy Operations—Chapter 10
  Preventing and Managing Medication Errors—Chapter 12
  Customer Service—Chapter 26
• Supervise the employees providing the service
  Performance Appraisal Systems—Chapter 20
• Marketing the service
  Marketing Fundamentals—Chapter 24
  Marketing Applications—Chapter 25
• Obtaining payment for services
  Third-Party Considerations—Chapter 23

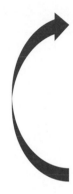
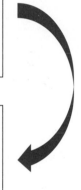

Step 6—Evaluate the service to determine how it is performed against predetermined goals, which may entail:
• Evaluate financial performance
  Financial Reports—Chapter 21
  Budgeting—Chapter 22
• Evaluate personnel performance
  Performance Appraisal Systems—Chapter 20
• Evaluate quality and other outcomes
  Ensuring Quality in Pharmacy Operations—Chapter 10

Step 7—Use what was learned in Step 6 to revise actions taken in Step 5. Repeat as needed, setting goals to either further grow or to discontinue the service

Figure 2-3. *(Continued)*

REFERENCES

Daft RL. 2018. *Management*. Boston, MA: Cengage Learning.

Drucker PF. 1999. *Management Challenges for the 21st Century*. New York, NY: Harper Collins.

Kaiser Family Foundation. 2019. http://kff.org/other/state-indicator/total-retail-rx-drugs/. Accessed January 2, 2019.

Merriam-Webster. 2019. http://www.merriam-webster.com/dictionary/manage. Accessed January 2, 2019.

Nelson B, Economy P. 2010. *Managing for Dummies*, 3rd ed. New York, NY: Wiley.

Tootelian DH, Gaedeke RM. 1993. *Essentials of Pharmacy Management*. St. Louis, MO: Mosby.

U.S. Bureau of Labor Statistics. 2019. http://www.bls.gov/webapps/legacy/cpsatab13.htm. Accessed January 2, 2019.

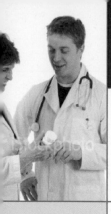

3

LEADERSHIP IN PHARMACY PRACTICE

Kyle M. Turner and Todd D. Sorensen

About the Authors: Dr. Turner is an Assistant Clinical Professor at the University of Utah College of Pharmacy and is a practicing clinical pharmacist in primary care at University of Utah Health. Dr. Turner earned his Doctor of Pharmacy (PharmD) degree at the University of Utah and completed the 2-year Pharmaceutical Care Leadership Residency at the University of Minnesota. Dr. Turner co-leads the University of Utah's Student Hotspotting program, designed to engage interprofessional teams in reducing cost and improving outcomes of patients with high health care utilization. Dr. Turner's leadership efforts include enhancing clinical practice through Comprehensive Medication Management implementation, developing interprofessional teams to improve care and enhance resilience, and engaging in clinic and system-level quality improvement projects. Dr. Turner teaches leadership and management courses and advises student professional organizations. His scholarship interests include leadership development, pharmacy practice innovation, interprofessional education, and building effective health care teams.

Dr. Sorensen is a Professor and Associate Head, Department of Pharmaceutical Care and Health Systems at the College of Pharmacy, University of Minnesota. He also serves as the Executive Director of the Alliance for Integrated Medication Management, a non-profit organization that engages health care institutions in practice transformation activities that support improved medication use. Dr. Sorensen received his PharmD from the University of Minnesota and has had professional experience in a range of professional settings, including acute care (critical care), community pharmacy, managed care, and academia. His academic work concentrates on identifying strategies that facilitate clinical practice development and developing leadership skills in student pharmacists, pharmacy residents, and practitioners. His research and service activities have focused on working with health care organizations to implement strategies that improve health outcomes associated with chronic illness, specifically identifying leadership strategies that allow organizations to integrate and sustain medication management services delivered by pharmacists within interprofessional teams. Dr. Sorensen has been highly active in state and national pharmacy organizations, including service as the President of the Minnesota Pharmacists Association and President of the American Association of Colleges of Pharmacy.

■ LEARNING OBJECTIVES

After completing this chapter, readers should be able to

1. Define leadership and determine its essential role in health care and pharmacy practice.
2. Determine the role of positional and non-positional leaders in creating change.
3. Compare and contrast the roles of and activities of leaders and managers.
4. Describe Kotter's eight steps for leading change.
5. Consider the role of strengths and values in enhancing self-awareness.
6. Identify the essential strategies and practices of effective teams.
7. Determine the next step in one's own leadership journey.

■ SCENARIO

Jane Nguyen is a recent pharmacy graduate working in her first job at a community pharmacy owned by a local non-profit health system located within an ambulatory care clinic. As a student, Jane was active in student organizations, holding several formal and informal roles. She enjoyed the leadership work she participated in as a student and has been looking for ways to apply what she learned now that she has begun her career. She does not hold a formal title within the hospital pharmacy, which employs 4 full-time pharmacists, 2 pharmacy interns, and 10 pharmacy technicians. Last year, her health system negotiated a value-based contract where the system would receive enhanced compensation for improving the A1c values of its patients. Mary Avilla, her dedicated but overworked manager, has been put in charge of the pharmacy's role in this diabetes project. Mary recognizes that the pharmacy needs to contribute but lacks the time and energy to lead the effort. Jane sees an opportunity to utilize her experience and continue to develop her leadership skills, contribute to the mission of the system, and ultimately enhance the success of the pharmacy.

■ CHAPTER QUESTIONS

1. Why will leadership skills be important for me in my career as a pharmacist?

2. How can my daily work improve practice and lead to a more effective health system?
3. What steps can I take now to be a more effective leader?
4. How do I create change within my organization and the profession?
5. How will I contribute to creating high functioning health care teams?
6. What types of leaderships efforts are pharmacists currently engaged in?
7. What additional resources are available to enhance my own leadership development?

Getting to WHY: The Need for Leadership in Pharmacy and Health Care

In his book, *Start with Why*, author Simon Sinek (2013) explains that successful leaders who truly make an impact in the world around them begin all efforts with a deep understanding of "why" which always precedes the "who" or "what" of any endeavor. In the spirit of that idea, this chapter considers the "why" behind the need for more influential leaders in health care and pharmacy practice. Once the "why" has been determined, the chapter delves into the true work of any leader—creating meaningful change—and describes how one can become an influential leader in pharmacy.

Health care is complex set of systems witness to constant change and interplay between providers, patients, and payers across public and private institutions. Due to the complexity and diversity in the way health care is delivered, the system is in a constant state of flux, and factors such as policy changes, emerging payment models, and education and training costs continually impact delivery, cost, and quality. These dynamics seem to be moving at an ever-increasing pace, thus requiring organizations to alter and innovate to stay competitive. Past mechanisms for providing care may not be sufficient for health care providers and health systems to deliver effective care at a low cost. The need to learn, adjust efforts, and align individuals and organizations has never been greater and will require skilled leaders to navigate through the complexity of these health care changes. The most effective organizations will rely on frontline practitioners to learn, adapt, and lead others to succeed in this environment. The work and experience of these clinicians will inform the decisions of managers, directors, and executives in delivering high-quality care.

One example of a major disruptive change in health care is the shift in payment from fee-for-service to value-based reimbursement—a system where professionals are paid not primarily on the number of visits, procedures, or medications provided, but rather on the quality of the outcomes for patients. To make the successful shift in payment models and help rescue a health care system that delivers poor quality at a high cost (Avendano & Kawachi, 2014; Papanicolas et al., 2018), policymakers introduced a concept called Triple Aim (Berwick et al., 2008), where care is provided with better outcomes at a lower cost through an exceptional patient experience. This principle, as a means to produce greater value in the health care system, is guiding health care transformation today and for the foreseeable future (Burwell, 2015). The ability to accomplish goals like those of the Triple Aim and manage dynamic changes in health care such as workforce change, evolving practice roles, and complicated financial systems will be driven by the leadership capabilities of health professionals, including pharmacists, across the spectrum of practice settings.

One key component of improving the delivery of health care and ensuring positive health outcomes is the appropriate use of medications. It has been estimated that the cost of suboptimal medication use in the US health system is $500 billion (Watanabe et al., 2018). Given this high dollar figure, the work of pharmacists to ensure that all medications are indicated for a given condition, maximally effective to treat that condition, safe to use given patient-specific factors, and able to be taken as prescribed has never been more important. Applying the unique knowledge and skills of a pharmacist in a patient-centered way to emerging practices and improving the care currently being delivered will require the vision and leadership of pharmacists across practice settings and positions.

Additionally, the pharmacy profession is not immune to change and disruption common to other health care industries. There have already been significant changes in medication delivery systems such as the rise of automation, mail delivery of prescriptions, and shrinking reimbursements on prescription goods and services. With these changes and the increasing complexity of medication regimens, pharmacists' clinical skills rather than their ability to distribute medications have taken on enhanced importance (American College of Clinical, 2000). The work of adapting the existing work of pharmacists to directly contribute to improving the health care system now and in the future will require an emphasis on frontline and systems-level leadership over traditional personnel and operations management.

Chapter Purpose and Goal

In transitioning from the "why" of leadership in pharmacy to the "how," it is important to acknowledge that the amount of research and writing that exists describing the work of leaders and how one most effectively prepares themselves for this role is immense. The goals of this chapter are not merely to provide a comprehensive review of leadership work, leadership styles, the various traits that support one in becoming an effective leader, or the many strategies one can pursue to develop their leadership abilities. Attempting to do so would provide little help to most early career pharmacists beginning to consider the leadership roles they may assume. Thus, the approach taken here is that of "surveying the landscape," where several key themes and concepts are introduced so as to provide a reasonably broad perspective on leadership and leadership development. The chapter introduces several ideas and resources that are critical to an aspiring leader. It is the intent to create a storyline that provides connections between these concepts and provides an introduction to key leadership concepts. These concepts will provide context for and synergize with other coursework, workshops, mentorship, and self-exploration of leadership development resources, many of which are cited throughout the chapter.

Leadership vs. Management

Leadership and management are not mutually exclusive concepts, although the terms are often used interchangeably, with neither one being more important than the other. It is important, however, to note the differences for clarity in discussing how to become more effective pharmacy leaders. In the book, *The 7 Habits of Highly Effective People*, Stephen Covey (Covey, 2013) compares leadership and management. He states that management is concerned with how to accomplish certain activities, while leadership determines which activities should be performed in the first place. To illustrate this concept, Covey details a group of producers, or problem-solvers, making their way through the jungle. Their managers are working with them to ensure their cutting tools are sharp, creating standardized policies and procedures, and implementing new technologies in order to maximize their effectiveness in moving through the jungle. Covey explains that, in contrast, the leader is the person who climbs the tallest tree, surveys the landscape, and yells down, "Wrong jungle!"

This story highlights the concept that leadership is focused on the proper direction to head (and if that is the right direction) while management is focused on how to get there. These two essential roles are not in competition with each other; rather, they work synergistically to accomplish important tasks. In his landmark article, "What Leaders Do," John Kotter (1999) describes the key difference between leadership and management. He argues that management is centered on bringing order to complexity, while leadership involves setting the vision for the direction that the organization needs to follow. Another key contrast relates to the jobs and people within an organization where management is focused on creating roles and job descriptions and filling those with qualified individuals, while leadership involves aligning people to the organizational vision. Lastly, Kotter states that managers focus on problem solving and controlling through meetings, reports, and others tools while the work of leaders is to inspire and motivate others through an appeal to their emotions, needs, and values. A summary of these key differences between leadership and management is found in Table 3-1.

These concepts could be captured in a community pharmacy that dedicates significant time and resources to improving workflow efficiencies to speed prescription delivery but fails to recognize that the pharmacy serves patients with multiple medications,

Table 3-1.	Comparison of Leadership and Management
Leadership	**Management**
Determines the vision for team or organization	Deals with how to accomplish the vision or objective through budgeting and planning
Creates inspiration and motivation	Enhances efficiency and encourages problem solving through policy and process
Aligns people to organizational mission and vision	Creates job description and seeks to fill roles and positions
Manages the change process	Manages organizational complexity

health and social complexities, and limited ability to get to the pharmacy and obtain essential prescription medications. With all the attention on managing operation and workflow, the pharmacy has neglected to consider that the focus must be on increasing access to medications for their specific population, which would ultimately enhance the financial sustainability of the pharmacy. This particular pharmacy requires leaders who can see that the mission and vision of the work being done needs to change to get medications to patients in need rather than merely being efficient in filling prescriptions only to see them never be picked up. The managers would then determine the staff, supplies, and process needed to deliver medications to these patients at optimal efficiency. Thus, both leadership and management skills are needed to achieve success.

When considering the concept of leadership, it is important to have a clear definition of the concept. There are many definitions of leadership, but for the purposes of this chapter, an excellent one from which this chapter is based was proffered by Harvard professor Marshal Ganz who stated, "Leadership is accepting responsibility to create conditions that enable others to achieve shared purpose in the face of uncertainty" (Nohria & Khurana, 2010). This definition encompasses the essential elements of leadership: taking responsibility, inspiring others, and setting and accomplishing a compelling vision despite unknowns.

Positional and Non-Positional Leadership

Effective leadership is essential for pharmacists at all levels of an organization irrespective of a formal title. This is often referred to as "big L" (leaders with a formal role or title) vs. "little l" (those who lead from where they stand) leadership (White, 2006). Both types of leaders are required for meaningful change within an organization. Positional leaders are key in determining the vision for the organization and focusing on how to mobilize people to accomplish that vision. Non-positional leaders recognize that both large and small changes need to occur in their teams and departments and work to build influence with others to see those changes come to pass. This

type of grass-roots leadership is often underutilized and desperately needed by today's pharmacy practitioners. The rest of the chapter will focus on the key attributes, skills, and actions of leaders, with a focus on non-positional leadership, although the concepts apply to all types of leaders.

Referring back to the chapter scenario, recall Jane and the project she is considering undertaking in her pharmacy and then contemplate the following questions as they relate to her as a leader.

Questions to Ponder:

- How do Jane's feelings demonstrate her role as a leader?
- Is Jane a "Big L" or a "little l" leader?

Finding Passions

Before leadership work can begin, one must first search out, reflect on, and engage in areas of practice that they are passionate about. Once a practitioner finds a setting and role that are engaging and motivating, they will be better suited to lead others and find places to grow personally, practice areas to improve, and a profession to advance. Howard Thurman, an American author and philosopher said, "Don't ask what the world needs, ask what makes you come alive, and go do it, because what the world needs is people who have come alive." Many thought leaders have discussed the idea of determining mission in life's work. Greg McKeown (2014), author of *Essentialism: The Disciplined Pursuit of Less,* argues that each of us must determine our area of maximal impact—where we devote the majority of our time and energy for the greatest benefit of others rather than bowing to the tendency to say yes and believe we can do it all.

Similarly, in the book *Good to Great,* Jim Collins (2001) relates the story of the fox and the hedgehog. In this anecdotal tale, the sly and cunning fox spends its days devising ways to catch the hedgehog. Each time the fox has created a trap or thinks it has its prey in its grasp, the hedgehog rolls into a perfectly protective ball. The hedgehog preserves itself because it knows the one big thing that makes it supremely successful. While this idea was originally designed by Collins for successful organizations, the principles are also applicable to individuals. Each person must determine their personal hedgehog concept—what they are deeply passionate about, what they can be best in the world at, and what drives their resource engine. In essence, each pharmacist must consider the roles and practice settings they care deeply about and enjoy engaging in, work to enhance our knowledge and skills to become experts in that area, and then seek a position where that passion and expertise can be put to use for the benefit of patients and the health care system.

When engaged and motivated in daily work, practitioners will naturally and perhaps effortlessly begin to see those practice or system elements in need of our attention as leaders. They will become inquisitive and innovative due to a genuine motivation to improve. From that solid foundation will grow the leadership work that will meet the health care needs of the future.

Adaptive Leadership: Learning to Lead Change

At its core, leadership is about creating change and improving outcomes for patients individually and for the health care system generally. Referring again to the chapter scenario, Jane likely does not realize that her pharmacy team is facing a unique type of problem that has been described by Heifetz and colleagues (2009) as an "adaptive challenge." Some problems faced by organizations are technical in nature—they may be large, complex problems, but they are challenges the organization has faced before and have relatively well-understood solutions. This is not to say these challenges are easy to address, but because there is an element of familiarity, the path to success is clear. In these situations, a top-down managerial approach that relies on direction from positional leaders is possible, often even welcomed by frontline staff.

However, adaptive challenges are the types of problems that present with less clarity for resolution. The positional leader does not have the answer; in fact, no one does. The path to addressing the challenge requires brainstorming, experimentation, and engagement of individuals at all levels of the organization. With this type of leadership challenge, the positional leader is a facilitator that partners with frontline staff to create engagement and collaborative problem-solving. Success is dependent on non-positional leaders bringing their own leadership abilities to the table—being open to testing new ideas, providing critical frontline perspective, and a commitment to work collaboratively with administrators to produce a new way of working that accomplishes the goals of the organization. This is precisely the leadership opportunity facing Jane at this time.

Like Jane's situation, solving adaptive challenges requires engaging others in creating meaningful and positive change. In their book, *Strengths-Based Leadership* (Rath & Conchie, 2008), Gallup researchers asked what qualities of a leader create engagement and compel others to follow. One answer was a hopeful vision of the future. Effective leaders must communicate a hopeful and compelling vision of the future and share that vision with others to motivate them to action. They must work collaboratively and garner the necessary buy-in and effort of all involved to solve adaptive challenges.

This concept of vision, and other key elements to producing change, was highlighted in *Leading Change* by John Kotter (1996), which identifies the following steps to create lasting change in organizations:

1. Establish a sense of urgency to address the challenge facing the organization.
2. Build a guiding coalition of individuals from different perspectives who will lead the efforts to create change.
3. Develop a strategic vision and set of strategies that will guide efforts to adapt the way individuals and the organization as a whole operates.
4. Communicate the vision frequently and in compelling ways to enlist others from across the organization to contribute to the envisioned change.
5. Remove barriers to enable action, creating opportunities for frontline staff to effectively contribute to the leadership work.

6. Generate short-term wins that allow all to see that progress is being made so that motivation and energy for change remains strong.
7. Sustain acceleration to ensure that the true vision for change remains in focus.
8. Institute change in a way that creates a new culture that allows the instituted changes to thrive.

Given this framework, Jane now has concrete steps as she moves her pharmacy and colleagues forward in their diabetes initiative. One key change process beyond a hopeful and compelling vision is to create a sense of urgency for change. Leaders must work to overcome the inertia of the status quo which compels most individuals to resist change. Creating the context for the need to change, coupled with a strategic vision and communicating that important story to others is among the most important skills for any leader seeking to improve their team or organization. With these foundational steps, leaders have the footing to help overcome conflicts, remove inevitable barriers, and create the short-term wins that build momentum to lasting change. These steps provide a road map for creating long-term change, and aspects of Kotter's model are highlighted throughout this chapter.

To Be a Leader, Start with Self

Before leaders can influence others and create change, they must first know and understand how their talents and personality will influence their leadership style. Leadership is not a quality that one possesses at birth, but rather, is a process of combining individual traits with experiences that hone leadership skills and ultimately allow one to develop their leadership style. By investing in the development of a leadership style and enhancing self-awareness, leaders determine the best method for them to build influence and create change. Enhanced self-awareness then leads to a pattern of self-improvement and eventually self-mastery. There is no "correct" style, and every person, regardless of personality, can build themselves into an effective leader.

For Jane, and all individuals who aspire to lead, taking personal ownership of self-development is critical. Noted leadership expert Peter Drucker (1999)

has highlighted the importance of this responsibility, outlining four areas that one must commit time and energy to self-understanding and development in order to achieve excellence as a leader: determining strengths, connecting to values, considering how one best accomplishes work, and taking responsibility for relationships.

A Strengths-Based Approach

In the early 2000s, the Gallup organization created the StrengthsFinder (Rath, 2007) tool to help individuals identify their Signature Themes of talent. The 34 Signature Themes represent recurring ways of thought, feeling, or behavior and are associated with high-level performance in business settings (Rath, 2007; Rath & Conchie, 2008). Inherent in the research that produced the StrengthsFinder instrument is an assertion that society generally focuses on "improving weaknesses" rather than harnessing each individual's talents or strengths. This mentality tends to spill over into personnel evaluations and disciplinary actions, which leads to dissatisfaction and decreased productivity.

To counter this problem, leaders need to learn for themselves what their strengths are, reflect on ways to regularly utilize those strengths to influence and benefit others, and connect those individual strengths to their leadership work. To be effective, leaders will gravitate to roles that naturally align with their strengths. They will ask, "What activities give me energy?" or "What type of work do I naturally gravitate toward and find success doing?"

Gallup has organized the 34 Signature Themes into four "leadership domains": executing, influencing, relationship-building, and strategic thinking. When leaders have more than one strength in a given domain, this tends to manifest as their natural leadership style. Categorized Signature Themes and the corresponding definitions of each domain are found in Table 3-2.

Questions to Ponder:

- Does the definition of one of the domains resonate with you more than others?

Table 3-2.   CliftonStrengths® Signature Themes by Domain (with Domain Definition)

Executing—high ability to get things done, problem-solve, and turn ideas into actual achievements	Influencing—naturally speak up and reach out, constantly selling ideas to internal and external stakeholders	Relationship Building—keep teams and organizations together, create synergy between individuals and groups leading to better outcomes	Strategic Thinking—consider ideas and concepts for the future, determine optimal solutions by analyzing data and options for action
Achiever®	Activator®	Adaptability®	Analytical®
Arranger®	Command®	Connectedness®	Context®
Belief®	Communication®	Developer®	Futuristic®
Consistency®	Competition®	Empathy®	Ideation®
Deliberate®	Maximizer®	Harmony®	Input®
Discipline®	Self-Assurance®	Includer®	Intellection®
Focus®	Significance®	Individualization®	Learner®
Responsibility®	Woo®	Positivity®	Strategic®

Gallup®, CliftonStrengths® and the 34 theme names of CliftonStrengths® are trademarks of Gallup, Inc. All rights reserved. To learn more about CliftonStrengths®, please visit www.gallupstrengthcenter.com.

- How have you perceived that your actions and behaviors are consistent with the domain definition(s)?
- Can you identify relationships between your perceived leadership domain and the leadership roles or styles you tend to assume?

When one begins to understand, apply, and develop their natural talents and the leadership style that is most comfortable, one will grow in their ability to become an authentic, effective leader. From the exploration of professional passions and the journey of personal talents, confidence in one's ability to influence and lead grows. This confidence, style, and authenticity are key elements in building influence with others and effectively leading change.

Again, recall Jane's project to improve diabetes control. Jane's employer asks each of its pharmacists to complete the StrengthsFinder assessment as part of employee orientation, and from this, she learned that her top five Signature Themes and descriptions are as follows:

1. Achiever: People exceptionally talented in the Achiever theme work hard and possess a great deal of stamina. They take immense satisfaction in being busy and productive.
2. Harmony: People exceptionally talented in the Harmony theme look for consensus. They don't enjoy conflict; rather, they seek areas of agreement.
3. Discipline: People exceptionally talented in the Discipline theme enjoy routine and structure. Their world is best described by the order they create.
4. Learner: People exceptionally talented in the Learner theme have a great desire to learn and want to continuously improve. The process of learning, rather than the outcome, excites them.
5. Communication: People exceptionally talented in the Communication theme generally find it easy to put their thoughts into words. They are good conversationalists and presenters.

Questions to Ponder:

- How might Jane leverage her strengths in leading the diabetes project?
- Where can she provide significant benefit?
- Where could she struggle or get bogged down?

Jane's strengths will naturally align to this project, as she will effortlessly begin to create long- and short-term goals for the project and develop the systems that will assist in seeing that those goals are accomplished. With her sights set on improving the diabetes-related outcomes of her patients, she will also have the ability to learn from others, ensure that those she works with understand the vision, and assist her team to move together in the right direction. She may need to be cautious to ensure that her drive for accomplishment and order does not move too quickly or produce results at the expense of her colleagues and their long-term buy-in to the project.

In considering the concept of harnessing individual strengths and the importance of this practice in the work of leadership, it is essential to remember that no strength is better or worse than another. All have a place and all contribute to the development of a personal leadership style. Avoid the tendency to see strengths as faults or to underestimate their value. In the work of providing exceptional care and leading change, all strengths are needed.

Determining Values

Learning and capitalizing on strengths is the first step in managing self, but not sufficient for effective leadership. Some of the most heinous leaders and dictators likely had potent strengths that they deployed, but to create change that is positive, leaders must have a sense of their core values—what they stand for and what shapes their hope and vision for the future. In *The Leadership Challenge*, Kouzes and Posner (2017) argue that values are like a compass that gives our work a sense of direction, serves as a guide to the hundreds of decisions we make each day, and provides motivation and empowerment. Clarity around our own values strengthens our ability to demonstrate them through words and actions, and then ultimately find shared values with others—a key component of the change work inherent in leadership.

While the list of potential values is exhaustive, it would be wise to pause and begin to explore which values resonate with you personally and have helped shape the person and leader you are today. Consider taking a few minutes to conduct an internet search to find a list of values. Once you have found a list, take a few moments and consider which of the listed values you align with naturally and write them down in a simple format such as that provided below.

My Core Values

1. _____
2. _____
3. _____
4. _____

Questions to Ponder:

- Where have these values appeared for you in the past?
- What core experiences have shaped who you are and how you see the world?
- How have those experiences defined your values?

Becoming aware of and being able to articulate our core values is pivotal in leadership work as these values, when aligned with others, will draw them to the important change work that needs to occur. In Jane's diabetes work, her core values of compassion and wanting what is best for her patients are driving her desire to be engaged in the project and help lower A1c values from a patient-centered approach. As she continues the work and seeks to engage others, this value will shine forward and invite others with similar values to join her in the effort.

Aligning Strengths and Values in Daily Work

Strengths and values are tied very closely to and incredibly influential in how to approach work as either a practitioners or a leader. They play a key role in our ability to be successful. Think of the last time you felt deeply engaged in a project or topic. What did that feel like? How long were you able to spend on the task without fatiguing or getting distracted? What was the quality of the end product your produced? Contrast this with times you have felt that you felt work to be mundane or draining. Were your strengths in play? Was the work aligned to your core values? To find both success and lasting satisfaction in daily work, we must utilize our strengths regularly and connect our work to our core values.

For an illustration of this concept, consider Jane's "achiever" strength and how that will influence the way she goes about her daily tasks. She will likely gain enhanced satisfaction from her work when she accomplishes goals, crosses off checklist items, or completes a project. Combined with her core value of trust, Jane will seek to complete her assigned tasks to build a reputation as someone who follows through. In contrast, she will grow frustrated if work piles up without adequate time to finish it, thus making her unable to follow through on her commitments. The loss of trust that results from letting down colleagues and patients will produce the trappings of failure and emotional exhaustion. If this becomes the norm rather than the exception, how engaged will Jane be in her work? How will she feel at the end of the day? How long will she stay in her position?

In this example, think of the difference for Jane personally, the team, and her patients if she is able to engage her team in providing optimal medication regimens and is able to take the time to learn the goals and desires of her patients. Through utilizing her strengths and aligning with her core values, she will become a more effective practitioner and have the potential to be a more influential leader. She will also have the resilience to come to work week in and week out with reserves to engage in the change work needed to improve patient care within her pharmacy and potentially the organization as a whole.

Thus, the alignment of strengths and values to daily work ensures that we can continue to capitalize on our passions and provides energy for our work. From that enhanced energy and effectiveness comes the enthusiasm to engage in the work of leadership and creating change.

Questions to Ponder:

- Am I able to utilize my strengths on a daily basis?
- Does my work and my approach to leadership align with my core values?
- What can I begin doing to leverage my strengths and align my values as a leader?

Responsibility for Relationships

Once leaders know the way their strengths and values impact how they perform, they are better able to turn their attention to developing relationships with others. Leaders must recognize the essential role of relationships in creating meaningful change and take responsibility for creating positive relationships. One key attribute of effective leaders is a high degree of emotional intelligence (EI), which includes awareness of and control over one's own moods and emotions and their effect on others, the ability to work with passion, motivation, deep empathy, and proficiency in building rapport and strong networks. Daniel Goleman (2004), a leading expert on EI, summed up the importance of EI as follows, "[Research], clearly shows that emotional intelligence is the sine qua non of leadership. Without it, a person can have the best training in the world, an incisive, analytical mind, and an endless supply of smart ideas, but he still won't make a great leader."

Another lens to use in considering a leader's responsibility in building relationships is the idea of considering our impact on others. The Arbinger Institute (Arbinger Institute, 2008, 2015, 2016) describes that our mindset, or the way that we view the people around us, has a tremendous impact on how others perceive us. The authors indicate that we can see others as people who have needs, objectives, and desires just like us or we can see others as objects—obstacles that we blame, vehicles that we use or irrelevancies that we ignore. This mindset of seeing others as objects, referred to as an inward mindset, then affects our behavior toward them and potentially their reciprocal behavior toward us. We then get stuck in this cycle of objectifying others and being objectified in return. This pattern of behavior causes energy to be spent in conflict rather than on achieving personal and organizational goals. With time, the underlying mindset of all parties and the behaviors driven from them, diminish our relationships and the ability to positively influence others and erode organizational effectiveness.

Thus, those who wish to lead must spend time and energy in developing their EI and mindset to create the type of relationships through which others will view them as a positive influence in the organization or on them personally. As Jane considers her role as a pharmacist, she must consider how she views the people around her and what impact she has on each of them and their ability to do their work.

Questions to Ponder:

- How might Jane begin to see people as objects—obstacles, vehicles, or irrelevancies?
- Could the view she has of others be the result of poorly controlled emotions or past conflict?
- How can she work to see each person she works with as a person with goals, objectives, and needs to impact them in a positive way?

Learning to improve and manage self is the first key step in becoming an effective leader and serves as the foundation for leading any change project. Once we have begun to recognize and develop our personal strengths and values, aligned them to our daily work, and combined this with the responsibility to positively impact others, we have created the foundation for our leadership work to begin. Through this process of self-management, we discover who we are and our own unique abilities and leadership style and we are ready to engage others in an authentic and effective way that inspires them to follow and join in our effort to lead change.

Teaming: You Cannot Lead Alone

After some time in self-reflection and consideration for why she feels compelled to provide leadership to the diabetes improvement project, Jane considers her next steps. She recognizes that her strengths most naturally align with the Executing domain from Table 3-1, meaning that she will naturally look to the accomplishment of tasks and goals in her leadership style. Her manager, grateful and relieved for her proactive desire to help, has given her approval to start working and suggested a few people she might contact, such as the medical director for the clinic where the pharmacy is located, the clinic manager (who has an MBA), and one of the pharmacy technicians who

has been looking for an additional project to work on. Jane also recognizes that another health care professional, such as a clinical nurse, may also be helpful to diversify the experience, training, and perspectives of the group. In considering diversity of talent as a benefit to team effectiveness, Jane will also consider the strengths of various team members and seek to include those with strengths in other domains. By bringing others to the table with complementary strengths, she will compensate for areas of work that may be difficult for her and increase the likelihood of team success.

With this in mind, Jane begins her work and quickly recognizes that she will need to meet with each person and learn more about them and their potential role in the project. They will also need to meet together to determine how they will work together and accomplish this quality improvement project. She recognizes that having an effective team, the guiding coalition identified in Kotter's change process, will be key to improving diabetes control rates in their patient population.

Once leaders have spent time learning to manage self, they can begin to consider how to engage others in leadership work. Health care's complexity and evolutionary nature require health care providers, support staff, and administrators to work together to be successful in achieving organizational goals and serving patients in the best way possible. Additionally, based on Ganz's definition of leadership, the practice of leaders cannot happen in a vacuum and requires individuals to work together in accomplishing a shared vision. Thus, leadership, by its very nature, involves motivating and influencing others to action. There are many theories and strategies for creating effective teams, and several chapters could be devoted to this topic alone. This chapter focuses the discussion on the application of self-awareness to teams and outlines a popular framework for creating effective teams.

Before exploring what effective teams do, consider that the word "team" is often used as a noun. To create teams that are successful in meeting the needs of the health care system, this concept must shift from a noun to a verb—"teaming"—as the key actions that effective leaders do to have high functioning teams. This idea is championed by Amy Edmunson, who defines teaming as "…a dynamic activity, not a bounded, static entity. It is largely determined by the mindset and practices of teamwork, not the design and structures of effective teams" (Edmondson, 2012). In this discussion of team, the focus is on action rather than structure to give concrete steps leaders can actually employ to create high functioning teams.

Peter Drucker (1999) notes that once leaders have become efficient self-managers they then develop the abilities to reach out to others, appreciate their strengths, values, and work preferences, and build meaningful and authentic relationships. To accomplish this, the same tools and strategies used to build self-awareness can be employed. Teams can determine the strengths of each member and discuss how those strengths can align for greater team and organizational success and enhanced team member satisfaction.

One strategy that can be effective in team development is to have members of a team explore their own Signature Themes and then begin to consider how those themes fit into the four StrengthsFinder Leadership Domains of Executing, Influencing, Relationships Building, and Strategic Thinking. The most effective teams will look to engage strengths across all four domains. Research has identified that most pharmacists are strongest in the Executing and Relationship Building domains (Ferreri et al., 2017; Janke et al., 2015; Yee et al., 2018). Without cognizant consideration, pharmacy teams may have gaps in Strategic Thinking and Influencing, two areas critical for producing effective change in organizations. In referring back to the chapter scenario, Jane may consider finding team members who complement her strengths, especially in the influencing domain, to be successful in her diabetes project.

Leaders must also guide others in the discovery of their values and then seek to find the common values that unite and motive the team. Leaders must create space for members to talk, share stories, and determine their core values. The team can then determine what values they share and utilize those to shape their activities and strategies. These activities will naturally lead to discussions about work preferences, including what activities play to each team member's strengths and contribute to increases in energy and performance. An overarching purpose of this dedicated time and intentional effort in strengths and stories will be the development of foundational relationships that will grow and develop over time.

Five Potential Dysfunctions of a Team

Another way for Jane to consider how her team can be most effective is to consider the ideas detailed in *The Five Dysfunctions of a Team* by Patrick Lencioni (2002). The author describes the key building blocks to team performance through a fictional story of an executive team filled with motivated and talented individuals that is on the brink of collapse because they have not learned how to work together effectively. They are displaying the "five dysfunctions," which include: (1) absence of trust, (2) fear of conflict, (3) lack of commitment, (4) avoidance of accountability, and (5) inattention to results. The opposite of each dysfunction is an "essential function" for teaming.

Trust

A discussion of the essential function of teams must begin with the foundational principle of trust. All members of a team must trust each other implicitly, or they will never be able to engage in the important work they tasked with completing. Trust is critical. With it, teams can synergize and accomplish amazing results. Without it, teams crumble and implode, and the work of leadership grinds to a halt.

Stephen Covey explored these issues in his well-renowned book, *Speed of Trust* (Covey & Merrill, 2008). At the center of his argument is the idea that when teams and organizations have deep levels of trust, the team becomes more effective and efficient. When trust is low, those efficiencies become stalled in policy, bureaucracy, and skepticism, which lead to increases in time and money expended. For example, consider the last time you navigated an airport to take a flight—a classically low-trust environment. How long did it take for you to make it from the curb outside to your seat on the plane? Because of the low level of trust, layers of screening and security bog down travel and increase cost. Consider your school setting. What policies and procedures have come about due to low levels of trust? Have these enhanced or hindered your effectiveness in learning? Leaders, both positional and nonpositional, must create an environment, or culture of trust. This includes building trust as a leader but also ensuring that people are encouraged to engage in high-trust behaviors and held accountable when they fail to do so. The consistent behavior of the leader as a role model in building trust and holding others accountable for trust-building begins to create a culture within a team or organization. To be successful in creating a high trust environment, leaders much maintain a high degree of EI by promoting equity, staying calm when challenged, and making altruistic decisions for the good of the organization. In an effort to provide concrete steps to build this culture, key trust-building practices from *Speed of Trust* are listed in Table 3-3.

Table 3-3.	Trust-Building Behaviors from *Speed of Trust*
Talk straight	Be honest and straightforward. Do not dance around hard facts or truths in order to please others. Give helpful and constructive feedback.
Demonstrate respect	Honor the dignity of each individual and show respect for all, including those who offer you no benefit. Care for those around you.
Create transparency	Remove hidden agendas and speak the truth in an open and authentic way where people can measure your words and actions against facts and information.
Right wrongs	Be humble and apologize quickly when mistakes are made or feelings are hurt. Make up for wrongs through restitution and giving more than was taken.
Show loyalty	Acknowledge the work and contribution of others in your own successes and give credit where due. Do not talk or gossip about others who are not present. Advocate for those who can't speak for themselves.
Deliver results	Do what you say you will do when you will do it. Be a person who delivers without excuses.
Get better	Seek to learn, grow, and improve. Seek for and act on feedback from others. Recognize the constant need to adapt and grow with changing internal dynamics and external forces.
Confront reality	Tackle the tough issues head on. Do not sweep problems under the rug. Be the person willing to have discussions about real problems.
Clarify expectations	Establish and seek clear expectations for yourself and others. Continually discuss and reaffirm what is expected for you and ensure the same with others.
Practice accountability	Take responsibility for outcomes and ensure you and others are held accountable for those results. Avoid the tendency to blame or deflect.
Listen first	Seek to understand through listening and observing. Ask others what is important to them. Don't make assumptions.
Keep commitments	Make commitments that you intend and are able to keep. Be thoughtful about what you agree to and then ensure you have done what you said.
Extend trust	Learn to extend trust as abundantly as possible. Honor those who have demonstrated trust with more and give judiciously to those who are still earning trust.

Data from Covey, 2008.

As can be observed from the list above, building trust requires time and is not achieved overnight. Trust is built day by day and decision by decision, and leaders must be diligent to ensure they are fostering trust amongst team members. Another way to enhance trust is to create what has been called psychological safety or "a climate in which people feel free to express relevant thoughts and feelings…[and] give tough feedback or have difficult conversations without the need to tiptoe around the truth" (see Chapter 16). In psychologically safe environments, people believe that if they make a mistake other will not penalize or think less of them for it. These teams become environments where team members can be innovative, challenge each other, and make mistakes without fear of retribution and in service of their ultimate goal (Edmondson, 2012). Others have sought to determine the role of psychological safety on teams. When Google sought to better understand what makes the most effective teams through their Project Aristotle, they found that one of the key components was psychological safety—a team member's perception of the consequences of taking risk and willingness to be vulnerable with others (Duhigg, 2016).

The essential role of leaders in creating trust is to engage in trust-building behaviors themselves in an authentic way, ensure that others engage in these behaviors, and create the safety needed for team members to innovate, ask questions and explore new solutions to complex problems. When done consistently, these actions create a culture that fosters and reinforces trust almost imperceptibly. From this foundation, teams can begin to tackle challenge and achieve results.

Questions to Ponder:

- Which trust-building behaviors will be especially important for Jane and her team?
- If you were Jane, which behaviors or ideas would you focus on first?

Attention to Results

Once a team's foundation of trust is building, the next essential function is to determine what results the team is striving to achieve. Stephen Covey (2013)

Table 3-4.	A Pharmacy Student's Essential Leadership Reading List

Leadership Models
The Leadership Challenge by James Kouzes & Barry Posner
Leadership Made Simple by Ed Oakley & Doug Krug

Organizational Change
The Speed of Trust by Stephen M.R. Covey
Good to Great by Jim Collins
Heart of Change or Our Iceberg Is Melting by John Kotter
Outward Mindset by the Arbinger Institute

Personal Development
StrengthsFinder 2.0 by Tom Rath
The Seven Habits of Highly Effective People by Stephen M.R. Covey
Strength-Based Leadership by Tom Rath & Barry Conchie
Emotionally Intelligent Leadership by Marcy Levy Shankman, Scott Allen, & Paige Haber-Curran
Essentialism: The Disciplined Pursuit of Less by Greg McKeown
The Servant by James Hunter
Leadership and Self-Deception by The Arbinger Institute

Teaming
Teaming by Amy Edmunson
The Five Dysfunction of a Team by Patrick Lencioni
Team of Teams by Stanley McChrystal

called this idea "begin with the end in mind" or determine the ultimate goal. By starting out with a deep discussion and determination of what the team is looking to achieve, there is always a centering point or measuring stick to come back to in assessing progress and achieving success. Additionally, as teams focus on results that unify and bind them rather than differences that distinguish them, conflict can be reduced and problem solving can focus on removing barriers and addressing issues rather than people-centered dust-ups. Truly, if leaders and teams never determine their destination, they will wander aimlessly and fail to reach their potential.

In the case of Jane's newly formed Diabetes Improvement Team, the group spends time learning from each other's stories and determining their strengths and now begins to consider the task at hand. They determine that their goal is to improve diabetes control by 75% in patients with a hemoglobin A1c value of greater than 8% over the course of 1 year. They consider their roles in patient care, their diverse practice experience, and each person's particular interest in the details of the project. Jane helps the team divide roles and assignments, and they plan to reconvene in a few weeks' time.

Engaging in Productive Conflict

Once a team has developed trusting relationships, they effectively engage in conflict. For most of us, the word conflict does not engender happy and positive feelings. Conflict is often regarded as a negative, something to be avoided, or hushed until it blows up in everyone's faces. But conflict, like the other essential functions is not, in and of itself, always negative. When handled productively and built on a foundation of trust and psychological safety, conflict can help achieve better results. Productive conflict draws on the power of diversity of thought and experience rather than surrendering to divisiveness. When leaders have fostered an environment where team members can disagree and push back, then true innovation and positive change can occur. The skill as the leader, then, is to find ways to surface conflict, invite opposing opinions, and focus all team members back to the ultimate goal discussed previously. When the focus becomes what we are trying to accomplish and not who is involved or getting the credit, our success and satisfaction as leaders and team members will improve. Thus, productive conflict can be the launching point of successful teams.

Questions to Ponder:

- Think back to the makeup of Jane's diabetes improvement team. Where might there be conflict given the background of participants on the team?

- How can the team utilize their diverse experiences and skills to enhance the project?

Enhanced Commitment & Shared Accountability

Consider the type of team described thus far with high trust and focused on a common goal. Picture yourself as a member or leader of this team. What do meetings look like? How do people respond to each other? This is a team that knows each other's strengths and values in a meaningful way. That knowledge allows them to assume the best in each other and recognize why people behave the way they do and where they excel or sometimes are challenged. The team recognizes that they are unified in values and purpose, and their goal is the same. When barriers or challenges come (as they always do), the team has the culture and ability to brainstorm and problem solve.

With these positive underpinnings, team members cannot help but be deeply committed to the cause and unwilling to let each other down. When someone begins to stray from the culture or destination, team members must hold them accountable and invite them back. Team members have become not only deeply invested in the work but also in each other and recognize that the only way to achieve meaningful and lasting change is together. They have become the guiding coalition and volunteer army in Kotter's change process.

It is worth noting that following these steps to form teams is indeed challenging. The process requires an investment of time and energy. It sometimes requires letting go of certain individuals or inviting them to move on to work that is more in line with their ideas and values. This can be difficult, emotionally taxing, and slow in its development. Because of the endurance needed, it is all the more critical to find team members with shared values and aligned vision for just such difficult moments. In that case, when the weight and pressures of the work bear down, the leader can turn to trusted and faithful team members for strength and encouragement to continue the work.

Additional Leadership Frameworks

The chapter has focused on a strengths-based approach to leadership in the context of creating change through teaming. In the leadership literature, however, there are many models and frameworks. A few are worth noting for those who wish to pursue additional study and development. Each model or framework carries principles and concepts that will assist clinicians in becoming better leaders and can be adopted based on the leadership challenge at hand or the current state and needs of the practitioner.

The Leadership Challenge (Kouzes & Posner, 2017). This model of leadership serves as a guide for those wishing to get people, teams, and organizations to accomplish extraordinary objectives. Through researcher on the practices of successful leaders, the authors developed the Five Practices of Exemplary Leadership: model the way, inspire a shared vision, challenge the process, enable others to act, and encourage the heart. These concepts are not necessarily novel; rather, they have stood the test of time and remain relevant for aspiring leaders today and serve as guidance for leading effective change across areas of pharmacy practice.

The Servant Leader (Hunter, 1998). In some leadership models, the focus in on strategy, whereas in servant leadership, the focus is to enhance one's own positive attributes to better serve the needs of others. Through the development of qualities such as humility, honesty, kindness, and empathy, leaders begin to care for those with whom they work, serve, and sacrifice for them, and thus gain influence in accomplishing shared objectives.

Reframing Leadership (Bolman & Deal, 2013). All leaders have tendencies in their style and in the way they approach their work. This model details four common "frames" that leaders utilize. Rather than using what each leader deems to be the "right" frame, the authors note that frames can be used like maps to see how best to move forward, each with pros and cons. The four frames are structural (leader as the architect), human resource (leader as the coach), political (leader as peacemaker), and symbolic (leader as storyteller). Each of these frames can be used strategically to play the role needed to lead change efforts.

Thomas–Kilmann Conflict Mode (Thomas & Kilmann, 2007). While not an explicit leadership model, this tool helps the leader identify their own style and reaction to conflict, each with its inherent strengths and weaknesses. Once leaders recognize their most commonly used modes, they can confront the conflict or challenge with more intentionality and a better chance of finding a resolution to find collaborative "win-win" situations for all parties involved.

Leadership Context in Pharmacy Practice

The need for leadership in pharmacy is not novel, and innovative change makers within the profession have long recognized the need for enhanced leadership at all levels of organizations. In her 2015 Whitney Award speech, Sharon Murphy Enright (2015) called for more "small-l leaders [to] own…change and run with it." Pharmacists in a variety of practice settings have answered that call by leading projects and initiatives within their own institutions and communities.

For example, pharmacists within a large chain of pharmacies determined to address the public health needs of their communities can initiate a project to respond to the opioid crisis by providing drug disposal kiosks, expanding access to naloxone, and educating patients on the risk of opioid overdose (Shafer et al., 2017). In another project, pharmacists were able to decrease patients' use of high-risk opioid medications, which led to safer practices and improved patient satisfaction and financial outcomes (Phatak et al., 2016). Pharmacists have also successfully led efforts to reduce 30-day readmissions (Shaver et al., 2019) and improve adherence to COPD medications (Abdulsalim et al., 2018). In line with the value-based reforms discussed previously, a group of pharmacists across multiple ambulatory clinics partnered with physician colleagues to improve care of chronic diseases such as diabetes, hypertension, and hyperlipidemia. resulting in improved patient outcomes at a lower cost (Matzke et al., 2018).

These pharmacists, and many others who lead where they stand by addressing organizational and societal needs, are creating the impact and improvement essential to improving the health care system and its resultant outcomes. These clinicians are "owning the work" of leadership and provide excellent role modeling and examples to follow.

Revising the Scenario

Over the course of the year, the team met regularly to discuss progress and determine next steps. Jane, as the leader of the team, engaged with each team member individually and ensured buy-in and accountability with the team collectively. When issues of unexpected increased costs and ambiguity around reimbursement surfaced between the clinic and pharmacy managers, she was able to intervene, bringing the two parties to the table to talk through solutions. After 1 year of effort, the team has improved the A1c results of the patients by 65%, short of their goal but above the 60% threshold required by the insurance provider for their enhanced compensation. Jane generated short-term wins to show the value of an interprofessional team leading a care improvement project.

In addition to the patient and financial outcomes of the project, Jane also recognizes that the capacity of the organization, both the clinic and the pharmacy, for working collaboratively and improving care increased. She created the momentum that will lead to further collaboration and a culture of change that will allow leaders like herself to thrive and create better outcomes for the organization and for the patients she and her colleagues serve.

Next Steps in Your Leadership Journey

Leadership is not a destination, but rather, is a lifetime journey and is needed at all levels of an organization. This chapter has focused on many key aspects of leadership development and presented theories, concepts, and skills that will be vital to creating the change needed for a better health care system, for better pharmacy practice, and for better results for patients. Leaders are not simply "born." Leadership style and competency come from a combination of experiencing one's own personality and talent combined with purposeful learning experiences.

The chapter began by asking "why," that is, why we need leaders now more than ever. It closes with an invitation. Each of us must determine our own personal "why"—why are we called to the work of leadership? Why do we choose to step up when others might step back? What are we called to do, and who can we influence along the way?

Reading this chapter is just the beginning and serves as a launching point in your own leadership development. The world needs individuals who lift where they stand and seek to improve and assist regardless of title or setting. The most important message to take away from this chapter is that leadership is a choice. It is not a mystical trait granted only to a few. The ability to lead starts with the choice to believe that each individual can be an effective leader. The ability to lead then is rooted in the multitude of choices one makes to pursue learning opportunities, seek mentorship, and commit to engaging in experiences that may push you outside your current level of comfort. The concepts and ideas presented in this chapter are intended to aid your leadership journey to find greater satisfaction and success.

■ QUESTIONS FOR FURTHER DISCUSSION

As you consider the choices you will make in your leadership journey, you might reflect on the following questions:

- What passion in health care will drive my desire to serve as a source of influence early in my career?
- What action will I take as a result of reading this chapter to advance my leadership journey with purpose?
- What leadership concept from this chapter do I want to explore with more depth?
- What resonated with me in this chapter that I want to explore further with an instructor, mentor, or peer?
- Who can I look to as a mentor or coach to help me on my journey?

REFERENCES

Abdulsalim S, Unnikrishnan MK, Manu MK, Alrasheedy AA, Godman B, Morisky DE. 2018. Structured pharmacist-led intervention programme to improve medication adherence in COPD patients: A randomized controlled study. *Res Social Adm Pharm* 14(10):909–914.

American College of Clinical Pharmacy. 2000. A vision of pharmacy's future roles, responsibilities, and manpower needs in the United States. *Pharmacotherapy* 20(8):991–1020.

Arbinger Institute. 2008. *Leadership and Self-Deception: Getting Out of the Box*. ReadHowYouWant.

Arbinger Institute. 2015. *The Anatomy of Peace Resolving the Heart of Conflict*. Oakland, CA: Berrett-Hoehler Publishers.

Arbinger Institute. 2016. *Outward Mindset: Seeing Beyond Ourselves*. Oakland, CA: Berrett-Koehler Publishers.

Avendano M, Kawachi I. 2014. Why do Americans have shorter life expectancy and worse health than do people in other high-income countries? *Annu Rev Public Health* 35:307–325.

Berwick DM, Nolan TW, Whittington J. 2008. The triple aim: care, health, and cost. *Health Aff (Millwood)* 27(3):759–769.

Bolman LG, Deal TE. 2013. *Reframing Organizations: Artistry, Choice, and Leadership*. San Francisco, CA: Jossey-Bass.

Burwell SM. 2015. Setting value-based payment goals—HHS efforts to improve U.S. health care. *N Engl J Med* 372(10):897–899.

Collins J. 2001. *Good to Great: Why Some Companies Make the Leap ... and Others Don't*. New York, NY: Harper Collins.

Covey SR. 2013. *The 7 Habits of Highly Effective People: Powerful Lessons in Personal Change*, 25th anniversary ed. New York, NY: Simon & Schuster.

Covey SR, Merrill RR. 2008. *The Speed of Trust: The One Thing That Changes Everything*. New York, NY: Free Press.

Drucker PF. 1999. *Managing Oneself*. Cambridge, MA: Harvard Business Review.

Duhigg C. 2016. What Google Learned from Its Quest to Build the Perfect Team. *New York Times*. Retrieved from https://www.nytimes.com/2016/02/28/magazine/what-google-learned-from-its-quest-to-build-the-perfect-team.html.

Edmondson AC. 2012. *Teaming: How Organizations Learn, Innovate, and Compete in the Knowledge Economy*. San Francisco, CA: Jossey-Bass.

Enright SM. 2015. Lean back, listen, and own up. *Am J Health Syst Pharm* 72(16):1393–1402.

Ferreri SP, Cross LB, Hanes SD, Jenkins T, Meyer D, Pittenger A. 2017. Academic pharmacy: Where is our influence? *Am J Pharm Educ* 81(4):63.

Goleman D. 2004. What makes a leader?(Best of HBR) (Reprint). *Harvard Business Review* 82(1):82.

Heifetz RA, Grashow A, Linsky M. 2009. *The Practice of Adaptive Leadership Tools and Tactics for Changing Your Organization and the World*. Boston, MA: Harvard Business Press.

Hunter JC. 1998. *The Servant: A Simple Story About the True Essence of Leadership*. Rocklin, CA: Prima Pub.

Janke KK, Farris KB, Kelley KA, et al. 2015. Strengths-Finder signature themes of talent in doctor of pharmacy students in five midwestern pharmacy schools. *Am J Pharm Educ* 79(4):49.

Kotter JP. 1996. *Leading Change*. Boston, MA: Harvard Business School Press.

Kotter JP. 1999. *John P. Kotter on What Leaders Really Do*. Boston, MA: Harvard Business School Press.

Kouzes JM, Posner BZ. 2017. *The Leadership Challenge: How to Make Extraordinary Things Happen in Organizations*. Hoboken, NJ: John Wiley & Sons.

Lencioni P. 2002. *The Five Dysfunctions of a Team: A Leadership Fable*. San Francisco, NC: Jossey-Bass.

Matzke GR, Moczygemba LR, Williams KJ, Czar MJ, Lee WT. 2018. Impact of a pharmacist-physician collaborative care model on patient outcomes and health services utilization. *Am J Health Syst Pharm* 75(14):1039–1047.

McKeown G. 2014. *Essentialism: the Disciplined Pursuit of Less*. New York, NY: Random House.

Nohria N, Khurana R. 2010. *Handbook of Leadership Theory and Practice: A Harvard Business School Centennial*. Boston, MA: Harvard Business Press.

Papanicolas I, Woskie LR, Jha AK. 2018. Health care spending in the United States and other high-income countries. *JAMA* 319(10):1024–1039.

Phatak A, Prusi R, Ward B, et al. 2016. Impact of pharmacist involvement in the transitional care of high-risk patients through medication reconciliation, medication education, and postdischarge call-backs (IPITCH Study). *J Hosp Med* 11(1):39–44.

Rath T. 2007. *Strengths Finder 2.0*. New York, NY: Gallup.

Rath T, Conchie B. 2008. *Strengths Based Leadership: Great Leaders, Teams, and Why People Follow*. New York, NY: Gallup Press.

Shafer E, Bergeron N, Smith-Ray R, Robson C, O'Koren R. 2017. A nationwide pharmacy chain responds to the opioid epidemic. *J Am Pharm Assoc* 57(2S): S123–S129.

Shaver A, Morano M, Pogodzinski J, Fredrick S, Essi D, Slazak E. 2019. Impact of a community pharmacy transitions-of-care program on 30-day readmission. *J Am Pharm Assoc* 59(2):202–209.

Sinek S. 2013. *Start with Why: How Great Leaders Inspire Everyone to Take Action*. London: Portfolio/Penguin.

Thomas KW, Kilmann RH. 2007. *Thomas-Kilmann Conflict Mode Instrument*. Mountain View, CA: CPP.

Watanabe JH, McInnis T, Hirsch JD. 2018. Cost of prescription drug-related morbidity and mortality. *Ann Pharmacother* 52(9):829–837.

White SJ. 2006. Leadership: Successful alchemy. *Am J Health Syst Pharm* 63(16):1497–1503.

Yee GC, Janke KK, Fuller PD, Kelley KA, Scott SA, Sorensen TD. 2018. StrengthsFinder® signature themes of talent in pharmacy residents at four midwestern pharmacy schools. *Curr Pharm Teach Learn* 10(1):61–65.

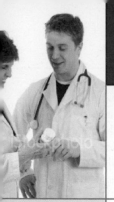

4

ETHICAL DECISION-MAKING, PROBLEM-SOLVING, AND DELEGATING AUTHORITY

Michael L. Manolakis and Evan T. Robinson

About the Authors: Dr. Manolakis is Vice President, Pharmacy Consulting for Aon. He received his Doctor of Pharmacy from the University of Southern California and his PhD in Philosophy with a concentration in bioethics from the University of Tennessee, Knoxville. Prior to joining Aon, he served as Associate Professor and Director of Interprofessional Education at Wingate University School of Pharmacy where he taught courses in bioethics, leadership, and the US healthcare system. In addition to his career in pharmacy education, he has practiced as a community pharmacist and a managed care pharmacist. His research interests include empathy development and leadership development.

Dr. Robinson is a Dean at the Creighton University School of Pharmacy and Health Professions. Prior to joining Creighton University he was Dean at the Western New England University College of Pharmacy and Health Sciences, where he has served since 2008. As the founding dean for the College of Pharmacy, Dr. Robinson has been involved in a variety of the foundational considerations of the program's development and implementation. He served as the Associate Provost for Academic Affairs from September 2016 to July 2018. Prior to his position at Western New England University, Dr. Robinson participated in the development of two new schools of pharmacy.

■ LEARNING OBJECTIVES

After completing this chapter, readers should be able to:

1. Identify key steps in the Markula Model for ethical decision-making (EDM).
2. Describe the difference between the rationalist and nonrationalist approaches to EDM.
3. Describe what is meant by sensemaking as it applies to problem-solving.
4. Explain the relationship between organizational culture and ethical problem-solving.
5. Explain the relationship between empowerment and delegation with problem-solving.
6. Describe how influence relates to leadership/management.

■ CHAPTER QUESTIONS

1. Do you reason first and then make an ethical decision, or do you make an ethical decision and then reason? The significance of this question will become clear as you work through the chapter, and your answer will inform how you approach EDM.
2. What is the significance of the development of a pharmacist's professional identity as it pertains to making ethical decisions?
3. How does sensemaking relate to problem-solving and ethical considerations?
4. How do ethical considerations relate to the tenets of management and leadership?
5. How do the tenets of management and leadership relate to problem-solving?

■ SCENARIO

Lynn Smith enters the hospital for an ailment that, at the time of her admission, was as yet unidentified. Lynn undergoes a battery of tests; after a few days her ailment is identified, and inpatient therapy begins. Soon thereafter, she receives the good news that she is discharged with a positive prognosis. Unfortunately, she is soon to learn that her ability to be treated, however, may be more complicated than she was told upon discharge. To be treated as an outpatient she begins to acquire one of her medications from a specialty pharmacy owned by a regional health system to get the product appropriately prepared and compounded.

Unfortunately, Lynn is subjected to a challenge that has begun to plague the U.S. health care system; drug shortages. The one product being prepared by the specialty pharmacy has limited availability, and as such, Lynn is faced with the situation that she cannot be assured of appropriate access to her medication. To access the product, the pharmacist-in-charge for the specialty pharmacy, Jackie Wu, seeks to access the medication from the "gray market."

Gray markets involve the trade of drugs that are less available and may have been stockpiled by whole-sale distributors. The activities that have created the gray market, while legal, are unofficial and unauthorized, thus creating consequences that were unintended by the original manufacturer. The presence of shortages may ultimately result in price-gouging as well as other problems as a result of wholesaler processing, which can involve drugs moving between multiple vendors, repackaging, relabeling, storage under improper conditions, or even being replaced by counterfeits (Cohen, 2014).

The situation faced by Jackie is far from unique and is resolvable, but to do so necessitates individuals within the organization to both lead and manage this situation, and not just the logistics of the situation but the ethics of it, as well.

■ INTRODUCTION

The situations and decisions faced in health care delivery are seldom black and white. More often than not, these decisions are shrouded with ethical and moral complexities that not only influence the decisions made at that time but also future decisions through the process of learning, reflection, and contextual leadership development. Put another way, what we do today shapes what we do tomorrow. While learning through experience via decisions and actions is natural, the ethical dilemmas faced may lead to more profound and significant changes over time. The ethical implications represent the common thread for each of the considerations presented in this chapter.

These ethical implications, combined within the management and leadership, represent challenges faced all who are in roles in which others look to them for vision, guidance, direction, or reaffirmation. They represent a compass that allows us to understand our direction and to help provide comfort to others seeking affirmation that the right things are being done for themselves and the organization.

The interesting part of leadership is that our jobs, and for that matter our lives, are often filled with questions for which we think we know the right answer, but whose actual solution involves considerable nuance and might lack a clear-cut solution.

Decisions exist in a gray space where there is not always a right or wrong answer. This can be further complicated when the decisions of those above us in a reporting structure help create that gray space. This chapter delves into the process of making difficult, ethical decisions, and the implications and outcomes linked with these decisions.

PROBLEM-SOLVING THROUGH ETHICAL DILEMMAS

In the chapter scenario, Dr. Wu is facing an ethical dilemma and a problem to be solved. Should she pursue the purchase of the drug in short supply from the gray market? In this case the purchase may be legal, but is it ethical? In other words, is it the right decision, or even a good one? If we understand a dilemma as a situation where we must make a choice between two competing alternatives, then we can think of an ethical dilemma as a situation where we make a choice between competing ethical standards in an effort to determine the decision or action that is morally appropriate. The act of making the choice requires cognitive effort through assessment, reflection, and critical thinking. Additionally, the outcome of Dr. Wu's decision will be judged in terms of pharmacy's professional norms of ethically appropriate behavior.

Pharmacists must make choices to resolve ethical dilemmas on a daily basis. Consider the situation of a patient who is loud and grabbing much attention at the prescription counter through their interactions with the cashier and the technicians. As the pharmacist who just filled the prescription for an antipsychotic medication, and having confirmed their diagnosis and prescription with the physician's office, you know that this individual is likely suffering the effects of their disease and has difficulty controlling their emotions in a manner deemed socially acceptable. Counseling and payment are made, and the patient leaves the pharmacy, wherein the cashier turns to you and asks "What is wrong with that person?" At this point you encounter an ethical dilemma; share the diagnosis in an effort to explain the behavior or tell the cashier to move on with their day and get to the next customer. It is a choice between maintaining or violating the release of patient-specific confidential information, which has legal implications, but through its release in this situation is a violation of our profession's Code of Ethics (APhA, 1994). Specifically, we are bound through Code provision II to "promote the good of every patient in a caring, compassionate, and confidential manner." The profession has established ethical norms for behavior in our role as the pharmacist; namely, respect the patient's privacy and the privacy of their confidential health information. Choosing the other horn of the dilemma and breaching the patient's confidence results in satisfying the curious cashier, but is a violation of this norm and of the law.

This example helps us to understand patient-specific ethical dilemmas, but pharmacy practice is further complicated by the myriad patient care and business concerns encountered on a routine basis. Just as we can discuss and debate what a pharmacist should do in a patient-specific situation, we can also discuss and debate behavior norms for pharmacists in business situations. These norms are behaviors that we expect from pharmacists. Often the two may intersect, which is the situation this example bears out. A decision to dispense a drug purchased from the gray market may compromise patient safety, as the integrity of the drug supply chain may have been violated and the product becoming susceptible to tampering (see Chapter 27). Additionally, the business practice of purchasing from a secondary wholesaler might increase costs and create a budget overrun that has to be explained and justified (ASHP, 2009). Noting that cost is already going to increase, Dr. Wu might consider stockpiling the drug in short supply to offset further patient-specific shortages. What initially may have been viewed as a business decision to provide product for a specific patient has been complicated by the fact that the product costs more. Dr. Wu now faces an ethical dilemma that must balance appropriate patient care with normative issues relating to the business of pharmaceutical product purchasing.

Norms can guide problem-solving efforts, and while they may align with laws or regulations, they may conflict when patient interests become the justifiable priority.

Pharmacy managers must provide ethical leadership to navigate their teams through dilemmas; however, ethical leadership, while necessary, may not be a sufficient deterrent for unethical behavior. The ethical pharmacist may be praised for the appropriateness of their behavior in the workplace, but EDM transcends routine practice behavior and describes a process whereby a leader/manager recognizes and subsequently responds to an ethical situation (Thiel, 2012).

■ EDM MODELS

Models provide a framework for making ethical decisions. Efforts to create models for making such decisions are common, as evidenced by the fact that a Google search on "EDM models" yields well over 50 million results! While not possible to review all ethical models, this chapter focuses on four of them to show similarities and differences that can be beneficial to the pharmacist as they go through the EDM process in the midst of solving problems.

The Markula Center Framework for EDM

The Markula Center for Applied Ethics provides a "framework for EDM" (Markula, 2015). It works under the assumption that ethics "refers to standards of behavior that tell us how human beings ought to act in the many situations in which they find themselves…." The roles that fall within the situations under consideration include businesspeople and professionals, so an analysis of the ethics of practicing pharmacy would be incorporated. A key assumption made in the Markula framework is what ethics is not. Ethics is not the same as (i) feelings; (ii) religion; (iii) following the law; (iv) following culturally accepted norms; nor (v) science. Each of these phenomena can inform ethical decisions, but in and of themselves do not necessarily provide the clear answer on what should be done in a particular practice situation.

For example, a law or a socially accepted norm could be corrupt and vary from what is ethical or right to do in a particular situation. The framework poses a list of 10 questions to work through to determine an ethically appropriate answer to an ethical question (Figure 4-1). These questions include:

1. Could this decision or situation be damaging to someone or to some group? Does this decision involve a choice between a good and bad alternative, or perhaps between two "goods" or between two "bads"?
2. Is the issue about more than what is legal or what is most efficient? If so, how?
3. What are the relevant facts of the case? What facts are not known? Can I learn more about the situation? Do I know enough to make a decision?
4. What individuals and groups have an important stake in the outcome? Are some concerns more important? Why?
5. What are the options for acting? Have all the relevant persons and groups been consulted? Have I identified creative options?
6. Evaluate the options by asking the following questions:
   a. Which option will produce the most good and do the least harm? This is the utilitarian approach.
   b. Which option best respects the rights of all who have a stake? This is the rights-based approach.
   c. Which option treats people equally or proportionally? This is the justice-based approach.
   d. Which option best serves the community as a whole, not just some members? This is the common good approach.
   e. Which option leads me to act as the sort of person I want to be? This is the virtue-based approach.
7. Considering all these approaches, which option best addresses the situation?
8. If I told someone I respect—or told a television audience—which option I have chosen, what would they say?

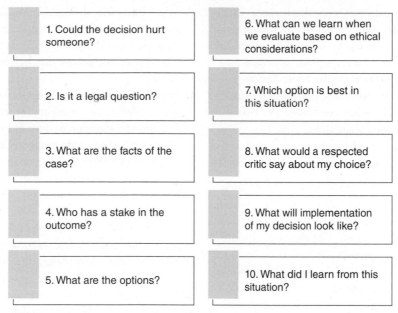

Figure 4-1. Evaluative questions for decision-making through the Markula framework.

1. Could the decision hurt someone?

2. Is it a legal question?

3. What are the facts of the case?

4. Who has a stake in the outcome?

5. What are the options?

6. What can we learn when we evaluate based on ethical considerations?

7. Which option is best in this situation?

8. What would a respected critic say about my choice?

9. What will implementation of my decision look like?

10. What did I learn from this situation?

9. How can my decision be implemented with the greatest care and attention to the concerns of all stakeholders?
10. How did my decision turn out and what have I learned from this specific situation?

The sixth question incorporates a philosophical perspective into the framework for evaluating options. Utilitarianism considers the consequences of our actions and determines the ethical choice to be the one that produces the greatest amount of good or positive benefit as opposed to the choice that produces more harm. A pharmacist might point out to a prescriber that Drug A, which is very effective, will produce significant adverse effects in a given patient; however, while the alternative Drug B might be slightly less effective, it will not produce any side effects. The utilitarian could argue that Drug B is the ethically appropriate choice, all other things being equal, as it produces more good than harm. The rights-based approach considers the ethical choice to be the one that protects the moral rights of the individuals involved in a situation. What exactly is a right is a question that can lead to much debate and controversy, as can the question of to whom rights are given, but if one simply considers a patient's right to privacy of their health information, then one can begin to appreciate how a rights-based approach can apply in pharmacy practice. Consider the patient, Lynn, in the chapter scenario. Does she have a right to be treated fairly by the health care system and the pharmacy when it comes to distribution the drug? Are her chances of receiving the drug in short supply maximized in a fair way? (Rosoff, 2012) This leads to consideration of the justice-based approach, which considers the question of how we treat people with a specific focus on equality or fairness. In pharmacy, we can think of providing all patients with access to the same level of medication therapy management regardless of the economic background as an example of equal treatment. The common good approach considers that we all are in relationships with each other as part of a community and ethical choices reflect compassion and respect for others. The U.S. health care system strives to provide access to the most vulnerable but does not always succeed in this endeavor.

The fact that hospital emergency departments often provide care for individuals, even when they are unable to pay, reflects our society's relative agreement on this goal. The virtue-based approach considers how pharmacists act in this role. Are we being compassionate and caring, or are we being callous? The virtues of compassion and care are considered the ethically appropriate actions of a pharmacist.

The PLUS EDM Model

The ten-question Markula Framework invites decision-makers to undertake the cognitive work of generating awareness and evaluating alternative approaches when considering the best action. The thorough breadth and scope of the ten questions is evidenced by comparing it to the PLUS EDM Model developed by the Ethics & Compliance Initiative (Markula, 2015). While the Markula Framework focuses on individual decision-making, the PLUS Model provides the context of doing so within organizations, such as Dr. Wu's dilemma to purchase a gray market drug under the auspices of the specialty pharmacy that employs her.

The PLUS Model is comprised of seven steps which recognize that employees have decision-making authority and that these decisions should be vetted against organizational policies and procedures, as well as against applicable laws.

- Step 1 is to define the problem. It is helpful to define "the problem in terms of outcomes," as this ensures that the problem is stated clearly.
- Step 2 is to seek relevant assistance, guidance, and support. These resources can be people, as in coworkers or an outside consultant, or in written resources such as a policy and procedure manual or a Code of Ethics.
- Step 3 is to identify available alternative solutions to the problem. This is a critical thinking step where one envisions as many solutions as possible, trying to get well beyond just two discrete choices, only.
- Step 4 is to evaluate the identified alternatives. This is a judgment phase in the model, as one is considering facts and assumptions, and envisioning future states with various alternatives implemented.

- Step 5 is to make the decision. Following the evaluation is the decision, which is either made by the individual or the team in organizational decisions.
- Step 6 is to implement the decision. It is time for action!
- Step 7 is to evaluate the decision. At this point, the decision-maker is asking if the solution identified solved the problem. If so, did it go well and/or what is to be learned from having implemented, or proceeded with the decision made?

There are clear parallels between the PLUS Model and the Markula Framework. Both begin with establishing awareness of the problem as the critical first step. The models both rely on consultation, although the PLUS Model incorporates this in Steps 2 and 4. This expansion is consistent with decision-making within an organization where policies and procedures play a significant role. Both models then incorporate moral reasoning activities in stepwise sequencing to reach a decision point. Moral reasoning is reasoning represents a type of development, or processes that shape our EDM. It is with moral reasoning where the PLUS Model varies from Markula. Whereas Markula points to classic philosophical theory in evaluating actions, the PLUS Model incorporates "ethical filters" that serve to bring out the ethical elements of the analysis to ensure they are not ignored or bypassed in the evaluation. The filters are applied at steps 1 (define the problem), 4 (evaluate alternatives), and 7 (evaluate the decision). An explanation of these filters uses the following PLUS mnemonic:

Policies—is it consistent with the organization's policies and procedures?

Legal—is it consistent with the law and applicable regulations?

Universal—does it align with universal principles and values that my organization has adopted?

Self—does it satisfy my definition of right, good, and fair?

The filters serve a critical function in this model by ensuring that ethical elements are not lost in the decision-making process. They do not guarantee an ethical decision, but they ensure consideration. For example, they allow for consideration of ethical trade-offs in evaluating alternatives, as the "universal" values are suggested to include empathy, patience, integrity, and courage. In the scenario facing Dr. Wu, the following questions might be raised. Will the purchase of the gray market drug diminish the pharmacist's or the pharmacy department's integrity in an effort to get the drug to the patient? Is courage by the pharmacist required to argue against the purchase, which might result in a delay of treatment and the potential for resulting patient harm from the delay? These are the ethical elements that the filters ensure are included in the deliberation. The authors of the PLUS Model urge organizations to set these agreed-upon values or principles, that they communicate the process to employees along with the relevant laws, and that they provide mechanisms for employees to work through this process. This aligns with the culture that the leader sets within their pharmacy department.

■ RATIONALIST OR NONRATIONALIST MODEL IN MORAL REASONING

The first two models discussed rely on moral reasoning that follows a stepwise process where a moral code is applied to help resolve an ethical situation. This model, which is labeled the rationalist-based theoretical model for EDM, has roots that trace back to research done by James Rest (1986). Rest adapted a theory of moral development initially defined by Jean Piaget and later researched and refined by Kohlberg and Hersh (1977). Kohlberg identified six stages of cognitive development that correspond with their ability to reason ethically. The six stages are shown in Figure 4-2. The model assumes that you always move forward in your development and not backward, and that thinking on the stage above incorporates thinking from the stage below. At its core, moral development for Kohlberg was more than knowing cultural

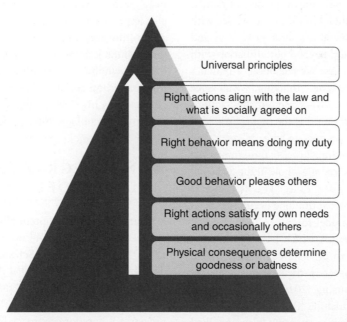

Figure 4-2. Kohlberg's stages of moral development. (Reprinted from Kohlberg L, Hersh RH. 1977. Moral development: a review of the theory. *Theory Pract* 6(2):53–59.)

values that might lead to ethical relativism; moral development is about a change in the way an individual structure how they think. We progress in our ability to judge ethically, which informs how we solve problems.

Stages 1 and 2 make up a level that Kohlberg labels "preconventional." In stage 1, goodness or badness is determined by physical consequences without a focus on meaning or value. This can be thought of a "do as you are told." Stage 2 introduces the idea that right actions are those that satisfy our own needs, which introduces egoism. It is akin to "you scratch my back and I'll scratch yours" to describe this stage. The conventional level includes stages 3 and 4. Stage 3 begins to consider behavior in terms of the approval of others. Think of the phrase "he meant well" or "she is such a nice girl" as characteristic of this level. At stage 4, ethical behavior aligns with the law and doing our duty. The post-conventional level includes stages 5 and 6. These stages incorporate something new, namely that what we value ethically is independent of what individuals or groups think and independent of what individuals within a group think. Consider the respect pharmacists have for the privacy of patient information. This is defined in the law as we see with HIPPA (level 4), but we also respect privacy in and of itself as individuals and beyond our affiliation with the profession of pharmacy. We talk about a patient's right to privacy, which is level 5 thinking. We all agree on the value we place on privacy and our right actions follow this agreement. Level 6 is the highest order of ethical thinking where we operate with universal and abstract principles of action. Level 6 thinking prioritizes what is best for society as a whole in the decision. An example is the "Golden Rule." This is the level where rational and impartial thinking occurs.

Rest described a model for EDM that includes four components or stages, which has been applied by nurses in an effort to evaluate day-to-day ethical issues they may encounter in their professional role (Advanced Practice Nursing, 2014). The four components of the model include (i) a developed awareness of an ethical problem or situation (also described as having an ethical sensitivity); (ii) the drawing of

a moral judgment or evaluation which may require drawing on a profession's Code of Ethics or principles of ethics; (iii) these lead to moral motivation or moral intent, which helps distinguish knowing what the right thing to do is and actually doing the right thing; and (iv) acting on these intentions through a behavior. In summary, Rest's model like the theoretical rationalist EDM models that followed it, posit that in becoming aware of experiencing an ethical problem, we attempt to bring it to resolution through a deliberative, cognitive, and rational approach that considers and weighs moral standards which may or may not conflict as we reach an end point of an ethical action. The Markula Framework and PLUS Model follow in this tradition, but there is another research approach to consider.

The nonrationalist approach, which is also called the intuitionist or sentimentalist approach, has been described by Jonathan Haidt (2001) as a social intuitionist approach. Haidt argues that his model is an alternative to the rationalist approach which has dominated the literature. It is different in that moral reasoning is seen as happening after a judgment has been reached, which stands in contrast to the rationalist approach where the reasoning leads to the judgment. Intuitive and emotive processes generate initial, quick moral judgments. Private, individual reasoning loses its emphasis in Haidt's theory, with emphasis now placed on social and cultural influences. Haidt characterizes his work as aligned with research findings from psychology, anthropology, and primatology.

■ AN INTEGRATED EDM MODEL

A separate model that potentially resolves the conflict between the rationalist and nonrationalist approaches to EDM just described (Schwartz, 2016). Schwartz describes an approach to EDM that has two key components; the first being the EDM process and the second being moderating factors that can influence the process. Of note for pharmacy leaders is the incorporation of antecedent elements and subsequent actions into the model discussed in greater detail later in the chapter.

The elements of the EDM process draw upon the work done by Rest and other rationalists. There is awareness or recognition of the problem that is followed by an evaluative or judgment phase which leads to intention (a commitment to action) and the behavior or action. The parallels between this aspect of Schwartz' integrated EDM approach and the Markula Framework and the PLUS Model should be clear.

The inclusion of the moderating factors reflects the fact that (i) different individuals can approach EDM in different ways and (ii) that situational (or contextual) variations can cause a person to reach a different conclusion when circumstances change. Specific to individual factors, Schwartz (2016) describes an individual's moral capacity as "based not only on one's level of moral maturity and the core ethical values they possess, but the extent to which they will cling to those values when faced with pressures to act otherwise". Consider a wrinkle to the scenario where Dr. Wu had previously been indirectly involved in a decision to purchase a gray market product that resulted in serious harm to a patient. The impact of being so close to this situation, perhaps so close that she felt remorse for not stopping it when it just seemed wrong, could inform how she approaches solving the problem in the next gray market purchase situation. This ability to withstand pressures is built off one's "moral character disposition" and their "integrity capacity." Character speaks to personal values that the pharmacist will bring into the EDM process while integrity reflects the maintenance of that character when it is put to the test. In pharmacy, the developing student or resident is transitioning through a socialization process from a purely personal identity to a professional identity that is inclusive of their personal and professional identities (Cruess et al., 2015) Professional identity can also be lost or diminished as a Canadian study showed when the researcher looked at foreign-trained, migrant pharmacists who went through the process of becoming licensed to practice (Austin, 2007). It is through the dynamic development of one's

professional identity, including conscious reflection and unconscious knowledge acquisition from mentors and learning experiences that we find our professional identity ready and able to withstand ethical challenges as to what is right or wrong in a particular situation. The seasoned, experienced pharmacist whose professional identity is secure maintains the integrity and character to assess any ethically challenging situation in complete alignment with their values.

Situation factors include three components: the issue, the organization, and personal factors. Schwartz argues that anyone of these three could come into conflict with one's moral character or integrity and thus lead to a poor ethical decision. The issue itself is understood through its moral intensity, its importance, and its complexity. As the moral intensity increases, so might the expectation that a pharmacist could violate the profession's Code of Ethics or other laws or promises. Issue importance reflects how the pharmacist thinks the issue is important to her or himself. If they detach from the issue through the perception that it doesn't having any bearing on them, or if importance is disregarded, then worry arises that moral awareness may be lacking. Issue complexity serves to identify situations where the decision-maker finds the issue difficult to understand or resolve. The worry associated with complexity is that perceived difficulty could become so overwhelming for the pharmacist that a type of moral paralysis results where no action is taken.

The organization component refers to the infrastructure that supports EDM. Pharmacists can rely on the Code of Ethics, as well as policy statements (e.g., conscientious objection) (APhA, 1998) and guideline documents that address ethically challenging situations such as gray market drug purchases (ASHP, 2009, 2018). The personal factor considers what the pharmacist perceives they have to gain (e.g., they are in significant debt), which can reflect how vulnerable they are within a particular dilemma to making a poor ethical decision.

The process of making the ethical decision begins with the behavioral norms that are in place for a certain community. In pharmacy, this can be regarded as "obvious and unresolvable red flags" observed by the pharmacist during the dispensing process, such as a patient's traveling long distances to get an opioid prescription filled, or for drug "cocktail" prescriptions. Recognizing these red flags as against the norm of the pharmacy profession has been upheld in court, despite the challenge they raise for pharmacists (Brushwood, 2018). The behavior that results turns on moral judgment, which is informed by emotion, intuition, reason, rationalization, and consultation. This is where the integration of the rational and non-rational models occurs.

Emotion may include an initial response of anger to an ethical situation, which is what pharmacists might feel when they read "The Toxic Pharmacist" (Draper, 2003). Knowing that the pharmacist in this true story diluted medications for thousands of individuals, including chemotherapy agents, for personal gain is abhorrent. Emotions can lead to an intuition (or sense) that something is wrong. Moral intuitions are less deliberative and can lead to a judgment that is acted upon. Reason (or reflection) can follow, as it is more deliberative and allows for resolution of conflicts that may remain between standards. Reflection has value in that it allows one to learn from experience, which can lead to better decisions in the workplace (Castleberry, 2016). It is a practice that managers can practice for their own improvement and can encourage among staff members. Rationalization follows reason or reflection, and it can be associated with either positive or negative outcomes. Schwartz sees its relationship with the cognitive EDM process as important and includes it in the model. Finally, consultation is incorporated into the integrated EDM, as discussion with colleagues, technicians, or members of a patient care team can provide guidance that can impact ethical judgments.

Two other aspects of the integrated EDM model merit attention for pharmacy leaders and managers. The first has to do with the individual who has a lack of awareness of an ethical issue, and the second has to do with the learning that comes from an ethical action that follows the EDM process. Specific to awareness, this is required for the EDM process to occur. When a pharmacist convinces herself or himself that the ethical standards of the profession do not apply to them, then the process of moral disengagement can occur. Other ways a lack of awareness can occur is when the pharmacist loses their sense of personal responsibility, or perhaps they engage in self-deception that what they are doing is somehow proper. Alternatively, one can limit their focus to the business side of the decision and lose focus on the ethical elements. This lack of awareness can be compounded by an organizational culture that discourages ethical issues from surfacing or being actively discussed and resolved (see Chapter 16). This is the opportunity for the pharmacy leader to keep ethical issues at the level of awareness for the individual and organization. Setting the example of the mindful leader can help individuals avoid negative rationalizations, promote ethical awareness, and foster a culture of consultation leading to positive EDM. These aspects of leadership tie directly with the learning aspect of the model. Learning is one of two feedback loops within the integrated EDM process. Lessons learned that are either positive or negative can be used to inform and improve individual moral capacity through retrospection and self-awareness. The second feedback loop links the behavior with the awareness of the issue that starts the process. The recognition of aspects of an ethical situation that were not considered can exert positive effects on how future situations should be addressed. These feedback loops highlight mentor opportunities for leaders with their colleagues or staff where negative outcomes can be turned into individual growth opportunity, ultimately benefiting the individual, and fostering a culture of ethical awareness.

■ SENSEMAKING AS AN ALTERNATIVE

The term "sensemaking" is used to describe the cognitive process associated with making sense of situations. The roots of sensemaking can be traced to Karl Weick (1995). Weick's description of situations where sensemaking is needed, which are situations many pharmacy leaders face, can help to understand the concept. He writes, "In real-world practice, problems do not present themselves to the practitioners as givens. They must be constructed from the materials of problematic situations which are puzzling, troubling, and uncertain. In order to convert a problematic situation to a problem, a practitioner must do a certain kind of work. He must make sense of an uncertain situation that initially makes no sense" (Weick, 1995). Consider the uncertainty of situations within a pharmacy department where the complexities of financial viability, which are integrally related to the financial viability of the entire health system, put pressure on product recommendations for formulary placement. This situation can be both a business and an ethical challenge for the pharmacist leader where unethical behavior could surface because the complexities of the situation are more than the pharmacist can comprehend. The leader cannot resolve an ethical dilemma that does not make sense.

This chapter previously reviewed the transition from the rationalist to the nonrationalist models for EDM. Recall that the crux of this discussion is the claim by the nonrationalists that the rationalist approach, whereby awareness of ethical situations and the reasoned application of ethical principles serve as the basis for resolving ethical dilemmas, is not complete. Theil et al. (2012) make the point that if the rationalist approach was viable, the ethical indiscretions and poor decisions seen in business today might simply be result of leaders who either cannot identify an ethical problem, or their set of principles is "less ethical" than required. Thiel et al. extend the nonrationalist discussion noting that (i) intuition must be accounted for in EDM and (ii) that constraints on action must be factored into the model, as they may interfere with resolving the ethical dilemma. Sensemaking is employed to incorporate these two elements, as the mental models individuals form during sensemaking allow for recognition of the problem, evaluation of the situation, and they serve as a framework for re-evaluation. In this way, sensemaking is contextual because it provides the leader with a means to recognize and build interpretations of uncertain circumstances. It provides for the unique connecting of environmental elements in ill-defined situations, which is where pharmacy leaders may find themselves in ethical dilemmas. The challenge for the pharmacy leader is to maintain their professional ethics and hold true to their professional identity while making high quality, ethical decisions, which may be aided by sensemaking.

Noting that sensemaking is a cognitive process occurring prior to EDM. Factors that might constrain sensemaking must be accounted for because they potentially change the relationship between sensemaking and the resulting EDM activity. Constraining factors can change the mental models created by the pharmacist leader through inadequate interpretation and a resulting lack of an ability to make sense of the situation. Thiel identifies these constraining factors as personal, situational, or environmental. Personal constraints can include bias or errors in judgment that can lead to ineffective sensemaking. Situational constraints can include time, stress, resource issues, interpersonal conflicts, or adverse financial incentives that can impact sensemaking. Environmental constraints can be found either inside or outside an organization and can include an unethical work culture or a code of ethics. These constraining factors resemble the "moderating factors" proposed by (Schwartz, 2016). These moderating factors, one individual and the other situational, can impact the EDM process at any point in a positive or negative manner depending on their strength. Whether understood as moderating or constraining factors, it is argued that these individual or environmental differences must be accounted for when making ethical decisions. Schwartz argues that when sensemaking is used in making an ethical decision—the cognitive process of making sense of a complex, perhaps ambiguous ethical situation—constraining factors must be prevented or minimized, as they can have a negative effect on the sensemaking and consequently a negative effect on the ethical decision. Think back to Dr. Wu for a moment. What might happen to her EDM process if her pharmacy department did not have clear policies and procedures in place for handling drugs in short supply? This factor could constrain her decision-making, likely resulting in a negative effect for either her current patient or a future patient.

Improving Sensemaking

If given that ethical sensemaking plays a part in the EDM process and that constraining factors can impede EDM, then the process of resolving ethical dilemmas must incorporate strategies for minimizing or eliminating these factors. The models built through sensemaking must be accurate and complete representations of the ethical dilemma being faced. As requirements for sensemaking, it has been said that it ". . . requires that leaders have emotional intelligence, self-awareness, the ability to deal with cognitive complexity, and the flexibility to go between the "what is" of sensemaking and the "what can be" of visioning" (Ancona, 2012).

Pharmacy leaders face uncertainty, as is demonstrated in this seemingly all-too-real hypothetical situation (Ancona, 2012):

> You are the pharmacist on call and receive an early morning page to the critical care unit. You know the patient from rounds the prior day. He is exceptionally difficult to manage, with multiple co-morbid conditions that are complicated by IV drug abuse, a lack of financial resources and no social support structure. Treatment plans have considered the use of a new drug, Curitall, which can cost up to $750,000 for an entire course of therapy. There are less costly alternatives, but none are expected to work as well. You enter the unit.
>
> "What's the situation?" you ask.
>
> "We are running out of options," the physician responds. "With no intervention, I am certain he will die very soon."
>
> "Is there a plan?" you ask.
>
> "I believe we need to use Curitall," says the physician. "Can you order it?"
>
> "It's not in stock here or in any local hospitals. I can get it from a secondary wholesaler, but the cost goes up," you say.
>
> "Do we know that it will be safe for this patient?" the nurse asks.

> "We will not know until it is infused," you say.
>
> "Can the pharmacy budget absorb the cost?" the physician wonders.
>
> "I don't know," you say.
>
> "Is it safe for this patient?" the nurse asks.
>
> "The trials don't include patients like this, so I can't say," you reply.
>
> "We don't have any other choices," responds the physician. "This is a drug therapy issue. What do you want to do?"

This hypothetical situation reflects the unpredictable, complex environment that a future manager might find themselves in where clinical expertise is expected and a given, decision-making authority and autonomy are secure, and what is most clearly seen is the unseen. Making ethical sense of this situation is incumbent on the pharmacist. Should significant financial resources be spent on a patient who is a known IV drug abuser with no social support system? Should the pharmacy department procure the product from the gray market via a secondary wholesaler? With safety knowledge lacking, are we creating a situation where we do more harm than good? The sensemaking model developed by Thiel et al. added to the literature on EDM by discussing tactics to improve sensemaking. These tactics attend to the constraints that can adversely impact sensemaking and therefore negatively impact the ethical decision. These tactics include: (i) emotional regulation, (ii) self-reflection, (iii) forecasting, and (iv) information integration.

Refer back to the story of "The Toxic Pharmacist" as a source of substantial negative emotional response. Assuming the response in this situation is anger, managing down and regulating the anger response is important for improving judgment and subsequently EDM. Strategies for regulating emotional responses include relaxation techniques or cognitive reappraisal, which can be learned through training. Self-reflection provides the leader with the opportunity to learn from past experiences, whether they be positive or negative, ultimately using this information and self-awareness to make sensemaking more accurate. This self-reflection can focus on outcomes, but also on the process used to achieve the outcome. Forecasting is deployed by the leader to generate multiple solutions to complex problems. Generating multiple solutions potentially offsets bias, minimizes disengagement from complex issues where the task is deemed too large to solve, and identifies the tactics to arrive at a high quality, ethical solution. Information integration is the process of continuously assessing and reassessing information into the mental models we form and reform as part of sensemaking. As such, it can impact how the model depicts the situation and the resulting EDM. Tactics for enhancing information include perspective taking, such as taking a broad perspective rather than a narrow one in considering an issue, and framing ethical problems so that we consider individual and organizational frames as we make sense of complexity.

Summary of EDM Models

The models presented in this chapter highlight both rationalist and nonrationalist approaches to EDM. Also included is a model that strives to integrate key elements of these two models. A fourth model builds on the integration of reason and intuition and posits sensemaking as the cognitive activity that precedes the EDM process. In this model the leader is presented with tactics that can be used to sharpen their sensemaking ability, which ultimately will improve EDM.

■ APPLYING SENSEMAKING TO LEADERSHIP

Sensemaking can help leaders understand, plan, and act. The steps to accomplish this (Weick, 1995) are as follows:

1. Learn
   a. Seek out as many types and kinds of data as possible, albeit numerical, verbal, etc.
   b. Involve others in trying to make sense of the situation or instance in question
   c. Seek to understand the nuance of the situation as opposed to making a predetermined assessment of what is occurring
   d. Seek to understand the situation from those closest to it as opposed to only trusting your view from potentially afar
2. Plan
   a. Consider new schema(s) for situation resolution as opposed to continuing to apply previous/old schema
   b. Apply a new, or potentially new, framework to the situation via the application of stories, metaphors, etc. that allow others within the organization to gain better context
3. Act
   a. Take steps to address a situation, but consider starting small and learning from the outcomes to see how to grow the application
   b. Be attentive to the impact of actions and individuals on a situation and how it impacts organizational environment/culture

■ LEADERSHIP IN CONTEXT

Leadership (and management) are multifaceted concepts, with many models and approaches (see Chapter 3). In any model or approach, EDM is an important facet. Four constructs of leadership serve as examples of how ethical considerations relate to the role of a manager/leader within any organization. Two of them are macro considerations of leadership (vision and mission, organizational culture), and two are micro considerations of leadership (empowerment and influence) (see Chapter 16).

In addition to considerations of leadership and management, there is another construct that is uniquely linked to both, that of problem-solving. Pharmacy education is guided by the Center for the Advancement of Pharmacy Education (CAPE) 2013 Educational Outcomes, which were revised from previous versions of CAPE (Medina et al., 2013). The CAPE Outcomes were created in an end-outcome approach by what an entry-level graduate should be able to do, and then identifying the relevant knowledge, skills, and abilities needed. In the end, four domains were identified: (1) Foundational

Knowledge; (2) Essentials for Practice and Care; (3) Approach to Practice and Care; and (4) Personal and Professional Development. This chapter deals with the critical elements of problem-solving within Domain 3's leadership and professionalism (as relates to EDM) within Domain 4. Problem-solving can be regarded as a process in which one identifies a problem, identifies possible outcomes, explores possible solutions, and selects one to act on, and implements the chosen solution (Oderda et al., 2010). The problem-solving process should always include an ethical lens when identifying outcomes as well as exploring and implementing solutions. When considering the situation of Dr. Wu in the chapter scenario, it is clear that she is faced with applying problem-solving through a critical ethical lens in order to reach the best possible outcome.

Considerations of Vision and Mission

Vision and mission are extremely important within any organization. Before individuals will buy into and support the vision and mission, they first need to buy into and support the organization's leadership. Consider the example of a sailing ship during the 1800s out at sea. The ship was a city, if not a country, unto itself. Its only resources were those it possessed or could obtain through the efforts of the crew. The mission of the ship, articulated by the captain and the other officers, was what defined success and in some instances was defined by issues of life and death. While achieving the mission and vision was more likely to occur when everyone was doing what was necessary within their roles, it was also more likely to occur when the individuals on the ship (aka, the organization) had confidence in the leadership to make the right decisions and to enact successful practices.

So how does EDM come into play with respect to vision and mission? If the ethical or moral compass is broken either within the organization or is broken within leadership, chances for success are limited. Even if success does initially result, that does not ensure its likelihood over the long term. The organization will

begin to show strain that will ultimately lead to mission failure.

Consider the situation of the sailing ship just mentioned and how problem-solving with ethical considerations could be applied. Given that the officers and crew had to be self-sustaining and to obtain or make anything that was needed, the ability to identify an issue and work through to a solution is quite germane. Obtaining drinking water for the occupants of the ship is a matter of life and death. If it rains then the issue is relatively easily resolved by capturing the rain as it falls. But what if it does not rain? In this instance the officers and crew have to find land and assess how close they can approach before sending a landing party ashore. If it is land unfamiliar to them, then safety is a concern, and the decision of whom to send depends on the crew member's experience in leading or participating in a landing party capable of finding water, assessing quality, and then transporting it back to the ship. What if the officers did not think through whom to send ashore or selected the wrong individuals? It could lead to a situation for the organization (aka the ship) that subsequently impacts the goals and ultimately the success of the organization's mission.

Regarding Dr. Wu, if the pharmacists in the clinic decide to take shortcuts in their tasks or lack the ethical and moral conviction to do what is right, the patient suffers as does the organization. Consequently, if organizational leadership lacks the moral conviction to support the vision and mission, the organization suffers from top value issues, which manifest in leadership espousing one thing, yet supporting another. It is possible for incongruence to exist within the organization and still achieve the organizational outcomes, but the likelihood of success is diminished compared with a situation where everyone buys in and engages with the mission and vision (see Chapters 6 and 16).

Applying sensemaking to the vision and mission, it is important for leadership to truly understand how the vision and mission are understood by those within the organization as well as how it is enacted. This is where the aspect of learning within sensemaking can be considered as a continuous and transparent assessment within the organization. In this manner, the management/leadership team, and for that matter everyone within the organization, can assess and benchmark progress toward the achievement of the organizational vision and mission.

When viewed through the lens of EDM, it is possible to see how both management and leadership can be impacted by ethical situations and circumstances within the contexts of either rationalist or nonrationalist approaches (Schwartz, 2016). From the management perspective, the chapter scenario could be perceived in the simplistic perspective of whether the product in question can or cannot be obtained by Dr. Wu. Once the product is available, then everything else falls into place; product preparation is possible, and the patient's treatment can continue unabated, and the best efforts are being put forth for positive and optimal patient outcomes.

This differs, however, from the leadership perspective. There are now considerations to being a participant in the gray market for product procurement. How does it impact the mission and vision of the organization? If it is assumed that the mission and vision of the organization support providing the best possible care to each patient in an individualized patient care approach, the willingness to treat the patient with a gray-market product is then mission-specific. But how does that relate to the next time this occurs, and does the situation represent an aberrant situation or shift in the organization's approach to patient care? Does this now have an impact on the culture of the organization and how employees now look upon enacting the mission? What about the organization's fiscal considerations? Will paying steeper procurement costs become an accepted norm, and what happens when the organization is no longer in as fiscally sound a position? Will it now decide participation in the gray market case by case and how does this relate to patient care?

The steps outlined above for sensemaking (learn, plan, act) are applied within both leadership and management approaches, just from different perspectives and working toward the same goal, albeit from slightly different paradigms. The actions from leadership will tend to be more holistic and performed at the 10,000-foot level versus the actions of management which will be front-line and conducted at ground level. So in regard to the scenario, the leadership approach to the issue may be how to address the situation within the organization and how to create systems to ensure a consistent and persistent approach to Dr. Wu's situation. The management approach would be creating policies and procedures to enact a consistent and persistent approach to handling this type of situation. In other words, both leadership and management are seeking to address the dilemma, but their approaches are different due to their perspectives.

■ EMPOWERMENT AND DELEGATION

Empowerment and delegation not only help the organization succeed via the successes of others, but it also helps those individuals grow and reach their potential, which is actually vital to the entire organization's success. They are essential to leadership because they represent the means by which employees who are more engaged at the point of customer service/care act in a manner that can lead to a successful outcome. Empowerment and delegation can help impart many skills, not the least of which is effective decision-making and problem-solving.

Consider the following situation from a community pharmacy perspective. A patient enters the store with four prescriptions for her son that are extremely expensive and require prior authorization as well as one requiring compounding. The pharmacist on duty (Sarah), a seasoned and experienced pharmacist, receives the prescriptions and after a lengthy conversation with the patient begins the process of preparing the medications. When Sarah asks the two technicians and intern to begin processing the prescriptions, she is asked by the senior technician if these prescriptions should be filled or if the store owner should be contacted. Sarah smiles and politely explains that ownership has given her the authority to decide on matters such as this and that she has a clear understanding of what her authority does and does not permit her to do.

Sarah has been empowered by management to use her judgment and is trusted to act in the best interests of the patient and the business. Imagine what could have happened had Sarah not been empowered to make these decisions. The patient would have left dissatisfied, the technicians and intern may have wondered about Sarah's authority, Sarah may have begun to question her role within the organization and her scope of responsibility, and ultimately it could have adversely impacted the patient's outcomes as well as the pharmacy's outcomes (see Chapter 26). Sarah's empowerment translates into her ability to address situations (problems) as they arise. One important consideration is where problem-solving can intersect with job satisfaction. Problem-solving can sometimes have a poor connotation in that problems are by their nature are potentially negative situations. Problem-solving, however, can be conducted proactively to create positive change. An even greater proactive problem-solving approach would be if Sarah, upon consideration of the situation she was in, put forth ideas to improve things and to minimize challenges going forward. The key is that problem-solving, whether reactive or proactive, is dependent upon individuals feeling empowered to address issues and even have been delegated the authority to make the changes.

Simply put, delegation and empowerment are essential within any organization in that leadership cannot be everywhere and involved in every decision. But to provide this level of autonomy and authority to an employee is not an easy thing and can only occur when a variety of elements are present, such as demonstrated proficiency, demonstrated judgment, accountability, trust, a willingness to accept the outcomes, and a willingness to let go. The first three relate to the employee and the second three relate to leadership.

For an employee to be viewed as someone to whom authority can be delegated and to be empowered, leadership will want to make sure they demonstrate proficiency regarding assigned and unassigned activities as well as show sound judgment. How can these things be understood? Perhaps it only happens after a few review cycles or after a certain period of time. Or maybe it happens as a result of observed outcomes that leadership sees and lets the employee work through.

One way that leadership can ascertain the best candidates for delegation is through inquiry when the opportunity presents itself. For example, an employee walks into the office of his/her supervisor with a question regarding a dilemma and is looking for the answer to the question. Instead of answering the question though, the supervisor says to the employee "*Sounds like an interesting question. Talk to me about how you would suggest addressing the issue.*" This not only allows the supervisor to learn about this individual's thought processes and judgment, but it also encourages the employee to develop confidence and to feel like the supervisor values his/her opinion. It also allows for a teachable moment to occur, irrespective of whether the employee's view is right or wrong. If the employee is right, the supervisor's response could be something like "*Great answer, and sounds like you already knew the right approach!*" If the employee's response is not on target or only partially on target, the supervisor's response could be something like "*That is an interesting idea. I wonder if there is a better solution that perhaps you could consider… Good job!*" The key is regardless of the answer, to continue to motivate the employee to try and stretch him or herself and to strive to grow. This inquiry approach also relates very well to creating a problem-solving approach to the opportunities that present themselves within the workplace.

As noted earlier, for empowerment and delegation to work requires the supervisor to release some control and to lets things take place within micromanaging the situation. Trust is essential to successful empowerment in that leadership has to have that level of comfort with the employee, and the employee has to feel like he/she has the trust and confidence of leadership to make decisions. The development of trust will take time and the approach outlined above about asking the employee to talk through his/her approach is a good way to develop bilateral trust.

Problem-solving and acting upon identified solutions is only possible in a trusting environment.

The supervisor must also be willing to accept the outcomes of delegating, which can be challenging. This is more relevant after the employee has been empowered to make decisions. Referring back to the example in which Sarah felt empowered to act, ownership cannot go back and change what Sarah did after the fact unless it wants to disempower Sarah and put her in the position of not wanting to make decisions for fear of being overturned again. The outcome needs to be accepted. The outcome, however, does not have to be completely agreed with and again, this could represent a teachable moment about how things could be handled in the future via a discussion on the pros and cons of the outcome versus an outright reversal of the decision or overturning it. Empowerment is not carte blanche to allow employees to do whatever they want to do at any time, nor is it an opportunity for leadership to second guess or micromanage the decisions that are made.

Another component, the willingness to let go, is challenging for many persons, including those in leadership/managerial positions. For you to be effective as a leader, it is important to have the self-awareness that you are not capable of doing everything. The only way to accomplish this is through the empowerment of others in a manner that frees up leadership to do what is required. Put a different way, the empowerment of others, or the delegation of authority, cannot occur in a micromanaged environment. If the empowerment results in the employee constantly checking-in, then leadership is not letting go of the activity and is not trusting the employee's judgment. Letting go can indeed be more difficult than it sounds!

What happens when a leader is unwilling to empower others? It can stifle change and innovation as well as create an environment in which individuals perceive less ownership, less involvement, become less engaged, all of which have a negative impact on the culture. Finally, it can create an environment in which no one makes decisions or accepts responsibility for things they perceive will be micromanaged or overturned.

In revisiting the conundrum with Sarah, she was placed in a situation that requires less in terms of sensemaking but does relate to ethical considerations, and this is where judgment and trust are extremely important. The situation in which Sarah found herself having to make a decision about filling the prescriptions or not filling the prescriptions was in a confusing space regarding pharmacy practice. The decision Sarah has to make, and the ethical situation she finds herself in, is reconciling the needs of the patient in terms of positive humanistic, economic, and clinical outcomes versus the expectations of ownership, which while including positive patient outcomes also focus on profitability. The previously mentioned EDM models represent ways in which Sarah can approach the issue.

Referring back to the definition of EDM, or "standards of behavior that tell us how human beings ought to act in the many situations in which they find themselves….," Sarah was put in the position of having to engage her personal ethics to discern right from wrong in terms of filling the prescriptions and the implications that could come from that.

■ INFLUENCE

Regarding leadership, it is important to consider the constructs of influence and inspiration, because without those, leaders have a difficult time getting anything accomplished. There is an age-old maxim which states that you are not a leader unless someone is following you. Put another way, "He who thinks he leads, but has no followers, is only taking a walk" (Maxwell, 2002). An individual can follow a leader for a variety of reasons, but two of the positive reasons are that the leader influences and/or inspires him or her.

Leaders/managers are often appointed to positions whereby the new title is some sort of reward. That being said, everything beyond the designation of title has to be earned. The granting of a title does not mean that the leader will be successful, but through influence and inspiration, it is far more likely that success will be the outcome.

So how do leaders generate influence, and subsequently how do they inspire? Readers of this chapter should take a few moments to reflect upon a leader/manager with whom they recently worked and whether that person had any attributes that helped influence the actions or activities of others.

Leaders possess various characteristics that help them create or generate influence within an organization, and through this influence they are able to better facilitate the success of the organization. Some of these attributes include: personal character and how he or she acts; the ability to create new and sustain existing relationships; is self-aware regarding personal strengths and weaknesses; is knowledgeable and credible about the field in which they work; has practical experience that relates to the field; and has good judgment regarding the field (Maxwell, 2007). Trust is very important. But with empowerment, the trust was considered more from the standpoint of the leader to employee; within the context of influence, it is a matter of the trust that employees have in the leader.

Taken another way, Covey (1989) considers developing or sustaining influence and subsequent success as being associated to the actions you take as an individual, being situationally aware and caring about others, and finally listening, learning, and empowering and/or delegating. Each of these areas has several components and steps.

First, the actions you take should relate to staying positive. This includes being patient with those whom you work, differentiating the outcome from the personal, being proactive instead of responsive, and honoring your commitments to others. Second, we must strive to assume the best in individuals, which means knowing the situation and caring. This means we must first seek to understand and be a good listener, to reflect back what you learn, reward honesty, be candid about your mistakes and own them, value one-on-one communication, listen and learn from colleagues, and remember your common sense of purpose.

Third is listening, learning, and delegating. To accomplish this, one must be open-minded, not get defensive, recognize when you can or cannot educate others, seek the best possible outcome, and when appropriate, delegate/empower and hold others accountable, involve others in meaningful projects with meaningful outcomes, and seek to avoid quick fixes.

■ REVISITING THE SCENARIO

As Dr. Wu explains the limited availability of the product to the patient, Lynn becomes very anxious and concerned about her future. Dr. Wu has been out of pharmacy school for less than five years, all of which has been spent working in this specialty pharmacy. She knows that to get the medication in question the pharmacy will have to pay a high price for the medication on the gray market and that she also will be faced with explaining to her supervisors that she made a decision in the best interests of the patient. Considering what has been discussed throughout this chapter, how would you advise Dr. Wu, and what considerations, both ethical and leadership-related, do you think will come into play?

Dr. Wu, as the pharmacist-in-charge, is placed in the unique situation of being a decision-maker, but as is always the case, is responsible to others. Several of the constructs identified in the chapter collide within this case. One is the issue of financials and patient outcomes and how to rationalize a decision knowing that it is not a simple binary choice, but one with a variety of considerations. This may lead to tension between the ethical considerations of patient care and the organizational vision and culture. It is also where Dr. Wu's ability to solve problems, both in real-time as well as proactively to minimize similar events in the future, intersects with the organizational vision, mission, and values. Is Dr. Wu solving problems for profits or patient outcomes? If the organization has a "patient-first" culture and that is imbedded in the mission and vision, then Dr. Wu should feel empowered to do whatever is necessary to treat the patient. If, however, there exists ambiguity within the organizational vision and culture, then she is faced with the dilemma of what to do and how to advocate for her patient. This may involve using one of the models for EDM or perhaps sensemaking as an activity prior to EDM. For the sake of this case, Dr. Wu decides that even beyond the organization's vision and culture, she views it as her personal mission to meet the patient's needs. Her decision to advocate for the patient leads her to seek to influence her superiors based on her feeling empowered.

■ CONCLUSION

As explained throughout this chapter, pharmacist managers/leaders must provide ethical leadership, but this may not be enough to deter unethical behavior within an organization. The efforts of the manager/leader must include the consistent application of an EDM process. They must be able to solve problems and address issues with an eye to the ethical aspects or nature of the dilemma before them.

There are numerous ways to ensure decisions factor in ethical components, and four have been highlighted. The model chosen for an organization must be incorporated into the culture, and EDM must be an element of the mission and the vision. Perhaps this could be accomplished by incorporating value statements for the organization as a part of the organization's mission and vision. This could be accomplished through the inclusion of a statement that highlights the value the organization places on integrity in decision-making. Eventually, the manager/leader must consider his or her actions at the visionary and operational levels. How an individual leads will impact the quality of the decisions they make. Will they feel empowered to make critical decisions and to exercise personal judgment? Will their decisions align with the mission and vision? Will they strive to be ethical in all instances? How will they approach problem-solving, and how will they model it for employees to demonstrate how to successfully address both patient and organizational issues? These are the choices the manager/leader must make.

The choices are never easy, but acting as an ethical pharmacy leader is a worthy goal that demands attention, perseverance, and consistency. Finally, it is important to remember that all leaders/managers learn from their successes and from their mistakes.

No one who takes the mantle of responsibility upon their shoulders does so without making some mistakes along the way. Every decision and action, albeit by employees empowered to act upon the best information they have or the manager/leader who acts on behalf of others is seeking to make a difference via addressing problems. Problem-solving can create a negative connotation that something needs to be fixed. While this is clearly not the case, the need for ethical understanding of problems and for appropriate sensemaking of situations is a must. But if the leader/manager understands the ethical issues associated with those decisions as well as learn from both the good and bad outcomes, they will continue to grow and improve.

■ QUESTIONS FOR FURTHER DISCUSSION

1. How can you connect empowerment and delegation to organizational culture?
2. How would ethical considerations influence your problem-solving when in a management or leadership role?
3. Kohlberg's theory of moral development has been criticized for an emphasis on rights or justice, which has roots in our Western culture. Some critics claim that the focus should be on the broader community while other critics claim that Kohlberg should focus more on caring rather than justice. What are your thoughts on Kohlberg's theory? Can you defend it?
4. Can you recall a situation where a pharmacist, resident pharmacist, or student pharmacist made a high-quality ethical decision while holding true to their professional identity? What do you recall about the decision-making process? What can take from that situation that you would share with a colleague who needs assistance with making an ethical decision?

REFERENCES

Advanced Practice Nursing. 2014. Rest's Four-Component Model. Available at https://ebrary.net/8251/education/rests_four-component_model#935. Accessed December 31, 2018.

American Pharmacists Association (APhA). 1994. Code of Ethics. Available at https://www.pharmacist.com/code-ethics. Accessed December 30, 2018.

American Pharmacists Association (APhA). 1998. APhA Policy Manual; Pharmacist Conscience Clause. Available at https://www.pharmacist.com/policy-manual?key=pharmacist%20conscience%20clause. Accessed December 31, 2018.

American Society of Health System Pharmacists (ASHP). 2009. ASHP Guidelines on Managing Drug Product Shortages. Drug Distribution and Control: Procurement—Guidelines: 101–109. Available at https://www.ashp.org/-/media/assets/policy-guidelines/docs/guidelines/managing-drug-product-shortages.ashx. Accessed December 30, 2018.

American Society of Health System Pharmacists (ASHP). 2018. ASHP Guidelines on Managing Drug Product Shortages. *Am J Health Syst Pharm* 75(21):1742–1750.

Ancona D. 2012. *The Handbook for Teaching Leadership*. Thousand Oaks, CA: SAGE Publications, Inc.

Austin Z. 2007. Geographical migration, psychological adjustment, and re-formation of professional identity: The double-culture shock experience of international pharmacy graduates in Ontario (Canada). *Globalisation, Societies and Education* 5(2):239–255.

Brushwood DB. 2018. Pharmacists face murky legal territory over concept of unresolvable 'red flags'. *PharmacyToday*. April. Available at https://www.pharmacytoday.org/article/S1042-0991(18)30491-2/pdf. Accessed January 1, 2019.

Castleberry AN, Payakachat N, Ashby S, et al. 2016. Qualitative analysis of written reflection during a teaching certificate program. *Am J Pharm Educ* 80(1):10.

Cohen HE. 2014. Black is the new gray in pharmaceuticals. *U.S. Pharmacist* 39(7):1.

Covey SR. 1989. *The Seven Habits of Highly Effective People*. New York, NY: Simon & Schuster, Inc.

Cruess RL, Cruess SR, Boudreau D, Snell L, Steinert Y. 2015. A schematic representation of the professional identify formation and socialization of medical students and residents: A guide for medical educators. *Acad Med* 90(6):718–725.

Draper R. 2003. The Toxic Pharmacist. *NY Times*, June 8. Available at https://www.nytimes.com/2003/06/08/magazine/the-toxic-pharmacist.html. Accessed January 1, 2019.

Haidt J. 2001. The emotional dog and its rational tail: A social intuitionist approach to moral judgment. *Psychol Rev* 108(4):814–834.

Kohlberg L, Hersh RH. 1977. Moral development: A review of the theory. *Theory into Practice*. 16(2):53–59. Available at http://links.jstor.org/sici?sici=0040-5841%28197704%2916%3A2%3C53%3AMDAROT%3E2.0.CO%3B2-%23. Accessed March 13, 2019.

Markula Center for Applied Ethics. 2015. A Framework for Ethical Decision Making. Available at https://www.scu.edu/ethics/ethics-resources/ethical-decision-making/a-framework-for-ethical-decision-making/. Accessed December 31, 2018.

Maxwell JC. 2002. *Leadership 101: What Every Leader Needs to Know*. Nashville, TN: Thomas Nelson Publishers.

Maxwell JC. 2007. *The 21 Irrefutable Laws of Leadership: Follow them and People Will Follow You*. Nashville, TN: Thomas Nelson Publishers.

Medina MS, Plaza CM, Stowe CD, et al. 2013. Center for the Advancement of Pharmacy Education 2013 Educational Outcomes. *Am J Pharm Educ* 77(8):162.

Oderda GM, Zavod RM, Carter JT, et al. 2010. An environmental scan on the status of critical thinking and problem solving skills in colleges/schools of pharmacy: Report of the 2009–2010 Academic Affairs Standing Committee. *Am J Pharm Educ* 74(10):S6.

Rest JR. 1986. *Moral development: Advances in Research and Theory*. New York, NY: Praeger.

Rosoff PM. 2012. Unpredictable drug shortages: An ethical framework for short-term rationing in hospitals. *Am J Bioethics* 12(1):1–9.

Schwartz MS. 2016. Ethical decision-making theory: An integrated approach. *J Bus Ethics* 139:755–776.

Thiel CE, Bagdasarov Z, Harkrider L, Johnson JF, Mumford MD. 2012. Leader ethical decision-making in organizations: Strategies for sensemaking. *J Bus Ethics* 107:49–64.

Weick K. 1995. *Sensemaking in Organizations*. Thousand Oaks, CA: Sage Publications Inc.

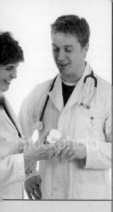

5

CREATING AND MANAGING VALUE

Greg L. Alston and Peter T. Bulatao

About the Authors: Dr. Alston is an Associate Dean and professor at Savannah Campus, South University School of Pharmacy. He has over 30 years of experience in community pharmacy management, both as a chain pharmacy administrator and an independent pharmacy owner. He earned a Doctor of Pharmacy (PharmD) degree from the University of the Pacific and has published three best-selling management books, *The Bosshole Effect—Managing People Simplified*, *The Ten Things A New Manager Must Get Right From the Start*, and *Own Your Value—The Real Future of Pharmacy Practice*. His passion lies in teaching the next generation of pharmacists how to create value for the stakeholders they serve.

Dr. Bulatao is an Associate Professor at Savannah Campus, South University School of Pharmacy. Dr. Bulatao received his BS degree in Pharmacy from Duquesne University, MS degree in Pharmacy from the University of Texas at Austin, MMAS from the Command and General Staff College, and PharmD from the University of Minnesota at Minneapolis. He completed an ASHP-accredited PGY1 residency and is dually board certified in Pharmacotherapy and in Ambulatory Care. Dr. Bulatao has approximately 30 years of experience in health system pharmacy management, serving in ambulatory, inpatient, and clinical supervisory positions, in addition to having been a pharmacy director and regional pharmacy consultant. His research interests range from clinical practice to operational management and strategic planning.

■ LEARNING OBJECTIVES

After completing this chapter, readers should be able to

1. Describe how value is created.
2. Describe the relative value theorem (RVT).
3. Describe the stakeholders in the health care marketplace.
4. Apply the RVT to pharmacy practice.
5. Apply the RVT to guide your personal life.

■ SCENARIO

James Deaux recently graduated with a PharmD degree, earning a 3.90 GPA. He had leadership roles in Rho Chi and Phi Lambda Sigma and was actively involved in several other student organizations. James performed well in his experiential rotations and generally received high marks from his preceptors.

James decided to apply for a clinical pharmacist position at The Ideal Hospital, located in the same city as his pharmacy school. He has crafted an impressive resume and was invited by Dr. Frank Stein, Director of Pharmacy, to interview for the position. After greetings and a few minutes of chit-chat, Dr. Stein gets right to the point, "James you seem like a fine young man. Your credentials are impeccable. But we have had over 100 applicants for this position. In the interest of not wasting time, I have only two questions to ask you. What do you have to offer me that the other 99 applicants do not? What are you going to do for me and The Ideal Hospital that should make me want to pay you $120,000 per year?"

How should James respond to Dr. Stein in order to portray his value most appropriately?

■ CHAPTER QUESTIONS

1. What is the current state of the health care marketplace?
2. What is the status of the pharmacist job market? Why is postgraduate training (residencies, fellowships, and graduate school) required for some pharmacist positions, but not for others?
3. What is the role of the pharmacist regarding management of drug therapy for individual patients? For organizations? For society? How successful have pharmacists been in these roles?
4. What is the concept of "value"? How can pharmacists add value to their patients, organizations, and to society?

■ INTRODUCTION

The health care marketplace continues to evolve. The Patient Protection and Affordable Care Act (ACA) signed into law in March 2010 illuminated the role of pharmacists in integrated care models, transitional care models, and Medicare Part D medication therapy management (MTM). The American Pharmacists Association (APhA, 2015) reported that 38 states designated pharmacists as providers, but that scope of practice and payment for services remained as challenges. And the nation's governors (National Governors Association, 2015) implored states to better integrate pharmacists into the delivery of quality health care. However, significant challenges exist in paying for this expanded coverage. The Congressional Budget Office (CBO) estimated that as of December 2018 the total public debt held by the United States was 15.7 trillion dollars and projected continued budget deficits through 2028 (CBO, 2018). Researchers (Blumenthal & Collins, 2014) suggest that the sustainability of coverage expansions will depend on the ability of the United States to control the overall costs of health care. Therefore, these competing demands of expanding opportunity for pharmacists to assume new clinical roles while at the same time ensuring that resources are available to pay for these services create an interesting predicament. Demand for pharmacist labor has dropped from a peak of 4.31 in 2006 to 32.92 at the end of the 3rd quarter of 2018 (Pharmacist Demand Indicator, 2018), indicating that a shortage of pharmacists does not appear to exist. Some researchers (Covvey et al., 2015) have expressed concern that too many graduates and slowing job growth will lead to an oversupply of pharmacists. Europeans (Martini, 2014) have expressed similar concerns. And the continued expansion in number of pharmacy schools coupled with a less than projected growth rate in pharmacist employment threatens to cause a downtrend in pharmacist earnings (Lebovitz & Eddington, 2019).

Given the realities of the market for pharmacist positions, resource constraints, a changing landscape in health care, and the knowledge and skills that pharmacists and students gain across their education and work experience, all pharmacists and students should ask two critical questions:

1. How will I distinguish myself to get the position I want with the salary I desire?
2. How will the profession of pharmacy serve the needs of patients, health care professionals, the health care system, and society?

Pharmacy students often focus much of their time and efforts mastering the clinical skills required to be a good pharmacist. Students tend to judge courses such as pharmacy management as having a lower priority than more clinically oriented courses such as pharmacology and therapeutics. It is important to remember that the key to one's success as a pharmacist is not, and never will be, what he or she knows, but rather what that pharmacist can do with what he or she knows. A critical component of learning to become a pharmacist is to do something useful with one's knowledge to create value for those who will be impacted, including their patients, coworkers, organization, profession, and society at large.

Anecdotal evidence suggests that pharmacists are not hired by employers in rank order of their pharmacy school grade point average. Factors such as past work experience, communication skills, problem solving, and the ability to work effectively with others, also influence hiring decisions. The Hiring Intent Reasoning Examination Survey surveyed over 3000 pharmacists nationwide to identify the relative importance of character traits versus academic success markers when making hiring decisions for entry level pharmacist jobs. The results suggest that employers value aspects of a person's character ahead of academic markers of success. The results were similar across all practice settings (Alston et al., 2018). This suggests that employers believe that success in the workplace requires a different set of attributes and behaviors than how success may have been measured in the classroom. The workplace requires pharmacists to translate knowledge into useful actions. Pharmacists who can do this successfully are rewarded, while pharmacists who cannot may find themselves with limited opportunities in the workplace.

An essential skill that distinguishes any individual from others is the ability to create value for those with whom they interact and serve. A pharmacist must not only create value but also must clearly articulate the value to others to thrive as a professional in today's health care environment. This chapter will explore how to create value using an approach known as the RVT. This approach borrows from the literatures in neuroscience, marketing, and economics to create a model that is simple to understand and easy to apply to decisions pharmacists make on a daily basis (Alston & Blizzard, 2011).

■ THE RELATIVE VALUE THEOREM

Pharmacy students and pharmacists cannot increase their value to the constituencies they serve unless they understand conceptually how value is created and utilized. Zeithaml has defined the concept of value, suggesting that value is a function of our desire to obtain high-quality goods and services that meet our needs and wants, as well as what we need to sacrifice to obtain them (usually, but not always, money or some other resource). The perceived value (PV) of a good or service has been defined as a balance between what one gets relative to what they must give up to obtain that benefit (Zeithaml, 1988). For example, the "value" of a drug product can be assessed by comparing the benefits that a patient obtains from using a drug (e.g., lower blood pressure, increased quality of life) relative to the costs of obtaining the drug (e.g., money, time, effort). The services that a pharmacist provides to a patient or an employer can be assessed in the same way. What benefits does that pharmacist bring to their patients or employer relative to what the patients or employer must pay to receive the pharmacist's services?

The RVT is a conceptual model that attempts to illuminate the key factors that a "buyer" uses to decide which goods or services to select for "purchase" from a list of possible alternatives. Whether a "buyer" is buying a tangible good at a store, or agreeing to use a professional service from a health professional, the mental process used to decide whether or not to make a purchase is the same. The "buyer" can be an individual patient, another health care professional, or an organization, such as a business, insurance company, or government agency. This decision to purchase a good or utilize a service is made by comparing the options available in the marketplace of choices. The person or entity considering the purchase must make a choice by comparing what they get, versus what they have to give up, to satisfy their needs and wants (see Chapter 24). Understanding how value is created can guide pharmacists in their decisions of what goods to sell in their pharmacies, and in the development of patient-care services. Understanding how value is created also can assist pharmacy students in creating their own career value strategies for potential employers. By understanding how they can translate their knowledge, skills, and experience to help meet the needs of potential employers, pharmacy students can market their value in an effort to obtain a position. Because just as any consumer likes a good bargain (when the benefits obtained from a good or service outweighs their costs), any employer would hope to obtain the same from their employees (the benefits of having the employee outweigh the costs of employment).

Let's revisit the potential hiring of James Deaux. Based on his historical performance, there is little doubt that he will be a capable employee at The Ideal Hospital. However, he needs to depict to Dr. Stein how he will create this bargain or value, whether through objective parameters such as productivity or through intangibles such as work ethic and conceptualization of ideas. After all, while James Deaux is likely to be capable, so will most of the other 99 applicants for the same position he has applied for.

Value, and specifically relative value (RV), can be expressed as a mathematical equation (RV = [P + S] × PV), where P is the price, S is the service, and PV is the perceived value. The relationships between these concepts can also be described graphically as they are in Figure 5-1.

As will be further described in Chapters 24 and 26, there are links between customer service, quality, and purchasing habits (Bloemer et al., 1999; Bolton & Drew, 1991; Caruana et al., 2000; Churchill & Surprenant, 1982; Cronin et al., 2000; Oliver, 1993). Additionally, customer loyalty and profitability of a business over the long term are improved by service quality as perceived by the customer (Reichheld, 1996; Venetis & Ghauri, 2004; Woodruff, 1997). Therefore, quality, customer service, and price matter in the mind of the purchaser of goods and services. Purchases are based not just on the amount of money sacrificed to obtain the good or service but also on the other factors including the quality of the good or service, the expected outcomes associated with using the good or service, the reputation of the vendor offering the good or service, the other "costs" of obtaining the good or service (physical, social, time), and the overall benefits the consumer perceives by having the good or service. The RVT model organizes these factors into three component groups listed as price (P), service (S), and PV. When combined in algebraic form, these components determine the overall RV of a good or service in the mind of the buyer.

The RVT is moderated by a fundamental question that buyers must ask themselves at some point: "Do I have the resources available to make the purchase at this time?" If the answer is yes, the buyer performs the mental calculations in determining if they are willing to sacrifice their resources given the benefits they perceive that they will obtain by making the purchase. If the answer is no, the mental calculations inherent in the RVT are not altered in any way. A buyer still can consider if they would sacrifice the resources if they had them. On the other hand, the buyer must delay making an actual purchase decision until the resources are available. Note that decisions that buyers make when they have resources to make a purchase may be different from those made when they do not.

Price (P)

The first element of the RVT is the price (P) component. The pricing element of the equation is the

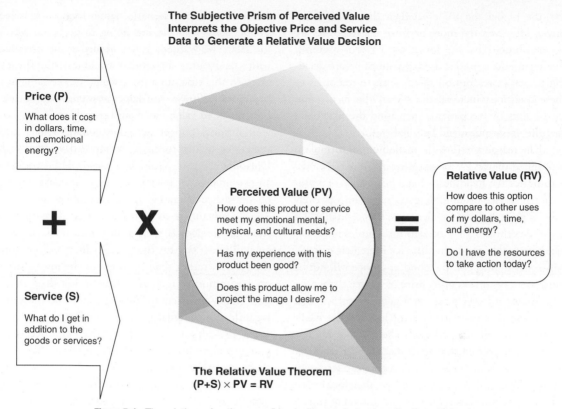

Figure 5-1. The relative value theorem. (Used with permission from Dr. Greg Alston.)

component in which the consumer analyzes the cost to acquire a product or service. Cost can include monetary and nonmonetary factors. Since we know that a variety of products exist in the marketplace, and that not all products are identically priced, there must be something besides price alone that buyers consider (Alston & Blizzard, 2011).

Service (S)

The concept of service (S in the RVT equation) widens the consumer thought process beyond the price/cost comparison. Service factors are those things the provider could market or use to distinguish their good or service from competing products. When developing a new good or service, pharmacists should consider these distinguishing features and purposefully build them into the overall design of their product.

Pharmacists can continue to highlight these extra benefits in their communications and marketing efforts to create perceptions of value in the minds of their consumers over and above a low-price strategy.

Perceived Value (PV)

PV, the third element of the RVT equation, is defined as the cognitive trade-off between perceptions of quality (what I get) versus the sacrifice (what I have to give up) (Teas & Agarwal, 2000). Buyers considering a purchase ask themselves several questions about any good or service. They include: (1) How well does this good or service meet my emotional, mental, physical, and cultural needs? (2) How well does this good or service allow me to project the image I desire to project? (3) How satisfactory has my experience with the good or service been? The more positive the responses are, the higher the PV created in the mind of the buyer. However, the more negative the responses are to these questions, the lower the PV. For example, many patients consider these questions before deciding to get a prescription filled. Positive responses to these questions increase the PV of the medication in the eyes of the patient, increasing the likelihood that the prescription will be filled.

The reason the (P + S) portion of the formula is multiplied by the PV component in the RVT model is to reflect the hypothesis that a buyer's PV of a professional service or tangible good can trump or overrule its price and service elements. Conceptually, if a buyer determines a PV of zero for a professional service or tangible good, then the RVT predicts that RV will equal to zero and the good or service will not be purchased, regardless of its price or service elements.

Setting a lower price on a good or service does not necessarily make it better or increase the likelihood that it will be purchased. The risk in using low price as a marketing strategy is that another marketer may be able to provide a similar good or service at an even lower price. The market risk therefore is that a good or service could become a commodity (e.g., a good or service that has no qualitative differentiation within a market), with sales that go up or down depending solely on how the competition is priced. A low-price strategy is only successful if the marketer will *always* be the low-price leader, and then only if the price generated covers the costs of producing the goods and services.

Many pharmacists fail to understand that even if they do not want to become business owners or managers of a business, they need to be able to offer value to their employer. By understanding RVT an individual pharmacist can create a personal value strategy that will make him or her competitive against other employees that could be hired. The employee pharmacist who wants to earn a higher salary, get a job promotion, or avoid being downsized during an economic downturn must learn to market their own value in order to ensure job security. The key to career success is to create value for those you serve. Wealth flows directly from value.

In the chapter scenario, James Deaux was asked by Dr. Stein what he was going to do to be worth the salary he wanted. James needed to be prepared with a compelling answer that would earn him the job offer. In this case, no answer would be the same as a bad answer. However, if James answered with a carefully reasoned value-based answer such as, "I can save your hospital budget over one million dollars next year alone by instituting a program I developed with Doctor Smartguy at Well People Hospital," he would be a top candidate for the job, so long as he could actually offer evidence or a rationale that he could really do so.

An advantage to pharmacies that develop professional services is their ability to attract customers willing to pay for the benefits they receive from the service, rather than seeking out the lowest price on a commodity such as a prescription drug product. While amoxicillin 500 mg should be the same regardless of the pharmacy, the services that a pharmacy provides to accompany that product (e.g., patient counseling, prescription delivery, therapeutic drug monitoring) can help shift consumer attention away from the price of the drug and toward the benefits of the services. A high-service strategy will succeed if a high-quality service is consistently delivered at a fair price. This high-service strategy allows a pharmacist to stand apart from the competition and offer a clear alternative to the low-price strategy so long as the service is provided on a uniform basis. An additional benefit of creating a service-based business is that it is more difficult for competitors to copy a successful business model. Professional service success is based upon the service provided, not solely the price charged. The challenge for continued success in a high-service business strategy is to consistently deliver great service and promote the business to distinguish their offerings from less expensive alternatives.

There are numerous products that consumers purchase due to their personal preferences, even though less expensive alternatives exist in the market. A good example is purchasing a car. A pharmacy student may want a nice car that he or she cannot afford. If the student values paying tuition more than buying a nice car (PV), the student may shop for a lower-priced car (P) that will not break down and will be inexpensive to maintain (S), such as a Honda Civic. Once the student graduates and starts earning a higher income, the same student may prefer a vehicle that reflects his or her new status. In this situation, the PV of the Honda Civic may become zero if it does not reflect the high-end image the student wishes to project. The fact that the Civic sells for $20,000 less than a BMW or Lexus is not important in the eyes of a purchaser seeking status over function. Honda may offer Civic at bargain prices, but the purchaser may not buy one if he or she has graduated to a luxury car mindset. Interestingly, once the graduate starts a family, he or she may find themselves back in the economy car mindset, as one's values often change with their priorities. The RVT does not predict the future, it simply suggests what is likely to happen using given set of conditions.

The RVT predicts that any professional service must have potential for generating a high PV in the minds of potential buyers if they are to succeed in the marketplace. The RVT predicts that if consumers do not perceive any value for a particular good or service (PV = $0), they will not assign it an RV regardless of the price or level of service provided, and will not make a purchase because there will be no RV. Conversely, high PV not only leads to purchase behavior, but can build high customer loyalty and result in higher profitability (Reichheld, 1996). As will be discussed in Chapter 26, high emotional customer satisfaction correlates with higher loyalty levels, and ultimately, higher profitability because PV exists in the mind of the consumer. Marketers such as pharmacies and pharmacists can attempt to influence PV by offering competitive pricing, enhancing the quality of their service offering, and adding additional service elements to their offer. But the only true metric for success is sufficient marketplace response.

For many years the pharmacist shortage created market conditions that favored the pharmacist with rising wages. As the labor supply has increased, the pressure is downward on wages. If a pharmacist wishes to see their personal income increase, they must continue to find ways to create more value for their employer than they consume in wages and benefits. When James Deaux was being interviewed by Dr. Stein he communicated that he was not just a pharmacist, but a pharmacist who would be able to help the hospital operate more efficiently and free up budgetary dollars that were currently being wasted. Instead of expecting to get the job solely because he had a PharmD degree with good grades, James took the time to research hospital waste and budgetary restrictions to determine how he could help them run the hospital pharmacy more efficiently. The key to creating this value-based answer is understanding how to create and market value.

Given the decreased profitability associated with dispensing prescriptions (see Chapter 23), pharmacists are increasingly developing professional services with the intention that consumers pay to obtain the benefits they can offer. Pharmacists must note that they are not the only professionals capable of providing services such as immunizations, smoking cessation, disease state management, drug regimen reviews, or even dispensing prescription medications. Pharmacists' failure to demonstrate that they can provide services at a competitive price, with better outcomes, or with high PV in the eyes of consumers may find consumers turning to other providers to obtain these services (e.g., physicians, nurses, respiratory therapists, etc.) (Alston & Blizzard, 2011). If pharmacists allow their professional services to become a commodity, other providers will find a way to offer a similar service for a lower price. In the same sense, what if Dr. Stein has another potential candidate who is willing to accept the job at a lower salary than James Deaux, though seems to have fewer qualifications? Dr. Stein would have to ask himself if the professional services The Ideal Hospital provides are essentially that of a commodity, or one that provides PV in the mind of the buyer. If so, does the PV offset the additional salary expense he would incur? Pharmacists must also seize upon opportunities availed to them by having a highly trained, competent, yet less expensive support staff (pharmacy technicians, see Chapter 19) to leverage and offer services employing these technicians that are that much more cost-effective when compared to services potentially offered by other professionals.

FUTURE CHANGES TO THE HEALTH CARE SYSTEM

Recent events indicate that substantial changes in the markets for health care, including the markets for pharmacies, pharmacists, and professional pharmacy services, are about to be seen in the coming years. These events include efforts to increase the quality, decrease the costs, and improve access to health care such as the passage of the Patient Protection and Affordable Care Act (ACA) in 2010 and the movement toward the patient-centered medical home model (PCMH). At the same time, a worldwide economic slowdown and budget deficits at all levels of government (a major payer of health care in the United States and other countries) limit resources available to pay for health care goods and services. These events point to stakeholders in the health care marketplace demanding even more value for their dollar. Pharmacists and other health care professionals are not guaranteed a future role in our nation's health care system. Pharmacists must prove they deserve a role by demonstrating that they bring value to all stakeholders in the health care system (Kaldy, 2010). An example of where pharmacists must demonstrate their value is the issue of medication adherence.

Medication adherence, which describes medication taking behavior, is defined according to three operational, quantifiable parameters: initiation, implementation, and discontinuation (which encompasses persistence) (Lehman et al., 2014)

Adherence can be measured using calculations such as the medication possession ratio and proportion of days covered. It is not the intent of this chapter to establish superiority of one calculation over the other, but in general, each depicts a snapshot of a patient's adherence to a given medication. It would be natural to assume that if patient counseling and follow-up is performed adequately and routinely, a majority of patients would be adherent with their medications. Unfortunately, that is not the case.

Poor medication adherence in the treatment of chronic diseases is a serious problem. The consequences of poor adherence grow as the prevalence of chronic disease grows worldwide. These consequences include poor health outcomes and increased health care costs. Improving adherence enhances patients' safety, and effective adherence interventions may have a far greater impact on the health of the population than any improvement in specific medical treatments. In the United States, poor medication adherence affects Americans of all ages, genders, income levels, and education levels. It has been estimated that this lack of medication adherence leads to unnecessary disease progression, disease complications, reduced functional abilities, a lower quality of life, and premature death. The total cost of suboptimal medication adherence has been estimated at $177 billion annually in total direct and indirect health care costs (National Council on Patient Information and Education [NCPIE], 2007).

The costs and consequences of medication nonadherence represent a wakeup call to all of health care, and particularly to pharmacy given the profession's desired role in MTM. Medication adherence represents an area where pharmacists truly do add value to the health care system, yet questions exist as to just how well that benefit is perceived by other stakeholders in health care. Moreover, while pharmacists have added value, they can certainly do more to improve the adherence of their patients to their medications.

As stated earlier in this chapter, goods and services that create value are not only the keys to success for any health professional or business; they drive the success of today's economy. Pharmacists can create value by engaging with patients to such a degree and in such ways that patients embrace medication adherence as something truly "valuable" (PV). Once this has been done, patients would recognize the PV inherent in taking medications in an effective manner, and would therefore take their own actions to this effect. This engagement would result in improved medication adherence and health outcomes.

It is not enough for a highly trained pharmacist to know relevant clinical therapeutics and applied pharmacology. Pharmacists must be able to motivate patients to achieve desired outcomes. Clinical knowledge is important, but understanding how to create value in the eyes of each of our stakeholders is equally, if not more, important. By utilizing the RVT, pharmacists may understand how to better motivate stakeholders to "buy in" to our recommendations.

Consumer purchasing decisions are driven by their perceptions of value of the goods and services they are offered. When thinking about patient decisions to accept, or "purchase" medication adherence services, pharmacists must learn to ask questions and listen to patients to understand their resistance to adherence. Are patients able or willing to spend the money, time, or effort on their medications or adherence (P)? Do they understand what they get for the expenditure of time, money, or effort (S)? Or, do they inherently value their medication therapy (PV)? While the rational mind computes the price and service components, PV is controlled by emotions and feelings. It is not uncommon for an adult male patient to refuse to take blood pressure medications because he believes the side effects can negatively impact his sexual performance. For some people, the PV of male pride can be much more of a motivator than the risk of a heart attack (S).

■ HOW WILL PHARMACISTS CREATE VALUE FOR HEALTH CARE STAKEHOLDERS

The process of developing patient-care services that will succeed in a competitive marketplace requires pharmacists to apply the concepts inherent in the RVT. Pharmacists must embrace the economic, business, and marketing concepts necessary to define the nature of the work that they are expected to perform in professional practice. Many student pharmacists, pharmacy practitioners, and even leaders in our profession have underemphasized the importance of business and management knowledge in creating

value for health care stakeholders. Given the realities of a market-based economy, the transition from dispensing services to patient-care services, a tightened job market for pharmacists and changes resulting from health care reform, all pharmacists will need to sharpen these skills to remain competitive in the marketplace. In short, to get a rewarding job or continue to get paid a competitive salary, pharmacists will need to demonstrate that they can create value and provide benefit to an employer that are worth their salaries.

■ HEALTH CARE INDUSTRY STAKEHOLDERS

Evidence suggests that there are five distinct groups with an economic, clinical, or humanistic stake in the health care marketplace (see Figure 5-2). These groups each have different perspectives on their role in today's health care marketplace. Many pharmacists overlook the professional service opportunities that exist outside of direct patient care. Each stakeholder group has a unique role in the health care system, and entrepreneurial pharmacists can greatly expand the universe of potential market niches by designing professional services custom tailored to the targeted needs of a stakeholder tier (Figure 5-2).

First-Tier Stakeholders

First-tier stakeholders are patients, their extended families, and unpaid caregivers who provide custodial assistance for daily living activities, such as bathing, wound care, shopping, child care, and meal preparation. This tier's primary focus is on receiving quality care, improved health, and a better quality of life for the patient at an affordable price.

Second-Tier Stakeholders

Second-tier stakeholders are the professional caregivers trained in a medical specialty that permits them to legally diagnose and/or treat disease or provide wellness services. This group includes physicians, pharmacists, nurses, physician's assistants, nurse practitioners, licensed caregivers, dentists, podiatrists, physical therapists, osteopaths, and chiropractors that provide

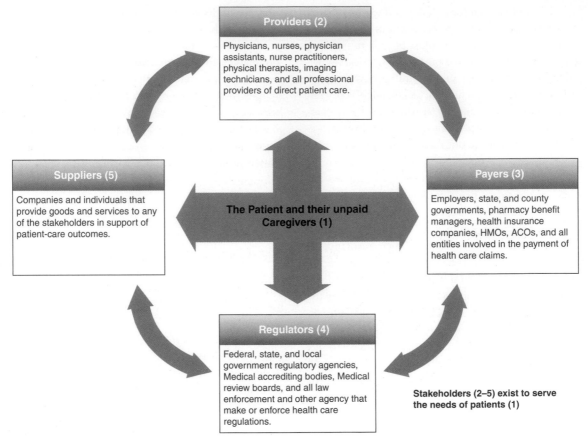

Figure 5-2. The health care industry stakeholders. (Used with permission from Dr. Greg Alston.)

direct patient care. These stakeholders seek value not only for their patients but also for their business operations. Because their professional practices treat or prevent patient illness, their interests are aligned with those of the primary stakeholders outlined above but expand to include additional factors such as the profitability of their professional practice and their compliance with industry standards.

Third-Tier Stakeholders

Third-tier stakeholders in the health care marketplace include employers, insurers, governmental agencies and programs, and taxpayers who, through the actions of their elected representatives, ultimately decide which bills get paid. The interests of these stakeholders

logically include all of the economic, clinical, and humanistic outcomes of the primary and secondary stakeholders, but from a different vantage point. Third-tier stakeholders typically focus less on individual patient treatment and more on managing the overall costs of providing care to a group of patients. This can create situations where a patient's therapeutic goals and the provider's clinical plans are not perfectly aligned with the payer's budget. Payers must be concerned with utilization rates, the cost-effectiveness of outcomes, fairness, and remaining solvent.

Fourth-Tier Stakeholders

Fourth-tier stakeholders include state, federal, and international agencies that regulate health care.

Regulators develop, write, revise, and enforce rules, regulations, and laws governing the practice of health care, the licensing of health care professionals, and the prosecution of criminal behavior. Fourth-tier stakeholders typically focus on preventing fraud, waste, and abuse more than improving the quality of health care outcomes for individual patients. Their role in the health care marketplace is characteristically to protect the public interest rather than optimizing individual patient care.

Fifth-Tier Stakeholders

Fifth-tier stakeholders are ancillary providers of goods and services to any of the other stakeholders. This tier includes drug wholesalers, drug and device manufacturers, office equipment suppliers, payroll services, raw materials suppliers, and numerous support services that add value to the supply chain. Not traditionally considered members of the health care team, these stakeholders can affect both the cost and productivity of health care providers' work. A thoughtful analysis of all elements that increase costs and decrease effectiveness must include all links in this value chain to produce the best result possible.

■ EXAMPLES OF PHARMACIST-CREATED VALUE

A large body of published research beginning nearly five decades ago reveals that patient-centered clinical services positively influences not only patient outcomes but also health care costs (Giberson et al., 2011; Perez et al., 2008; Schumock et al., 1996; Schumock et al., 2003; Touchette et al., 2014; Yap, 2015). These clinical services and their demonstrated economic value included a variety of practice sites representing health care systems, community pharmacies and clinics, health maintenance organizations, ambulatory care clinics or physician offices, long-term care, and home care. The clinical pharmacy services broadly ranged from general pharmacotherapeutic

or medication therapy management, disease state or drug-specific programs, and patient education.

Today, the value of pharmacists and pharmaceutical care continues to build on our history. For example, a recent Institute of Safe Medication Practices white paper noted that pharmacists are perhaps best suited to serve as institutional medication safety officers (ISMP, 2018). Regardless of provider status, pharmacists performing chronic care management involving non-face-to-face patient visits through contractual agreements with medical offices are receiving reimbursement for those services as a result of improving provider quality metrics. Pharmacists working within the Food and Drug Administration and other organizations protect patients and pharmacies ensuring supply chain security (i.e., prevent counterfeit or substandard drugs from entering the US Supply chain, see Chapter 27). Other colleagues work to ensure therapeutic alternatives are available to compensate for numerous drug shortages. Community pharmacists serve among the front line of defense to treat opioid use disorder, manage contraceptive care, provide immunizations and injectable medications (e.g., long-acting antipsychotics), and provide assistance/oversight of pharmacogenetic and point-of-care testing. Specialty pharmacists manage complete drug regimens for debilitating conditions, and clinical pharmacy specialists working as credentialed providers in the Veterans Administration continue to advance, expand, and demonstrate the value of pharmacists on patient-care teams (Groppi et al., 2018).

Given pharmacists' changing professional roles from a product-centric to a patient-care–centered profession, identifying a niche to provide value to any one or more of the five distinct health care industry stakeholders begins with one's imagination. However, not every idea produces a positive return on investment or a positive value to the same extent as another. Understanding how to evaluate the market for value-added services (see Chapter 29) and successfully implementing those services (see Chapter 30) is equally, if not more important, to determine what value-added services to pursue and provide.

■ REVISITING THE SCENARIO

After James Deaux processes what was just asked of him, he begins to think how he can create PV in the mind of Dr. Frank Stein. James wisely asks a series of follow-up questions to determine what Dr. Stein values in the position. This step is important in any attempt to conclude how to create PV in the "buyer's" mind. One must never assume what he or she believes to be of utmost importance, but rather, find what motivates the other party. It is not uncommon that several factors may increase PV. Whether in this scenario, or in trying to develop new revenue streams for your business, determining what positively influences the PV to your target audience, and subsequently fulfilling that value will aid you in your journey to distinguish yourself as a pharmacist.

■ CONCLUSION

The discussion of value is increasingly critical in the health care marketplace due to resource limitations, the complexities of medical practice, and health care reforms efforts as drivers of institutional change. Regardless of one's personal political philosophy, costs must be controlled, outcomes must be improved, and resources must be used wisely.

The RVT is a simplified model to guide pharmacists through the process of deciding what will be valuable to a stakeholder. An individual practitioner can use the RV theory to create value for his or her stakeholders and carve a successful niche in the American health care system.

Student pharmacists can apply the RVT to help them make decisions that will impact their careers. Students should consider the price or cost of a decision (P), the benefits they receive for making the decision (S), and if making this decision allows them to project the image they wish to project (PV)? There is no insurmountable barrier to success other than one's own desire to make a difference.

■ QUESTIONS FOR FURTHER DISCUSSION

1. What type of professional service could you develop that would create value for a first-tier stakeholder?
2. What type of professional service could you develop that would create value for a second-tier stakeholder?
3. What type of professional service could you develop that would create value for a third-tier stakeholder?
4. What type of professional service could you develop that would create value for a fourth-tier stakeholder?
5. How could you use the value creation theory to create a personal career plan for the first 3 years after graduation from pharmacy school?

REFERENCES

Alston GL, Blizzard JC. 2011. The value prescription: Relative value theorem as a call to action. *Res Soc Admin Pharm* 8:338–348.

Alston GL, Marsh W, Castleberry AN, Kelley KA, Boyce EG. 2018. Pharmacists opinions of the value of specific applicant attributes in hiring decisions for entry-level pharmacists. *Res Social Adm Pharm* pii: S1551–7411(18)30149–30149.

American Pharmacists Association (APhA). 2015. *More States Address Pharmacists' Provider Status Recognition.* Available at https://www.pharmacist.com/more-states-address-pharmacists-provider-status-recognition. Accessed August 31, 2015.

Bloemer J, de Ruyter K, Wetzels M. 1999. Linking perceived service quality and service loyalty: A multidimensional perspective. *Eur J Mark* 33:1082–1106.

Blumenthal D, Collins SR. 2014. Health care coverage under the Affordable Care Act—a progress report. *N Engl J Med* 371:275–281.

Bolton RN, Drew JH. 1991. A multistage model of customers' assessment of service quality and value. *J Consum Res* 17:375–384.

Caruana A, Money AH, Berthon PR. 2000. Service quality and satisfaction: The moderating role of value. *Eur J Mark* 34:1338–1352.

The case for medication safety officers (MSO). Horsham, PA: Institute for Safe Medication Practices; 2018.

Churchill GA, Surprenant C. 1982. An investigation into the determinants of customer satisfaction. *J Mark Res* 19:491–504.

Congressional Budget Office (CBO). 2018. *Budget Projections*. Available at https://www.cbo.gov/topics/budget/outlook-budget-and-economy. Accessed December 31, 2018.

Covvey JR, Cohron PP, Mullen AB. 2015. Examining pharmacy workforce issues in the United States and the United Kingdom. *Am J Pharm Edu* 79(2):17.

Cronin JJ, Brady MK, Hult GT. 2000. Assessing the effects of quality, value, and customer satisfaction on consumer behavioral intentions in service environments. *J Retail* 76:193–218.

Giberson S, Yoder S, Lee MP. Improving patient and health system outcomes through advanced pharmacy practice: A report to the US surgeon general. Office of the Chief Pharmacist. US Public Health Service. December 2011.

Groppi AM, Ourth H, Morreale AP, Hirsh JM, Wright S. 2018. Advancement of clinical pharmacy practice through intervention capture. *AJHP* 75:886–892.

Kaldy J. 2010. Medical home 101: The pharmacist's role in this growing patient-centered care model. *Consult Pharm* 25(8):468–474.

Lebovitz L, Eddington ND. 2019. Help wanted: Trends in the pharmacist workforce and pharmacy education. *Am J Pharm Educ* 83(1):7051.

Martini L. 2014. With no control on student numbers, tomorrow's pharmacists will have a bleak future. *Public Health* 16:46.

National Council on Patient Information and Education (NCPIE). 2007. Enhancing prescription medicine adherence: A national action plan. Available at http://www.talkaboutrx.org/documents/enhancing_prescription_medicine_adherence.pdf. Accessed October 3, 2011.

National Governors Association. 2015. States look to expand pharmacists' role in health care delivery. Available at http://www.nga.org/cms/home/news-room/news-releases/2015–news-releases/col2-content/states-look-to-expand-pharmacist.html. Accessed August 31, 2015.

Oliver RL. 1993. A conceptual model of service quality and service satisfaction: Compatible goals, different concepts. *Adv Serv Mark Manage* 2:65–85.

Pharmacist Demand Indicator. 2018. Pharmacy Demand Indicator. Available at https://pharmacymanpower.com/index.php. Accessed January 3, 2019.

Patient Protection and Affordable Care Act. 2010. Patient protection and affordable care act. Public Law 111–148.

Perez A, Doloresco F, Hoffman JM, et al. 2008. Economic evaluations of clinical pharmacy services: 2001-2005. *Pharmacotherapy* 28:285e–323e.

Reichheld FF. 1996. *The Loyalty Effect: The Hidden Force Behind Growth, Profits and Lasting Value*. Boston, MA: Harvard Business School Press.

Schumock GT, Meek PD, Ploetz PA, Vermeulen LC. 1996. Economic evaluations of clinical pharmacy services—1988-1995. *Pharmacotherapy* 16:1188–1208.

Schumock GT, Butler MG, Meek PD, Vermeulen LC, Arondekar BV, Bauman JL. 2003. Evidence of the economic benefit of clinical pharmacy services: 1996-2000. *Pharmacotherapy* 23:113–132.

Teas RK, Agarwal S. 2000. The effects of extrinsic product cues on consumers' perceptions of quality, sacrifice, and value. *J Acad Mark Sci* 28(2):278–290.

Touchette DR, Doloresco F, Suda KJ, et al. 2014. Economic evaluations of clinical pharmacy services: 2006-2010. *Pharmacotherapy* 34:771–793.

Venetis AK, Ghauri NP. 2004. Service quality and customer retention: Building long-term relationships. *Eur J Mark* 38(11–12):1577–1598.

Woodruff RB. 1997. Customer value: The next source for competitive advantage. *J Acad Mark Sci* 25:139–153.

Yap D. 2015. Data prove the point: Pharmacists provide value at Tripler in Hawaii. *Pharm Today* 21:50–53.

Zeithaml V. 1988. Consumer perception of price, quality and value: A means end model and synthesis of evidence. *J Mark* 52:2–22.

SECTION II

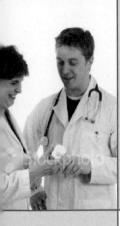

MANAGING OPERATIONS

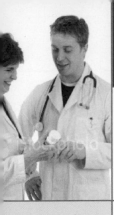

6

STRATEGIC PLANNING IN PHARMACY OPERATIONS

Andrew J. Donnelly and Glen T. Schumock

About the Authors: Dr. Donnelly is a graduate from the University of Illinois at the Medical Center (BPharm) and the University of Illinois at Chicago (MBA, PharmD). He is currently Director of Pharmacy Services at the University of Illinois Hospital & Health Sciences System and Clinical Professor and Associate Dean for Clinical Affairs at the University of Illinois at Chicago College of Pharmacy; where he is responsible for planning, organizing, and directing the activities of the pharmacy department. Dr. Donnelly's areas of interest include pharmacy administration as well as technology and automation as it relates to the medication use process. He lectures on strategic planning, leadership, and reimbursement issues in the College and has presented internationally on topics related to pharmacy administration and innovative pharmacy services. Dr. Donnelly is a Fellow of the American Society of Health-System Pharmacists (ASHP).

Dr. Schumock is a graduate from Washington State University (BPharm), the University of Washington (PharmD), and the University of Illinois at Chicago (MBA, PhD). He also completed a residency and a research fellowship. Currently, Dr. Schumock is Professor and Dean of the College of Pharmacy at the University of Illinois at Chicago. He has taught courses in pharmacy management, pharmacoeconomics, and business planning for pharmacy services. He has published over 200 articles, book chapters, and books; and is on the editorial boards of the journals *Pharmacotherapy* and *PharmacoEconomics* and is Associate Editor of the *Journal of Comparative Effectiveness Research*. Dr. Schumock is a Fellow of the American College of Clinical Pharmacy.

■ LEARNING OBJECTIVES

After completing this chapter, readers should be able to

1. Provide an overview of planning activities conducted by pharmacy and health care organizations.
2. Describe the general process common to all types of planning.

3. Describe the purpose of strategic planning and illustrate the specific steps to develop a strategic plan.
4. Differentiate a vision statement from a mission statement.
5. Highlight examples of strategic planning in pharmacy organizations.
6. Identify barriers and limitations to planning.
7. Identify and describe the different people involved in the strategic planning process, and what roles/functions they play.

■ SCENARIO

Ted Thompson graduated from pharmacy school magna cum laude 2 years ago with a Doctor of Pharmacy degree and successfully passed the licensing examination, making him a registered pharmacist. After graduation, Ted completed a pharmacy practice residency at a prestigious teaching hospital with a reputation for having an excellent pharmacy department and advanced clinical pharmacist services. Following his residency, Ted took a job as a clinical pharmacist in a community hospital in his hometown. In hiring Ted, the hospital pharmacy department fulfilled an interim objective toward its goal of advancing its pharmacy practice model in alignment with the ASHP Practice Alignment Initiative (PAI), formerly known as the Pharmacy Practice Model Initiative (ASHP, 2011).

The hospital is located in a town of approximately 100,000 people, and a large portion of the population is older adults. Partly because of both the favorable payer mix (mostly Medicare) and the fiscal savvy of the Chief Financial Officer (CFO),[1] the hospital has done very well from clinical and economic perspectives. The pharmacy department has a good drug distribution system and a Director of Pharmacy

(DOP) who, while not trained clinically, understands the value of these services.

The hospital is growing rapidly and, as such, has become increasingly reliant on pharmacy services. Because of the many opportunities that confront the pharmacy department, the DOP has decided that the department should develop a plan to guide its priorities over the next 3 to 5 years. To accomplish this, the DOP has determined that over the next several months, the department will undergo a strategic planning effort. This effort will begin with a selected group of individuals from within the department, each representing key functions and constituencies. Ted was asked to be part of this group because of his expertise related to clinical pharmacist services provided by the department and the increasing importance such services will have on patient outcomes and the financial performance of the hospital. As such, these services will be part of this strategic plan.

Having no real management training or experience, Ted recognized the need to learn more about the purpose of strategic planning and the process that will be required to develop the departmental strategic plan.

■ CHAPTER QUESTIONS

1. What are the different activities that pharmacies and health care organizations engage in when they plan for the future?
2. What is the purpose of strategic planning and how is it different from other types of planning?

---

[1]In a business or organization, the CFO is the individual who is responsible for the financial decisions and investments made by the company. In a hospital or health system, the CFO is likely to have several departments and functions reporting to him or her, including general accounting, accounts receivable and accounts payable, payroll, budgeting, procurement, and finance.

3. What are the steps typically taken by a pharmacy organization when developing a strategic plan?

4. What is a vision statement and for whom is it written?

5. What is a mission statement and for whom is it written?

6. What are the barriers or limitations associated with planning that should be kept in mind while undertaking this process?

7. Who are the people involved in the planning process and what roles/functions do they play?

■ INTRODUCTION

The scenario illustrates an important activity within pharmacies and health care organizations that is rarely considered by new pharmacists. In this scenario, Ted is asked to participate in the development of a strategic plan. Strategic planning is one of the most common types of planning that is conducted by health care organizations. However, strategic planning is not unique to pharmacies or health care organizations; in fact, it represents a core management activity that is employed by all businesses.

This chapter begins with a general discussion of management planning by pharmacy organizations. Pharmacies and health care organizations, like many businesses, are involved in or should be involved in, many different types of planning for different purposes within the organization. This chapter provides an understanding of where the responsibility for planning lies within organizations and the general structure or process involved in planning efforts. These general concepts are applicable to all types of planning in all different types of organizations, including pharmacies.

Next, this chapter discusses one specific type of planning—strategic planning. The intent of this discussion is to provide a general understanding of the role of strategic planning and to identify its key steps or components. While the material in this chapter is applicable to almost any type of organization, examples pertinent to the profession of pharmacy or pharmacy practice within health care organizations are provided. For readers interested in a more complete understanding of planning, there are many options for obtaining information beyond what is presented here. There are literally hundreds of textbooks addressing both general and specific topics within this field. Several good texts are included in the reference list at the end of this chapter (Allison & Kaye, 2015; Grünig & Kühn, 2011; Haines & McKinlay, 2011; Harrison, 2010; May, 2010; Nolan et al., 2008; Zuckerman, 2012).

■ PLANNING IN GENERAL

In the broadest sense, *planning* represents the purposeful efforts taken by an organization (for our purposes, a pharmacy organization) to maximize its future success. Planning, as it is referred to here, is sometimes called *management planning* because it is typically part of the duties of managers. Planning has been described as one of the four key functions of managers (along with organizing, leading, and controlling). In fact, of the four functions, planning is crucial because it supports the other three (Stoner et al., 2007). However, planning may involve more than just managers at high levels; in fact, in smaller companies or in companies with fewer levels of management, frontline employees are often involved in planning.

Many different types of planning activities occur within pharmacy organizations. The most common types include business planning, financial planning, operational planning, organizational planning, resource planning, emergency planning, and strategic planning. The purpose of each type of planning is different. It is not the intent of this chapter to cover all these types of planning. Instead, a brief description of the purpose and characteristics of each is outlined in Table 6-1. Some of these types of planning activities have subtypes within them. For example, one type of resource planning deals specifically with human resources (Bechet, 2008; Ward et al., 2013; Young, 2009). Another type of resource planning that has gained increasing importance is information

Table 6-1. Types of Planning

Type	Purpose	Characteristics
Strategic planning	To ensure that the organization is doing the right things. Addresses what business the organization is in, or ought to be in, provides a framework for more detailed planning and day-to-day decisions.	Long term (5–20 years); scope includes all aspects of the organization; viewpoint is external—how the organization interacts with or controls its environment.
Operational planning	To ensure that the organization is prepared, performs the immediate tasks and objectives to meet the goals and strategy of the organization. To ensure that the organization is doing things right.	Short term (1–5 years); scope is specific to the immediate actions that need to be taken to move the organization forward; viewpoint is internal—day-to-day accomplishment of tasks.
Business planning	To determine the feasibility of a specific business or program. Business planning is used to make a decision about investing in and moving forward with a program.	Short term (1–5 years); can be used to make decisions to start a new business, expand a business, or terminate a business.
Resource planning	To ensure the resources necessary to achieve the goals and strategy of the organization. Resource planning can be comprehensive (all resources needed to achieve goals and strategic plan of the organization) or can focus on a specific type of resource.	Midterm (1–10 years); scope is specific to the resource or resources defined in the plan—specific resources may include human resources, information/technology resources, financial resources, capital and facilities, and others; viewpoint is internal—the resource needs of the organization.
Organizational planning	To ensure that an organization is organized appropriately to meet the challenges of the future. Key elements include reporting relationships, definition of responsibilities, and definition of authorities.	Midterm (1–10 years); scope specific to the structural aspects of the organization, including divisions, reporting relationships, coordination, control; viewpoint is internal—how the company organizes itself.
Contingency planning	To provide a fallback option or direction should the original strategy of the organization fail or something unexpected occur. Contingency planning can occur for a specific anticipated situation, the most common of which are business-related crises (such as a labor strike) and changes in management personnel.	Short- to long term (1–20 years); scope is specific to the particular situation that may occur; viewpoint is both external (if the situation is created in the environment) and internal.
Emergency planning	To address emergencies that may be expected in the workplace. These can include fires, tornadoes, floods, and "active shooter" situations. Plans should be in place that describes what staff at the workplace should do in emergency situations.	Midterm (1–10 years); scope specific to the particular situation that may occur; viewpoint is both external and internal.

technology planning. This type of planning focuses specifically on the present and future information needs of an organization and the technologies and systems to meet those needs (Cassidy, 2006; Chew & Gottschalk, 2009).

Because of the importance of effective planning, many organizations invest significant time and resources in these efforts. Ultimately, the Chief Executive Officer (CEO) or President of a company is responsible for making certain that the organization is successful—ensuring that success largely depends on planning that occurs within the organization.[2] However, in large companies, given the scope of planning activities that must take place, much of the work involved in planning is delegated to a special department dedicated entirely to planning. Often, outside consultants are employed to assist organizations in their planning efforts.

The actual process of planning may vary by the type of planning being conducted and by the size of the organization or system. Here, the term *system* refers to the entity for which planning is being conducted. That entity may be the entire pharmacy organization or a program or function within it. Programs can be considered subunits or specific services within an organization. An example of a program within a pharmacy organization would be a clinical pharmacist service program, such as what Ted is responsible for in our scenario. A *function* is an activity that cuts across different subunits of an organization. An example of a function within a pharmacy organization would be the function of information management.

Regardless of the system for which planning is being conducted, planning varies in terms of sophistication. In some cases, planning can be relatively simple and straightforward. In other cases, it may involve extensive analyses of data with complicated forecasting, decision-making models, and algorithms. Nevertheless, all planning processes share a few basic

Table 6-2.	Steps in the Planning Process

1. Define or orient the planning process to a singular purpose or a desired result (vision/mission).
2. Assess the current situation.
3. Establish goals.
4. Identify strategies to reach those goals.
5. Establish objectives that support progress toward those goals.
6. Define responsibilities and timelines for each objective.
7. Write and communicate the plan.
8. Monitor progress toward meeting goals and objectives.

characteristics. Specifically, the eight steps shown in Table 6-2 define the general process that is followed in most planning efforts. These general steps in some cases may be expanded or condensed depending on the situation or presented in a slightly different fashion. Nevertheless, the key components of understanding the purpose, assessing the situation, establishing goals, and devising a method to accomplish those goals should be common to all planning activities.

As shown in the table, the planning process should begin with consideration of the purpose of the organization or system and of the planning effort, itself. This is followed by an analysis of the present situation or status of the system. Next, specific future goals are determined, and then a strategy for bridging the gap between the present and future is developed. Interim objectives that measure progress toward the goals are then identified, and responsibilities and timelines for each objective are assigned. The plan then needs to be communicated, implemented, and monitored.

■ STRATEGIC PLANNING

The purpose of strategic planning is to ensure that the organization is doing the right things now and in the future. Strategic planning addresses what business

---

[2]The CEO is the top executive and the key decision maker of an organization, reporting only to the Board of Directors. The CEO, together with the Board of Directors, is responsible for the overall success of the organization.

the organization is in or ought to be in and helps to determine long-term goals for the organization. For example, what is the business of a particular community pharmacy? Does the pharmacy want to be in the "prescription business" or the "health care business"? Does a health system want to be in the "hospital business" or a "business that provides a continuum of care"? Obviously, how pharmacy leadership answers these questions, no matter the setting, provides a framework for more detailed planning and day-to-day decisions.

Strategic planning has been defined as the process of selecting an organization's goals, determining the policies and programs (strategies) necessary to achieve specific objectives in route to those goals, and establishing methods necessary to ensure that the policies and strategic programs are implemented (Martin, 2019). More broadly, strategic planning can be considered as an effort that enables the optimal deployment of all organizational resources within current and future environmental constraints. The result of this optimization is to increase the likelihood that the organization will survive, and preferably thrive, in the future.

Before further discussion on strategic planning, the differences between strategic and *business planning* should be noted. These are the two most common types of planning, and while they are very different, people often confuse the two. Table 6-1 helps to clarify the differences, the most important being their purpose. While strategic planning is about achieving a long-term vision and making sure the organization is doing the things necessary to ensure overall success, business planning focuses on the feasibility of a specific program (usually a new initiative). Business planning, like all the other types of planning listed in Table 6-1, must occur within the context of the strategic plan of the organization. As such, the strategic plan can be viewed as the overarching effort that should guide all other types of planning and even the day-to-day activities of the organization.

In evaluating the performance of a company, it is often informative to look at its strategy historically over time. While many factors can influence organizational performance, companies that engage in long-range strategic planning are often more successful than those that do not. Again, this is true for pharmacy organizations as well as other types of businesses. Strategic planning can be either reactive or proactive. Reactive strategic planning is not the ideal, but it is often necessary, especially in industries that are changing rapidly (such as health care). Preferably, proactive strategic planning enables an organization to control its environment instead of vice versa.

Beyond proactive planning, organizations that are able to think and plan in an "out of the box" manner may position themselves not only to control the business environment but also to actually create or recreate the business environment. This type of strategic thinking has been considered the pinnacle of planning efforts by organizations—ideal for companies to position themselves to be most competitive. Using strategy to create an environment that puts the company at an advantage compared with its competitors is integral to this effort (Porter, 2008). An example outside the health care industry is Apple, Inc., and its evolution of electronic products and services that respond to customer needs and reshape the digital environment, from the iMac and MacBook, to the iPhone and iPad, to the Apple Watch and now the iCloud. Other examples include the social networking and sharing services, Facebook, Twitter, and Instagram. These businesses have developed new markets and customer interactions via the Internet that did not exist previously.

The time horizon of strategic planning helps to distinguish it from other types of planning. Strategic planning has also been called *long-term planning*. The actual timeline used by organizations may vary or in some cases may not be known. Because the future is unknown, it is often difficult to predict with any accuracy the amount of time it will take for an organization to reach its long-term goals. Nevertheless, a key component of strategic planning is to identify time periods within which goals are to be reached.

The time horizon for strategic planning may be as long as 10 to 20 years or as short as 2 years. In a survey conducted by the Net Future Institute, managers were asked what time period they considered to be long term (Martin, 2002). The most common response was 2 years (40.2%), followed by 5 years (32.7%), and 1 year (17.9%). Admittedly, many of the companies involved in this survey were in high-tech industries, where rapid change may impair longer term planning. However, health care is also an industry of rapid change, and thus planning must be done similarly to that in other fast-growing industries.

The problem with strategic planning, even in 5-year time period, is that it is not likely to result in any truly sustainable competitive advantages or a significant organizational metamorphosis. Further, because strategic goals are based on the company's vision for the future, goals that incorporate new paradoxes or visionary changes may be difficult for employees to believe if the time period for accomplishing those goals is too short. Nevertheless, these are the types of goals that should be created in strategic planning, so it is the time period that must be congruent with these goals, not vice versa. The worst mistake would be to "dumb down" the goals to make them consistent with a shorter time period.

Vision and Mission

An important part of the process of strategic planning is to create momentum and to motivate personnel within the pharmacy organization. Strategic planning has a lot to do with defining what a company is all about and creating a "story" about the organization. The communication of the organization's story occurs across a number of different statements that may be products of strategic planning. Most essential of these statements are the vision and the mission.

The *vision* is what the pharmacy organization wants to be at some future time point. The vision may be complex and multidimensional, while at the same time it must be concise. The *vision statement* should make people think and motivate them, especially employees, to create a different and better future for the organization. For example, the vision of Walgreens Boots Alliance is "Be the first choice for pharmacy, wellbeing and beauty—caring for people and communities around the world"

(see http://www.walgreensbootsalliance.com/about/vision-purpose-values/). This vision sets a clear goal that serves to inspire the organization and its employees.

The vision of the organization is used in the strategic planning process as both the beginning point and the end point. That is, once the vision is set, then strategic planning is about how to reach that end point. The vision is also used to define the mission of the organization. For example, the vision statement of Cleveland Clinic in Cleveland, OH, is to ". . . be the world's leader in patient experience, clinical outcomes, research and education" (see http://my.clevelandclinic.org/about-cleveland-clinic/overview/who-we-are/mission-vision-values). This vision drives both the mission of the organization and its values, and presumably, these together guide the daily business decisions made by Cleveland Clinic.

The *mission* is the purpose of the company. The *mission statement* defines what the company does or is. It is a statement of the present going ahead into the near future. It is a document written to create a sense of purpose for customers and employees. The mission statement should be short—usually no more than two sentences. It focuses on the common purpose of the organization and may draw from the values or beliefs held by the organization. The mission statement should help to differentiate the company from others that provide the same products or services. Some organizations include in the mission statement not only what the company does but also how it does it—essentially the differentiating point. The Cleveland Clinic's mission statement is "to provide better care of the sick, investigation into their problems, and further education of those who serve" (see http://my.clevelandclinic.org/about-cleveland-clinic/overview/who-we-are/mission-vision-values).

The following elements have been suggested in developing a mission statement for a community pharmacy: the intended (or target) customers, the core values of the pharmacy (such as compassion, respect, and confidentiality), the key services and products provided by the pharmacy, the benefits incurred by customers (such as improved health and improved safety), and the desired public image of the pharmacy (Hagel, 2002). All pharmacy organizations should have a mission statement.

CVS Caremark is the largest dispenser of prescription drugs with greater than 9,600 pharmacies, as well as the biggest operator of health care clinics in the United States. The organization provides a good example of a mission statement that focuses on the customer's experience—"Above all else . . . our mission is to improve the lives of those we serve by making innovative and high-quality health and pharmacy services safe, affordable and easy to access" (see http://www.makingafortune.biz/list-of-companies-c/cvs-caremark.htm). As noted earlier, the mission statement creates a sense of purpose for both the employees and customers of the organization. Employees of CVS Caremark know that their customers are a first priority and that the varieties of services they provide are intended to improve the overall health of their customers. Later in this chapter, we discuss how pharmacies such as CVS that have well-defined missions and that engage in strategic planning are more likely to be successful.

In addition to the mission statement, some businesses use a *company slogan* to convey a message to customers about the organization. The company slogan generally is more marketing driven than is the mission statement, but in some cases the company slogan serves a similar role. Like the mission statement, the company slogan sends a message to both customers and employees, and it must be congruent with the actions of the organization or else it will not be credible. A great example of a company slogan is that of the Nike Company. The slogan "Just Do It!" has energy and a sense of action. It is easy to see how the slogan and the company's mission, "To bring inspiration and innovation to every athlete in the world," combine to create a powerful image of what this company is all about (http://about.nike.com/). Other memorable slogans are "I'm Loving It" of McDonalds, "Finger Lickin' Good" of Kentucky Fried Chicken, and "Fly the Friendly Skies" of United Airlines. Again, these slogans are brief yet convey meaningful messages.

The vision, mission, and other statements that form the company story are critical elements in strategic planning. If these elements already exist in the organization, then the process of strategic planning starts with these as its foundation or modifies them as necessary. If these elements do not already exist, then the process of strategic planning must include their conception. What do you think the vision and mission for the hospital pharmacy department in our scenario should be?

Process of Strategic Planning

Structuring, facilitating, and implementing the process of strategic planning is an important consideration for any organization (Fogg, 2010). The process of strategic planning does not vary significantly from the process used in other types of planning. This chapter highlights only the aspects of the steps shown in Table 6-2 that are distinctive to strategic planning compared with other types of planning efforts.

Preplanning Phase

Preplanning can be defined as the steps necessary to organize the strategic planning effort—or "planning for the planning." Strategic planning is a significant undertaking that consumes much time and energy. A pharmacy organization choosing to engage in a strategic planning effort should not take this lightly. Strategic planning is a financial investment—in the personnel time required and in the payment of consultants, if used. These costs should be weighed against the value to be gained by the effort. If strategic planning is performed correctly, its value will greatly exceed any costs. On the other hand, if strategic planning is done in a superficial or hurried manner, its costs will exceed its benefits. Preplanning should include a careful assessment of this balance.

Preplanning should define the objectives of the planning efforts and the procedures that will be used to accomplish those objectives. Preplanning will define who should be involved, where the planning process will occur, and how much time will be allotted to the effort. Preplanning should also consider any political purposes and ramifications of the undertaking. In laying out the scope of the planning effort, preplanning should orient the activity to the vision of the organization, if one exists.

Among the preplanning activities, determining who should be involved in strategic planning is most important. The type of organization and level of the strategic planning effort will dictate who should be involved. For example, if the plan is at the highest level within a large corporation then planning must start at the Board of Directors. Conversely if a plan is designed for a department within an organization, such as is the case in our scenario, then participation may be limited to the department leaders and managers, key staff, and perhaps important stakeholders.

For example, the strategic plan for the hospital pharmacy department in our scenario will need to include the DOP. He or she would also want to be sure to communicate with the senior leadership of the hospital so that the planning process includes consideration of issues pertinent to the hospital-wide vision and strategic goals. Participation in the planning effort should include key managers and staff within the pharmacy department who will be involved in day-to-day implementation of the proposed plan, including Ted because he is responsible for a major component of the pharmacy's clinical services. Other important stakeholders might also be involved. These might include influential medical staff, managers from other departments (such as nursing), and perhaps individuals from the finance department, human resources, and/or marketing. For most strategic planning of any significant scale or impact, some outside consultant or advisor will be brought in to provide an external perspective and to ensure that the process is complete and objective. This may or may not be necessary for departmental planning.

Planning Phase

In the *planning phase* of strategic planning, ideas are actively generated for the pharmacy organization. This may be referred to as *strategizing*. As in any planning process, it is usually best to start with the destination in mind, such as viewing a map while planning a trip. Once the destination is clear, one must find the starting place on the map. The next step is to determine the different routes or options to get from here to there. Among the different routes, one should select the one that best meets the needs within the constraints of limited resources. If speed is important, then one selects the quickest route. If scenery is important, then one selects the most scenic route. Besides the route, the mode of transportation needs to be determined. Options might include taking a train, driving a car, or flying in an airplane (or a combination of any of these). Once the route and method of transportation are known, one selects key milestones, or places to stop, along the way. Knowing these intermediate points helps to keep the journey on track. The process of strategic planning is very similar. Moreover, just like going on a trip, the decisions should be a group effort of everyone involved (i.e., those engaged in strategic planning are involved at all levels of the organization).

In strategic planning, the "destination" is the vision of the organization in the future. It is also necessary, though, to identify where, what, and how the organization is in the present. This is called *situation analysis*, and it should consider both the past performance and the current situation. This is the starting point of the journey. Based on the vision (destination), along with the present situation (starting point), planners should next identify the goals for the organization. These goals could be considered synonymous with the things considered important in the map example, such as speed and scenic beauty.

For example, goals developed by the pharmacy department at Brigham and Women's Hospital in Boston for their fiscal year 2018 strategic plan included to (1) evaluate and restructure the department's organization, workflow, and clinical duties to enhance employee productivity while supporting safe and optimal clinical care to patients and (2) understand and communicate important departmental quality metrics to support patient care and improve overall efficiency (see https://www.brighamandwomens.org/assets/bwh/patients-and-families/pharmacy/pdfs/pharmacy-services-annual-report.pdf). Similarly, the pharmacy department at Ohio State University

Wexner Medical Center in their 2017–2024 strategic plan developed goals which included to (1) create innovative health care delivery models that deliver high-value care with unparalleled patient experience and access and (2) be a responsible steward of all resources (see https://wexnermedical.osu.edu/about-us/strategic-plan). Finally, in the most recent strategic plan for the pharmacy department at the University of Illinois Hospital, goals included (1) ensuring that the practice model is relevant, efficient, innovative, and sustainable in an ever-changing health care environment and (2) improving pharmacy technician recruitment, retention, and professional development.

Once the goals are identified, the course is plotted to get from the present to the future. For this, it is crucial to identify and select preferred strategies that will accomplish the goals. Strategies are synonymous with the routes and the modes and costs of transportation in the travel example. Last, one should determine SMART objectives (Table 6-3) (see https://simplified-strategicplanning.com/what-is-a-smart-objective/) that will help to reach the goals. Objectives are like

Table 6-3.   SMART Objectives

S – Specific
  • State exactly what is to be achieved.
M – Measurable
  • Capable of measurement; can determine if it is achieved.
A – Aggressive but Attainable
  • Should challenge but should not demand the impossible.
R – Results-oriented
  • Should specify a result, not just an activity.
T – Time-bound
  • Specify a time frame for meeting objectives; deadlines need to be realistic.

the intermediate points, or places to pass through on the map. These objectives provide a short-term milestone and, in implementation, help to measure progress toward the goal.

The relationship between vision, goals, strategy, and objectives is shown graphically in Figure 6-1.

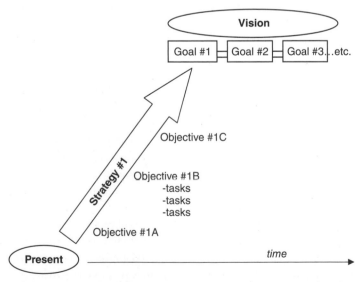

Figure 6-1. Relationship between vision, goals, objectives, strategy, and mission. To reach a certain vision, or future state, the organization must set and reach one or more goals. Each goal is associated with a specific strategy or method of reaching that goal. The strategy can be defined by the objectives that are necessary intermediate accomplishments toward the goal. A set of tasks, or actions, may be associated with each objective. Collectively, these tasks are also called *tactics* that the organization employs to meet an objective.

Considering the preceding overview, the steps in the planning process can be examined more closely. After crafting a vision statement, Ted and others in our scenario must analyze and define the current situation. As is the case with any system, history helps to define the present. Therefore, part of the situation analysis is to evaluate the past performance of the organization. This evaluation should include all measures of performance, including customer satisfaction and financial indicators.

The situation analysis also should define the present. A common method for conducting the situation analysis is to evaluate the internal strengths and weakness of the organization and the external opportunities and threats to the organization. This is known as a *SWOT (strengths, weaknesses, opportunities, threats) analysis.* Strengths and opportunities are generally considered to be positive attributes of the company/program or characteristics of the environment that may bode well for the success of the business. Weaknesses and threats are negative attributes or characteristics, as shown in Figure 6-2.

Categories of internal strengths and weaknesses to consider when conducting a SWOT analysis may include profitability, quality of pharmacy service, customer service, competence and ability of pharmacy staff, and the efficiency of the pharmacy operations. Categories of external opportunities and threats to consider may include the extent of competition from other pharmacy organizations, the availability of technology, regulations that may help or hinder the business, the availability of reimbursement for services provided (i.e., clinical pharmacist services), costs incurred by the pharmacy organization, political issues having an impact on health delivery, and changes in the market and types of customers served by the organization. A more detailed example of a SWOT analysis for a pharmacy program is provided in Chapter 7.

By comparing the results of the situation analysis with the desired future state (vision), the extent and nature of the gap between the two begins to become clear. The next steps in the planning phase attempt to bridge that gap. First, strategic planning serves to define goals for the organization that are consistent with the vision. These goals should capitalize on the organization's strengths and opportunities while minimizing the threats and mitigating the weaknesses.

The last part of the planning process deals with organizing to *operationalize* the strategy. Because the goals and vision are a desired future state that may be unachievable in the short term, intermediate objectives are needed to help advance toward that target. In the planning process, the objectives pertinent to each goal are identified and usually accomplishable in the short term (1 year), whereas goals are in the longer term (3 to 5 years). Because objectives are short term, a budget, schedule, and responsibility can be assigned to each.

There is no common or standard way to organize the written strategic plan. However, most contain the following key elements: (1) the organization's vision and mission, (2) strategies, (3) goals for each strategy, (4) objectives required to meet those goals, and (5) tasks or action plans to complete the objectives. Examples of strategic plans for pharmacy organizations can be found in the references listed at the end of this chapter, and Table 6-4 provides an example of a strategic plan for Ted Thompson's pharmacist services scenario at the beginning of this chapter. Note that the tasks listed should also include a planned date for completion of the task and a party responsible for each task.

	Positive	Negative
Internal	S	W
External	O	T

Figure 6-2. Conceptual diagram of the elements of a SWOT analysis. Strengths, weakness, opportunities, and threats are the elements that comprise a SWOT analysis. These elements can be characterized with respect to both their place in the environment, for example, either internal or external to organization, and based on their desirability, for example, either positive or negative from that standpoint of the organization. These relationships are shown here.

Postplanning Phase

Once the major pieces of the planning phase have been developed, the *postplanning phase* begins. This phase includes three vitally important steps:

Table 6-4.   Example Strategic Plan

Mission: To improve patient lives by providing comprehensive, contemporary clinical pharmacist services, utilizing a well-trained work staff of pharmacists and technicians, and taking advantage of technology and automation to ensure an efficient and safe medication distribution system.

Vision (future): To become the preeminent pharmacy in the system by providing the highest quality of patient-focused pharmacist services, helping to optimize outcomes while being fiscally responsible.

Strategy: The department will align its services to be consistent with the hospital's initiative to become part of a multihospital system.

Goal: Develop and implement specific clinical pharmacist services that help to deliver care, improve patient outcomes, reduce spending, and/or generate revenue.

Objectives:
- By the beginning of the next fiscal year, identify three gaps in care delivery, quality, and/or spending where pharmacist services can lead to a reduction in medication cost per discharge, a reduction in length of stay, and/or a reduction in sepsis mortality.
- By the end of the current quarter, select one clinical pharmacist service to implement that will lead to a reduction in medication cost per discharge.

Tasks/action plans:
- Perform a situation analysis of the hospital, and pharmacy department, including a SWOT analysis.
- Prepare a list of clinical pharmacist services that can be developed and implemented to meet the needs of the organization, and compare the services on the basis of feasibility and impact.
- Select the most appropriate service and develop a business plan for the service.

(1) communicating the plan, (2) implementing the plan, and (3) monitoring progress and assessing results once the plan is implemented.

While strategic planning is a process, the strategic plan is a document that communicates the plan. The strategic plan should be written such that it communicates all aspects of the plan effectively.

The actual implementation of the strategic plan requires managers and executives of the pharmacy organization to understand the long-range goals while at the same time determining and taking the steps necessary to accomplish the shorter-range objectives. The process of mapping out the actions necessary to accomplish short-term objectives is called *operational planning*, which focuses on determining the day-to-day activities that are necessary to achieve the long-term goals of the organization. One can differentiate strategic planning from operational planning by viewing the primary focus of each. Strategic planning focuses on doing the right thing (effectiveness), whereas operational planning focuses on doing things right (efficiency). In other words, strategic planning defines what to do and operational planning defines how to do it.

The operational plan is an outline of the tactical activities or tasks that must occur to support and implement the strategic plan—sometimes called *tactics*. The relationship between tasks or tactics (operational planning) and the key elements of strategic planning is shown in Figure 6-1. Managers in an organization focus their day-to-day work on tactics. Their perspective tends to relate to the short term. Yet it is important that, on a periodic basis, an attempt be made to step back from day-to-day activities and reorient oneself to the bigger picture (the vision, goals, and strategy of the organization). For example, a pharmacy manager may receive a request from a physician or a nurse to have the department begin to provide a new service in a hospital. Before agreeing to do so, it is important that the manager considers how this new service fits into the vision and goals of the pharmacy department.

Another key element of the postplanning phase is *monitoring*. A plan for monitoring should be created. This monitoring should evaluate the extent of implementation in comparison with the planned schedule and the effectiveness of the organization in meeting its goals, especially in the deployment of limited resources, both human and financial. In other words, have both the plan and its implementation been effective? Intrinsic to this monitoring process is the possibility that changes to the plan may be necessitated by changes in the environment or by changes in the organization. As such, the strategic plan should be considered a fluid document.

■ STRATEGIC PLANNING EXAMPLES IN PHARMACY ORGANIZATIONS

There is a variety of literature related to strategic planning in pharmacy, including some in both the community and hospital pharmacy environments (Sanborn et al., 2009; Vermeulen et al., 2019; Weber et al., 2015; Westerling et al., 2010). However, it should be noted that for chain drug stores, independent pharmacies, or other for-profit pharmacy organizations, it may be counterproductive to publish the company strategy and objectives. Rather, these plans are frequently guarded fiercely so that they do not fall into the hands of competitors. Below we highlight some of these.

A series of studies on strategic planning in community pharmacies has been published by Harrison (2005), Harrison (2006), and Harrison & Ortmeier (1996). For community pharmacies that conduct strategic planning, an average of 5.9 (of 7) different steps in the strategic planning process were used (Table 6-5). The authors also reported that community pharmacies that conducted strategic planning had significantly higher organizational performance based on self-rated performance on clinical services, dispensing services, and financial performance—suggesting that strategic planning can improve

Table 6-5.   Steps Used in the Strategic Planning Process by Community Pharmacies

Step	Percentage[a]
Develop mission statement	76.9
Identify strengths and weaknesses	94.2
Identify threats and opportunities	90.2
Formulate and select strategies	83.8
Review pharmacy structure and systems	60.1
Implement strategies	86.1
Evaluate implemented strategies	76.3

Adapted from Harrison DL, Ortmeier BG: Strategic planning in the community pharmacy. *J Am Pharm Assoc* 1996;NS36(9):583–588.
[a]*N* = 173 community pharmacies that reported use of strategic planning; values represent the percentage that incorporate each specific step of the strategic planning process.

organization success. Also, as might be expected, owners and managers of independent community pharmacies who participated in a formal strategic planning education program were more likely to conduct strategic planning, and had greater comprehension of strategic planning concepts, when compared to those who did not participate (Harrison, 2007).

There is also literature on the subject of strategic planning in the hospital pharmacy environment. A survey was conducted by the University HealthSystem Consortium and found that strategic planning occurs routinely in pharmacies associated with academic medical centers. In fact, 88.6% of the pharmacy directors who completed the survey reported that their departments had a strategic plan (University HealthSystem Consortium, 2011). Further, these plans most commonly encompassed a timeframe of 3 to 5 years.

A study of pharmacy directors at hospitals in the United States was conducted to determine if more sophisticated planning resulted in improved departmental outcomes (Birdwell & Pathak, 1989). Pharmacy departments were categorized into levels of strategic planning sophistication based on different steps that were employed in the planning process. In departments with high levels of planning, outcomes such as satisfaction by hospital administrators, professional image among hospital administrators, number of clinical pharmacy programs, and the quality of clinical pharmacy programs were rated higher by pharmacy directors than in departments with lower levels of sophistication in planning. Although the study is somewhat dated, it is expected that similar results would be seen today if it was repeated. In other industries, strategic planning has also been shown to improve company performance and has yielded positive results (Hodges & Kent, 2006).

In another study examining the impact of strategic planning for a hospital-based clinical pharmacy section, more than 70% of the targeted objectives were achieved or exceeded. The number of clinical pharmacists doubled from 6 to 12 as did the number of board-certified clinical pharmacists (4 to 8). Research within the clinical pharmacist group increased substantially in addition to lectures to the medical staff. Further, they were able to make inroads with respect to clinical pharmacy services in the ambulatory setting (Abulezz et al., 2018).

Strategic planning in pharmacy is particularly important when there are changes that occur in the practice environment. The Medicare Modernization Act (MMA) of 2003 is a good example of such a change. This legislation, which went into effect in 2006, created the Medicare prescription drug benefit (also known as Medicare Part D) and established the requirement that medication therapy management (MTM) be provided to high-risk Medicare beneficiaries (see Chapter 28). Successful pharmacy organizations used strategic planning to predict the impact of the MMA and to develop practice plans for provision of MTM (Lewin Group, 2005).

Another example of a more recent change in the pharmacy practice environment is the increased emphasis on drug diversion, which is partially a result of the opioid crisis. By monitoring the literature, successful hospital pharmacy departments were able to be proactive in predicting the need for an institutional drug diversion programs. These departments then

strategically developed and implemented plans to ensure that there were sufficient resources and technology to support such programs (O'Neal & Siegel, 2007).

A third example of change in the pharmacy practice environment that has required strategic planning is the rapid uptake in use of specialty medications. This trend shows no signs of slowing down, and these drugs are used in a variety of therapeutic areas—including hepatic disease, multiple sclerosis, oncology, and inflammatory conditions. Hospital pharmacy departments strategically recognized the need to keep these products in-house to prevent fragmentation of care and optimize patient outcomes, and developed specialty pharmacy programs to ensure that this occurred (Hanson et al., 2014; Thompson, 2014).

■ BARRIERS AND LIMITATIONS TO PLANNING

Effective planning requires a serious commitment of time and resources. For a variety of reasons, organizations may not be successful in their planning efforts. Lack of success may stem from failure to recognize and minimize common barriers to planning efforts or failure to understand inherent limitations in planning.

Barriers

Organizations must overcome several barriers to ensure a successful strategic planning process, as shown in Table 6-6. The most serious barrier is lack of endorsement by the top executive(s). Buy-in and participation by top corporate executives and the Board of Directors are critical to strategic planning. Without these, the whole planning effort could be a waste of time and resources.

A frequent barrier to effective planning is failure to commit sufficient time to the planning process. Good planning requires significant management and staff time. Ideally, some of the more creative aspects of planning should be accomplished during uninterrupted time. Pharmacy organizations commonly hold retreats, whereby those involved in the planning process meet in a location outside the usual work

Table 6-6.   Barriers to Effective Planning

1. Failure to commit sufficient time to the planning effort.
2. Interpersonal issues, such as struggles over power or politics and individual or group resistance to change.
3. Lack of planning skills.
4. Failure to plan far enough into the future.
5. Constantly changing environment.
6. Failure to implement owing to lack of time or lack of resources.
7. Failure to monitor progress.
8. Lack of support from top executive and/or board of directors.

environment. The time and expense associated with such events require a huge commitment on the part of both the organization and the personnel involved.

Sometimes interpersonal issues, such as organizational culture or struggles for power and politics, become barriers to effective planning. Individuals who are involved in planning or implementation may be resistant to change (for a variety of reasons) and thus consciously or subconsciously sabotage the planning effort. Likewise, if the organization or personnel lack the skills necessary to conduct planning, the results may be less than optimal and even harmful to the organization. In the same context, failure to plan far enough into the future can be problematic, especially for certain types of planning. Strategic planning in particular is intended to guide the organization over the long term.

The environment can also pose a barrier to effective planning. In an environment such as health care, where things are changing constantly or sometimes ambiguous, effective planning is more difficult and uncertain. For example, consider all the changes that may affect pharmacy organizations that make planning for the future difficult. These include changes in technology and automation, new drugs and therapies, changes in payment rates of prescriptions and availability of reimbursement for clinical pharmacist services, changes in regulations, and fluctuations in the labor market for pharmacists.

Organizations operating in rapidly changing environments may put off or avoid planning altogether. Unfortunately, failure to plan, even when it is difficult, may be even more detrimental in the long term.

Another barrier to the planning effort is failure to communicate the plan effectively to the employees of the pharmacy organization. Written plans must be drafted in such a way that the messages are communicated clearly to the appropriate audience. Plan documents sometimes have the tendency to use jargon or terminology, so-called plan-speak, that is not consistent with that which would be most beneficial to clear and accurate interpretation by the audience. Besides the written document, verbal presentations and other forms of communication are often important.

The most common barrier to effective planning is failure to implement, so-called "analysis but no action." Three causes of failure to implement plans include the unavailability of resources, lack of time, and failure to monitor or measure progress. Implementation of strategy often involves the mobilization of resources. If organizations do not have the necessary resources, or are unwilling to commit those resources, then implementation will be jeopardized. In today's ever-increasing speed of business, managers often cannot find the time to use adequately the results of planning already conducted to guide their daily activities. The term *management by crisis* is often used to describe the modus operandi of busy managers, meaning that their work is directed more by the problems they face at the immediate moment than by any careful consideration of the actual goals of the organization. In the long term, this may result in failure of the company to meet its goals (Martin, 2002). Finally, the failure to monitor, for whatever reason, the progress made toward goals developed in the planning process can be a significant barrier to success of the planning effort.

Limitations

Besides the barriers to planning just listed, certain limitations to planning must also be acknowledged. Managers are often caught up in the notion that planning is a magic bullet for the ills of an organization. They must acknowledge the fact that planning is no cure all.

First, planning is, to some degree, guesswork (but educated and experienced guesswork, hopefully). While decisions are based on evidence available about the past and the likelihood of events in the future, risk is still involved. Nothing is certain. Even with good data and good strategy, negative things may happen that were unpredictable and thus unavoidable.

Second, plans and predictions are only as good as the data and information that go into them. Poor data will result in poor strategy. What pharmacy organizations get out of the planning activity will be correlated directly with the degree of effort, creativity, time, and resources they put into it. Organizations that adopt boilerplate or "cookie cutter" approaches to planning most likely will not get the optimum results they would like to achieve.

Two additional limitations of planning deal with how an organization implements the plan. Planning is not a substitute for action. Organizations that are all about planning but neglect to take the actions dictated will not be successful. To the opposite extreme, the plan should not be considered as static or unyielding. Planning should be a continuous process, and plans should change as the environment dictates. To follow a plan blindly without consideration of changes in the environment that may make the plan obsolete is foolhardy.

■ CONCLUSION

The scenario of Ted Thompson that began this chapter illustrates how knowledge of planning-related concepts may be applicable to the work activities of a new pharmacist. Knowledge of concepts in the chapter should better position Ted to participate in the strategic planning initiative being organized by the DOP. Ted should now clearly appreciate the importance of this type of planning to the future of the hospital and to the pharmacy department. He should be able to anticipate the process that might be followed. Ted should also anticipate certain questions that will need to be addressed in the planning process. For example, given the pharmacy described in the scenario, what

might be a suitable vision for the department? What goals and objectives might the department establish during its strategic planning exercise?

The concepts discussed in this chapter become only more important as one advances through a career and assumes higher levels of leadership and responsibility in a pharmacy or health care organization. It is also important for students and new practitioners to understand the process involved in establishing and maintaining the viability of the organization for which they work. A good understanding of management concepts, and planning in particular, will allow the pharmacy practitioner to better appreciate the context from which management operates. This will then better enable pharmacy practitioners to have input into and be able to influence the direction and decisions of a pharmacy organization.

■ QUESTIONS FOR FURTHER DISCUSSION

1. Select a specific pharmacy practice setting (i.e., hospital practice, community practice, or managed care). What barriers do you believe would limit the ability of pharmacists and pharmacy managers to conduct effective planning in that setting?

2. Write a vision statement for a hypothetical pharmacy organization. Explain how you selected the language and message of the statement.

3. Conduct an Internet search of vision and mission statements of health care organizations. Identify and compare the statements from at least three different organizations. What are the strengths and weakness of these statements?

4. Describe changes that have occurred in the practice of pharmacy over the past 20 years. How would strategic planning have enabled a pharmacy organization to better position itself for those changes?

REFERENCES

Abulezz R, Alhamdan H, Khan MA. 2018. Use of a strategic plan for the clinical pharmacy section in a tertiary care center. *J Basic Clin Pharma* 289–293.

Allison M, Kaye J. 2015. *Strategic Planning for Nonprofit Organizations: A Practical Guide and Workbook*, 3rd ed. Hoboken, NJ: John Wiley & Sons.

American Society of Health-System Pharmacists. 2011. The consensus of the pharmacy practice model summit. *Am J Health-Syst Pharm* 1148–1152.

Bechet TP. 2008. *Strategic Staffing: A Comprehensive System for Effective Workforce Planning*. New York, NY: American Management Association.

Birdwell SW, Pathak DS. 1989. Use of the strategic-planning process by hospital pharmacy directors. *Am J Hosp Pharm* 46:1361–1369.

Cassidy A. 2006. *A Practical Guide to Information Systems Strategic Planning*. Boca Raton, FL: Auerbach Publications.

Chew EK, Gottschalk P. 2009. *Information Technology Strategy and Management: Best Practices*. Hersey, PA: Information Science Reference.

Fogg CD. 2010. *Team-Based Strategic Planning*. New York, NY: AMACOM American Management Association.

Grünig R, Kühn R. 2011. *Process-Based Strategic Planning*, 6th ed. Berlin, Germany: Springer.

Hagel HP. 2002. Planning for patient care. In Hagel HP, Rovers JP (eds.) Managing the Patient-Centered Pharmacy. Washington, DC: American Pharmaceutical Association.

Haines SG, McKinlay J. 2011. *Reinventing Strategic Planning: The Strategic Systems Approach*. Mumbai: Jaico Publishing House.

Hanson RL, Habibi M, Khamo N, Abdou S, Stubbings J. 2014. Integrated clinical and specialty pharmacy practice model for management of patients with multiple sclerosis. *Am J Health-Syst Pharm* 71:463–469.

Harrison DL. 2005. Strategic planning by independent community pharmacies. *J Am Pharm Assoc* 45:726–733.

Harrison DL. 2006. Effect of attitudes and perceptions of independent community pharmacy owners/managers on the comprehensiveness of strategic planning. *J Am Pharm Assoc* 46:459–464.

Harrison DL. 2007. Effect of strategic planning education on attitudes and perceptions of independent community pharmacy owners/managers. *Am J Pharm Assoc* 47:599–604.

Harrison DL, Ortmeier BG. 1996. Strategic planning in the community pharmacy. *J Am Pharm Assoc* NS36:583–588.

Harrison JP. 2010. *Essentials of Strategic Planning in Healthcare*. Chicago, IL: Health Administration Press.

Hodges HE, Kent TW. 2006. Impact of planning and control sophistication in small business. *J Small Bus Strategy* 17(2):75–88.

Lewin Group. 2005. Medication therapy management services: A critical review. *J Am Pharm Assoc* 45:580–587.

Martin BC. 2019. *Strategic Planning in Healthcare—An Introduction for Health Professionals*. New York, NY: Springer Publishing Company, LLC.

Martin C. 2002. *Managing for the Short Term: The New Rules for Running a Business in a Day-to-Day World*. New York, NY: Doubleday.

May GL. 2010. *Strategic Planning: Fundamentals for Small Business*. New York, NY: Business Expert Press.

Nolan TM, Goodstein LD, Goodstein J, Pfeiffer JW. 2008. *Applied Strategic Planning: An Introduction*. San Francisco, CA: Pfeiffer.

O'Neal B, Siegel J. 2007. Diversion in the pharmacy. *Hosp Pharm* 42:145–148.

Porter ME. 2008. *Competitive Advantage: Creating and Sustaining Superior Performance*. New York, NY: Simon and Schuster.

Sanborn M. 2009. Developing a meaningful strategic plan. *Hosp Pharm* 44:625–629.

Stoner JA, Freeman RE, Gilbert DR. 2007. *Management*, 6th ed. Englewood Cliffs, NJ: Prentice-Hall.

Thompson CA. 2014. Specialty pharmacy presents opportunities for hospitals, health systems. *Am J Health-Syst Pharm* 71:687–689.

University HealthSystem Consortium. 2011. *Best Practices for Pharmacy Strategic Planning*.

Vermeulen LC, Eddington ND, Gourdine MA, et al. 2019. Pharmacy forecast 2019: Strategic planning advice for pharmacy departments in hospitals and health systems. *Am J Health-Syst Pharm* 76:71–100.

Ward DL, Tripp R, Maki B. 2013. *Positioned: Strategic Workforce Planning that Gets the Right Person in the Right Position*. New York, NY: AMACOM, American Management Association.

Weber RJ. 2015. Issues facing pharmacy leaders in 2015: Suggestions for pharmacy strategic planning. *Hosp Pharm* 50:167–172.

Westerling AM, Haikala VE, Bell JS, Airaksinen MS. 2010. Logistics or patient care: Which features do independent Finnish pharmacy owners prioritize in a strategic plan for future information technology systems? *J Am Pharm Assoc* 50:24–31.

Young MB. 2009. *Implementing Strategic Workforce Planning*. New York, NY: Conference Board.

Zuckerman AM. 2012. *Healthcare Strategic Planning*. Chicago, IL: Health Administration Press.

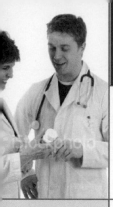

7

BUSINESS PLANNING FOR PHARMACY PROGRAMS

Glen T. Schumock and Andrew Donnelly

About the Authors: Dr. Schumock is a graduate from Washington State University (BPharm), the University of Washington (PharmD), and the University of Illinois at Chicago (MBA, PhD). He also completed a residency and a research fellowship. Currently, he is Professor and Dean of the College of Pharmacy at the University of Illinois at Chicago (UIC). Dr. Schumock has taught courses on pharmacy management, pharmacoeconomics, and business planning for pharmacy services. He has published over 200 articles, book chapters, and books. He is on the editorial boards of the journals *Pharmacotherapy* and *PharmacoEconomics*, and is Associate Editor of the *Journal of Comparative Effectiveness Research*.

Dr. Donnelly is a graduate from the University of Illinois at the Medical Center (BPharm) and the University of Illinois at Chicago (MBA, PharmD). Dr. Donnelly is currently Director of Pharmacy Services at the University of Illinois Hospital & Health Sciences System and Clinical Professor and Assistant Dean for Clinical Affairs at the University of Illinois at Chicago. He is responsible for planning, organizing, and directing the activities of the pharmacy department. Dr. Donnelly's areas of interest include pharmacy administration as well as technology and automation as it relates to the medication use process. He is a Fellow of the American Society of Health-System Pharmacists.

■ LEARNING OBJECTIVES

After completing this chapter, readers should be able to

1. Describe the purpose of "business plan" planning.
2. Discuss the important components of a business plan.
3. Review important aspects of communicating and implementing a business plan.
4. Highlight examples of business plan planning within pharmacy organizations.
5. Understand how to write a business plan for a pharmacy organization.

■ SCENARIO

The scenario begun in Chapter 6 continues here. In brief, Ted Thompson is a clinical pharmacist at a medium sized community hospital. Ted has just finished participating in the process of developing a strategic plan for the pharmacy department. Included in the 5-year plan is a goal for the department to develop and implement specific clinical pharmacist services that help to deliver care, improve patient outcomes, and reduce spending, which aligns with the American Society of Health-System Pharmacists (ASHP) Practice Alignment Initiative (PAI).

After his first year at the hospital, Ted has formulated several ideas for new clinical pharmacist services that the department could offer which might improve patient outcomes, reduce spending, and generate revenue. During his annual performance evaluation, he discusses these ideas with his boss, the Director of Pharmacy (DOP), who is happy that Ted has come forward with his ideas and encourages him to investigate these options further. One idea that is of particular interest is to develop an outpatient medication management service for patients with complex or chronic diseases who are prescribed high-cost and complex specialty medications. As a clinical pharmacist, Ted has developed a high level of interest and expertise in specialty pharmacy. His duties often involve determining the appropriateness of specialty medications and facilitating transitions in care, continuity of drug therapy, and the prevention of readmissions. Because of this, and because of his concern for patients, Ted has developed a good reputation with the medical and nursing staff not only in the hospital but also within the outpatient clinics. Ted tells the DOP that during his contacts with these clinics, he has heard that most are unhappy with the quality of the medication management currently provided by the hospital's outpatient pharmacy—where most patients get these medications. They have asked repeatedly if he or the hospital would consider providing an outpatient specialty medication management service.

The DOP indicates that he thinks that the specialty medication management idea is a good one and that it would likely be of interest to the hospital executives. The hospital can leverage the value of the service by expanding their dispensing of specialty medications from their outpatient pharmacy. He suggests that Ted develops a "business plan" in accordance with the strategic plan that was developed previously. Ted has heard of the term *business plan* before but really does not know what it entails. However, he is willing and prepared to learn and to do whatever is necessary to accomplish the proposed idea.

■ CHAPTER QUESTIONS

1. What is the primary objective of business planning in the pharmacy environment?
2. What are the important components of a business plan of a proposed pharmacy service?
3. What are the principal factors to include in an analysis of the potential financial performance of a proposed new program?
4. For whom is a business plan written?

■ INTRODUCTION

Chapter 6 discussed general concepts of planning by pharmacy organizations and reviewed a specific type of planning—strategic planning. This chapter discusses another key type of planning that is used by pharmacy organizations. The distinguishing characteristic of *business planning* is that it focuses on a specific program or business within the organization. Here the term *business* is used synonymously with *program*. For example, in a pharmacy organization, the business or program may be a new clinical service. In a large corporation, such as a chain pharmacy, the business or program may be a drive-through prescription service or a disease management program in selected stores. Business planning can also be used for start-up companies, where the proposed program or business comprises the totality of the organization.

The purpose of business planning is to provide data and proposed actions necessary to answer a business question, usually in the form, "Should we invest in the proposed business?" As this question illustrates, business planning is used most commonly when an organization wishes to predict the future risks and benefits of a proposed new business venture. For example, in the scenario faced by Ted, the business question relates to the proposed new outpatient specialty medication management service. However, business planning may also be used to make decisions about expanding or terminating an existing program.[1]

As with strategic planning, the process of business planning produces a written plan. A key point to clarify here is that the business plan needs to be written with the "audience" in mind. If the decision maker is the Chief Executive Officer (CEO), Chief Financial Officer (CFO), owner, or sponsor, then the plan should be written so that it is applicable to and appropriate for that audience. Business plans that do not consider the audience are less likely to be acted on favorably. A common mistake by authors of business plans (including pharmacists) is to write in a manner that is too technical or detailed, thus failing to hold the attention of executives, who might be the decision makers.

This chapter will discuss practical issues in the development of a pharmacy-related business plan. Because business planning is an activity that is commonly employed by organizations of all sizes, there are ample resources on this topic. Some excellent general guides to business planning are listed in the reference section of this chapter (DeThomas et al., 2015; McKeever, 2014; Pinson, 2014). There are also several references specific to business planning in pharmacy organizations (Chater et al., 2008; McDonough, 2007; Phillips & Larson, 2002; Schumock et al., 2004). A more detailed resource for business planning for pharmacy services is also available and may

be especially useful to those who are in the position of developing an actual business plan (Schumock & Stubbings, 2018).

■ THE BUSINESS CONCEPT

The practice of pharmacy is a unique combination of the provision of patient care and the running of a business, and there are many opportunities for pharmacists to create new and innovative services that both fulfill patient needs and generate profits. Pharmacists should not lose the "entrepreneurial" spirit that is necessary to promote and nurture the business side of pharmacy, as it is this that has driven many of the advances in the profession. Business planning is a means by which pharmacists can do this.

The place to start with any new business idea is to conduct a preliminary evaluation. This is also called *exploring the business concept*. The purpose of this preliminary exploration is to determine if the idea merits the development of a complete business plan. As with other planning processes, business planning is not a trivial undertaking. For this reason, it is advisable to be sure that the concept is one that is reasonable prior to investing time and energy into developing the business plan.

The preliminary evaluation usually begins with a literature search. Literature searches yield the best results when conducted using electronic databases such as that of the National Library of Medicine, which can be searched using PubMed. Other databases, such as International Pharmaceutical Abstracts, and search engines are also available in most medical libraries. Search terms should be consistent with the area of interest. For example, to identify articles that describe specialty medication management, Ted (from the scenario) might use the following search terms: *specialty pharmacy, specialty pharmacy services, specialty medications,* or terms associated with any of the disease states that would be the focus of the proposed specialty medication management business plan, such as *oncology* or *rheumatology*. Literature searches can be made more specific by limiting the search to certain date ranges, types of articles (i.e., reviews or

---

[1]Here it may be useful to distinguish the terms *business plan, business planning,* and *"business plan" planning*. Business plan planning culminates in the development of a business plan and is the primary topic of this chapter. Business planning encompasses not only the development of the business plan but also the ongoing monitoring and review of the success of a program.

descriptive reports), or specific journals of publication (i.e., pharmacy journals), if appropriate.

Another way to identify primary literature of interest is to obtain systematic literature reviews that have been published. These reviews usually provide extensive citations and may categorize articles based on types of pharmacist services or other classifications that are of interest. A number of very comprehensive reviews have been published and are included in the reference list of this chapter (Chisholm-Burns et al., 2010; Perez et al., 2009; Schumock et al., 2003; Touchette et al., 2014).

A further source of information is the Internet. Using the search terms listed earlier, it is possible to identify additional resources pertinent to the subject of interest. For example, by typing *specialty pharmacy services* into a search engine such as Google, Ted will identify the website of the ASHP or the American Pharmacists Association (APhA), which will lead to a host of resources available on this topic. However, as most experienced web users will recognize, Internet searches can produce an inordinate amount of "noise" in the form of unrelated sites or references and, from that standpoint, may be inefficient. However, some websites will have links to other related sites that are very helpful.

Primary and secondary literature identified in these searches can provide a variety of information to assist in exploring the business concept. First, some publications will serve primarily to describe the experiences of others in providing the program or service. Other publications may provide an actual evaluation of the program or service being proposed in the business plan. For example, an article may evaluate the impact of the service on the health outcomes of patients or may provide evidence of the financial impact of the program. Obviously, this type of information will be extremely valuable to anyone proposing to implement similar services. In fact, part of the process of exploring the business concept may include the generalization of results found in the literature. For example, it is possible to combine the results of published studies and estimate the clinical and economic outcomes that may be expected if the service

were to be implemented in a different setting (Schumock, 2000; Schumock & Butler, 2003).

Resources are also available for developing and establishing certain types of pharmacy services, including those in ambulatory care (American College of Clinical Pharmacy, 2008; Kliethermes & Brown, 2012; Sachdev, 2014), consulting pharmacy (Schumock et al., 2004), and medication therapy management (Chater et al., 2008; Lofton, 2012). The American College of Clinical Pharmacy (ACCP) has a number of resources on its website for assisting pharmacists in developing clinical pharmacy services—including a paper titled "Developing a business-practice model for pharmacy services in ambulatory settings" (ACCP et al., 2008).

As mentioned, both APhA and ASHP has a Specialty Pharmacy section on its website with links to articles, business plans, presentations, webinars, and podcasts, and these may be of particular interest and benefit someone like Ted from our scenario at the beginning of this chapter (American Society of Health-System Pharmacists, 2016).

Besides gaining experience from literature, exploration of the business concept should consider the size and receptivity of potential customers of the service. A preliminary analysis of the demand that may exist for the service should be conducted. This should include a clear description of the need for the service and the number of potential customers that may exist in the market. Information about the market can come from a variety of sources. Demographic data related to trends in the population in the community are usually available from county or city websites or from the U.S. Census Bureau. Local, state, and federal public health agencies will be able to provide information on disease patterns and statistics. Information can even be gathered from existing or potential customers by conducting interviews or surveys. Consulting companies may also be available to assist in assessing the market for the proposed program.

Once information on the market is obtained, it can then be used to consider the revenue that may be generated by the program. It should be noted that some programs will not generate revenue; rather, they may reduce costs, which can be equally important. Further, while most programs are expected to provide a financial benefit, in some other cases, nonquantifiable benefits may be considered of equal or greater importance (i.e., clinical benefits).

Given that the proposed program appears to have a potential market and that it may create a financial benefit (or some other form of benefit) for the organization, the remaining issue is the ability of the program to address a specific goal(s) in the organization's strategic plan. For example, if a hospital's strategic plan includes a goal of expanding vertically into related health care markets, such as specialty pharmacy, then the pharmacy's proposal to initiate a specialty medication management service would be consistent with and supportive of that goal.

Having conducted the preliminary exploration of the business concept, it is probably prudent to seek the advice of others before moving forward with the complete business planning process. Here, Ted may consider discussing the idea with key stakeholders in the organization, including the individual or individuals who will make the ultimate decision to move forward with the concept. For example, Ted should solidify support from DOP, and together, broach the idea of the specialty medication management service proposed in the scenario with executives in the hospital, beginning with DOP's supervisor, onward to the CEO and CFO. Ted may also wish to get input from key stakeholders in the outpatient specialty clinics, such as physicians, nurses, or physician assistants. If the reception to the concept is positive, the development of a complete business plan can begin.

■ STEPS IN THE DEVELOPMENT OF A BUSINESS PLAN

The process of business planning is similar to other types of planning and, as such, is consistent with the general steps discussed in Chapter 6. This section describes the usual steps taken in the business planning process.

Define the Business or Program

As with other types of planning, the initial step of business planning is to define the business or service proposed. After exploring the business concept (see above), Ted likely already will have developed a clear idea of the business proposal. To formalize a definition of the business, he should develop a specific statement of the purpose of the program. This statement is also called a *mission statement* and was discussed in Chapter 6. The mission will crystallize the aims of the program and help to determine the direction taken in other steps of the planning process.

Conduct Market Research and Analysis

The next steps in business planning (evaluating the market, evaluating competitors, and assessing clinical and quality requirements) are part of the situation analysis described in the general planning process (see Chapter 6). The term *market* refers to the customers of the program. An analysis of the potential customers of the business is clearly an important exercise, and this can be done in a number of ways. First, the market can be described geographically. For example, the organization may collect data that would give projections of the number of customers in different local regions. In the scenario, Ted would want to identify the demographics of the population served by the hospital. Ted will want to know the number of people in the hospital's service area and the trends with respect to the age of the population, health status, and major diseases. He will also need to analyze the demographics of the current customers (patients) of the hospital. The hospital administration department usually keeps these data, such as number of outpatient visits by clinic type. Ted should align the customer data with the need for medication management in outpatient clinics such as transplant, oncology, liver, rheumatology, neurology, or others.

It is important to note that the term *customers* is not always synonymous with *patients* when speaking of health care programs. In particular, the customer of a pharmacy program may be something or someone other than the patient. In many cases, the customers of pharmacy programs are providers such as physicians or other health care professionals, or payers such as the health plan or employer group. In the scenario, the customers are the providers in the outpatient specialty clinics because they will incorporate the specialty medication management services in their clinics and the health plans that pay for the patients' medical care and prescriptions. Ted must "sell" his services to the providers and payers before he can start delivering the service to patients (see section on *Develop a Marketing Strategy*).

Identify the Target Market

After analyzing all the potential customers, Ted should identify one or more segments of the market to which the program or business is most apt to appeal. This is commonly known as the *target market*. The target market may be based on a special market niche that the program fulfills and/or a special customer need. For example, Ted identifies that the hospital has 15 outpatient clinics, six of which treat patients that often receive specialty medication prescriptions. The *target market* is the six specialty clinics.

Conduct Competitor Analysis

A key component of analyzing the external environment is to identify and gauge potential competitors. The goal of the competitor analysis is to understand the characteristics of other providers so that the business can be positioned favorably compared with competitors. Data about competitors are sometimes difficult to obtain. Surveys of customers, price comparisons, and publicly available information (i.e., websites) should be investigated.

A comparison should be made of the characteristics and market share of each competitor with those of the proposed program. Characteristics such as years in business, number of customers, percentage of the market (i.e., market share), and product or service niche should be compared. The strengths and weaknesses of each competitor should also be reviewed and compared with those of the proposed business. Categories of strengths and weakness to consider include

service quality, staff competence and credentials, customer service, customer access, price, technology or innovation, and delivery mechanisms.

In health care, the definition of *competitors* sometimes has to be broadened beyond that which is most obvious. For example, in the hospital environment, a new pharmacist program might compete with other professions within the hospital. Many of the advanced clinical services that pharmacists provide replace functions of other health care professionals, especially physicians. This is true even in the outpatient environment. For example, a pharmacist-run immunization clinic may compete with physician offices that also administer vaccines.

In the case of the proposed specialty medication management service (scenario), Ted should consider as competitors any other organizations that provide the same service such as outside specialty pharmacies. Some outside specialty pharmacies are owned by payers (health plans), so Ted's competitor will be a payer. It will be a challenge for Ted to convince the health plan to pay for his service if it is also a competitor (see section on *Develop a Marketing Strategy*). One could consider other competitors to be nurses or physicians in the outpatient clinics who are already providing the services, but in the scenario we understood that these were some of the chief proponents of the new service. The outpatient clinic providers may be more open to Ted's service, especially if they are not paying for the service. It is important in developing a business plan to understand customers and competitors, and their role in paying for the service.

Assess Clinical and Quality Requirements

The health care industry is highly regulated. Anyone proposing a new business in a regulated environment must be aware of these regulations and have a plan to comply with them. Thus, part of the business planning process is to analyze applicable regulations and requirements. This analysis should extend beyond just the mandatory legal rules or requirements. It should include voluntary standards, such as those endorsed by professional organizations and societies; it should also include standards of accrediting bodies and any other guidelines or expectations with respect to the service proposed. On the legal side, there are federal, state, and city/county ordinances, laws, statutes, and regulations that must be followed when applicable.

In the proposed specialty medication management service (scenario), there are many different sources of regulatory guidelines. First, the Food and Drug Administration regulates the utilization of high-risk medications through its Risk Evaluation and Mitigation Strategies (REMS) program. Some specialty medications have REMS requirements. Second, pharmacists that practice in specialty clinics often have specialty certification, which is administered by the Board of Pharmacy Specialties. Finally, because the practice of pharmacy is regulated primarily at the state level, the state pharmacy practice act must be complied with. Each state has a different approach to pharmacist provider status and collaborative practice agreements. Adherence to state and federal regulations will inform the framework for the proposed pharmacy service.

Ted's proposal for a specialty medication management service is to benefit the hospital's outpatient pharmacy where these medications are being dispensed. Pharmacies that dispense specialty medications (also called "Specialty Pharmacies") are subject to some unique regulatory and quality considerations. In particular, there are a number of organizations that accredit specialty pharmacies, including the Utilization Review Accreditation Commission, the Accreditation Commission for Health Care, The Joint Commission, and Center for Pharmacy Practice Accreditation. It is likely that the proposed specialty medication management service will be able to help the outpatient pharmacy meet these rigorous accreditation requirements.

Assessing clinical and quality requirements of the proposed program also means planning for how to comply with these standards. Compliance should be considered both on an initial basis and over the long term. Clinical and quality requirements may necessitate the hiring of certain (qualified) staff, the development of work processes to monitor quality, and the implementation of technology or procedures to ensure compliance.

Define Processes and Operations

The business planning process shifts from the initial situation analysis to more of a projection and goal-setting approach in the next four steps. Defining the details associated with the planned operations of the business is the first of these steps. This step includes planning of the optimal organizational structure (with a link to the larger organization), the staffing levels, personnel requirements, and the reporting relationships of the program. Personnel job titles, job descriptions, and the number of full-time equivalents[2] (FTEs) needed in each position should be determined.

Planning also should elicit the physical structure, equipment, and resources required to operate the program. This includes planning for the types of equipment, physical layout, furniture, and information systems. Finally, the work processes should be planned. This can be done using flowcharts and other tools to design the customer interface and delivery of the proposed service. An example of Ted Thompson's proposed workflow for the outpatient specialty medication management service is shown in Figure 7-1. It shows how the pharmacists in the specialty clinics interact with the outpatient/specialty pharmacy. The planned operations should be sufficient to determine the workload capacities of the program. From this, strategies should be devised to deal with extremes in demand (either insufficient or excess workload).

Planning of the processes and operations helps to clarify the practical, day-to-day activities that will occur in the program. This type of planning provides critical information needed in later steps of the business planning process (i.e., for development of financial projections).

---

[2]A *full-time equivalent* (FTE) is a value used to measure the actual or budgeted work hours in an organization. One FTE is equal to 2,080 hours per year (or 40 hours per week, 52 weeks per year). Part-time employees are counted as less than a full FTE. For example, an employee who works 20 hours per week is equal to 0.5 FTE.

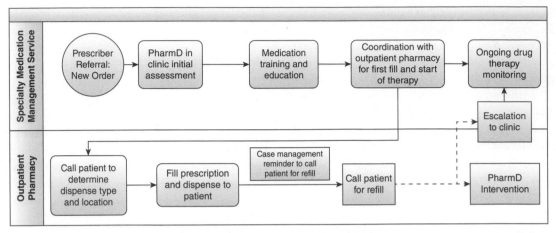

Figure 7-1. Workflow for the outpatient specialty medication management service. This figure shows the workflow that might occur within the proposed specialty medication management service. Pharmacists employed by the hospital would receive referrals for new specialty medications. They would perform initial clinical assessments, medication training and education, coordination with specialty pharmacy for first fill and start of therapy, and ongoing drug therapy monitoring. The dotted lines in the diagram show how the clinic-based pharmacist would interact with the hospital's outpatient/specialty pharmacy.

In the outpatient specialty medication management proposal given in the scenario, planning of processes and operations will include estimation of the number and types of pharmacists (or other staff) that will be needed to provide the proposed services. Ted will also need to determine the job requirements (i.e., must have achieved board certification) and have a rough idea of the job descriptions for each position. With respect to the organizational structure, he will need to determine to whom the pharmacist(s) should report and where within the hospital pharmacy department organizational structure this service will reside. The work processes of the pharmacists will need to be defined, along with any work aids that may be required in this process (i.e., electronic drug information or documentation systems). Important policies or procedures that govern the scope of work and decision making of the program and staff also should be determined. Methods for communication between the pharmacist(s) and the other clinic providers should be defined. This planning process should also include identification of a system for workload monitoring and for billing for the services provided. Many other details of the operation will also need to be developed in this planning process.

Develop a Marketing Strategy

The second of the goal-setting steps is to define a marketing strategy. The marketing strategy should be based on information gathered in the previous steps of the business planning process, especially the market and competitor analyses. The marketing strategy should identify the target market for the program and develop a plan for gaining the business of that market. This plan should include the means of communicating to customers and the message that should be communicated to them. The strategy for a new business should be separated into the initial marketing plan and the ongoing marketing plan. The initial marketing plan defines the promotional activities and market goals for the period directly before and immediately after implementation of the new program. The ongoing marketing plan defines the promotional and market goals over the longer term. Resources are available to assist in the development of pharmacy-related marketing plans (Doucette & McDonough, 2002; Holdford, 2007).

The marketing strategy for the outpatient specialty medication management service (scenario) will largely depend on the perceived value of the pharmacist in the target clinics. Value, simply defined as benefit/cost, is how much benefit the customers receive compared to how much the service costs. Typically the marketing message should be directed at the group that is paying for the pharmacy service. In the case of Ted's proposed service this could be the health plan. The customers should understand that the benefit they will receive from the service exceeds its cost, therefore providing value to the health plan. The hospital may negotiate with the health plan for payment for the pharmacy service, based on the pharmacist's ability to reach performance metrics such as clinical outcomes or total cost reduction. If the health plan already owns a specialty pharmacy (see section *Conduct Competitor Analysis*), they will need to be convinced of the added value provided by the pharmacists in the outpatient clinics. Ted can communicate the value of the pharmacist by providing outcomes data for his specialty medication management service. The best method of communicating information about the program and payment likely will be well-designed, face-to-face presentations by Ted with those administrators responsible for the clinic and the health plan. The marketing plan may call for obtaining contracts with only a couple of health plans in the first 6 months of the program but then will increase gradually by one plan in every 6 months. The ongoing marketing strategy would be in accordance with this.

Develop Financial Projections

Perhaps the most critical step in the business planning process is the development of financial projections for the program. Most programs that do not have a positive benefit-to-cost ratio usually will not be approved. That is, the program must be profitable. While it is preferable that programs generate revenue, it is possible that pharmacist services are justifiable based on reducing expenditures. For example, a clinical pharmacist antibiotic dosing service in a hospital may reduce expenditures on antibiotics and reduce patient length of stay but generate no revenue. If the financial benefit of the dosing service (i.e., reduced expenditures) exceeds the costs associated with providing the program (i.e., pharmacist salary), then the program

can be considered financially viable. Obviously, there may be additional benefits from the dosing service, such as improved patient outcomes, that also would favor its approval.

The business planning process must include an analysis of both the costs that will be incurred to provide the service and the financial benefits that may occur as a result of the program. The calculations involved in this planning process may be aided by the use of financial spreadsheets. More detailed descriptions of the methods and a set of financial spreadsheets designed for creating financial projections are available to those in the position of having to develop a business plan (Schumock & Stubbings, 2018). The revenue and expense statement, which lists revenue by category, expenditures by category, and net profit each year for a 3- to 5-year period, is the most useful of these. An example of a revenue and expense projection for the specialty medication management program (scenario) is shown in Table 7-1.

In developing the financial projections, revenue (if it exists) should be based on the anticipated volume of business, changes to that volume expected over time, and the income per unit of service. Information on billing for pharmacist services may be helpful in estimating potential revenue of the proposed service (Kliethermes, 2017; Sachdev, 2014; Stubbings, 2011). Also see Chapter 30 of this book, "Implementing Value-Added Pharmacist Services." Discounts to income (contractual agreements) should be factored into these calculations, as should future increases in the amount charged for the service. Expenditures must also be projected. If the program requires significant capital investment, those expenditures should be depreciated over the life of the item and accounted for appropriately. Other investments required to initiate the program should also be shown in the financial estimates. Ongoing costs, such as salaries and benefits, minor equipment, supplies, rent, and other overhead, should be categorized and accounted for. Costs that are considered variable should be increased proportionate to the changes in volume expected. All costs should be increased annually based on inflation, the consumer price index (CPI), or other evidence of

Table 7-1.   Example Revenue and Expense Projections for Outpatient Specialty Medication Management Program, Most Likely Scenario, Years 1–5

	Year 1	Year 2	Year 3	Year 4	Year 5	Total
Operating revenue						
Patient revenue	504,000	1,008,000	1,176,000	1,260,000	1,764,000	5,712,000
Deductions from revenue	0	0	0	0	0	0
Net patient revenue	504,000	1,008,000	1,176,000	1,260,000	1,764,000	5,712,000
Operating expenses						
Salaries	312,000	426,400	561,600	595,296	1,017,120	2,912,416
Employee benefits	81,100	110,900	146,000	154,800	264,500	757,300
Medical director	0	0	0	0	0	0
Medical supplies	6,000	6,890	7,420	7,950	8,500	36,760
Office supplies	0	0	0	0	0	0
Education and travel	0	0	0	0	0	0
Maintenance/repair	300	318	337	357	757	2,069
Consulting	0	0	0	0	0	0
Contracted services	0	0	0	0	0	0
Marketing	5,000	2,500	2,650	2,809	5,300	18,259
Dues and subscriptions	3,585	3,780	3,975	3,975	4,170	19,485
Rent	12,500	12,700	13,500	14,300	15,150	68,150
Postage	3,500	4,200	4,800	5,300	6,900	24,700
Equipment expense	13,000	1,272	1,348	0	1,515	17,135
Utilities/telephone	8,300	8,798	9,326	9,886	10,479	46,789
Insurance	900	1,166	1,248	1,323	1,826	6,463
Other expenses	16,500	3,090	3,285	12,423	8,894	44,192
Bad debt expense	0	0	0	0	0	0
Building depreciation	0	0	0	0	0	0
Equipment depreciation	0	0	0	0	0	0
Total operating expenses	462,685	582,014	755,489	808,419	1,345,111	3,953,718
Net income (loss)	41,315	425,986	420,511	451,581	418,889	1,758,282
Net assets at beginning	350,000	391,315	817,301	1,237,812	1,689,393	4,485,821
Net assets at end	391,315	817,301	1,237,812	1,689,393		

expected increases in the costs of goods or services. Additional resources are available on financial management in pharmacy organizations, which might be useful in developing the financial projects in a business plan (Carroll, 2007; Wilson, 2008).

Identify an Action Plan

The next step in the business planning process is to define major milestones and an action plan of implementation and operation of the program. This action

Step	Description	Duration	Month 1	2	3	4	5	6	7	8	9	10	11	12
1	Plan service	2 months	█	█										
2	Hire staff	1 month		█										
3	Implement information system for documentation and billing	2 months		█	█									
4	Contract with first health plan	1 month			█									
5	Provide service to first outpatient clinic	indefinite				█	█	█	█	█	█	█	█	█
6	Measure clinical and economic outcomes in first clinic	1 month					█							
7	Measure customer satisfaction in first clinic	1 month						█						
8	Market services to target clinics and health plans	indefinite						█	█	█	█	█	█	█
9	Contract with second health plan	1 month								█				
10	Provide service to second outpatient clinic	indefinite									█	█	█	█
11	Hire and train additional staff	1 month								█				
12	Contract with additional health plans (if available)	1 month									█			
13	Provide service to third—sixth outpatient clinics	indefinite										█	█	█
14	Compare performance of program to objectives	1 month											█	
15	Make decision to continue or discontinue program based on performance to-date	1 month											█	
16	If decision to continue, then expand to additional health plans or clinics if available	1 month											█	█
17	If decision is to discontinue, then inform clinics, notify staff, and discontinue	2 months											█	█

Figure 7-2. Example of a Gantt chart for implementation of proposed outpatient specialty medication management service. This figure shows the steps that should be taken in order to implement the proposed service. The chart includes when (month) each step should be initiated and when it would be expected to be completed. Gantt charts such as this often also include the party/person responsible for completion of each step (not shown here).

plan should detail the start and finish dates and list responsible individual(s) for each task necessary to accomplish the objectives of the business plan. The action plan should include periodic monitoring and assessment of the performance (i.e., clinical, financial, or other) of the program. A Gantt chart is one method to depict the action plan visually. An example of a Gantt chart for outpatient specialty medication management program is shown in Figure 7-2.

Assess Critical Risks and Opportunities

Another key step in the business planning process is to determine the critical risks and opportunities of the proposed program. Chapter 6 introduced the concepts of a *SWOT* (*strengths, weaknesses, opportunities, threats*) *analysis*. As part of the business plan, such an analysis should be completed for the proposed business/service. While it may seem more reasonable to conduct the SWOT analysis earlier in the business planning process, as was done in strategic planning,

because the program is in the proposal stage, some of the key considerations for this analysis must come from the previous steps, such as the financial analysis, and thus it is done later in the process.

An example of a SWOT analysis for the proposed outpatient specialty medication management service is shown in Tables 7-2 and 7-3. As mentioned in Chapter 6, strengths and weakness are internal characteristics, whereas opportunities and threats are characteristics of the external business environment. A number of factors can be considered when conducting this analysis. The factors considered will vary based on the nature of the business and the business environment.

Establish an Exit Plan

The last step of the planning process is to develop an exit plan. The *exit plan* is a formal protocol for determining when and why a decision would be made to terminate the program. The exit plan also defines the

Table 7-2.	**Internal Strengths and Weaknesses of Outpatient Specialty Medication Management Service**	
Factor	**Strength**	**Weakness**
Profitability	As a new program associated with a hospital, overhead expenses will be minimal and thus profitability could be high.	Profitability may be limited initially due to start-up expenses and small number of patients served.
Quality	Quality management is a strength of the hospital environment and this may apply to the outpatient specialty medication management service.	As a new program, the organization has limited experience specific to the outpatient specialty medication management environment. This may jeopardize quality initially.
Customer	Because the program is small (at least service initially), it may be able to provide more attention to customers and thus better customer service.	Because the hospital is the primary responsibility of the pharmacy department, it may not always be able to respond as quickly to outpatient customer needs.
Staff	Because the pharmacists included in the program have hospital experience, their level of clinical knowledge is beyond that of most competitors.	The pharmacists are new to the outpatient specialty medication management business so there may be a learning curve and lack of specialty medication knowledge initially.
Operations	Because the program is associated with a hospital, it can rely on the hospital pharmacy department for backup during off hours.	Because the program is small and new in this business, efficiency may be limited. It may also be difficult to establish relationships in the outpatient specialty clinics initially due to existing workflow patterns.

steps that would be taken if such a decision were to be made.

A decision to exit a program is usually based on failure of the business to meet predetermined goals (financial or otherwise). Typically, any new business is given a certain amount of time to meet its goals (18–24 months). Many organizations fail to have a mechanism in place to make a termination decision and instead let the business flounder and perhaps continue to lose money. It is much more preferable to have a definitive benchmark to which the program can be compared and a decision made promptly and decisively. This requires routine measurement of the ongoing performance of the business and comparison to those pre-established benchmarks or performance thresholds.

If a decision is made to terminate a program, then there should be clear actions for how the business will be dissolved. First, there should be a plan for when and how customers will be notified. Further, in some cases it may be important to provide customers with information about others who can provide the service and then schedule a seamless transition. Second, there should be a plan for how employees will be notified. The plan may include efforts to place employees in other areas of the organization or what, if any, compensation package may be available. Third, there should be a plan for how the facilities, equipment, and other capital (*capital* will be discussed in Chapter 22) will be sold or transferred. An exit plan for a program could involve transferring the control of the program from one organization or one administrative unit to another.

Table 7-3.   External Opportunities and Threats of Outpatient Specialty Medication Management Service

Factor	Opportunities	Threats
Competition	Because some health plans also own specialty pharmacies, they could be considered biased in the clinical recommendations they make—this may be an advantage for the proposed service which will focus only on the medication management.	Competitors (health plans) are well established, large, and financially sound. They may also dispense prescriptions through their specialty pharmacies, which may be desirable to the health plans. New competitors may enter the local market in the future.
Technology	The competitors do not have the same access to and understanding of technology as might already exist in the hospital (electronic medical records, bar coding, and other technology) and be advantageous to the outpatient clinics.	Competitors have advanced information systems and experience with these systems.
Regulation	Pharmacy services are mandated by state law. States with expanded pharmacist provider status will create new practice opportunities in outpatient specialty clinics.	There may be changes to regulations in the future that may alter the ability of the hospital to provide this service in the future.
Reimbursement	The proposed program will provide a new revenue stream for the outpatient clinics. If the hospital has an outpatient pharmacy, there will be additional revenue and profit from the dispensing of specialty medications.	Payers may not be willing to pay for pharmacy services, or payment may not be adequate. If the hospital does not have an outpatient pharmacy, they will not be able to realize any revenue or profit from dispensing specialty medications.
Costs	Competitors may not be able to use pharmacists as efficiently as the proposed program.	Competitors may use nurses or other health care providers to lower costs.
Market/ customers	The specialty pharmacy market is one of the fastest growing health care markets, and treatment is becoming increasingly complex.	Payers may mandate that medication management be done by competitors such as outside specialty pharmacies.

While the exit plan implies termination of the program, there are actually several possibilities for how a business may be disposed. These include: (1) closing the program, (2) merging the business with another program, (3) selling the business/program, and (4) taking it out of its current arrangement and operating it as a separate and individualized entity.

■ COMMUNICATION OF THE BUSINESS PLAN

Typically, there are two key components to communicating the work accomplished in planning. The first is to create a written document—the actual business plan. The second is to present the business plan orally, usually as part of a formal decision-making process.

Table 7-4.	Typical Table of Contents of the Business Plan

1. Executive summary
2. Background and description
3. Market analysis and strategy
4. Operational structure and processes
5. Financial projections
6. Milestones, schedule, and action plan
7. Critical risks and opportunities
8. Exit strategy
9. Conclusion
10. Supportive documents (include financial pro forma statements, letters of support)

Writing the Business Plan

As stated previously, writing the business plan is an extremely important part of business planning. The business plan should be informative and balanced in its presentation of the proposal. The document should be written with a specific audience in mind (the financial decision maker). It should be both easy to read and easy to understand and therefore must possess proper organization, grammar, punctuation, and sentence structure.

The contents of a business plan typically follow a sequence of items that are unique to this type of planning. An example of the table of contents of a simple business plan is shown in Table 7-4. It should be noted that the contents of the business plan will vary based on the industry, the business proposed, and the needs of the organization. More detailed plans may be required in certain industries.[3]

---

[3]As another example, the proposed contents of a business plan for a for-profit venture could include executive summary, introduction/synopsis, venture idea, overall industry, market research/competition, production/sourcing plan, service/delivery plan, marketing/sales plan, management plan, human resources plan, ownership/organization plan, financial plan, financing plan, growth/exit plan, implementation plan, contingency plan, and assessment/evaluation plan.

The business plan should begin with an *executive summary*. This summary should be short (one to two pages) but should hit the main points of the proposal. The executive summary needs to capture the attention of the reader. In a poorly written business plan, the reader may form a negative opinion of the program and read no further than the executive summary. This illustrates the importance of a writing style that is engaging and error free. Because of its position in the document, the executive summary is clearly the most critical section of the plan. In addition to the executive summary, the plan should also begin with a *table of contents*. This will both help the writer organize the plan and assist the reader in navigating the document.

The second section of the business plan is the *background and description*. Here, in a logical sequence, the plan should define the rationale for the program or service (i.e., the patient care need) and provide an explanation of why the organization is prepared to fill this need. The *service opportunity* provides the reader with a picture of the purpose of the proposed program and should lead directly to a description of the formal *mission of the business*. Finally, this section should provide other details that will help to illustrate the service, including data that may have been obtained from literature or other sources.

The next section of the business plan is the *market analysis and strategy*. In some cases, the market analysis is presented as a separate section from the marketing strategy. In either case, the market analysis is part of the situation analysis conducted during planning, whereas the marketing strategy is part of the goal-setting and strategy development elements of planning. In the business plan document, these are sometimes presented together because they address the same general topic.

The fourth major section of the business plan is the *operational structure and processes*. In brief, this section describes how the program will be run. This section of the document should provide details on how the service will be provided and by whom—in other words, the work processes that will occur. It should include information on how customers will interface with the program. The organizational structure, number and types of employees, and equipment and other resources used in operation of the program should be described. This section should also include definitions of the regulatory, clinical, and quality requirements that may be applicable to the business and a description of how these requirements will be met.

The fifth major section of the plan is the *financial projections* or *financial pro forma*. This section identifies the estimated expenditures and revenue over the first 3 to 5 years of the program. Investments required to begin and operate the program should be described as either start-up costs or ongoing costs (or operating costs) and should be organized by cost categories (e.g., salaries, equipment, capital, etc.). The financial data are best presented in a revenue and expense statement (sometimes referred to as the *profit and loss statement*), as shown in Table 7-1.

The sixth section of the business plan defines the *milestones, schedule,* and *action plan* for the program. A timeline should be defined that includes the major accomplishments and goals of the program for implementation and through the first 3 to 5 years and may include long-range growth and expansions objectives. The action plan may also include responsibility assignments and is often presented as a Gantt chart. For an example see Figure 7-2.

The next section of the business plan defines the *critical risks* and *opportunities* of the business. Here, the plan should outline the major strengths and weakness of the proposed business and describe the opportunities and risk associated with the program if implemented (as formulated in the SWOT analysis). This information, both positive and negative, must be presented in an unbiased manner so that an informed decision can be made about moving forward with the program.

The business plan should include a brief discussion of what will happen if the business should fail, or alternatively become very successful. This *exit strategy* or *contingency strategy* should define specifically when and how a decision would be made to exit the business. The section then should outline a plan for exiting the business. This plan might include issues such as what to do with existing patients or customers (i.e., refer to other providers), what will happen with existing staff (i.e., reassign to other divisions of the organization or terminate), and how equipment and resources may be disposed of.

The last section of the business plan is the *conclusion*. The conclusion should be brief in summarizing the document. Most importantly, the conclusion should provide a recommendation with respect to the proposed business decision. Following the conclusion are any *attachments* or *additional materials*. Supportive documentation, tables, figures, financial statements, and/or letters of support should be attached to the business plan to corroborate the written text or present the material in a more detailed fashion.

Presenting the Plan

The oral presentation of the business plan may be as important as the written document. In most organizations, those seeking to implement new programs must present the business plan before a group, usually consisting of senior leaders in the company.

A good oral presentation can go a long way toward garnering positive support for the business plan. The personal nature of the oral presentation may add dynamics to the decision-making process that do not exist with the written document. These issues, which include politics, group dynamics, and personal interactions, can be either positive or negative. In either case, these dynamics should be anticipated and either reinforced or pre-empted depending on the situation.

■ CONCLUSION

After reading this chapter, Ted Thompson should be prepared to address the charge given him in the scenario. Ted will recognize quickly that developing a business plan for the proposed specialty medication management service will be a significant undertaking. Ted would be well advised to seek assistance from others as he begins this planning process. For example, he might want to establish a team that would include representatives from the hospital finance department, other pharmacists who might be involved in the program, and perhaps even a physician or nurse with experience in managing specialty medications. Then the assembled team could begin the business plan planning process as outlined in this chapter. When this process is complete, Ted and his boss (the DOP) will need to follow the appropriate administrative channels within the organization to gain approval from key hospital decision makers.

Obviously, business planning is an important tool for gaining further acceptance and penetration of contemporary pharmacist services. New pharmacists must understand and be able to write business plans that will justify new or continued investments in these services. It is very likely that most new pharmacists will be expected to develop or help to develop a business plan for a pharmacy program at some point in their careers. Clearly, the ability to do so will benefit the pharmacist, the employer, and patients. If accepted, the new program may be an opportunity to provide new or unique services—thus heightening job satisfaction. Likewise, the new program may generate revenue or save costs elsewhere in the system, thus benefiting the employer. Patients, physicians, nurses, and others who are the recipients of the program will also benefit.

■ QUESTIONS FOR FURTHER DISCUSSION

1. Conduct a literature search to identify articles that may be pertinent to the business proposal described in the scenario. How many articles did you find, and how useful are they to understanding the business concept?

2. Conduct a hypothetical market and competitor analysis, and develop a marketing strategy for the specialty medication management program. What are the market segments that may be important to this business? What are the strengths and weaknesses of the proposed service compared with those of its potential competitors?

3. What are the important costs that would be incurred if the specialty medication management program were implemented? Classify these costs as fixed or variable.

4. Explain why you think an understanding of business planning is important for pharmacists. What changes are occurring in the health care environment that make business planning even more important?

REFERENCES

American Society of Health-System Pharmacists. ASHP Specialty pharmacy resource guide. 2016. Available at https://www.ashp.org/-/media/assets/pharmacy-practice/resource-centers/specialty-pharmacy/specialty-pharmacy-resource-guide.ashx. Accessed January 28, 2019.

Carroll NV. 2007. *Financial Management for Pharmacists: A Decision-Making Approach*, 3rd ed. Baltimore, MD: Lippincott Williams & Wilkins.

Chater RW, Moczygemba LR, Lawson KA, et al. 2008. Building the business model for medication therapy management services. *J Am Pharm Assoc* 48:16–22.

Chisholm-Burns MA, Kim Lee J, Spivey CA, et al. 2010. US pharmacists' effect as team members on patient care: Systematic review and meta-analyses. *Med Care* 48:923–933.

DeThomas AR, Derammelaere SA, Fox S. 2015. *Writing a Convincing Business Plan*, 4th ed. Hauppauge, NY: Barron's Educational Series.

Doucette WR, McDonough RP. 2002. Beyond the 4Ps: Using relationship marketing to build value and demand for pharmacy services. *J Am Pharm Assoc* 42:183–193.

Harris IM, Baker E, Berry TM, et al.; American College of Clinical Pharmacy. 2008. Developing a business-practice model for pharmacy services in ambulatory settings. *Pharmacotherapy* 28(2):285.

Holdford DA. 2007. *Marketing for Pharmacists*, 2nd ed. Washington, DC: American Pharmacists Association.

Kliethermes M. 2017. Understanding billing basics. *Pharmacy Today*. 2017;23(7):57–68.

Kliethermes M, Brown T. 2012. *Building a successful ambulatory care practice: A complete guide for pharmacists.* Bethesda, MD: American Society of Health-System Pharmacists.

Lofton J. 2012. *How to Start an MTM Practice: A Guidebook for Pharmacists.* Washington, DC: American Pharmaceutical Association.

McDonough R. 2007. Writing a business plan for a new pharmacy service. *The Dynamics of Pharmaceutical Care: Enriching Patients Health, Monograph 23.* Washington, DC: American Pharmacists Association. Available at https://www.pharmacist.com/sites/default/files/files/mtm_writing_business_plan.pdf. Accessed January 20, 2019.

McKeever M. 2014. *How to Write a Business Plan*, 12th ed. Berkeley, CA: NOLO Press.

Perez A, Doloresco F, Hoffman JM, et al.; American College of Clinical Pharmacy. 2009. Economic evaluations of clinical pharmacy services: 2001–2005. *Pharmacotherapy* 28(11):128.

Phillips CR, Larson LN. 2002. Creating a business plan for patient care. In Hagel HP, Rovers JP (eds.) *Managing the Patient-Centered Pharmacy.* Washington, DC: American Pharmaceutical Association.

Pinson L. 2014. *Anatomy of a Business Plan*, 8th ed. Tustin, CA: Out of Your Mind . . . and in to the Marketplace.

Sachdev G. 2014. Sustainable business models: Systematic approach toward successful ambulatory care pharmacy practice. *Am J Health Syst Pharm* 71:1366–1374.

Schumock G. 2000. Methods to assess the economic outcomes of clinical pharmacy services. *Pharmacotherapy* 20;243S–252S.

Schumock G, Butler M. 2003. Evaluating and justifying clinical pharmacy services. In Grauer D, Lee J, Odom T, et al. (eds.) *Pharmacoeconomics and Outcomes: Applications for Patient Care*, 2nd ed. Kansas City, MO: American College of Clinical Pharmacy.

Schumock G, Butler M, Meek P, et al. 2003. Evidence of the economic benefit of clinical pharmacy services: 1996–2000. *Pharmacotherapy* 23:113–132.

Schumock G, Stubbing J. 2018. *How to Develop a Business Plan for Pharmacy Services*, 3rd ed. Lenexa, KS: American College of Clinical Pharmacy.

Schumock G, Stubbings J, McBride SJ. 2004. Business planning and marketing. In *Developing a Senior Care Pharmacy Practice: Your Guide and Tools for Success.* Alexandria, VA: American Society of Consultant Pharmacists.

Stubbings J, Nutescu E, Durley S, Bauman J. 2011. Payment for clinical pharmacy services revisited. *Pharmacotherapy* 31:1–8.

Touchette DR, Doloresco F, Suda KJ, et al. 2014. Economic evaluations of clinical pharmacy services: 2006–2010. *Pharmacotherapy* 34:771–793.

Wilson A. 2008. *Financial Management Basics for Health-System Pharmacists.* Bethesda, MD: American Society of Health-System Pharmacists.

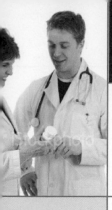

8

OPERATIONS MANAGEMENT

Greg L. Alston and William Wynn

About the Authors: Dr. Alston is an Associate Dean and professor, Savannah Campus, South University School of Pharmacy. He has over 30 years of experience in community pharmacy management, both as a chain pharmacy administrator and an independent pharmacy owner. He earned a Doctor of Pharmacy (PharmD) degree from the University of the Pacific and has published three best-selling management books, *The Bosshole Effect—Managing People Simplified, The Ten Things A New Manager Must Get Right From the Start*, and *Own Your Value—The Real Future of Pharmacy Practice*. His passion lies in teaching the next generation of pharmacists how to create value for the stakeholders they serve and learn the business skills they need to thrive.

Dr. William Wynn is a graduate of Medical University of South Carolina (B.S. 1997) and University of South Carolina (PharmD 1999), currently living in Blythewood, South Carolina. William was a Revco and CVS Pharmacist with a community pharmacy career from 1997 to 2009, serving as a staff pharmacist, pharmacist in charge, and pharmacy supervisor, managing up to twenty stores and hundreds of employees. As Assistant Professor, Experiential Education Coordinator, and Director of Interprofessional Education for the Columbia Campus of South University, most of his classroom time is dedicated to management, advocacy, leadership, our ever changing health care system, and pharmacoeconomics. William is a former President of the South Carolina Pharmacy Association (SCPhA), and currently serves on SCPhA's and South Carolina Society of Health-System Pharmacist's legislative committees. Nationally, William has served the American Pharmacists Association (APhA) House of Delegates for 9 of the past 10 years, the APhA House of Delegates New Business Committee for 1 year and the American Association of Colleges of Pharmacy (AACP) Faculty House of Delegates for 2 years. William is also an AACP Academic Leadership Fellow, the recipient of the Smith Drug Visionary Leadership Award, the Class of 2019 Teacher of the Year at South University, and the 2018 South Carolina Ken Couch Distinguished Mentor Award.

■ LEARNING OBJECTIVES

After completing this chapter, readers should be able to:

1. Define the role of the business in society and the role of profits in business.
2. Define the role of operations management within a business.
3. Describe the concept of command intent.
4. Describe how operations managers accomplish the command intent of an organization.
5. Describe the essential operations management tasks.
6. Illuminate differences between a production worker and a knowledge worker.
7. Describe Human Sigma as a model for customer service operations.
8. Equate the management process to the Pharmacists' Patient Care Process.

■ SCENARIO

Trey Smith, PharmD, is the pharmacy manager at Smith's Drug, a small independent pharmacy. His pharmacy performs regular dispensing, custom compounding, and sells a line of durable medical equipment. Trey has recently lost one of his senior technicians to a competitor and has since hired a new associate, Lisa. It is Trey's responsibility to ensure that every member of Smith's Drugs staff is adequately trained in the pharmacy's workflow. Lisa has no prior experience in pharmacy, but is willing to give a great effort and wants to be well trained so that she can be an asset to the pharmacy team. Trey has outlined a plan with Lisa to get her up to speed on how to count and label prescriptions, how to compound medications, and perform third-party billing procedures. One of the most experienced technicians at Smith's Drug, Bill, often handles the position in the pharmacy that offers the greatest challenge—that is, where the patients drop off their prescriptions for entry into the computer system. As part of the training plan for Lisa, Trey has decided to let her train at the drop-off position on Wednesday afternoons when the pharmacy's business is slower so that she can work on inputting prescription and insurance information. This plan has worked quite well for the past 2 weeks, but on this particular Wednesday there happens to be a festival going on just up the street from the pharmacy. This

had led to an influx of customers, and prescriptions are beginning to pile up at Lisa's station. Customer waiting time for prescriptions has increased from 10 minutes to 25 minutes. What is the most appropriate course of action for Trey to take to ensure the success of his business?

■ CHAPTER QUESTIONS

1. What is the role of a business in society?
2. What is the role of profits in a business?
3. What do operations managers do to help their business achieve its goals?
4. What is command intent? How can it be applied to pharmacy operations?
5. What is Human Sigma? How can it be applied to pharmacy operations?

■ INTRODUCTION

The first two chapters of this book described the domains of patient-oriented pharmacy practice and its intersections with the managerial sciences. This chapter will deal with the domain of business management and the science of operations.

When most people think of the concept of management and what it is that managers do, they are envisioning operations managers. Operations managers are often referred to as "front-line" managers, as they typically are involved in directly overseeing a business' major functions (e.g., dispensing prescriptions in a community pharmacy, preparing medication orders in a hospital). While operations managers typically have input with the executive team on all phases of the management of a company, this chapter will focus on those functions that are the primary responsibility of the operations manager.

After the executive team creates the vision and mission statements for a business, it is the responsibility of operations managers to execute the vision and mission in compliance with the values of the organization. Operations managers must make the daily decisions required to keep the business moving in the right direction. Operations management involves a variety of tasks that managers perform to control, organize, and lead the work team to fulfill the goals and objectives of the organization.

All business processes require that management effort be routinely applied to remain effective. Pharmacy dispensing and professional services are no different. Whether you see yourself in a formal administrative position (e.g., chief pharmacist, pharmacy director, assistant or associate director, clinical coordinator) or as a staff pharmacist, the reality is that the highest ranking pharmacist on duty must play the role of the professional operations manager to ensure the provision of quality patient care.

■ THE ROLE OF BUSINESS IN SOCIETY AND THE ROLE OF PROFITS IN A BUSINESS

It is important to first discuss the role of a business in society, especially a professional business such as pharmacy. The profession of pharmacy exists in society to provide a variety of goods and services related to optimizing medication and health outcomes. These goods and services provide an array of benefits to patients, health care providers, and society at large.

The primary role of any pharmacy in society should be to benefit those that they serve, not necessarily to make money for pharmacy owners. Yet, if *any* pharmacy fails to bring in enough revenue to cover their expenses, the pharmacy will not be able to continue to provide goods and services that create benefits for others. And for a for-profit organization in a market-based economy (e.g., most community pharmacies in the United States), pharmacies must be able to generate a profit (the excess of revenues over expenses) large enough to justify an owner's investment in the organization. If pharmacies cannot generate profits, owners will lack incentives to invest in pharmacies, leaving patients and society without the benefits they provide.

Management expert Peter Drucker echoes this idea of businesses existing to serve society. A company should focus on serving its customers, and profits are simply a required resource for the company to continue to serve society (Drucker, 1973). Money and profits do play a role in a pharmacy, and that is to keep the pharmacy solvent so that it can continue to provide its highly needed goods and services to society.

A good way to demonstrate how this principle works is to ask the following question.

Why Did You Choose Pharmacy as a Career Path?

While interviewing for admission to a PharmD program, students are often asked why they would like to become pharmacists. Prospective students are afraid to mention money and income as a motivator to enter the profession because they fear this motivation will appear unprofessional. The typical response from a prospective student is something like, "I want to help people" in an effort to appeal to the sense of altruism commonly found among health care professionals.

Now ask another question. If pharmacists were paid only minimum wage, would people still be so inclined to enroll in pharmacy school? Over the course of their professional education (not including pre-pharmacy studies), the average pharmacy student with debt will accumulate over $164,000 of student loan debt (American Association of Colleges of Pharmacy, 2017). If the minimum wage was $15 an hour, a full-time pharmacist working 2080 hours per year would only earn $31,200 per year. A total of $164,000 of student loans paid back at 7% interest over 10 years would cost $22,850 a year in student loan payments alone. That would leave a pharmacist making minimum wage with less than $695 a month to live on. Most pharmacists, like almost everyone who pursues a higher education, would like to seek a greater return on investment of their time, effort, and financial resources.

What this points out is that there are economic and financial realities to any business and any profession. If the external mission (that is seen by the public) of any business is to serve society, and the internal mission (what is vital to the organization itself) is to provide income for the operators of the business, then it is not just the business owners that benefit from an organization's profits. Society benefits by having a valuable service provided. And all employee salaries, benefits, and professional development activities are paid out of the income generated by any business. Whether the business is a for-profit organization (like most community pharmacies) or a not-for-profit organization (like many hospitals and organizations which provide care as a charity) the rules do not change, someone has to pay the bills.

The Role of Operations Management within a Business

It is the role of operations managers in any business to ensure the smooth functioning of the business unit to achieve both its public and private missions. This was expertly outlined by Peter Drucker (1973):

> And the manager in public-service institutions faces the same tasks as the manager in a business: to perform the function for the sake of which the institution exists; to make work productive and the worker achieving; to manage the institution's social impacts and to discharge its social responsibilities [p. 32].

An operations manager must understand the vision, mission, and goals of the organization to direct his or her workforce. The management structure of an organization requires multiple roles to be played. Typically large public corporations will have a chief executive officer (CEO) whose responsibility is to direct the strategic planning of the organization, a chief financial officer (CFO) who directs the budget and financing activities of the organization, and the chief operating officer (COO) who is responsible for the day-to-day operations of the business. In a small business (e.g., an independent community pharmacy, a consulting firm), a single person (e.g., a pharmacy owner, a consultant) may play all of these roles.

The operations manager focuses the energy and intent of the organization on what must be done today to accomplish the long-term goals of the business. These focused activities must align with the vision, mission, and values of the organization. The executive team creates the goals or "marching orders" for the organization. An operations manager must understand the intent of the orders and the results of potential actions to avoid disaster and ensure success.

At the most basic level, operations managers decide:

1. What must be done right now?
2. Who needs to be doing it?
3. What resources do they need?
4. When is the work finished?

It may be helpful to think of operations management in terms of the critical decisions that need to be made by operations managers. The ten decisions under the purview of operations management are described by Heizer and Render (1999) in Table 8-1.

Not all tactics and directives employed by operations managers are equally successful. However, operations managers are ultimately responsible for modifying their directives until the results are successful. All business tactics and directives must occur within the framework of the values held by the business. Tactics and directives that contradict the company's ideals, even though they may achieve financial goals, are not acceptable. For example, suppose that a pharmacy condoned the selling of cigarettes to teenagers without identification. The pharmacy could make a lot of money selling cigarettes to teenagers. But at the same time, this tactic would be illegal

Table 8-1. Decisions under the Purview of Operations Managers

Designing goods and services	What should be offered for sale and at what price? How should the business arrange the price and service component of the product to maximize perceived value using the relative value theorem?
Process strategies	What is the best workflow methodology to ensure productivity?
Managing quality	How do we provide sufficient productivity while maintaining impeccable quality?
Location strategies	Where is the best location for this service to be offered?
Layout strategies	What is the best physical layout to ensure productivity? Does this layout fit with the pharmacy's workflow process?
Human resources	How do you motivate and inspire people to do excellent work? How can you develop engaged employees that represent your brand and develop relationships with your customers?
Scheduling	When and where should each employee be when our customers need service?
Supply chain management	Which suppliers will best help the company meet the needs of our customers?
Inventory management	How does the business insure that it will have enough without having too much or too little inventory?
Maintenance	How can the business keep all the equipment and facilities in good working order?

Data from Heizer J, Render B. 1999. *Operations Management*, 5th ed. Upper Saddle River, NJ: Prentice-Hall.

as well as contradict the health and wellness missions held by most pharmacies.

The Theory of Command Intent

It could be argued that the most challenging component of managing a pharmacy's operations is managing its human resources. A manager cannot supervise what every employee is doing all day long. The manager must find a way to ensure that employees are working on the right tasks at the right time. In addition to understanding the fundamentals of human resources management (see Chapters 16–18, 20), operations managers must develop plans and communicate them effectively. The business has no hope of achieving its goals without a clearly communicated plan of action.

A useful strategy to ensure that this is accomplished is known as *command intent* (Shattuck, 2000). The U.S. Army has determined that the most successful battlefield commanders are the ones who

are able to think critically and change tactics during a mission, while still working toward the ultimate goal of capturing a strategic location, cutting off a supply line, or achieving a military objective. Good leaders are aware of the command intent of their orders and understand that circumstances constantly change while in battle or in a pharmacy. As conditions have changed the military has clarified the differences between intent, commander's intent, and command intent. Merriam Webster's dictionary definition of Intent: a usually clearly formulated or planned intention is contrasted with the department of defense description of commander's intent as, "a concise expression of the purpose of the operation and the desired end state that serves as the initial impetus for the planning process. It may also include the commander's assessment of the adversary commander's intent and an assessment of where and how much risk is acceptable during the operation," (Hieb & Schade, 2007).

Command intent gives a description of what the desired outcome is in relation to the current mission. That is, the command intent focuses on the endpoint, and does not summarize how to achieve that endpoint. The idea being that it will focus subordinates on what needs to get done, even when monumental change is encountered on the battlefield and the original plans are no longer able to be applied. The U.S. Army General George S. Patton summarized this philosophy by stating, "Never tell people how to do things. Tell them what to do and they will surprise you with their ingenuity." The commander who gives very precise battle plan orders, but does not communicate the command intent to his or her subordinates is at risk of exposing soldiers to disastrous consequences. The battle never goes exactly as planned, so if the troops are not able to adjust to the constantly shifting tide of battle, they could be more easily defeated.

The concept of command intent can be applied to pharmacy operations management. An example of a vision statement for a community pharmacy may be "To be a recognized leader in customer service by providing affordable, timely, and effective drug therapies to improve our patients' lives." There are many tasks involved in the day-to-day operations of a pharmacy to strive to accomplish its vision and achieve success. These include ordering medications and supplies, stocking shelves, receiving and entering patients' prescriptions, printing labels and filling vials, verifying accuracy of orders, checking out customers, counseling patients, and offering a variety of patient care services. These tasks should be accomplished as efficiently and effectively as possible. But how does a manager know when to change the priority of the tasks? In a busy pharmacy, circumstances may change at any given moment, making it difficult for technicians and service employees to know the best task to perform at any given moment.

To continue this example, assume that the pharmacy's order of medications and over-the-counter goods from their warehouse normally arrives on Tuesday mornings. The pharmacy manager may plan to have additional clerks scheduled to work Tuesday mornings, ensuring that technicians have clear access to shelves, preventing delays in filling prescriptions and improving inventory control. If on any Tuesday morning one of the additional clerks calls in sick, the priorities of the pharmacy manager and other employees may need to shift. Even if the pharmacy manager is off duty and is not directly supervising associates, the command intent of his or her orders needs to be followed. If the pharmacy manager has communicated his or her command intent properly, the employees will immediately recognize the priority of customer service and cease putting away the order to help meet customer demand. The staff should be able to adjust the command from "put away the order" to "serve the customers" without facing discipline.

Managers who give orders without providing a command intent context may unintentionally imply that putting away an order from the warehouse is more important than customer service. This type of rigid top down order giving can make employees feel powerless to make changes regarding how key tasks are accomplished. It also psychologically relieves employees of any responsibility that they might have felt to rectify a faulty directive and do what they know to be the real mission of the business. This ultimately creates inefficient operations. When an operations manager communicates command intent to associates and subordinates, the statement should be brief, and it should promote flexibility so that resources can be most efficiently utilized to accomplish tasks.

How Do Operations Managers Carry Out Command Intent?

Once the operations manager knows the command intent and how to communicate it, how do they use this knowledge to guide their daily actions? An operations manager must set specific goals for what needs to be accomplished at the pharmacy. These goals must be set in real time based on an accurate assessment of the situation.

Examples of operational goals can be seen in Table 8-2.

Regardless of the work environment, any list of operational goals should be formulated with feedback

Table 8-2.   Example Operational Goals for a Pharmacist Manager

Goal 1—Improving the speed and efficiency of patient service.
a. Are there bottlenecks in the workflow?
b. Is the pharmacist's time being used efficiently?
c. Is the business meeting its productivity goals?

Goal 2—Offering more services to patients.
a. Is there a service that a pharmacy's customers want or need that they are not currently providing?
b. Can they provide this service at their traditional standard of quality?
c. Do they have the expertise and talent to make it work?

Goal 3—Creating and maintaining a collegial work environment for employees.
a. Do employees enjoy working at the pharmacy?
b. Are they challenged to excel?
c. Does the team work well together when it matters?

Goal 4—Improving the knowledge of health care team members.
a. Can the pharmacy staff use their talents to improve the efforts of others?
b. By identifying problem areas and resolving those problems, can the pharmacy improve their efficiency?
c. Can the pharmacist positively influence patient outcomes by educating others?

from employees, customers, and management. The list should be clear, concise, and align with the overarching vision of the business.

Executive-level management sets the vision and mission for the long-term value strategy of an organization. Operations managers use this guidance to create the goals or command intents of the business. The operations manager then must turn these goals into actions that create results. While the executive team views the mental process as "set the goals to direct the actions," the frontline employees view the process as "complete the actions to achieve the goals."

The primary challenge for operations managers is to bridge the two points of view to create success.

In the context of the military, if the commanding officer is unable to continue in command, the next highest ranked officer takes over to ensure continuity of command. In the pharmacy world, if the pharmacy supervisor is not present or able to provide guidance at a particular time, a staff pharmacist must perform the operations management roles for the organization to be successful. This is a very common occurrence in pharmacies, in that there is no practical way in which an administrator can oversee or direct every event in a pharmacy. This is another of the many reasons why all pharmacists, from administrators to staff pharmacists, must have some degree of management skills (see Chapter 2).

When an administrator with a formal supervisory role (e.g., pharmacy manager, pharmacist in charge, director of pharmacy, etc.) is off duty or otherwise unable to perform his or her role, it must be clear to the work team who is in charge. In health care professions, the professional authority bestowed upon practitioners (e.g., pharmacists, physicians) does not allow them to abdicate their authority over the patient care process. When choices must be made to keep the daily activities (e.g., appropriate care of patients) aligned with the command intent of the organization (e.g., maximizing sales), the health care professional on duty should have the authority to make that call. For example, pharmacists must have the authority to refuse to fill a prescription if the prescription would harm the patient, even though the command intent of maximizing sales may not be met in this particular case. Good pharmacists and operations managers realize that there are alternative methods to meet the command intent that do not put patient care at risk.

What Tasks Do Operations Managers Actually Perform?

Once a list of goals is established for the pharmacy, operations managers are charged with coming up with specific plans of action to meet these goals. Each goal is likely to have a number of tasks associated with it. These tasks drive what pharmacy managers do on a day-to-day basis. These tasks will change depending on the circumstances of the day, and the ways to accomplish these tasks can change. The tasks are what employees must complete to accomplish the command intent of the pharmacy.

For example, the list of operational goals previously mentioned can be expanded into specific action tasks for a pharmacy manager to use to direct his or her staff. By focusing on action steps, in the context of the business mission, the command intent of the organization can be clarified for employees. General goals such as "improving sales" do not belong on an action list. When the action list items are completed, a natural consequence will be an increase in sales.

Action steps are clear, concise, and can be acted upon in a short period. Review the action steps in Table 8-3. Do you think the command intent is clear and unambiguous?

These are just a few examples of the types of tasks that pharmacy operations managers can develop. The tasks will change depending on the circumstances. The daily activities must change to meet the command intent of the organization. Operations managers must get the job done irrespective of the previously determined corporate plan.

For a business to operate successfully its employees must operate in alignment with the mission, vision, and values of the organization. Historically, management practices were built upon the industrial

Table 8-3.	Example Actions Steps to Drive Performance	
Goal #1: Improving the speed and efficiency of patient service. Many different tasks can be derived from this goal:	1. Cross train staff members to do each other's jobs. 2. Redesign the workflow to smooth out bottlenecks. 3. Upgrade the computer systems. 4. Add an additional computer terminal. 5. Take shorter lunch breaks to cover a staffing shortage.
Goal #2: Offering more services to patients. There are many different services that customers may want or need. Are there services that a pharmacy could add that would provide a good return on their investment?	1. Develop a customer survey to identify unmet needs. 2. Conduct a customer focus group with ten customers. 3. Ask every employee to identify profitable opportunities. 4. Get all pharmacists immunization certified. 5. Create a layout plan for a new private counseling room.
Goal #3: Creating and maintaining a collegial work environment for employees. There are many simple things that a manager can do to make work more enjoyable:	1. Create a professional development plan for each employee. 2. Take one employee out for a private lunch each week. 3. Catch employees doing something well and praise them immediately. 4. Develop a corrective action plan for the employee who is always late. 5. Rotate job assignments during slow afternoon hours.
Goal #4: Improving the knowledge of health care team members. One low-risk strategy for expanding a pharmacy manager's sphere of influence as a professional is to devote time and energy to improving the functional knowledge and skills of other providers:	1. Provide educational seminar on new drug developments. 2. Provide educational seminar on Medicare Part D annual plan changes. 3. Provide a lunch meeting for physician office staff to explain formulary changes. 4. Create a drug chart to assist prescribers in selecting the preferred drug for their patients.

factory model that came into vogue with the development of the industrial revolution in the 19th and early 20th centuries (see Chapter 2). As the economy moved from one of industrial production to one based on service jobs, Peter Drucker (1973) formalized the concept of a new type of worker distinct from a production worker that he called a knowledge worker:

> The basic capital resource, the fundamental investment, but also the cost center of a developed economy, is the knowledge worker who puts to work what he has learned in systematic education, that is, concepts, ideas, and theories, rather than the man who puts to work manual skill or muscle. [p. 32]

Drucker envisioned the importance of the knowledge worker in today's society. He hypothesized that the knowledge worker cannot be productive unless he or she is allowed to figure out how they work best, and to modify their routine accordingly.

There are some key differences between a production job and a knowledge worker job. Factory production lines are optimized to control every step of the process to produce identical products of consistent quality. Knowledge jobs typically revolve around customer service. Customer service "production" is different from factory line production because the end product is different depending on the customer.

To manage a customer service "production line," the employee must be empowered to figure out what the customer needs, and then modify the process to deliver the correct product. Knowledge workers now far outnumber factory workers in the US economy. Knowledge workers need to be managed differently than production line employees (see Chapter 2).

Health care in general, and pharmacy in particular, cannot be effectively managed using production line management techniques because health care is essentially a customer service business. While many of the activities that pharmacists perform on a daily basis mimic a factory production line, there are critical distinctions that must be made. These distinctions are not based on the processes used, as the dispensing activities performed in pharmacies physically resemble a process-driven assembly line. Nevertheless, pharmacists do not just assemble prescriptions accurately; they are also responsible for knowing when prescriptions should not be filled, how medications should be appropriately used, and what to tell patients and their caregivers to help them get the most from their medications. The critical distinctions are that a pharmacist's professional license demands that they evaluate whether the prescription order is appropriate for the end-user and that they modify the order to achieve the intended outcome. Practically speaking, they must use their professional knowledge to deliver, or refuse to deliver, the proper product to the correct patient.

The professional knowledge component of what pharmacists do is the personification of a knowledge worker. Even though prescriptions are written and dispensed correctly the vast majority of the time, the time one could not lead to potentially devastating complications. One of the roles of the pharmacist is to ensure that medication errors and their sequelae are avoided. The efficient production of prescriptions must always be tempered with a healthy dose of professional judgment.

Pharmacy is not simply a production job where the same product has to be provided in the same fashion to every customer. The command intent of any pharmacy will involve providing high-quality patient care. Pharmacy is a customer service-driven profession that requires tailored approaches to each individual. A pharmacist needs to be able to apply their years of advanced training and knowledge to ensure that the right patient receives the right dose, of the right medication, at the right time, and in the right way.

Principles of Human Sigma

As mentioned earlier, it would not be difficult to argue that the most important aspect of managing a pharmacy is managing the people who work there. A pharmacy's employees are providing the myriad of goods and services to patients and customers. Many service-oriented industries have tried to apply quality control principles that were designed for production line models. Perhaps the most famous of these models is the Six Sigma program originated by the Motorola Corporation. Six Sigma assumes that output quality improves by eliminating defects in the production of the product (Pyzdek, 2003). The primary approach to performance improvement is based on the model known as DMAIC (Gygi et al., 2005):

1. *Define*
2. *Measure*
3. *Analyze*
4. *Improve*
5. *Control*

The intent of the Six Sigma approach is to create high quality, identical outputs from standardized inputs. Many hospitals and health care systems use the Six Sigma approach to improve the quality of patient care. However, recent evidence suggests that this type of quality improvement process breaks down in a customer service enterprise. Unlike a production line, consumers of services desire and need different outputs, and those desires and needs are framed by the circumstances of that specific encounter. For example, no two patient encounters are identical, even if they are getting the same medication for the same condition.

The Gallup organization recognized this potential inability of Six Sigma to address a customer service environment effectively, and consequently spent a great deal of time and energy researching customer service encounters. The insights gathered from their research led to the development of the Human Sigma project.

The Human Sigma is based on the five fundamental principles.

- *Rule 1: You cannot measure and manage the employee and customer experiences as separate entities.* This essentially means that employee and customer experiences should be measured and managed under the same department. The employee-customer experience is directly linked, and to manage them separately would be inefficient.
- *Rule 2: Emotion frames the employee-customer encounter.* This suggests that the customers that contribute

the most loyalty, and therefore the most business, to a company are the ones that feel an emotional connection with it. Customers that passionately advocate for the company through word-of-mouth advertising are the backbone of any successful business. Employees should be managed to develop this kind of deep relationship with customers, and performance metrics should be oriented toward measuring these emotional connections.

- *Rule 3: You must measure and manage the employee-customer encounter at a local level.* In an environment where there are multiple locations run by the same management, it would be easy to assume that all locations will achieve the same results. This assumption could not be farther from the truth. Even if all locations have the same process strategies, policies, regulations, and expectations, there will still be a significant variance between their outputs. This is primarily due to differences in the "who" factor. Who is managing the location that is not performing? Who is working there as the face of the brand to the public? Engaging these people and giving them the command intent that they need will improve local performance.
- *Rule 4: We can quantify and summarize the effectiveness of the employee-customer encounter in a single performance measure—the Human Sigma metric— that is powerfully related to financial performance.* This rule suggests that there is one performance metric that strongly predicts the success and future organic growth of a company. It is known as the Human Sigma metric, and it involves the levels of customer and employee engagement. The evidence has shown that, when combined together, high levels of customer and employee engagement achieve synergy. The sum of the two is greater than the parts. Just having high levels one or the other will provide a degree of success, but balance between the two should be striven for.
- *Rule 5: Improvement in local Human Sigma performance requires deliberate and active intervention through attention to a combination of transactional and transformational intervention activities.* Managers should gather the correct data in order to

efficiently evaluate their company's performance and set goals. Improvement strategies should be custom tailored to each department's (or individual's) level of engagement. Finally, rewards and recognition should be designed to promote an increased sense of pride in employees' responsibilities and encourage improvement.

It is important for pharmacists to understand that business management of the health care enterprise is essentially identical to the Pharmacists' Patient Care Process as described in the literature (Joint Commission of Pharmacy Practitioners, 2014) (see Table 8-4). Because of pharmacy's rich history as a community-based business the pharmacy has a unique role in the health care system. The pharmacist must balance the commercial interests of the operation with the obligation to act in the best interest of the patient. This adds complexity to business decisions and challenges the pharmacist to be a health care provider first and a business owner second.

Human Sigma data helps explain why scripting employee and customer relations does not work well and has the potential to backfire. Consider the following example of a production line Six Sigma management style mistake made at a pharmacy operation.

John is a pharmacist at a large chain pharmacy. The company has a library of training resources that are provided to each new employee. Among these resources are scripted strategies to deal with a customer when a medication error has been made. The scripts are designed to placate the customer and decrease the likelihood of losing them as a patron or being sued. A key strategy for addressing the issue involves waiving the patient's co-payment and providing them with a gift card as compensation.

Marie calls the pharmacy after noticing that her new prescription looks different from previous orders. John takes Marie's call, and after some research, discovers that Marie's prescription was filled for hydralazine 25 mg instead of hydroxyzine 25 mg. John follows the steps outlined in his training manual, explaining the mistake and letting Marie know that he would call her doctor. John then follows his corporate script and offers to refund her co-pay and give her a gift card.

Table 8-4.   Patient Care versus Business Care Process

Pharmacists' Patient Care Process Step	Example in Clinical Practice	Example in the Business Process
Goals	Process Goal: Improve patient outcomes	Process Goal: Improve business outcomes
Collect	History of present illness, Labs, Blood pressure, Weight	Income, Cash flow, Balance sheet
Assess	Is the patient improving toward their treatment goal?	Is the business performing on its key performance indicators?
Plan	What has to be modified to create improvement?	What has to be modified to create improvement?
Implement	Execute the plan	Execute the plan
Follow-up, Monitor, and Evaluate	Check progress, monitor the right markers, and adjust as needed	Check progress, monitor the right markers, and adjust as needed

Data from Joint Commission of Pharmacy Practitioners. Pharmacists' Patient Care Process. May 29, 2014. Available at: https://jcpp.net/wp-content/uploads/2016/03/PatientCareProcess-with-supporting-organizations.pdf. Accessed Feb 1, 2019.

However, Marie does not respond the way the corporate script outlines and anticipates. She becomes offended by the suggestion that her problem can be bought off with a gift card. She didn't want money, she just wanted someone to fix the mistake and deliver it to her home. The mechanical use of the script made her feel like the company was trying to buy her off. She was insulted and transferred all of her prescriptions to another pharmacy.

This connects back to the earlier discussion of command intent in pharmacy management. It is important that pharmacy operations managers emphasize the desired outcome and not try to micromanage every aspect of pharmacy associates' jobs, especially the encounters they have with customers. Fleming and Asplund (2007) mention that inefficiencies may result when policies take away too much of employees' flexibility in engaging customers:

> Once an employee becomes accustomed to ignoring customer comments or behaviors because they don't conform to the steps in the script the employee is required to follow in a given situation, employees will be primed to ignore customers in all situations. [p. 178]

If John had been given more freedom, he could have listened to Marie and determined her desired outcome and then made the effort to fix the mistake for her in a more engaging manner. Even though an error had been committed and Marie was displeased, John had an opportunity to take care of her and through the outcome, instill a sense of deeper connection between Marie and the pharmacy. When training associates on customer service, operations managers should emphasize flexibility and the outcome desired, and then let the employee with the most intimate knowledge of the situation develop the best approach to achieve the desired outcome. This begins to explain a key difference between a transactional-based customer service model and that of a relational-based model. There will likely be instances during high volume moments that a transaction will need to occur in an expedient, yet professional nature. In the short term, this may suffice to retain a customer, but for the long-term relationship that every organization strives for, a more personal and emotional interaction needs to consistently take place, which defines the characteristics of a relational-based model.

Human Sigma data also suggest that to form long-lasting relationships with customers and make them value a company above its competitors, the company must go beyond simply trying to achieve customer satisfaction. Companies must try to engage their customers on a deeper level. Engaging customers on an emotional level is what will gain their trust and loyalty. Rationally satisfied customers are those who can logically justify that the service they received was satisfactory but are not necessarily emotionally invested. Emotionally satisfied customers feel a strong emotional commitment to the company and people who have given them excellent service.

In fact, Gallup research shows that little difference exists between the behavior of rationally satisfied customers and dissatisfied customers, but the behavior of emotionally satisfied customers is strikingly different. Emotionally satisfied patrons frequently visit more often and tend to spend more money with each visit (Fleming & Asplund, 2007).

How could a pharmacy operations manager engage his or her pharmacy's customers at a deeper, emotional level? Operations managers should start by recognizing that most customer engagement occurs at the level of their frontline employees, those that directly interact with customers. Ongoing coaching sessions with frontline employees will help improve employee-customer engagement. Operations managers and frontline employees should recognize that every interaction is a potential opportunity to further enhance the emotional connection of the customer. Employees that are also engaged directly with a company will want the company to succeed, and will more actively pursue tactics and directives to achieve mutual success. In addition, they will have a more thorough understanding of a company's short- and long-term goals.

The quality of the local operations manager is a critical ingredient in creating a highly productive workplace. Managers who consistently keep their employees engaged produce superior results for their organization.

The four dimensions of employee engagement as defined by Gallup suggest that employees base their engagement level at work on these dimensions. They essentially want answers to the following questions: (1) What do I get as a result of working here? (2) What do I have to give to be of value? (3) Do I belong in this organization? (4) How can I grow and excel as a part of this team?

As a manager, what you do and how you act is more important than what you say. If a manager tells employees what he or she are going to do for them, but then they never get around to doing it, they have unintentionally communicated to their employees that they are not important. If a manager threatens to discipline an employee who is always late, but the manager never gets around to it, the manager has unintentionally communicated that he or she does not really care if employees are always late. If a manager criticizes employees when they do something wrong, but does not praise them when they do something right, the manager has unintentionally communicated that giving extra effort is not important. However, if a manager treats everyone fairly, refuses to accept less than everyone's best effort, and delivers on his or her promises, the manager and their organization are much more likely to be successful.

■ REVISITING THE SCENARIO

As the prescriptions start to back up at the drop off station, Trey must recognize that the operational goals have suddenly shifted, and he must compose and deliver new command intent to his associates. Trey needs to associate tasks with the goal, and to determine which tasks should be delegated to Bill and Lisa. Bill and Lisa should both recognize the new directive, and Bill should reassume the spot where he has more expertise than Lisa. This will ensure that customers are taken care of in a timely fashion. It is important that Trey not try to manage how his technicians handle the situation. Once he gives the new tasks, Trey

must trust Bill and Lisa to do what is necessary in the way that best suits their individual strengths and weaknesses. When they are given the freedom to make decisions and direct their own success, Trey's employees will develop a closer connection and sense of pride in their jobs. This is especially true if the appropriate recognition is provided for a job well done. An increase in the quality of customers' experiences and their engagement level with Smith's Drug is to be expected once Trey's employees become more concerned with the pharmacy's success.

■ CONCLUSIONS

The primary role of operations managers in a pharmacy environment is to manage the human resources and tasks derived from the pharmacy's goals to produce quality customer service. This transformation of human resources and physical goods into a custom solution for each individual patient is what distinguishes pharmacy from most "production worker" styles of business. Goals should be derived from the overarching vision of the pharmacy, and daily tasks are developed from these goals. Tasks should be clear, concise, and measurable. Operations managers must prioritize tasks for completion, realizing that not everything can simultaneously be accomplished and that circumstances may change the order in which tasks need to be approached. Operations managers should communicate clear and unambiguous command intent to employees and allow them appropriate flexibility to best accomplish these specific tasks. Finally, the operations manager should understand that inspiring engaged employee is the key to creating engaged and loyal customers.

The daily work of the operations manager is to get the tasks:

1. Done right
2. In a timely fashion
3. Consistent with the values of the organization
4. In a way that creates long-term value for all the stakeholders in the business

■ QUESTIONS FOR FURTHER DISCUSSION

1. Write an imaginary mission statement that outlines the reasons that your pharmacy exists.
2. As a community pharmacy operations manager, develop a command intent statement to deliver to your staff to accomplish the following goal: Educate local prescribers on the various compounding services offered at the pharmacy.
3. Identify specific tasks that can be derived from the following operational goal: Increase the efficiency of the pharmacy's drive-through service.
4. Identify operational strategies that can be used to more deeply engage customers.

REFERENCES

American Association of Colleges of Pharmacy. Graduating Student Survey 2017 National Summary Report. 2017. Available at https://www.aacp.org/sites/default/files/2017-10/2017_GSS_National%20Summary%20Report.pdf. Accessed April 13, 2019.

Drucker PF. 1973. *Management: Tasks, Responsibilities, Practices.* New York, NY: Harper & Row.

Fleming JH, Asplund J. 2007. *Human Sigma: Managing the Employee—Customer Encounter.* New York, NY: Gallup Press.

Gygi C, DeCarlo N, Williams B. 2005. *Six Sigma for Dummies.* Hoboken, NJ: Wiley Publishing, Inc.

Heizer J, Render B. 1999. *Operations Management,* 5th ed. Upper Saddle River, NJ: Prentice-Hall.

Hieb MR, Schade U. 2007. Formalizing command intent through development of a command and control grammar (i-069). In *12th International Command and Control Research and Technology Symposium.*

Joint Commission of Pharmacy Practitioners (JCPP). 2014. Available at https://jcpp.net/wp-content/uploads/2016/03/PatientCareProcess-with-supporting-organizations.pdf. Accessed Feb 1, 2019.

Pyzdek T. 2003. *The Six Sigma Handbook.* New York, NY: McGraw-Hill.

Shattuck LG. 2000. *Communicating Intent and Imparting Presence.* Fort Leavenworth, KS: Army Combined Arms Center Military Review.

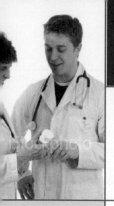

9

MANAGING TECHNOLOGY THAT SUPPORTS THE MEDICATION USE PROCESS

Brent I. Fox and Mark H. Siska

About the Authors: Brent I. Fox is an associate professor of Health Outcomes Research and Policy at the Harrison School of Pharmacy at Auburn University. He received his PharmD from Auburn and then worked in the software development industry prior to returning to Auburn, where he earned his PhD. Brent's education, outreach, and research efforts focus on improving medication-related outcomes through health information technology.

Mark H. Siska is the Chief Pharmacy Informatics Officer at the Mayo Clinic. Mark is the past Chair of the American Society of Health-System Pharmacists Section of Informatics and Technology and has served or continues to serve on a number of health care information technology advisory committees and workgroups, most recently the Pharmacy Health Collaborative. He received his Bachelor of Science in Pharmacy degree from the University of Illinois, College of Pharmacy in 1980, completed his Hospital Pharmacy Resident training at Mayo Clinic Rochester in 1981, and completed his MBA in technology management in 2007.

■ LEARNING OBJECTIVES

After completing this chapter, readers should be able to

1. Describe key drivers for technology and automation in pharmacy practice.
2. List and describe the domains of the pharmacist's role in health information technology.
3. List the technologies involved at each step in the medication use process.
4. Describe the goal of closed-loop medication management systems.
5. List the elements of a request for proposal (RFP) as it relates to vendor selection for procuring health information technology resources.
6. Describe four ways to manage change related to health information technology.
7. Describe the types of backup options for pharmacy information management systems (PIMSs).
8. List five questions to consider when planning a backup procedure for a PIMS.
9. Describe the role of best practices for PIMSs.
10. Describe the role and future implications of interoperability for pharmacy practice.

■ SCENARIO

Charlie Chodavarapu completed his PharmD training several years ago and accepted a staff pharmacist position with a local community pharmacy. Charlie recently started spending some of his free time staffing in the local hospital pharmacy. Despite these experiences, Charlie is reminded of the distinct differences between his primary practice in the community and his periodic practice in the institutional setting. The most obvious difference is that his role in the hospital does not involve reconciling prescription claim issues. Charlie also misses directly interacting with patients in the community. Despite these differences, Charlie was most surprised by the similarities found between the two practice settings.

Unexpectedly, Charlie found similarities in the use of technology between the two practice settings. Charlie's community practice is completely reliant on a number of technologies to perform administrative, clinical, and distributive functions. Through his work in the hospital, Charlie has had the opportunity to experience the daily workflow of a hospital pharmacist, and the extraordinary reliance on technology and automation to perform core practice responsibilities. Charlie's experiences in these two settings prompted reflection on how the integration of practice and technology can significantly impact the patients' experience and outcomes.

■ CHAPTER QUESTIONS

1. What is the pharmacist's role in health information technology management?
2. What are the primary health information technologies at each step of the medication use process?
3. How can health information technology positively impact pharmacy practice?
4. How can pharmacists actively improve the medication use process through their use of health information technology?
5. What is the pharmacist's role in the technology vendor selection process?
6. How can pharmacy leaders minimize resistance to health information technology-related change?
7. How can pharmacists use downtime and backup policies and procedures to support patient care and administrative functions?
8. How can pharmacy leaders utilize best practices to positively impact health information technology use?
9. What does the future hold for pharmacists and their use of health information technology?

■ KEY DRIVERS FOR AUTOMATION AND TECHNOLOGY IN PHARMACY PRACTICE

The use of automation and information systems in pharmacy practice evolved in the early 1960s and 1980s, respectively. Limited resources, regulatory and legal requirements, end-user satisfaction, the need to streamline operational costs, financial reimbursement, and point of sale prescription benefit adjudication were the predominate drivers for early adoption of technology and automation in pharmacy practice. Changes in the professional practice model, primarily the transition from traditional distributive and dispensing roles to patient-centered pharmaceutical care (1990s) and medication therapy management (MTM) in the early 2000s, dramatically increased the demand for utilizing automation and technology to free the pharmacist from traditional preparation and dispensing roles.

An Institute of Medicine (IOM) report significantly influenced the medication management technology and automation landscape (Kohn et al., 1999). Although operational efficiency remained an important driver for technology adoption, the IOM report heightened the awareness of technology's importance for enabling medication use process continuous quality improvement and safety. The report made it clear that to improve medication safety, health care organizations must "implement, manage, and optimize proven medication safety practices and technologies to reduce reliance on memory, standardize terminology, minimize data handoffs, and utilize constraints and forcing functions, protocols, and checklists." The report referenced several emerging technologies and systems that may be used to effectively reduce medical mistakes. It called for automation of patient-specific clinical information within the context of an integrated electronic health record (EHR) and included tightly connected applications supporting electronic ordering, drug distribution, preparation, administration, and monitoring. These systems ideally would work together within and across organizational boundaries and episodes of care sharing real-time, patient-specific clinical information, providing timely and relevant clinical decision support (CDS) across the continuum of care, and creating an environment for robust data mining and analytics (Kohn et al., 1999).

The American Recovery and Reinvestment Act (ARRA) of 2009 and the Health Information Technology for Economic and Clinical Health (HITECH) Act provided the necessary financial incentives for health care organizations to implement certified EHRs and avoid significant federally mandated penalties. To be eligible for these payments, hospitals and physicians were required to demonstrate *meaningful use* of HIT, be able to exchange electronic health information across organizational boundaries and the continuum of care. The recommendations in the IOM reports and the federal government's financial commitment through the HITECH Act were significant drivers for advancing HIT in pharmacy practice specifically and in the broader landscape of health care delivery in the United States (111th Congress, 2009).

■ ROLE OF THE PHARMACIST IN HEALTH INFORMATION TECHNOLOGY

Pharmacists are responsible for patient safety throughout the medication use process and should take a leadership role at all levels of health care to ensure that HIT supports safe medication use. This includes the following:

- Data, information, and knowledge management
- System selection, development, and design
- System implementation, maintenance, and optimization
- Education and quality improvement
- Practice analytics

Data, Information, and Knowledge Management

Pharmacy practice is a data and information intensive discipline requiring the best evidence to support optimal decision-making. Pharmacists must take a leadership role in assuring that medication data, information, and knowledge management best practices (i.e., processes that lead to a desired result) are utilized across all supporting systems (Table 9-1). The most common approach for effectively managing medication content in the HIT environment is through the use of a commercial drug knowledge and database vendor (e.g., First Databank, Cerner Multum, or IBM Micromedex), who provides reliable, authoritative, evidence-based information to support clinical decision-making. Medication management supporting systems are able to leverage the integrated content to assist in therapeutic decision-making, alert for harmful drug–drug interactions, drug disease contraindications, potential duplicative therapies, and dose range checking, among a list of over 20 CDS modules. Although the commercial drug database vendors' approach is commonplace in today's practice, pharmacists should continue to evaluate their efficacy and consistency to identify shortcomings and opportunities for optimizing these systems in clinical practice.

System Selection, Development, and Design

When new medication management supporting technologies are being discussed and/or evaluated, the pharmacist should play a leading role in the RFP process to ensure that the technology supports safe medication use, but more importantly that it is effectively aligned with the ideal HIT-enabled medication use process. The RFP process allows potential vendors to

Table 9-1.	Data, Information, and Knowledge Management Best Practices

Data Quality Management Best Practices

- Accessibility—easily obtainable
- Accuracy—correct and valid values
- Comprehensiveness—all applicable data are included
- Consistency—the value of data are reliable
- Recency—the data are current
- Definition—clear definitions, following a standard vocabulary
- Granularity—attributes and values of data are defined at the correct level of detail for the application
- Precision—data values should be large enough to support the application
- Relevancy—data are meaningful to the performance of the process
- Timeliness—data are used in appropriate context

Information and Knowledge Management Best Practices

- Adoption of standard formats, human and machine interpretable
- Readily and rapidly understood and accessed in the context of the workflow
- Centrally managed, collaboratively developed, and easily disseminated and maintained
- Platform independent
- Controlled terminology for interoperability
- Assign responsibility for different content areas to individuals with domain expertise
- Validation and audit trail maintenance
- Measurement and evaluation of content
- Use of tools to support data, information, and knowledge management

submit formal proposals detailing information about their company, the cost, and other requested information pertaining to the purchase, installation, and support of a medication management technology. The pharmacist should work closely with vendors, application programmers, and medication management system users to develop system requirements while understanding system capabilities and limitations. Pharmacists must translate clinician requirements (i.e., features and functions that clinician users need) into specifications for clinical information systems, identify and prioritize system enhancements, and design safe and effective medication workflows across the medication use continuum (American Society of Health-System Pharmacists, 2016).

System Implementation, Maintenance, and Optimization

The pharmacist should lead medication management supporting system deployments, maintenance, and optimization efforts. Leadership efforts begin with active involvement in creating the project charter, identifying the project vision and objectives along with scope, deliverables, organizational structure, roles and responsibilities, budget, and risks. The pharmacist should serve in a project leadership role across the entire project lifecycle, including project initiation, planning (analysis, design), execution (build, test, train, activate), and closure. They should take responsibility for expected system benefits, integrity of the process design, information and knowledge management, risk management, trouble shooting, and production maintenance. They must collaborate with stakeholders to assist with system analysis, identifying opportunities for optimization (American Society of Health-System Pharmacists, 2016).

Education and Quality Improvement

Pharmacists should assist with providing HIT educational road maps and competencies for pharmacy staff development programs. Additionally, to support preparing future pharmacy informatics professionals, pharmacists should also engage colleges of pharmacy in their HIT and informatics educational efforts. This is especially relevant as current accreditation standards require informatics education (Accreditation Council for Pharmacy Education, 2015). Core curriculum should focus on the role of technology and automation in medication management, how it can improve medication safety and quality, the inherent risks and negative aspects of implementing medication use technologies, and the pharmacist's responsibility for the end-to-end systems supporting safe and efficacious medication use. Other curriculum content should focus on the following (American Society of Health-System Pharmacists, 2007):

- Best practices surrounding the storage, retrieval, and analysis of health information.
- Key issues affecting human–computer interaction.
- IT-enabled closed-loop medication management.
- Principles for the development of decision support tools to solve patient-related problems.
- The structure and key elements of an EHR.
- The impact of alerts on workflow and patient outcomes.
- Project and change management principles and best practices for technology projects.

Pharmacists have responsibility for performing quality improvement activities that involve the core issues of medication management supporting systems. Quality improvement efforts should include the use of controlled medication vocabularies, usability, interoperability (the ability to meaningfully exchange information in electronic format), and demonstrate value involving efficiency, safety, and quality (see Chapter 10). The pharmacist should assist in determining the balance of clinical informatics and health care system reengineering needed to optimize the medication use process and improve patient safety (American Society of Health-System Pharmacists, 2007).

Pharmacists must utilize their overarching knowledge of safe and effective use of medications and medication management systems. They should be able to efficiently and effectively translate and communicate the language of medication use bidirectionally across the continuum of care. They should be able to decipher system requirements into sound medication ordering system designs, assuring effective electronic exchange of prescription and prescription-related information. Their understanding of core pharmacy operations and skills to manage the business as well as clinical aspects of medications across the continuum of care make them an invaluable resource for system development and ongoing system maintenance (American Society of Health-System Pharmacists, 2016).

Practice Analytics

Data are traditionally considered to be discrete elements, while information is often described as data that has meaning. In today's health care environment, health care organizations, including pharmacy departments create, share, and manage large amounts of data. The challenge these organizations face is turning data into information that provides "concise, timely, descriptive, predictive, and prescriptive insight" into their business and clinical practices (American Society of Health-System Pharmacists, 2016). Business intelligence (BI) and analytics (BA) are processes and technologies that organizations use to transform data into information, providing insight for organizational leadership to improve overall performance and maintain their competitive advantage—based on their own data. With their foundational knowledge of pharmacy practice, pharmacy informaticists understand the end-to-end business and clinical processes involved with medication management. Other skills related to medication information systems and data management are important tools that enable pharmacy informaticists to play an important role in BI and BA activities within their organization. These activities focus on optimizing outcomes of care while increasing organizational efficiency. Suggested pharmacy informatics roles and responsibilities in BI and BA must include the following (American Society of Health-System Pharmacists, 2016):

- Ensuring data are standardized, structured, and modeled to support a data-driven BI and BA culture.
- Creating effective analytics tools that allow for multiple formats and layers of analysis, from summary reports for a population of patients to a practice and at the individual patient-encounter level.
- Development, maintenance, and quality assurance of clinical, operational, and financial dashboards,

scorecards, screening, and surveillance tools to guide achievement of treatment and strategic goals.

- Driving analytics to the front line by creating greater end-user accessibility to BI and BA tools.
- Monitoring effectiveness of tools and information to deploy or further develop point of care or analytical systems."

■ TECHNOLOGIES SUPPORTING MEDICATION USE PROCESS

The medication use process as depicted in Figure 9-1 consists of six domains: (1) selection and procurement, (2) storage, (3) ordering and verification, (4) preparation and dispensing, (5) administration, and (6) patient monitoring and assessment. The processes within these domains are exceedingly complex, involving numerous handoffs and regulations in widely diverse health care arenas, including pharmaceutical manufacturing, insurers, community pharmacies, long-term health care facilities, hospitals, and clinics. These processes also involve numerous stakeholders, including patients and family members, physicians, nurses, pharmacists, and other allied health care workers. They frequently require multiple methods of communication, documentation, and manual as well as automated sources of data with the goal of providing safe and effective medication management (California HealthCare Foundation, 2001).

Leape et al. (1995) outlined where errors are most likely to occur and their corresponding rates for

Table 9-2.	Medication Use Process Errors	
Medication Use Step and Common Type of Error	**Distribution of Errors by Step**	**Errors Intercepted**
Prescribing	39%	48%
• Wrong dose		
• Wrong choice		
• Known allergy		
Transcribing/ Verification	12%	33%
• Wrong dose		
• Wrong frequency		
• Missed dose		
Dispensing	11%	34%
• Wrong dose		
• Wrong drug		
• Wrong time		
Administering	38%	2%
• Wrong dose		
• Wrong choice		
• Wrong drug		

Data from Bates DW, Cullen DJ, Laird N, et al. 1995. Incidence of adverse drug events and potential adverse drug events: Implications for prevention. *JAMA* 274(1): 29–34; Leape LL, Bates DW, Cullen DJ, et al. 1995. Systems analysis of adverse drug events, *JAMA* 274(1):35–43.

being detected prior to reaching the patient (Table 9-2). Pharmacists should use this and similar research as a road map for developing medication management technology strategic plans. Table 9-3 provides a list

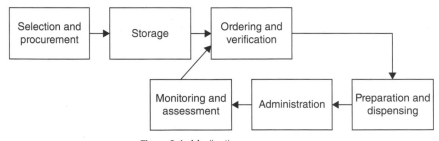

Figure 9-1. Medication use process.

Table 9-3.	Medication Use Process Technology and Automation Strategies

Prescribing
- Computerized prescriber order entry systems
- Clinical decision support systems

Transcribing/Order Verification
- Order management systems
- Pharmacy information management systems

Preparation and Dispensing
- Solid dosage form robotics
- Workflow management systems
- Inventory management systems
- Automated dispensing devices
- Tablet counters
- Bar code packagers
- Sterile compounding robotics

Administration
- Electronic medication administration records
- Bar code medication administration systems
- Smart pumps

Data from the California HealthCare Foundation.

of automation and technology solutions that address common causes of medication errors within the medication use process. Although this list is not exhaustive, it is intended to present those technologies widely adopted by health care organizations across the country. It is important for pharmacists to understand both the positive effects and the limitations for technology and automated systems and the variability in their actualized benefits from one organization to the next.

The core medication use process supporting technologies include the following:

- Computerized prescriber order entry (CPOE) and CDS systems
- PIMSs
- Preparation and dispensing systems
- Medication administration systems

CPOE is an integrated application allowing clinicians to create orders with the benefit of CDS tools that provide guidance within the context of a patient's electronic medical record (EMR) ensuring that they receive the most appropriate medication therapy. The software incorporates a variety of tools to help prescribers, including alerts, checks, reminders, and best practice guidelines. CPOE is generally regarded as difficult to implement and costly; however, it is considered one of the most important HIT investments an organization can make to improve safety and quality (California HealthCare Foundation, 2001).

An e-prescribing or ambulatory CPOE system provides a standardized, secure, and safe vehicle for transporting and sharing information across the health system and community pharmacy environment. E-prescribing allows for the transmission of prescription or prescription-related information between prescribers, community pharmacies, and pharmacy health plans. By adopting a nationally established electronic messaging standard (NCPDP SCRIPT) and a third-party pharmacy health information exchange network (e.g., Surescripts), e-prescribing allows medication use process stakeholders to access secure, low-cost electronic prescription fill and history information from payers and pharmacies across the country. This connection offers the needed technical framework to improve medication communication failures at interfaces and transitions in care and assists providers in making more informed medication-related decisions. Conversely, community pharmacy practices have the potential to receive pertinent medication-related information from health systems, including laboratory data, allergy, and diagnosis information. This information allows pharmacists to more effectively manage medicines and unlocks the door to developing convergent pharmacy practice models (Siska, 2011). Features of CPOE and e-prescribing systems that contribute to safety and quality include the following:

- Legibility
- Structured menu-driven orders
- Real-time patient information at the point of care
- Embedded drug information, including dose checking, drug–drug interaction checking, and allergy alerts

PIMS have been in place for more than two decades and are often considered the backbone of medication use process technologies. These systems can function as independent ordering systems requiring verification, or they ideally can be tightly integrated with CPOE systems to reduce the potential for errors in verification. These systems effectively control access to medications prior to administration, and through their integration with medication documentation systems, they direct the creation of the electronic medication administration record (eMAR). PIMS can also be used to assist in managing inventory, point of sale, and prescription benefit reimbursement (Siska, 2006). Features of PIMS that contribute to safety and quality include the following:

- Verification of prescribed orders
- Structured ordering
- Online drug information support (dose checking, drug interactions, allergy alerts)

Preparation and dispensing automation is widely utilized in both the hospital and community pharmacy environments. The goals for use of automation include improving patient care, customer service, and resource utilization. Technologies include the following:

- Drug purchasing and supply chain management systems
- Automated drug distribution systems
  - Automated dispensing cabinets (ADCs)
  - Robotic cart filling systems
  - Automated medication storage systems
- Preparation systems
  - Sterile compounding devices
  - Unit dose and bar code packaging systems
  - Medication counting and labeling devices

The key benefits of pharmacy automation in the dispensing and preparation processes go well beyond safety. The advent of computer-controlled equipment to automate processes that were traditionally performed by pharmacists has allowed technicians to play a more active role in medication dispensing. This allows pharmacy administrators to maximize their resources and move pharmacists into patient care roles. This redesigned practice model enables hospitals and community pharmacies to utilize the pharmacist's expertise in MTM and the provision of patient-centered clinical services.

Point-of-care medication administration systems, sustained by data produced from upstream-integrated CPOE and pharmacy systems, provide important medication information at the bedside and allow nurses to electronically document medications administered. Bar code medication administration (BCMA) technologies combine several hardware and software components to perform important safety checks within a process that is highly vulnerable to error. BCMA systems perform a number of safety checks that include the Five Rights: right patient, right medication, right dose, right time, and right route. Before administering a medication to a patient, the nurse scans a bar code on their identification badge, a second bar code on the medication package, and a third bar code on the patient's wrist band. These three scans allow the nurse to verify that the medication they are about to administer is intended for that patient. Nurses are alerted of any discrepancies via a visual and/or audible alert that requires acknowledgement prior to administration (California HealthCare Foundation, 2001).

eMARs manage data throughout an organization and provide valuable, accurate, real-time medication information for all health care providers. The eMAR is a multidisciplinary application that provides an important solution for medication documentation, therapeutic assessment and treatment, monitoring, and quality and compliance measurements. Of all the electronic tools currently used in the medication use process, the eMAR is most likely to be utilized by virtually every member of the health care team. Pharmacists should ensure that an eMAR is integrated clearly and concisely with the organization's primary order entry and pharmacy systems, including any ADCs, point-of-care BCMA systems, infusion pumps, or other disparate medication documentation applications. The eMAR also must have the capability of integrating with the organization's billing and financial services systems as linking administered medication records can improve compliance with billing regulations (Siska, 2005).

Medication infusion devices (i.e., sterile compounding devices) play an important role in delivering medication infusions to patients in both inpatient and outpatient settings. Intravenously (IV) administered medications pose the greatest risk to patients and often result in medication-related events causing harm. Smart infusion devices provide precise delivery of medication, and when configured with CDS guidelines, they have the potential to prevent severe or even fatal medication errors. The pump can be programmed with user-defined soft and hard lower and upper limits for each medication visible to the clinician before final confirmation is requested. These hard and soft limits are at the heart of the pump's ability to avert fatalities.

■ CLOSED-LOOP MEDICATION MANAGEMENT

A closed-loop medication management system (Figure. 9-2) is developed to feed outcomes from medication processes back into the system to enable the deployment and development of improved practices and to effectively monitor patient care across the continuum. Through the automation of all medication-related processes, closed-loop medication management reduces many steps in the complex process, significantly reducing the number of opportunities for error (Kilbridge & Classen, 2002). The transition between each step in the process is seamless, information is exchanged and used by all systems involved, and it remains intact as it is handed off from

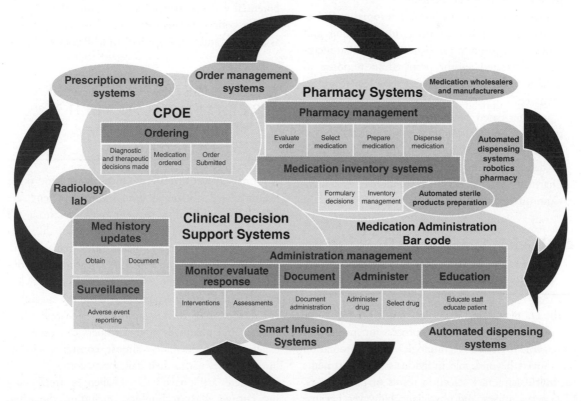

Figure 9-2. Closed-loop medication management. (Data from Kilbridge P, Classen D. A Process Model of Inpatient Medication Management and Information Technology Interventions to Improve Patient Safety. VHA 2001 Research Series Volume 1. © VHA Inc. All Rights Reserved.)

one application to the next. Closed-loop medication management technologies help prevent medication errors by organizing information and making it easily available, linking discrete pieces of information, and performing repetitive tasks including monitoring for problems. The closed-loop system includes technologies that enable clinicians to make the most appropriate decisions about patient care at each step of the process.

Ideally, a closed-loop system would have a succession of systems that are all interconnected and can share data fully in real time. Such an automated infrastructure should minimally consist of the following:

- An electronic patient health record.
- A provider order entry process.
- CDS systems that evaluate not only orders as they are entered but also evaluate all orders as changes in patient condition may demand.
- A preparation and distribution automation infrastructure that uses automatic identification and other information technologies to verify that medications selected and/or prepared in response to specific orders were appropriately selected and/or prepared.
- Computer-based bedside verification of medications at administration that is tolerant to the variety of products and dose forms that might be used to deliver a medication dose (ASHP Section of Pharmacy Informatics and Technology Executive Committee, 2009).

■ PHARMACISTS AND TECHNOLOGY VENDOR SELECTION

In the era of system integration and its known complexities, the vendor selection process for medication management-related technologies and automation has moved beyond sole individuals or departments to multidisciplinary selection teams of pharmacists, IT experts, nurses, and physicians. However, because of their expertise and knowledge of best medication management practices, the pharmacist is responsible for ensuring that proper technology vendor selection takes place. Pharmacists are the most qualified to perform a proper assessment of the potential clinical, operational, and safety features and functionalities available in a system. Pharmacists must participate in the vendor selection processes for all medication management-related systems, including ordering and prescribing, as well as medication documentation and administration systems. The pharmacist must articulate the ideal vision and strategy for the ideal IT-enabled medication use process and ensure that technology solutions are aligned with institutional goals and ideal HIT strategic objectives (Siska & Tribble, 2011).

A number of steps are required in selecting a medication management supporting technology, including the development of technical and functional requirements, a comprehensive analysis of potential vendors, benchmarking with other organizations, contractual requirements, a system readiness assessment, and the creation of an RFP (Bucki, 2011).

■ CHANGE MANAGEMENT RELATED TO HEALTH INFORMATION TECHNOLOGY

A primary driver of HIT use in pharmacy and other health-related disciplines is to improve patient care and, most importantly, patient outcomes from the care they receive. HIT supports clinician decision-making, workflow, and medication management. However, HIT is similar to the consumer electronics market in that change is constant. In both fields, innovation occurs at a rapid rate, although for different reasons. Due to this rapid rate of change, pharmacists and pharmacy staff members can expect to experience considerable—almost constant—change in the IT they use in their daily operations.

There are unavoidable challenges from staying current with technology, including the often expensive cost of replacing outdated technology or upgrading to completely new technology. Technical challenges also exist when moving to a new technology and frequently present as difficulties getting disparate technologies to "speak" to each other. This type of challenge is often beyond the skill set of most pharmacists and requires the expertise of a technology vendor and/or specially trained personnel; thus, it is not a focus of this chapter. A decidedly different challenge is the personnel aspect, that is, how to help people deal with technological change.

A simplistic way to view the difference between clinical practice and HIT is that a change in clinical practice impacts medication use (e.g., dose); whereas, implementation of HIT impacts the way someone does their job. New technology can actually change the daily workflow of a pharmacist and others involved in medication management, and it can even change their responsibilities. This type of change can have a significant impact on job satisfaction and performance. Adding potentially more difficulty to the change process is that decisions regarding technology selection and implementation can often occur without input from the person(s) ultimately impacted by the change. For example, ARRA continues to have substantial impact on the implementation of new technologies in hospitals and community pharmacies.

From a management perspective, the significance of HIT-related change should not be overlooked. Resistance to change is to be expected, but managers can draw on a variety of resources to help manage change. The research and experiences of many have produced several consistent themes in managing change, and these themes, described below, can be applied to managing change related to IT.

1. Leadership is critical to navigating any type of change. Leaders should be effective communicators that establish the need and a vision for change, convene a group to lead the change, and empower others to implement change. Leaders should identify anticipated tangible improvements due to change and should acknowledge those involved in the improvements. The connection between changes experienced and achievement of organization goals should be articulated by leadership (Kotter, 1995).

2. End-users should be involved in technology design and implementation decisions, since they know what best fits their workflow. This critical step is often overlooked.

3. Training is critical to acceptance of new technology. Training should be available in a variety of formats (in-person, written materials, video tutorials, etc.) and should be available at times that fit trainee schedules, and it should be available on-demand for supplemental uses. Training should be tailored to the specific needs of the trainee and conducted in a nonthreatening environment.

4. Theories of change demonstrate that users' acceptance of new technologies is strongly influenced by their perceptions of usefulness of the technology. Accordingly, users are more likely to adopt technologies that prove useful in their jobs (Davis et al., 1989; Kijsanayotin et al., 2009; Venkatesh et al., 2003).

5. Resistance to change is inevitable, should be expected, and can be overt and covert. Resistance is due to a sense of loss of control. Change that is more appealing leads to less resistance (Luo, 2006).

Pharmacists faced with leading technology implementation and adoption should consider the importance of their role as leaders, the importance of staff involvement, and the use of training as an opportunity to demonstrate the positive impact of change. In reality, technological change will likely bring about both positive and negative implications. Social influences within the pharmacy may also provide positive (and negative) support for acceptance.

Health Information Technology Essentials

Downtime and Backup

In August 2005, hurricane Katrina devastated the Louisiana and Mississippi gulf coasts. Images of flooded homes in New Orleans and cement foundations where homes once stood on the Mississippi coast are vivid reminders of the power of the storm. More recently, Hurricane Michael devastated sections of the Florida panhandle and southeastern Alabama. Unfortunately, natural disasters do not intentionally bypass health care facilities, as evidenced by reports from the aftermath of Katrina and Michael. Hospitals in New Orleans were flooded. Pharmacies in coastal Mississippi, Florida, and Alabama were washed away. In 2005, most hospitals relied on paper-based medical records, and although pharmacies in hospitals and the community rely on electronic patient records, records stored on computers submerged under or washed away by rising flood waters were not retrievable.

Hurricanes Katrina and Michael provide clear pictures of the worst-case scenario regarding pharmacy downtime and the loss of patient records. Fortunately, the devastation from such a storm does not occur very often. However, pharmacies are faced with the potential for downtime (a temporary outage of computing systems) and data loss (the permanent inability to access data) due to failed computing equipment, theft, fire, floods due to faulty plumbing, power surges, and a variety of other causes. Scheduled maintenance is another cause of downtime.

Scheduled downtime is most often seen in hospital pharmacies as community pharmacy downtime occurs when the pharmacy is closed or not busy. Unscheduled downtime occurs in both settings and is more likely to negatively impact pharmacy operations. To minimize the impact of either type of downtime, pharmacies should have a downtime policy in place that clearly defines how the pharmacy will transition to a manual process. Key concepts related to downtime planning and recovery are addressed later in this chapter.

Downtime planning should focus on ensuring uninterrupted pharmacy services in both planned and unplanned outages. A downtime *policy* designates who to call in the event of an outage. That person then determines what aspects of the downtime policy to enact. In general, downtime policies should clearly describe who is responsible for pharmacy operations, such as maintaining patient records, overseeing existing medication orders, handling new orders—including clinical review, label preparation, communicating with other providers and patients, and any differences in responsibilities across shifts. Downtime *procedures* describe the progressive steps that are to be followed to comply with the downtime policy, including

recovery. Recovery is a challenging, critical step that can lead to additional confusion due to uncertainty about the process and timing for reverting back to the original, electronic system. Therefore, it is important that downtime policies and procedures include the recovery phase (Lockwood, 2010; Miller, 2009). A sample downtime policy for an ambulatory pharmacy can be found on page 42 of this policy and procedure manual: https://www.stonybrookmedicine.edu/sites/default/files/manual1.pdf (Accessed December 29, 2018).

One of the most effective methods to minimize the impact of unplanned downtime is to have a backup procedure in place that routinely copies pharmacy files to another location. There are several approaches to backups. The local backup occurs when personnel within the pharmacy make a copy of their data on physical media that remains on site. Several years ago, this was the customary practice for backing up pharmacy records. After a predetermined period of time, the media was cycled through to overwrite a previous backup. As an example, a backup policy could call for having the last 6 days' worth of data available on external media.

Today's advancements in networking and storage provide additional options for performing backups. Two primary backup procedures today are (1) off-site backup with data stored internally and (2) data stored and backed up externally. In the first backup method, the PIMS vendor remotely connects to the pharmacy system and transfers data to an external location. This method provides a second backup location in case a backup made and stored locally in the pharmacy is not available. The second backup method is actually a result of a pharmacy's use of software as a service (SaaS), an approach to computing in which a technology vendor (PIMS, in this case) uses a secure network connection to provide software and manage associated data. The advantage of SaaS is that the pharmacy bears little responsibility for computing hardware and software because it is maintained by the vendor. From a backup perspective, data are already stored external to the pharmacy. Related, some vendors use a cloud-based model, which shares similarities to SaaS. As with SaaS, the cloud model allows data backups to occur external to the pharmacy's brick and mortar operations.

Considering that there are several backup methods, what are the desirable features? The primary goal of backing up is to safely and securely store critical data in an easily retrievable manner. At a minimum, backup processes should safely store patient data, including demographic data, allergy lists, medication histories, and insurance information (in community pharmacies) in compliance with Health Insurance Portability and Accountability Act (HIPAA) regulations. Other features that managers should consider include the following:

1. How frequently do backups occur? Does pharmacy management have input into the frequency of backups?
2. How are patient data secured? Data should be encrypted for transmission to and storage at the backup location.
3. Where are data backed up? Off-site backups should store data on robust media in multiple locations that are protected from fire, water, and temperature damage. Data centers should have redundant power supplies and 24/7 security. Backups that occur within the pharmacy using physical media should also be stored in locations protected from fire, weather, and temperature damage.
4. How quickly can backed up data be accessed in the event of an outage?
5. Does the backup process include application and/or operating system software, in addition to patient data?
6. Are automated notifications available to inform key personnel when backups occur, or more importantly, when scheduled backups do not occur?
7. Can incremental backups be performed to capture changes since the most recent backup?
8. For SaaS and cloud models, how reliable are network connections between the pharmacy and vendor for both backups and day-to-day operations?
9. For multisite pharmacies that share data, are data backed up such that a failure of the central server does not prevent access to backed up data by one or more pharmacies?

10. In the case of a catastrophic event at the pharmacy or hospital, is remote access to backed up data available from other sites?

Due to our natural inclination to mentally minimize the anticipated risks of natural disasters, downtime and backup procedures are likely not considered to be the most critical aspects of pharmacy operations. However, significant weather events clearly demonstrate the need for diligent downtime planning (Modern Healthcare, 2013). Once a planned or unplanned downtime event is over, restoration of pharmacy data from backups becomes critical to resumption of activities.

■ BEST PRACTICES

Although infrequent, the impact of downtime or the loss of data due to the absence of a backup storage method can have far reaching consequences on a pharmacy. The questions above address proven ways (i.e., best practices) to minimize the impact of downtime and perform secure backups. Best practices are often developed through a combination of research and real-world experience. In the domain of HIT, best practices define ways to use HIT to improve the quality of care as well as to enhance business functions. An important characteristic of best practices is that they are not legislated or regulated. Instead, best practices are benchmarks for self-assessment to attain a desired outcome, focusing on quality.

Best practices in HIT often focus on workflow, system design, and usage. For example, in hospital settings, despite calls for medication reconciliation best practice research and dissemination nearly a decade ago (Greenwald et al., 2010), work continues in the search for the ideal technology-assisted medication reconciliation process (Lesselroth et al., 2018). Siska and Tribble (2011) called for best practices to guide CDS within clinical information systems. They also identified a need for best practices to guide deployment of clinical information systems within hospitals. ADCs are frequently encountered in hospitals and are intended to increase the efficiency and safety of medication distribution. Due to the importance of ADCs

Table 9-4.	Sample Best Practices Resources for Pharmacy Manager	
Resource		**Web URL**
American Pharmacists Association		www.pharmacist.com
American Society of Health-System Pharmacists		www.ashp.org
Institute for Safe Medication Practices		https://www.ismp.org/
Leapfrog Group		www.leapfroggroup.org
Markle Foundation		www.markle.org/health
National Governor's Association Center for Best Practices		www.nga.org
The Joint Commission		www.jointcommission.org
The Office of the National Coordinator for Health Information Technology		www.healthit.gov

in the medication use process, the Institute for Safe Medication Practices (ISMP) published guidelines on ADC use, specifically focusing on safety (2019).

A systematic review identified barriers and facilitators to e-prescription implementation (Gagnon MP, 2014). More to the point of best practices, Rupp & Warholak identified 11 best practices for e-prescriptions in community pharmacies (2008). These best practices—that apply to both pharmacies and prescribers—focus primarily on workflow and are listed as follows:

1. Physicians should enter electronic prescriptions or closely review prescriptions entered by other providers.
2. CDS software should be enabled for prescribers.
3. The receipt of an electronic prescription in the pharmacy should trigger an obvious notification in the PIMS.
4. Pharmacy procedures should eliminate the process of printing and then re-entering prescriptions into the PIMS.
5. Electronic prescribing systems should allow pharmacists to request additional information from prescribers and for prescribers to respond to these requests.

This sample of e-prescribing best practices includes steps that likely seem logical and reasonable for anyone who has worked in a community pharmacy. While these best practices do focus on workflow, the underlying goal is to improve patient care. For example, enabling decision support is a workflow change for prescribers. The intent of this change in workflow, however, is to assist prescribers in making more informed prescribing decisions, resulting in medication use that is safer and more efficacious.

Best practices can be found for various aspects of HIT use in pharmacy practice. However, due to the wide range of HIT use and the variety of pharmacy practice environments, there is no single source for best practices. Accordingly, pharmacy managers who are tasked with implementing best practices within their pharmacy (hospital or community) have several potential sources to consider. In general, these sources include internal documents, published literature, HIT vendors, professional associations, patient safety groups, accrediting bodies, foundations, and other groups. Table 9-4 includes suggested resources for best practices.

■ THE FUTURE: PHARMACY PERSPECTIVES ON NATIONAL INITIATIVES FOR INTEROPERABILITY

Interoperability

Not too many years ago, PIMS operated in silos both in hospitals and in the community. In today's health care environment, significant emphasis is being placed on the ability of disparate computer systems to exchange data in a manner that allows the data to be used in a meaningful way (Brailer, 2005). This type of exchange is known as *interoperability*. Pharmacists are responsible for ensuring safe and effective medication therapy. Prescription drug utilization continues to be an important and substantial component of the overall US health care system (Kaiser Family Foundation, 2019). Due to the importance and widespread use of medications in patient care and the responsibility of pharmacists to manage medication therapy, pharmacists should be aware of and involved with interoperability efforts related to medication management.

The inability to use clinical and administrative information—including information related to medication use—that has been generated or is stored in another location leads to a variety of problems. These problems take the form of unnecessary repeat procedures, errors and delays in care, and providers making less than optimal decisions because they do not know the full story. There are obvious financial implications from repeating procedures or tests that were previously performed. One report projects an annual savings of over $77 billion due to interoperability between providers and laboratories, radiology centers, pharmacies, payers, public health departments, and other providers. This interoperability avoids repeat procedures or tests, the associated administrative work for such activities, and errors due to oral reporting of results (Walker et al., 2005). There are also costs and risks to patients who undergo an unnecessary repeat procedure or test. In addition, it is difficult to measure the financial impact of delays in care. We do know, however, that a lack of access to pertinent information does hamper clinical decision-making (Leape et al., 1995).

With nearly 70,000 community pharmacies, 1,000,000 practicing physicians, 5,000 hospitals, and 16,000 nursing facilities, there are, unfortunately, an abundance of opportunities for patient-related information to be created in one location but not be available in another location (Brailer, 2005; Kaiser Family Foundation, 2016, 2018; Qato, 2017). Adding to the complexity and challenge of sharing patient-related information is today's reality that 60% of the data related to a person's health is created external to the health care system throughout the person's life (Health Policy Brief, 2014). These data are extremely challenging to integrate into the clinical systems pharmacists and other providers use.

The practice of pharmacy provides a great example. A patient can have their prescription filled at Pharmacy A. If they then go to Pharmacy B, the pharmacists at Pharmacy B will not know about any medications filled at Pharmacy A unless the patient tells them. If this patient is then admitted to the hospital, there is a strong likelihood that their complete medication list will not follow them into the hospital. Consider the number of physician offices, hospitals, and hospital pharmacies, and the magnitude of the problem can be appreciated. Polypharmacy and drug interactions are two obvious outcomes of not sharing medication-related information across pharmacies. Due to the financial and humanistic significance of this problem, the federal government has devoted substantial resources to the creation of a nationwide interoperable health information network. The goal of this network is to allow patients' medical records to follow them wherever they receive care.

E-Prescribing and Electronic Patient Records

Interoperability efforts took a major step forward with nationwide implementation of e-prescribing. The ability of Pharmacy Health Information networks to connect prescribers, payers, and pharmacies to electronically exchange prescription-related information addresses safety and efficiency issues on both the prescribing and dispensing ends of the process. Within pharmacies, e-prescribing primarily impacts pharmacy workflow by creating a new method for prescription receipt and entry into the PIMS, and by providing a new method for requesting prescription refills. These are important areas of training for pharmacy staff. Patients should be informed that the use of e-prescriptions does not necessarily decrease the time to fill their prescription. A variety of unrelated factors impact filling time, and pharmacists should be careful to educate their patients to temper expectations. An important consideration for any independent community pharmacy manager is that the pharmacy is responsible for a transaction routing fee for each e-prescription. This fee varies across e-prescribing networks.

EMRs are software applications that are owned by a care delivery organization (e.g., hospital) or by a provider (e.g., physician) and serve to house the electronic history of the care that patients receive in that location. EHRs are also repositories for patient care information, but EHRs pull a patient's information from multiple EMRs to create a comprehensive record of all their care. Federal interoperability efforts focused on EMR design and functionality for physician offices and hospitals to ensure that information exchange occurred across EMRs to create EHRs for US citizens. A key term in the EMR/EHR domain is "meaningful use," which signifies that hospitals and providers must be able to demonstrate that their use of EMRs meets specific functional and technical benchmarks. Hospitals and providers who are able to demonstrate achievement of meaningful use are eligible for financial incentives to support the adoption of this new technology. A sample functional benchmark is that a minimum percentage of orders in the hospital setting must be entered using CPOE. To date, over 540,000 providers and 5,000 hospitals have received a portion of the $37 billion dispersed in the EHR meaningful use program (Centers for Medicare and Medicaid Services, 2017).

Medications are an important part of patient records and are addressed in current federal EMR, and EMR development efforts that include standards for medication and allergy information access, e-prescribing, formulary and benefits checking, and other transactions related to medication prescribing and dispensing (Hanson et al., 2012). Current federal efforts are largely focused on physicians and hospitals, not recognizing other health care professionals who play a significant role in the patient-centered multidisciplinary model of care. Recognizing this deficiency, nine pharmacy organizations formed the Pharmacy e-Health Information Technology (HIT) Collaborative in 2010. The two-pronged purpose of the Collaborative is (1) "to assure the meaningful use of standardized EHRs that supports safe, efficient, and effective medication use, continuity of care, and provide access to the patient-care services of pharmacists with other members of the interdisciplinary patient care team" and (2) "to assure the pharmacist's role of providing patient-care services are integrated into the National HIT interoperable framework" (Pharmacy Health Information Technology Collaborative, 2018a). The Collaborative developed a road map that defines pharmacy's priorities for HIT.

The road map, which has been updated several times since it was first published in 2011, lays out a vision for HIT as it relates to pharmacy in the evolving national infrastructure (Pharmacy Health Information Technology Collaborative, 2018b). The updated road map continues to reflect the Collaborative's longstanding mission of including pharmacists and pharmacy services in the national interoperable health information network. This includes pharmacists' ability to participate in bidirectional information exchange to support care delivery, health information exchange, and national quality efforts (Mackowiak, 2011). The road map's goals (Table 9-5) also reflect the importance of the Joint Commission of Pharmacy

Table 9-5.	Goals of the Pharmacy Health Information Technology (HIT) Collaborative's Roadmap for Pharmacy HIT Integration in US Health Care: 2018 to 2021 Update
Goal 1	INTEROPERABILITY: Advance the adoption by pharmacists of systems capable of standards-driven health information exchange.
Goal 2	WORKFLOW and USABILITY for systems and providers: Health IT supports the JCPP Pharmacists' Patient Care Process and the provision of patient care services.
Goal 3	QUALITY: Support national quality initiatives enabled by HIT.

Data from The Roadmap for Pharmacy Health Information Technology Integration in US Health Care: 2018 to 2021 update. Pharmacy Health Information Technology Collaborative (2018b).

Practitioners (JCPP) Pharmacist Patient Care Process (PPCP) as a shared structure and framework for pharmacy services, including the role of HIT systems as supporting technology for pharmacist's clinical services. The goals also align with existing efforts to advance pharmacists as providers recognized under Medicare. The Collaborative's website (www.pharmacyhit.org) provides a variety of additional resources, including guides for the use of SNOMED CT to document patient encounters and how to talk with PIMS vendors about pharmacy's needs in an EHR.

The JCPP PPCP example highlights the potential for exciting change on the horizon. The goal of the JCPP PPCP is to establish a consistent patient care process across the varied pharmacy practice settings. The PPCP is akin to processes of care followed by other professions. While the stepwise process articulated in the PPCP applies across all pharmacy practice settings, pharmacy *workflow* varies across practice settings. The opportunity and challenges articulated in the Collaborative's updated roadmap reflect the need for pharmacists to develop and use HIT that supports the JCPP PPCP.

To that end, pharmacists have the opportunity—and challenge—to engage standards development organizations to encourage the development of national standards that align with the PPCP workflow. Pharmacists should also collaborate with HIT vendors to design, build, test, and implement systems that advance pharmacists' patient care activities that are consistent with the PPCP. This development work should be driven by the systematic patient care process framework described in the PPCP. Related, significant education of current and future pharmacists will be necessary to catalyze widespread adoption of HIT systems that support the PPCP workflow.

The PPCP example reflects the importance of pharmacists' independent clinical activities to provision of quality patient care. Documentation of these activities should be incorporated in patients' EHRs, informing other providers. Similarly, pharmacists need access to EHRs to have a complete picture of their patients to enhance decision-making. These changes will bring new practice roles for pharmacists.

Pharmacists' documentation will become widely visible, increasing awareness of pharmacists' contribution to patient care. Challenges will exist. Professional and pharmacy business models will require significant reengineering to change the care delivery process. Community pharmacists could benefit from something as simple as a diagnosis, but the opportunity to review a patient's medical history can inform the pharmacist's activities. Unfortunately, today's community pharmacies face daunting prescription volumes that may not allow pharmacists to fully utilize the available information. Readers also might consider the opportunity for pharmacists to document the care they provide, especially in the community setting. This may be even more challenging than reviewing newly available information.

If the coming role of EHRs in pharmacy practice is likely to pull pharmacists away from actual reimbursable activities (i.e., dispensing), then how can these new activities be adopted? There is a growing movement in health care to focus reimbursement on the quality of care. For example, hospitals currently face decreasing reimbursement if patients are readmitted for a condition that they recently received treatment for. In many of these readmission events, poor medication adherence leads to the readmission. The Collaborative's longstanding efforts are intended to lead to—among many other things—community pharmacists having access to medication discharge information, allowing them to help ensure patients take the appropriate medications in an appropriate manner. This positions the pharmacist to be recognized for bringing quality to medication management by preventing readmissions.

The Centers for Medicare and Medicaid Services (CMS) created a star rating system that recognizes health plans for their ability to provide quality care. A component of the star ratings includes medication management practices. While pharmacists are not directly, financially incentivized by the star rating system, business agreements can be reached between pharmacies (or pharmacists) and health plans in which some of the monetary incentives a plan receives for a higher star rating are shared with those pharmacies that helped the plan achieve a high rating. Pharmacies are able to follow their performance on CMS quality measures as well as compare their performance to others using the Electronic Quality Improvement Platform for Plans & Pharmacies (EQuIPP).

The Collaborative's work and CMS' star rating system are important examples of change that is occurring in health care. While the future is uncertain regarding what will ultimately happen for pharmacists' documentation in the EHR and if approaches similar to CMS' star ratings for health plans will ever be developed for pharmacy, this is a dynamic time in which HIT plays a critical role in the support of health information. If the changes described above occur, everyone in the pharmacy will be impacted. New workflows will need to be established. Training will need to address responsibilities and policies for EHR use as well as components of medication management quality. New relationships between pharmacy staff and other providers will likely be established. Patients will need education regarding the changing dynamic between providers, as well as the patient's role as a contributor to their own EHR and in appropriate medication use. Pharmacists will need to adapt to the changing health care landscape, focusing on safe and effective medication use.

■ REVISITING THE SCENARIO

Charlie's experiences in community and hospital pharmacy practice settings have helped him appreciate the interaction and impact a pharmacist has with HIT, and how interoperable systems can dramatically influence patient care. These systems support the administrative and clinical aspects of his practice, but are not fully optimized until they can meaningfully exchange information. Charlie recognizes how health care and the practice of pharmacy may be mediated by technology. He is encouraged by having access to critical point-of-care information to assist in filling prescriptions in the community and having accurate, up-to-date medication information while working in the hospital. Charlie also recognizes

the significant change that these systems can have on how people work and the importance of leadership in guiding people through the change. Ultimately, pharmacy managers, supervisors, and other leaders will be responsible for implementing policies, procedures, and workflow to fully benefit from future HIT advancements.

■ CONCLUSION

Health care technology continues to play a significant role in pharmacy practice. The information and technology wave allows for abundant sharing of medication-related data while offering an unprecedented number of opportunities for remote monitoring, clinical advisories, and intervention. Pharmacists are experts in medication management systems and in medication therapy use. As such, pharmacists should be involved in any efforts impacting the medication use process, whether or not HIT is involved. When considering HIT, pharmacists should carefully evaluate the impact of HIT on pharmacy workflow and patient care, and provide leadership within all practice settings. Leadership can involve developing RFP

■ QUESTIONS FOR FURTHER DISCUSSION

1. How has the role of technology and automation in pharmacy changed over the last several years? What future changes do you anticipate?
2. What can pharmacy managers do to support the emerging role of pharmacists in HIT?
3. What is the PIMS vendor's role in assisting pharmacy leaders establish downtime procedures and backup services?
4. What are the potential negative consequences of not having pharmacy fully involved in national efforts for interoperability?

documents, planning system implementation, developing new policies due to emerging practice models, formalizing adoption of best practices related to medication management, and managing personnel respective to change. Pharmacists should follow national efforts related to HIT, as these efforts will impact practice. Furthermore, pharmacists should become directly involved in these efforts whenever possible.

REFERENCES

111th Congress of the United States of America. 2009. American Recovery and Reinvestment Act of 2009—Title XIII: Health Information Technology. Available at https://www.hhs.gov/sites/default/files/ocr/privacy/hipaa/understanding/coveredentities/hitechact.pdf. Accessed February 28, 2019.

Accreditation Council for Pharmacy Education. 2015. Accreditation standards and key elements for the professional program in pharmacy leading to the Doctor of Pharmacy degree. Available at https://www.acpe-accredit.org/pdf/Standards2016FINAL.pdf. Accessed February 28, 2019.

American Society of Health-System Pharmacists. 2007. ASHP statement on the pharmacist's role in informatics. *Am J Health Syst Pharm* 64:200–203.

American Society of Health-System Pharmacists. 2016. ASHP statement on the pharmacist's role in clinical informatics. *Am J Health-Syst Pharm* 72:410–413.

Bates DW, Cullen DJ, Laird N, et al. 1995. Incidence of adverse drug events and potential adverse drug events: Implications for prevention. *JAMA* 274:29–34.

Brailer DJ. 2005. Interoperability: The key to the future health care system. *Health Aff* (Suppl Web Exclusives):W5–W19–W5–W21.

Bucki J. 2018. 6-step vendor selection process. Available at http://operationstech.about.com/od/vendorselection/a/VendorSelectionHub.htm. Accessed February 28, 2019.

California HealthCare Foundation. 2001. Addressing medication errors in hospitals: A framework for developing a plan. Available at https://www.chcf.org/wp-content/uploads/2017/12/PDF-addressingmederrorsframework.pdf. Accessed February 28, 2019.

Centers for Medicare and Medicaid Services. 2017. December 2017 EHR incentive program. Available at https://www.cms.gov/Regulations-and-Guidance/Legislation/EHRIncentivePrograms/Downloads/December2017_SummaryReport.pdf. Accessed December 29, 2018.

Davis FD, Bagozzi RP, Warshaw PR. 1989. User acceptance of computer technology: A comparison of two theoretical models. *Manag Sci* 35(8):982–1003.

Figge HL. 2009. Reducing medication errors using technological innovations. *US Pharm* 34(3):HS–H15.

Gagnon MP, Nsangou ER, Payne-Gagnon J, Grinier S, Sicotte C. 2014. Barriers and facilitators to implementing electronic prescriptions: A systematic review of user groups' perceptions. *JAMIA* 21(3):535–541.

Greenwald JL, Halasyamani L, Greene J, et al. 2010. Making inpatient medication reconciliation patient centered, clinical relevant and implementable: A consensus statement on key principles and necessary first steps. *J Hosp Med* 5(8):477–485.

Hanson A, Levin BL, Scott DM. 2012. Informatics in health care. In McCarthy RL, Schafermeyer KW, Plake KS (eds.) *Introduction to Health Care Delivery: A Primer for Pharmacists,* 5th ed. Sudbury, MA: Jones & Bartlett Learning, pp. 315–335.

Health Policy Brief: The Relative Contribution of Multiple Determinants to Health Outcomes. *Health Affairs,* August 21, 2014.

Institute for Safe Medication Practices. 2019. Guidelines for the safe use of automated dispensing cabinets. Available at https://www.ismp.org/resources/guidelines-safe-use-automated-dispensing-cabinets. Accessed February 28, 2019.

Kaiser Family Foundation. 2016. Total hospitals. Available at http://kff.org/other/state-indicator/total-hospitals. Accessed February 28, 2019.

Kaiser Family Foundation. 2018. Total professionally active physicians. Available at http://kff.org/other/state-indicator/total-active-physicians. Accessed February 28, 2019.

Kaiser Family Foundation. 2019. What are the recent and forecasted trends in prescription drug spending? Available at https://www.healthsystemtracker.org/chart-collection/recent-forecasted-trends-prescription-drug-spending/#item-start. Accessed February 28, 2019.

Kijsanayotin B, Pannarunothai S, Speedie SM. 2009. Factors influencing health information technology adoption in Thailand's community health centers: Applying the UTAUT model. *Int J Med Inform* 78(6):404–416.

Kilbridge P, Classen D. 2002. Surveillance for adverse drug events: History, methods, and current issues. *Volunt Hosp Am* 3:1–35. Irving, TX: VHA Inc. Research Series.

Kohn LT, Corrigan JM, Donaldson MS, eds. 1999. *To Err is Human: Building a Safer Health System*. Washington, DC: National Academy Press.

Kotter JP. 1995. Leading change: Why transformation efforts fail. *Harv Bus Rev* 73(2):59–67.

Leape LL, Bates DW, Cullen DJ, et al. 1995. Systems analysis of adverse drug events. *JAMA* 274:35–43.

Lesselroth BJ, Adams K, Church VL, et al. 2018. Evaluation of multimedia medication reconciliation software: A randomized controlled, single-blind trial to measure diagnostic accuracy for discrepancy detection. *Appl Clin Inform* 9(2):285–301.

Lockwood WA. 2010. Automation of ambulatory care pharmacy operations. In Fox BI, Thrower MR, Felkey BG (eds.) *Building Core Competencies in Pharmacy Informatics*. Washington, DC: American Pharmacists Association, pp. 299–310.

Luo JS, Hilty DM, Worley LL, Yager J. 2006. Considerations in change management related to technology. *Acad Psychiatry* 30:465–469.

Mackowiak L. 2011. The Pharmacy eHIT Collaborative: Its purpose and progress to date. Presentation at the American Society of Health-System Pharmacists Summer Meeting. Denver, CO.

Miller AS. 2009. Planning for downtime. In Dumitru D (ed.) *The Pharmacy Informatics Primer*. Bethesda, MD: America Society of Health-System Pharmacists, p. 195.

Modern Healthcare. 2013. Storm tests EHR. Available at https://www.modernhealthcare.com/article/20130525/MAGAZINE/305259978/storm-tests-ehr. Accessed February 28, 2019.

Pharmacy Health Information Technology Collaborative. 2018a. Primary focus. Available at https://www.pharmacyhit.org/. Accessed December 29, 2018.

Pharmacy Health Information Technology Collaborative. 2018b. The roadmap for pharmacy health information technology integration in US health care: 2018 to 2021 update. Available at https://www.pharmacyhit.org/pdfs/workshop-documents/PHIT_Roadmap_2018-2021_Final.pdf. Accessed December 29, 2018.

Qato DM, Zenk S, Wilder J, et al. 2017. The availability of pharmacies in the United States: 2007-2015. *PLoS One* 12(8):e0183172.

Rupp MT, Warholak TL. 2008. Evaluation of e-prescribing in chain community pharmacy: Best-practice recommendations. *J Am Pharm Assoc* 48(3):364–370.

Section of Pharmacy Informatics and Technology Executive Committee. 2009. Technology-enabled practice: A vision statement by the ASHP Section of pharmacy informatics and Technology. *Am J Health Syst Pharm* 66(17):1573–1577.

Siska MH. 2005. Organizational and functional requirements for eMAR selection. In *Pharmacy Purchasing & Purchasing*. Available at https://www.pppmag.com/article/96/September_2005/Organizational_and_Functional_Requirements_for_EMAR_Selection/. Accessed February 28, 2019.

Siska MH. 2006. Functional requirements for pharmacy information management systems. In *Pharmacy Purchasing & Purchasing*. Available at http://www.pppmag.com/article/107/November_2006/Functional_Requirements_for_Pharmacy_Information_Management_Systems/. Accessed January 21, 2019.

Siska MH. 2011. E-prescribing: One giant leap toward pharmacy practice integration. *Am J Health Syst Pharm* 68(5):380–381.

Siska MH, Tribble DA. 2011. Opportunities and challenges related to technology in supporting optimal pharmacy practice models in hospitals and health systems. *Am J Health-Syst Pharm* 68(12):1116–1126.

Venkatesh V, Morris MG, Davis GB, Davis FD. 2003. User acceptance of information technology: Toward a unified view. *MIS Q* 2003:425–428.

Walker J, Pan E, Johnston D, Adler-Milstein J, Bates DW, Middleton B. 2005. The value of health care information exchange and interoperability. *Health Aff* (Suppl Web Exclusives):W5–W8.

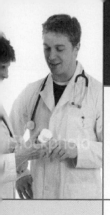

10

ENSURING QUALITY IN PHARMACY OPERATIONS

Terri L. Warholak, Patrick J. Campbell, and Mel L. Nelson

About the Authors: Dr. Warholak is a professor and Assistant Dean of Academic Affairs and Assessment at the University of Arizona College of Pharmacy. She earned BS, MS, and PhD from Purdue University, Indiana. Her professional pharmacy experience encompasses practice in both hospital and community pharmacies, including 5 years as a commissioned officer in the U.S. Public Health Service (Indian Health Service) and a short tour of duty with the Food and Drug Administration. Dr. Warholak has been recognized as a winner of the American Association of Colleges of Pharmacy Council of Faculties Innovations in Teaching Competition for her work titled "Application of Quality Assurance Principles: Reducing Medication Errors in 30 Pharmacy Practice Settings." This work formed the basis of a national quality improvement (QI) educational program (Educating Pharmacists in Quality) with the Pharmacy Quality Alliance (PQA). Dr. Warholak's teaching and research interests include medication error reduction, health information technology evaluation, and bringing pharmaceutical care to underserved populations. As such, she has substantial experience collaborating with pharmacists and other health care providers. She has participated in studies evaluating the quality of patient care, techniques for reducing medication errors, and health information technology assessment.

Dr. Campbell is the Director of Measurement Outcomes Research at the PQA. He earned a Doctorate of Pharmacy (PharmD) and a PhD in Pharmaceutical Economics, Policy, and Outcomes from the University of Arizona. He has worked in community pharmacy practice since 2010 and has experience with workflow processes, performance metrics, and business operations. Dr. Campbell has been involved with PQA since 2013, serving on workgroups and measure development teams.

Dr. Nelson is the Director of Research and Academic Affairs at the PQA. In this role, she is responsible for the advancement and coordination of PQA's research portfolio. She also directs PQA's student and post-graduate programs to support PQA's commitment to educate the next generation of health care quality leaders. Prior to her role at PQA, Dr. Nelson spent several years as a research assistant at the University of Arizona College of Pharmacy, with a focus on investigating health care QI and health professions education. During that time, she also earned her PharmD degree.

■ **SCENARIO**

Anita Katz was promoted to "pharmacy manager" at a community pharmacy last week. She was excited and wanted to make some positive changes. Among the charges assigned to her was to implement a QI program to decrease errors, increase efficiency, and improve store performance on pharmacy quality measures. The goals of the QI program were to improve patient satisfaction, decrease medication errors, and to improve performance on metrics that contribute to Medicare Part D plan Star ratings. However, she was overwhelmed but did not know where to start the QI process. Some questions she asked herself were: How should I begin? Who should I involve? How should I decide which quality issue to address first? What interventions have been successful in the past? What data will I need to collect? How will I assess if my interventions are successful? Are there "off the shelf" QI programs available that I could use? From which stakeholders do I need buy-in? Anita started researching on the Internet but also began to recall key concepts from her QI and Medication Error Reduction class in pharmacy school. Armed with this information, she began the planning process that would make her pharmacy truly exceptional.

■ **CHAPTER QUESTIONS**

1. How is *quality* defined within the context of pharmacy practice?
2. Define *health care quality* in layperson's terms.
3. How can the need for QI be justified to decision makers?
4. How can quality be measured?
5. What can pharmacy organizations learn from other industries concerning quality?
6. List the steps of a CQI model.
7. List four practical CQI suggestions for the pharmacist.

■ **WHAT IS QUALITY?**

Quality may appear to be a nebulous term. We know what quality is when we see it, but its definition might be subjective. In fact, there are quite a few definitions of quality. For example, *Webster's Dictionary* defines *quality* as a "degree of excellence" (Merriam-Webster, 2019a). While this definition provides a framework for quality in general, it is also helpful to examine the definitions of quality specific to health care.

The U.S. Office of Technology Assessment (OTA) has defined the *quality of medical care* as "evaluation of the performance of medical providers according to the degree to which the process of care increases the probability of outcomes desired by patients and reduces the probability of undesired outcomes, given the state of medical knowledge" (Congress of the United States & Office of Technology Assessment, 1988).

The Institute of Medicine (IOM), in a report entitled, "Medicare: A Strategy for Quality Assurance," stated that "quality of care is the degree to which health services for individuals and populations increase the likelihood of desired health outcomes and are consistent with current professional knowledge" (Lohr, 1990a), whereas Ovretveit (1992) simply states, "A quality health service/system gives patients what they want and need."

An amalgamation of these definitions may provide the best explanation of the concept of quality in health care. The OTA definition implies that the care offered to patients should increase the probability of positive outcomes (e.g., curing an infection) and decrease negative outcomes of care (e.g., death). The care offered to patients should be in line with current scientific knowledge. While the broadened perspective from Ovretveit has merit, patients may not be the best judges of the quality of medical care because even though they may know what they *want* from medical care, they may not have well-defined notions of what they *need* from medical care. Thus, it is up to the medical provider to offer quality care to benefit the patient even when the patient does not know what he or she needs. While this may appear paternalistic, it seems reasonable that any person who is not an expert in a field may not know all the best alternatives.

So, what is quality in pharmacy practice? Extrapolating from the preceding discussion, it can be said that quality in pharmacy practice

- Represents a degree of excellence;
- Increases the probability of positive outcomes;
- Decreases the probability of negative outcomes;
- Corresponds with current medical knowledge;
- Offers the patient what he or she wants; and
- Provides the patient with what he or she needs.

Understanding these aspects of quality will help Anita explain pharmacy quality to patients and will serve as the basis for pharmacy improvement.

■ HOW IS QUALITY MEASURED?

Historically, pharmacy practice quality has been measured by assessing its structure, process, and outcomes (Donabedian, 1969, 1991). Simply put, for a good or service

- *Structure* refers to the raw materials needed for production;
- *Process* is the method or procedure used; and
- *Outcomes* are the end result.

Each of the precedings (i.e., structure, process, and outcomes) has been used to measure quality. Traditionally, pharmacy quality has been measured by structure and process methods. This relies on a premise that a quality outcome is not possible without appropriate structure or process. Moreover, it is much simpler and less controversial to measure structure and process than it is to measure outcomes. Recently, however, measuring quality outcomes has become more prevalent.

In the realm of pharmacy, the raw materials or structures necessary for quality care are many and varied. Examples include number of pharmacists per shift, counter space, pharmacist credentials or licensing, pharmacy square footage, medication reference books, medication stock, and counseling facilities.

Since pharmacists are responsible for all phases of medication use, processes in the pharmacy can refer to any phase of the medication use process (e.g., prescribing, transcribing, dispensing, administering, or monitoring). Examples of process measures include, but are not limited to, adherence to clinical guidelines or pathways, percent of prescriptions assessed for appropriateness, and percent of patients counseled.

Outcomes are the driving force behind medication therapy management (MTM), which has pharmacists participating in patient education, medication review, and disease management. Through such activities, pharmacists have been able to improve patient care by: (1) increasing patients' control of their medical conditions (Bluml et al., 2014; Brummel et al., 2014; Bukhsh et al., 2018; Bunting et al., 2008; Chisholm-Burns et al., 2010; Dunn et al., 2015; Houle et al., 2012; Jokanovic et al., 2017; McAdam-Marx et al., 2015; Milosavljevic et al., 2018; Morgado et al., 2011; Murphy et al., 2016; Obreli-Neto et al., 2015; Pinto et al., 2018; Santschi et al., 2018; Skinner et al., 2015; Theising et al., 2015; Van Eikenhorstet al., 2017); (2) decreasing use of health care resources (Murray et al., 2007; Obreli-Neto et al., 2015; Pellegrin et al., 2017); (3) increasing patients' knowledge of their conditions, treatments, and medications (Bluml et al., 2014; Bukhsh et al., 2018; Dunn et al., 2015; Van Eikenhorst et al., 2017); (4) increasing adherence to and persistence with medication regimens (Chisholm-Burns et al., 2010; Milosavljevic et al., 2018; Moore & Smith, 2018; Morgado et al., 2011; Murray et al., 2007; Pinto et al., 2018; Pringle et al., 2014; Skinner et al., 2015; Stanton-Robinson et al., 2018; van Boven et al., 2014; Van Eikenhorst et al., 2017); (5) increasing patients' satisfaction with their care (Cardosi et al., 2018; Chisholm-Burns et al., 2010; Hatton et al., 2018; Schuessler et al., 2016; van Boven et al., 2014;); and (6) saving payers money (Brummel et al., 2014; Houle et al., 2012; McAdam-Marx et al., 2015; Murray et al., 2007; Ni et al., 2018; Pellegrin et al., 2017; Pringle et al., 2017); and (7) improving patients' quality of life (Mishra et al., 2017; Mohammed et al., 2016; Sakthong et al., 2018).

The systems engineering initiative for patient safety (SEIPS) model expands Donabedian's process concept from direct patient care to processes that support patient care (i.e., housekeeping) and indicates that these processes must also be designed to support safety. SEIPS is a multidisciplinary initiative applying systems engineering, human factors engineering, and quality engineering approaches. The research supporting this model examines systems design, quality management, job design, and technology implementations that affect safety-related patient and organizational and/or staff outcomes (Carayon et al., 2006, 2014; Wooldridge et al., 2017).

Pharmacists' ability to identify, resolve, and prevent medication-related problems, as well as take responsibility in disease management, is well-documented (Brummel et al., 2014; Chisholm-Burns et al., 2010; Dunn et al., 2015; Guignard et al., 2015; Hansen et al., 2006; Moczygemba et al., 2011; Obreli-Neto et al., 2015; Sakthong & Sang-thonganotai, 2018; San-Juan-Rodriguez et al., 2018). Thus, outcomes describe the ultimate goal of the care or therapy and answer the question, "What are we trying to accomplish?"

There are different ways to look at outcomes. One method, the ECHO model, purports three basic types of outcomes: economic, clinical, and humanistic (Kozma et al., 1993). Economic outcomes include direct costs and consequences, both medical and nonmedical, and indirect costs and consequences. For example, when assessing outcomes from a patient perspective, a medication copayment would be a direct medication cost, whereas gas money to pick up the medication from the pharmacy would represent a nonmedical direct cost. Lost wages from missed work as a result of a health condition could be regarded as an indirect cost.

Clinical outcomes measures can include morbidity and mortality, event rates, or symptom resolution (Mainz, 2003; Ovretveit, 2001). These measures directly assess outcomes but may be difficult to evaluate, especially in pharmacist interventions, where their onset could be years following a treatment or intervention (Chassin & Galvin, 1998; Shane & Gouveia, 2000). In these cases, indicators or markers can be used to assess outcomes. These indicators can be condition-specific (e.g., A1C for diabetes) or procedure-specific (e.g., rate of postoperative infection after hip surgery), or address an important issue of patient care. For example, blood pressure may be used as a marker to assess susceptibility to stroke because it is not practical, safe, or ethical to wait and measure the occurrence of stroke.

Humanistic outcomes include measures of the "human" aspects of care. Specific types of humanistic outcomes include patient satisfaction and health-related quality of life (HRQoL). For example, a survey concerning patient satisfaction with pharmacist services could be used to assess humanistic outcomes for patients receiving these services. Alternatively, a HRQoL assessment may be useful to assess the impact medication therapy has on the patient's life as a whole.

Measuring outcomes can seem to be a daunting task. Thus, the remainder of this chapter will present these concepts in an easy-to-understand manner and will include simple implementation tips.

■ WHAT CAN PHARMACY LEARN FROM OTHER INDUSTRIES?

Health care traditionally has lagged behind other industries in QI. It has been suggested that medicine should follow the lead of the airline and other industries by using quality management to decrease unnecessary variation and to improve quality (Leape, 1994). An IOM report supported this contention when the authors suggested that the American health care system can improve the quality of care by borrowing techniques used in other industries to standardize processes (Kohn, 2000). Many of these techniques are based on systems theory.

Systems theory, developed by von Bertalanffy (1968), has been used in engineering, medicine, and education to improve process efficiency and quality (Nagel, 1988; Sheridan, 1988). A systems approach involves defining the purpose and performance expectations of the system, examining the characteristics of the inputs, considering alternative mechanisms for achieving the stated goals, implementing the system, and adjusting the system based on feedback (Park, 1997; Sheridan, 1988).

There has been an emerging demand for leaders who are system-oriented thinkers, particularly in health care settings (Bleich, 2014a). "Skilled systems thinkers should be able to: (1) differentiate cause and effect algorithms and procedures with work design that encompasses awareness of systems; (2) determine downstream and upstream influences and processes that gives intention to decision making; (3) align human and material resource requirements for fitness and appropriateness within the system; and

(4) identify and set boundaries around systems that are nested within other interdependent systems" (Bleich, 2014b). Clinical, social, and economic perspectives are commonly employed to capture the health care system's complexity. A system-oriented thinker would solicit and utilize these diverse perspectives when making both current clinical decisions as well as decisions concerning long-term system efficiency (Bleich, 2014a).

Various organizations and regulators have turned to a systems view of QI termed *human factors principles* (FAA, 1993; Leape et al., 1998a). The human factors view of quality focuses on the relationship between quality problems and the system in which they occur (Rasmussen et al., 1994). "Human factors principles are concepts about the design of work that take advantage of the strengths and weaknesses of the human mind and compensate for its limitations" (Leape et al., 1998a). Human factors principles include: (1) reducing reliance on memory; (2) simplifying and standardizing; (3) using protocols and checklists; (4) using mechanisms to physically prevent error (constraints and forcing functions); (5) improving access to information; (6) decreasing reliance on vigilance; (7) differentiating; and (8) implementing automation (Kohn, 2000; Leape et al., 1998a).

In pharmacy practice, decreased reliance on memory can be accomplished by using decision-support systems. Drug monographs, interaction tools, and clinical guidelines are available in most community settings and can be referenced to support pharmacist clinical decision making. In-store computer systems to assist with Omnibus Budget Reconciliation Act of 1990—mandated (OBRA 90—mandated) prospective drug utilization review (DUR) are also widely used in community settings. These decision-support systems can also be used to decrease reliance on vigilance through alerting the pharmacist of potential problems. However, decision-support systems should be used wisely because they are not intended to supplant the pharmacist's clinical decision-making skills (Leape et al., 1998a; Nolan, 2000).

Standardization is thought to be one of the most powerful tools for improving quality and workflow efficiency (Leape et al., 1998b). If a person does something the same way every time, the chances that he or she will perform the activity incorrectly are greatly reduced (Leape et al., 1998b). Subsequently, many industries, including pharmacy, have adopted the principles of the Henry Ford Production System to create rules of work: standardized tasks, defined connections between workers, and simplified process pathways (Zarbo et al., 2009). Industry has long known that quality and variation are inversely related; quality improves as variation is reduced (Deming, 1986). In pharmacy, standardization is the simplest, most broadly applicable, and most effective method for QI (Leape et al., 1998b). In fact, the move to standardization has created the impetus for critical pathways that focus not only on error prevention but also on optimization of outcomes, cost reduction, and satisfaction (American Pharmacists Association, 2003; National Guideline Clearinghouse [NGC], 2000). The inclusion of clinical services like immunization administration and MTM programs in community pharmacies has demonstrated that successful programs require standardized processes (Gardner, 1996; Law et al., 2009).

Protocols and checklists serve as reminders of critical tasks, especially when an omission can have serious consequences, and are often recommended as mechanisms for increasing quality (Boeing, 1993). Policies and protocols decrease confusion, thus improving overall quality. A constraint that "prevents further action until some condition is met" (Leape et al., 1998a) can also be written into protocols to provide a quality check in a system. For example, a protocol on medication procurement and stocking may ensure that adequate quantities are maintained to support the prescription filling process. Or a dispensing policy may include constraints to prevent prescriptions from being dispensed until they have been approved by the pharmacist's final check.

Improving access to information leads to improved quality (Abelson & Levi, 1985; Weinstein & Fineberg, 1980). One study indicated that pharmacists make more appropriate prospective DUR decisions when they have access to more complete patient information, such as medication profiles, allergy information, patient age, and diagnosis (Warholak-Juarez et al., 2000). These pieces of additional information, in conjunction with decision-support systems, decrease the pharmacist's reliance on vigilance and should be considered before medication orders are processed.

Differentiation of products and the incorporation of automation in the medication dispensing process have been endorsed by the National Coordination Council for Medication Error Reporting (2007, 2015). An example of differentiation and automation technology in pharmacy practice settings is the use of barcode technology. Including product verification via bar code at strategic points of the dispensing and administration processes can reduce errors and the need to rework (Morriss et al., 2009; Poon et al., 2005; Siebert et al., 2014).

Moreover, improved quality produces a corresponding increase in productivity because less rework is needed and less waste is produced (Deming, 1986). In pharmacy, QI may produce improved clinical and humanistic outcomes such as improved HRQoL and customer satisfaction. Improved customer satisfaction can help make the workplace more pleasant and may produce a corresponding increase in employee satisfaction. This ultimately may lead to the pharmacy having a competitive edge and an image as a provider of high-quality pharmaceutical care and may allow the business to recruit and maintain the most highly qualified and desired personnel.

■ METHODS FOR ENSURING QUALITY IN PHARMACY PRACTICE

Quality Control

QC, as defined by *Webster's Dictionary*, is "the activity of checking goods as they are produced to make sure that the final products are good" (Merriam-Webster, 2019b). QC can be thought of as defect *detection*. Problems are addressed *after* they occur (Godwin & Sanborn, 1995).

Quality Assurance

QA has been defined as "a program for the systematic monitoring and evaluation of the various aspects of a project, service, or facility to ensure that standards of quality are being met" (Merriam-Webster, 2019c). QA aims to *prevent* defects.

CQI

CQI is "a philosophy of continual improvement of the processes associated with providing a good or service that meets or exceeds customer expectations" (Shortell et al., 1998). CQI has been referred to as the *QI process, total quality management,* and *total QC* (Lohr, 1990b).

CQI introduced two important ideas that transcend QA and QC. First, CQI represents a total systems perspective concerning quality; all workers within the health care system are interconnected (Godwin & Sanborn, 1995). When examined from a systems perspective, every action of a health care professional is performed to benefit the patient (Shortell et al., 1998). Therefore, all actions must be planned to improve care and should not focus on correcting individual mistakes after the fact (Godwin & Sanborn, 1995; Shortell et al., 1998). Thus, quality problems are not examined (or blamed) on an individual level (Blumenthal & Kilo, 1998). CQI promotes identification of the cause of problems via "fact-based management and scientific methodology, which make it culturally compatible with the values of health care professionals" (Shortell et al., 1998, p. 605).

Second, CQI demands that the QI process is continuous or never-ending (Blumenthal & Kilo, 1998). Improvement occurs by integrating information concerning quality into the cyclic redesign and improvement of care (Godwin & Sanborn, 1995). The changes can be quick and on a small scale but should be occurring constantly. In this manner, CQI empowers health care providers to improve quality on a daily basis (Shortell et al., 1998).

CQI is more than looking for things that could be wrong; it is a systematic process for continuously improving the quality of every aspect of a pharmacy practice setting from patient care to managerial responsiveness. In this manner, CQI is a much more positive process than QA or QC because the focus is on constantly making things better for all who work in and have contact with the practice. CQI is a method for constantly striving for improvement in every facet and every portion of the medication use system.

■ A CQI IMPROVEMENT MODEL

Many CQI models exist. Examples of specific models include the plan, do, check, and act (PDCA) model and the find, organize, clarify, understand, select, plan, do, check, and act (FOCUS-PDCA) model, and six sigma (Lazarus & Butler, 2001; Lazarus & Stamps, 2002). Most models include elements that reflect the following core concepts: (1) plan, (2) design, (3) measure, (4) assess, and (5) improve (Coe, 1998a).

CQI has been described as a practical application of the scientific method (Blumenthal & Kilo, 1998). Planning in both processes is similar. In this manner, one can think of the steps in the CQI cycle as parallel to the sections of a scientific article: background, methods, results, conclusions, and recommendations. Considering CQI in this manner diminishes the need to memorize additional terminology. See Figure 10-1 for a flowchart representation of the process.

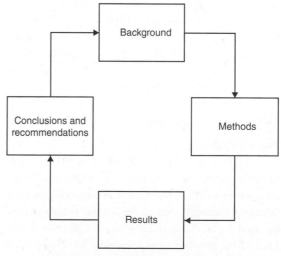

Figure 10-1. The CQI measurement cycle.

The steps to CQI discussed in this chapter are included in the CQI Cycle Checklist and Planning Worksheets in Appendices A and B, respectively. The CQI Cycle Checklist includes an abbreviated list of the actions needed for a successful CQI cycle. The Planning Worksheets are more detailed forms to assist in CQI cycle implementation. Worksheet 1 is intended for use during the first team meeting, Worksheet 2 should be used for the second meeting and reused through completion of data collection, and Worksheet 3 begins with data analysis and guides the user through the remainder of the CQI cycle.

Recruiting the CQI Team

The planning phase of CQI is essential. The first step in developing a cohesive plan is to assemble an expert panel. This panel should be interdisciplinary and include representatives of those who are part of or will be affected by the quality plan. The team also should include subject matter experts, decision makers, and frontline personnel. In a pharmacy setting, the entire staff should be invited to participate. This will stress the importance of the quality process and help to get staff support for the QI projects. The diversity of experiences, job roles, and perspectives from each team member contributes to effective team dynamics; diversity within groups promotes effective team functioning due to higher variability in ideas, creativity, and innovation (Knight et al., 1999). It is important to note that while buy-in will be increased by inviting staff participation and opinions, this effect will be lost quickly if staff members do not perceive that their participation is beneficial.

CQI Cycle Background

Focus Selection

The CQI cycle begins with the selection of a QI focus. Selection may be based on mandate, or the choice may be left to the team. If the team is given the latitude to choose, one of the several processes may be used to facilitate this decision. The team could brainstorm possible areas for study. In this case, all team members should provide ideas freely, and each

idea should be recorded. Ideas then may be ranked, and team consensus can be used for system selection. Examples of systems that have been shown to provide QI opportunities in health care settings include the following:

- Identifying and measuring the incidence of medication errors,
- Implementing methods to reduce medication errors,
- Measuring medication-filling time,
- Analyzing satisfaction with pharmacy services,
- Evaluating the effect of pharmacists' interventions,
- Analyzing adherence to requirements for documentation,
- Documenting the incidence of medication allergy,
- Auditing patient-controlled analgesia pumps,
- Assessing patient-specific medication errors in cart filling, and
- Analyzing hypertension control and guidelines compliance.

Alternatively, processes such as failure mode and effects analysis or root cause analysis can be used to identify systems ripe for QI activities. Failure mode and effects analysis is a prospective procedure used to identify areas for QI before they become a problem (Cohen et al., 1994; DeRosier et al., 2002; NCPS, 2011a). Once possible areas are identified, the investigators decide if the results will be tolerable or intolerable (Cohen et al., 1994).

Root cause analysis is a systematic process used to identify the exact or root cause of a problem (Coe, 1998b). It is used after a quality problem has been discovered (a retrospective procedure) to prevent recurrence (Coe, 1998c; NCPS, 2011b). The process begins with "triage questions" that help the team decide what issues (e.g., staff training, competency, human factors, equipment, and information) could have contributed to the quality problem (Gosbee & Anderson, 2003). Once these questions are answered, more detailed, specific questions are considered to identify ways to improve systems to reduce the chance of it recurring. The investigators create an action plan for implementing system improvements and

Table 10-1.   Two Tools for Identifying Quality Improvement Priority Areas

Prospective: Failure Mode and Effects Analysis (FMEA)

The Veterans Administration National Center for Patient Safety (NCPS) has translated this industrial and engineering procedure for health care. The NCPS has termed its adaptation *healthcare failure mode effects analysis* (HFMEA), and it offers live and videoconference training courses on use (DeRosier et al., 2002). Before doing FMEA, obtain a copy of the articles and worksheets that have been developed as a process guide (available from NCPS at http://www.patientsafety.va.gov/professionals/onthejob/ hfmea.asp). HFMEA can be performed for general processes (e.g., use of medications on the night shift) or for specific medications. Steps include the following:

Step 1: Define the scope or topic to be studied.

Step 2: Assemble a multidisciplinary team that includes a subject matter expert.

Step 3: Describe and narrow the focus.

Step 4: Conduct a hazard analysis.

Step 5: Select necessary actions and outcome measures and assign activities to specific persons and dates for follow-up.

Retrospective: Root Cause Analysis

A comprehensive root cause analysis guide is also available from NCPS (see https://www.patientsafety. va.gov/professionals/onthejob/rca.asp). This guide walks the pharmacist through every step of a comprehensive root cause evaluation of a quality problem. The guide focuses on system-level failures and is split into the following four sections

- What happened?
- Why did it happen?
- What action can we take to prevent it from happening again?
- How will we know if the action we took made a difference?

In the first section, the user is led through detailed questions that address various possible situations. These more detailed questions cover areas such as human factors, communication, training, fatigue, scheduling, environment, equipment, rules, policy, procedure, or barriers to quality. Each additional section serves to walk the user through the root cause analysis process by providing scenarios, descriptions, and step-by-step guidance.

improvements evaluation (Anonymous, 2002; Bagian et al., 2001). A more detailed account of these two processes is included in Table 10-1.

Focus Description

After the focus for QI has been chosen, it is important to make sure that it is clear to each team member. This can be accomplished by providing a detailed description of the area chosen for study, the setting in which the focus occurs, the portion of the medication use process affected, and baseline data, if applicable.

Flowcharts that explicitly represent all portions of the process can be helpful for system description. Flowcharts use standard symbols that represent all process steps (represented as rectangles), as well as decision points (represented by diamond shapes) and the direction of progression from one subprocess to the other (Coe, 1998a). Flowcharts are also useful because they can help the team recognize if the process chosen is too broad (i.e., represented by an unwieldy flowchart). An example of a flowchart is given in Figure 10-1.

Focus Importance

Next, the team should state why the focus is important. The selected focus should be important to the organization and have the potential to lead to the improvement. It should be considered high priority, high volume, high cost, or high risk. For example, a community pharmacy may choose to focus on prescription order-entry error if anecdotal evidence suggests that this may be an error-prone step in its dispensing process.

Literature Review

Relate the focus to the literature by investigating what is known and not known about similar situations. This step can save the team an enormous amount of time in the long run. A brief literature search will help the team to discover techniques, interventions, and other tools that have been successful in improving quality in similar situations.

Goals

Once the focus (i.e., process or problem) is chosen, the team should *determine the overall goal* (Leape et al., 1998c). Common overall goals include (1) discovery, (2) frequency estimation, and (3) measuring a change (Leape et al., 1998c). For example, after a pharmacy's CQI team has decided that it wants to focus on prescription order-entry error, team members must then decide *what* they want to know about it. They may decide that since this is their first CQI cycle, they will focus on frequency estimation of the problem. This will serve as baseline data for the assessment of improvements. The overall goal can be used to *choose specific goals for the cycle* (Leape et al., 1998c). Note that it is important to assess the practicality of the specific goal. The CQI team should examine the specific goal carefully to determine whether it is realistic. If the goal is not realistic, then it may need to be scaled back (Leape et al., 1998c). Choosing something reasonable for the first CQI cycle will provide the team with experience, improve its chances for success, and thus bolster team members' confidence for the next cycle.

CQI Cycle Methods

Intervention

Interventions discovered through a literature review should be included on a list of possible interventions. These may include QI techniques such as reducing reliance on memory, simplifying, standardizing, or automating processes.

Process and Outcomes Measures

Next, the CQI team must determine what measures will be used to assess progress toward goals (Leape et al., 1998c). Team members should list process and/or outcome measures necessary to determine if the goals were met. Usually, a mix of process and outcome measures is recommended (Leape et al., 1998c). Many measures have been developed, so keep the following in mind: do not invent a new measure if a good one exists; measure what is important—not easy; and do not measure things you cannot change or interpret (Ovretveit, 2001). Table 10-2 provides additional resources on selecting and developing measures.

Data Collection Procedures

If the required data are not already being collected, the CQI team should devise a plan to collect the appropriate data. The team can choose from several different data collection methods (Leape et al., 1998c), including inspection points, focus groups, monitoring for markers, and observation.

Data Analysis Plan

The planned statistical analysis should be thought out in detail to make sure that all necessary information will be gathered. It can be frustrating and time-consuming to gather forgotten data at a moment's notice. This seems self-evident but is a mistake that many people make.

CQI Cycle Results

Analyze Data

Most descriptive statistics (e.g., mean, median, and percentages) often suffice for data analysis. Some analyzes can be performed simply by plotting data onto

Table 10-2.   Health Care Process and Outcome Measurement Resources

Need help selecting a measure?

Many process and outcome measures exist, so there may be no need to develop one of your own. Measure selection can be expedited by examining the core critical literature, soliciting expert opinion, or using recognized guidelines such as those from The Joint Commission, The National Committee for Quality Assurance (e.g., Healthcare Effectiveness Data and Information Set or HEDIS), The Pharmacy Quality Alliance (PQA) or Healthy People 2020.

Other resources include the National Quality Measures Clearinghouse (NQMC). NQMC provides information on health care quality measures and measure sets and includes a glossary of terms and information on how to select, use, apply, and interpret a measure. Available at https://www.ahrq.gov/gam/index.html. Ready-to-use quality tools can be accessed via http://www.ahrq.gov/professionals/quality-patient-safety/quality-resources/index.html.

charts or graphs which can help to determine patterns and trends. For more sophisticated analysis, outside assistance may be required. If there is not a statistician on the CQI team, it may be beneficial to refer to statistics books to make sure that the chosen analysis is appropriate. Asking for outside help is also an option; the team should not hesitate to call the local college of pharmacy for a referral.

CQI Cycle Conclusions, Implications, and Recommendations

The final section in the process is describing the conclusions, implications, and recommendations that the team reached after examining the results. Since this is the "bottom line" of the process, it is important that this section be understandable to those outside the CQI team. This section should concisely explain the

conclusions and detail the actions that need to take place. The CQI process is iterative; thus, the team's recommendations for *this CQI cycle* and for the *next CQI cycle* must be included (Leape et al., 1998b). This will be good news to pharmacist Anita. Because CQI is a continuous improvement process, an understanding of the iterative nature of the process will take the pressure off her to "fix" all pharmacy system problems at once.

■ ACCREDITATION/ COMPLIANCE WITH QUALITY STANDARDS PROMULGATED BY AGENCIES OR ASSOCIATIONS

Often QI activities are necessary for accreditation. Earning accreditation indicates that an organization has met predefined standards. The accreditation process provides a framework to help organizations focus on providing safe, high-quality service and requires that the organization demonstrate to outside reviewers its commitment to continuous improvement (Ovretveit, 2001). There are several organizations in the US that offer accreditation services.

The Joint Commission

The Joint Commission is an independent, non-profit organization founded in 1951 by the American Medical Association and the American College of Surgeons (O'Malley, 1997). The Joint Commission was established to "continuously improve health care for the public, in collaboration with other stakeholders, by evaluating health care organizations and inspiring them to excel in providing safe and effective care of the highest quality and value" (Joint Commission on Accreditation of Healthcare Organizations, 2019a). This is accomplished by evaluation and accreditation of more than 21,000 health care organizations and programs, including, but not limited to hospitals, ambulatory care clinics, home health and behavioral health care practices, and independent clinical laboratories (Joint Commission on Accreditation of Healthcare Organizations, 2019b).

The Joint Commission initial accreditation process is conducted via an onsite survey (and regular follow-ups) to determine if organizations are meeting Joint Commission standards, which include a focus on continuous improvement. Although Joint Commission compliance is voluntary, many organizations view it as mandatory (O'Malley, 1997). Not obtaining Joint Commission accreditation can adversely affect an organization's prestige and reimbursement status (Coe, 1998c; Joint Commission on Accreditation of Healthcare Organizations, 2018; O'Malley, 1997). Key dimensions of performance evaluation have evolved over time but include efficacy, appropriateness, availability, timeliness, effectiveness, continuity, safety, efficiency, respect, and caring (Coe, 1998a).

The Joint Commission's annual patient safety goals often involve medication use and thus pharmacists can use these goals to help improve the quality of medication use throughout the health care system. For example, one of the recent Hospital National Patient Safety Goals was "Use medicines safely" that includes identifying the patient's home medications, making sure new medications are appropriate to add to the patient's regimen, providing a medication list to the patient's next caregiver during their health system stay, and then providing the medication list to the patient's regular physician and the patient upon discharge. The medication list should be explained to the patient (Joint Commission on Accreditation of Healthcare Organizations website, 2019c). These are roles for which the pharmacist is uniquely suited, and a pharmacist who can contribute in this way to the health system will not only improve the quality of patient care but will also help better integrate him- or herself into the interprofessional medical team.

National Committee for QA

The National Committee for QA (NCQA) was established in 1979 by two managed care trade associations in response to a call from a former federal agency (Office of Health Maintenance Organizations) for an organization to perform quality care reviews with standardized quality measurement and reporting (Marwick, 1997). Since 1990, NCQA has operated as an independent, non-profit organization that reviews and accredits a broad range of health care programs, such as health plans, patient-centered medical homes, preferred provider organizations, and even independent physicians (NCQA, 2019a). The NCQA maintains a publicly accessible, comprehensive listing of all their quality accredited organizations (NCQA, 2019b).

Quality Measurement

While health care accreditation organizations have existed for quite a while, quality data were not readily available to the general public until recently. These quality measurements (sometimes called "report cards") make health care quality indicators readily available to the public. This encourages health care organizations to compete on the basis of quality and creates markets where quality, not just cost containment, is rewarded (Blumenthal & Kilo, 1998; O'Malley, 1997).

HEDIS

The Health Plan Employer Data and Information Set (HEDIS) is a tool to measure performance created by NCQA that is used by more than 90% of America's health plans to measure performance (NCQA, 2019c). HEDIS standardizes health plan performance data and disseminates this information publicly so plans can be compared on a normalized basis (O'Malley, 1997). This allows health care purchasers and consumers to compare plans and make informed decisions and provides plans with data on where they could focus to improve quality. Specifically, HEDIS is made up of more than 90 performance measures across six domains including effectiveness of care, access and availability of care, experience of care, utilization and risk-adjusted utilization, health plan descriptive information, and measures collected using electronic clinical data systems. Many HEDIS measures involve medication management, thus providing an opportunity for pharmacists to help improve the quality of patient care (NCQA, 2019d).

Leapfrog Group

The Leapfrog Group was formed by a coalition of Fortune 500 companies and leading health care purchase organizations (Leapfrog, 2019a). The Leapfrog Group was developed to create a market that rewards quality, not just the lowest cost provider, by providing quality, safety, and efficiency information to consumers (Leapfrog, 2019a). They launched the hospital survey in 2001, which initially included 3 performance metrics, or "leaps". All 3 were structural measures, e.g., presence of computerized physician order entry and appropriate staffing. Since 2012, The Leapfrog Group has provided the Hospital Safety Grade, which utilizes both process and outcome measures to assign a letter grade to hospitals, allowing consumers to easily find a safer, high quality hospital (Leapfrog, 2019a). Beginning in April of 2019, The Leapfrog Group expanded to outpatient settings for the first time by collecting and reporting safety data for outpatient and ambulatory surgery centers. The first public report will be available in 2020 (Leapfrog 2019b).

PQA

The PQA is not an accreditation organization; however, PQA's quality metrics are used in a number of value-based programs, including the Centers for Medicare and Medicaid Services (CMS) Part D Star Ratings program. PQA is a leader in the development of quality measures that target appropriate medication use and safety. Established in 2006 as a public-private partnership with CMS shortly after the implementation of the Medicare Part D Prescription Drug Benefit, PQA's initial role was to develop quality measures specifically for the Part D Star Ratings program (PQA, 2019a). PQA's multi-stakeholder membership has engaged in a transparent, consensus-based measure development process ever since those early days. However, PQA has now evolved into a nationally recognized, non-profit quality organization with roles not only as a measure developer but also health care quality researcher, educator, and multi-stakeholder convener (PQA, 2019a). PQA's medication use performance metrics focus on six areas: adherence, appropriate medication use, medication safety, medication therapy management, and core sets in both opioid prescribing practices and specialty medications. Example of specific measures include dosing for specific conditions such as diabetes, suboptimal treatment of conditions such as hypertension, drug–drug interactions, inappropriate medication use in the elderly, and completion rate for comprehensive medication review by health plans (PQA, 2019b).

The Future

Since establishment of the Joint Commission, the scope of health care organizations that are eligible for accreditation has widened from hospitals to encompass health systems, pharmacy benefit managers, nursing homes, and now even independent health care providers (Joint Commission on Accreditation of Healthcare Organizations, 2019b). In some countries, such as Australia, pharmacies are even accredited (Quality Care Pharmacy Program, 2015). The National Association of Boards of Pharmacy (NABP) partnered with the American Pharmacists Association (APhA, 2003) and the American Society of Health-Systems Pharmacists (ASHP) to develop the Center for Pharmacy Practice Accreditation (CPPA) (NABP, 2014). This program develops and implements pharmacy practice site accreditation programs. Initially, this organization accredited community pharmacies, and in 2015 just 3 community pharmacies were accredited; however, it now accredits specialty pharmacies and telehealth pharmacy practices as well (CPPA 2019a). The accreditation process includes standards specific to each practice type; however, QI remains a domain for each and every one of them (CPPA 2019b). To achieve accreditation from the CPPA, pharmacy practices would have to implement and maintain CQI programs (CPPA, 2019b). The rapid transformation of pharmacy practice sites seeking accreditation over such a short period illustrates just how much the health care industry is focused on QI practices. The future of the QI process is becoming more focused on outcomes measurement. Eventually, health care report cards will be offered across all practice settings and will be both more accessible and easy to understand, thus helping to grow the market for quality. In some cases, pharmacy QI may be mandated by state and local governments. For example, the state of Arizona requires that every pharmacy participate in a QA program (Arizona Revised Statutes, 2007). The state of Virginia approved a similar rule, requiring pharmacies to establish a CQI program (NABP, 2015). So, what does this mean for pharmacy practice? More pharmacists must understand CQI and be able to develop, implement, and measure the outcomes of such a plan. This could provide an opportunity for a community pharmacy report card (quality measurement) system on which pharmacies can compete on the basis of quality. Such a system may provide a great opportunity for pharmacies to advertise quality outcomes to payers and patients. If such a system is successful, quality could drive patient choices and payer decisions. Ultimately, the pharmacies with the highest quality may get more market share or obtain higher reimbursement rates for certain services (pay-for-performance). In addition, work is progressing to develop a publicly reported pharmacy Star measure to help drive pharmacy QI and empower patient choice based on quality.

■ REVISITING THE SCENARIO

There are several things that Anita can do to improve quality in her pharmacy. First, she can promote a "systems view" of errors within her organization (Hume, 1999). Systems changes should be implemented only when the organization is ready for a culture shift and has capable leadership that supports a systems view of "no finger-pointing" (Shortell et al., 1994). Everyone in the organization should be informed of and invited to participate in any quality systems changes (i.e., the quality team) to foster a feeling of ownership among all team members. Personnel evaluations (i.e., performance appraisals) should comprise a QI component so that employees are rewarded for their efforts in such matters (Shortell et al., 1994).

Second, Anita and the QI team she creates should focus on high-leverage important systems changes (Hume, 1999; Shortell et al., 1994). For medication

safety, this could involve focusing on high-alert medications (e.g., fast movers, narrow-therapeutic-index medications, and medications that are available in multiple strengths), high-risk populations (e.g., pediatrics, older adults, and patients with multiple comorbidities and/or medications), or problem processes (e.g., e-prescribing). Significant opportunities for improvement can be gleaned from an analysis of intervention data, medication errors that get identified before they leave the pharmacy (near misses), medication error incident reports, patient comments, or employee feedback (Johnson et al., 2002; Rogers, 1997).

Third, Anita and her team should implement small changes in quick improvement cycles (Hume, 1999). The QI team should be given the opportunity to learn about quality by attempting small changes; it may be too frustrating to take on a large project for the first cycle. Team members should be allowed to experience a success and see how much improvement can be made with a relatively small change; then their enthusiasm will redouble.

Fourth, Anita and her QI team should implement interventions that have worked elsewhere (Hume, 1999). This improves the likelihood of success and reduces the amount of effort required in the process. It is worth noting that the most successful interventions changed *systems*, not *people* (Nolan, 2000; van Bokhoven et al., 2003).

If Anita's pharmacy organization does not want to develop its own CQI plan, help is available. Pharmacy Quality Commitment has developed the Sentinel System for community pharmacies. This system, which incorporates best practices, risk management techniques, and systematic procedures to increase quality, is ready to use and is available from the National Alliance of State Pharmacy Associations at www.pqc.net.

It is important to remember that QI in pharmacy is far reaching and that QI projects may take many shapes. That is, the pharmacist can be involved in many different type of QI projects such as the following: decreasing prescribing errors by educating physicians on principles of safe prescribing, improving patient medication compliance by providing a lower cost alternative, decreasing mortality by helping prescribers select appropriate antibiotics, decreasing medication dispensing errors by implementing dispensing technology, improving the identification of e-prescribing drop down menu selection errors by having prescribers transmit the diagnosis with prescriptions, helping patients better adhere to anticoagulant therapy by providing education, using "show and tell" patient counseling as a method to identify medication errors before they leave the pharmacy, or improving quality of medication use by adding pharmacist-performed medication reconciliation to an accountable care organization. The list—and the ways in which pharmacists can improve the quality of patient care—is endless.

CONCLUSION

Quality is an essential component of competent, professional pharmacy practice. Increasing quality can have many beneficial effects on any practice, such as minimizing rework and increasing productivity. Many QI changes are simple and can be implemented quickly but may have a large impact on the quality of patient care.

Health care quality finally has achieved a position of high visibility on the national agenda. Thus, pharmacists will be called on increasingly to ensure quality in all portions of the medication use system.

QUESTIONS FOR FURTHER DISCUSSION

Anita has begun to address quality in her pharmacy practice setting.

1. What other steps should she take?
2. How can a QI plan be sustained continuously?
3. How can the pharmacy use the QI plan for marketing?
4. Where can Anita go for additional information about QI?

ACKNOWLEDGMENTS

We would like to thank Dr. Tom Reutzel for his guidance and support in helping to write this chapter, and Jessica Reilly, PharmD Candidate, for her assistance.

REFERENCES

Abelson RP, Levi A. 1985. Decision making and decision theory. In *Handbook of Social Psychology*. New York, NY: Random House, p. 231.

American Pharmacists Association (APhA). 2003. *American Pharmacists Association Catalogue*. Washington, DC: APhA.

Anonymous. 2002. *Root Cause Analysis*. Washington, DC: VA National Center for Patient Safety.

Arizona Revised Statutes. 2007. Amending Title 32, Chapter 18, Article 3, Arizona Revised Statutes, by adding 32–1973, relating to the state board of pharmacy.

Bagian JP, Lee C, Gosbee J, et al. 2001. Developing and deploying a patient safety program in a large health care delivery system: You can't fix what you don't know about. *Jt Comm J Qual Improv* 27:522–532.

Bleich MR. 2014a. Developing leaders as systems thinkers—Part I. *J Contin Educ Nurs* 45(4):158–159.

Bleich MR. 2014b. Developing leaders as systems thinkers—Part II. *Contin Educ Nurs* 45(5):201–202.

Blumenthal D, Kilo CM. 1998. A report card on continuous quality improvement. *Milbank Q* 76:625–648, 511.

Bluml BM, Watson LL, Skelton JB, Manolakis PG, Brock KA. 2014. Improving outcomes for diverse populations disproportionately affected by diabetes: Final results of Project IMPACT: Diabetes. *J Am Pharm Assoc (2003)* 54:477–485.

Boeing. 1993. *Accident Prevention Strategies: Removing Links in the Accident Chain*. Seattle, WA: Boeing Commercial Airplane Group.

Brummel A, Lustig A, Westrich K, et al. 2014. Best practices: Improving patient outcomes and costs in an ACO through comprehensive medication therapy management. *J Manag Care Pharm* 20: 1152–1158.

Bunting BA, Smith BH, Sutherland SE. 2008. The Asheville project: Clinical and economic outcomes of a community-based long-term medication therapy management program for hypertension and dyslipidemia. *J Am Pharm Assoc (2003)* 49(1): 23–31.

Bukhsh A, Khan TM, Lee S, Lee LH, Chan K, Goh BH. 2018. Efficacy of pharmacist based diabetes educational interventions on clinical outcomes of adults with type 2 diabetes mellitus: A network meta-analysis. *Front Pharmacol* 9:339.

Carayon P, Schoofs-Hundt A, Karsh BT, et al. 2006. Work system design for patient safety: The SEIPS model. *Qual Saf Health Care* 15(Suppl 1):i50–i58.

Carayon P, Wetterneck TB, Rivera-Rodriguez AJ, et al. 2014. Human factors systems approach to healthcare quality and patient safety. *Appl Ergon* 45(1):14–25.

Cardosi L, Hohmeier KC, Fisher C, Wasson M. 2018. Patient satisfaction with a comprehensive medication review provided by a community pharmacist. *J Pharm Technol* 34(2):48–53.

Chassin MR, Galvin RW. 1998. The urgent need to improve health care quality. Institute of Medicine National Roundtable on Health Care Quality. *JAMA* 280:1000–1005.

Chisholm-Burns MA, Lee JK, Spivey CA, et al. 2010. US pharmacists' effect as team members on patient care: Systematic review and meta-analyses. *Med Care* 48:923–933.

Coe CP. 1998a. An overview of the Joint Commission's improving organizational performance standards. In *Preparing the Pharmacy for a Joint Commission Survey.* Bethesda, MD: ASHP, p. 189.

Coe CP. 1998b. Overview of the Joint Commission's Sentinel Event Policy. In *Preparing the Pharmacy for a Joint Commission Survey.* Bethesda, MD: ASHP, p. 200.

Coe CP. 1998c. Joint Commission on Accreditation of Healthcare Organizations. In *Preparing the Pharmacy for a Joint Commission Survey.* Bethesda, MD: ASHP, p. 1.

Cohen MR, Senders J, Davis NM. 1994. Failure mode and effects analysis: A novel approach to avoiding dangerous medication errors and accidents. *Hosp Pharm* 29:319–330.

Congress of the United States, Office of Technology Assessment. 1988. *The Quality of Medical Care: Information for Consumers.* Washington, DC: U.S. Government Printing Office, p. x.

Center for Pharmacy Practice Accreditation (CPPA). 2019a. *About.* Available at https://www.pharmacypracticeaccredit.org/about. Accessed January 25, 2019.

Center for Pharmacy Practice Accreditation (CPPA). 2019b. *Our Programs.* Available at https://www.pharmacypracticeaccredit.org/our-programs. Accessed January 25, 2019.

Deming WE. 1986. *Out of the Crisis.* Cambridge, MA: Massachusetts Institute of Technology, Center for Advanced Engineering Study.

DeRosier J, Stalhandske E, Bagian JP, et al. 2002. Using health care failure mode and effect analysis: The VA National Center for Patient Safety's prospective risk analysis system. *Joint Comm J Qual Improv* 28:209, 248–267.

Donabedian A. 1969. Quality of care: Problems of measurement: II. Some issues in evaluating the quality of nursing care. *Am J Public Health Nations Health* 59:1833–1836.

Donabedian A. 1991. Quality assurance: Structure, process, and outcome. *Nurs Stand* 7:4–5.

Dunn SP, Birtcher KK, Beavers CJ, et al. 2015. The role of the clinical pharmacist in the care of patients with cardiovascular disease. *J Am Coll Cardiol* 66(19):2129–2139.

Federal Aviation Authority (FAA). 1993. *Human Factor Policy.* Washington, DC: US Department of Transportation.

Gardner JS. 1996. A practical guide to establishing vaccine administration services in community pharmacies. *J Am Pharm Assoc* 6:683–692. quiz 692–693.

Godwin HN, Sanborn MD. 1995. Total quality management in hospital pharmacy. *Am Pharm* NS35: 51–60.

Gosbee J, Anderson T. 2003. Human factors engineering design demonstrations can enlighten your RCA team. *Qual Saf Health Care* 12:119–121.

Guignard B, Bonnabry P, Perrier A, Dayer P, Desmeules J, Samer CF. 2015. Drug-related problems identification in general internal medicine: The impact and role of the clinical pharmacist and pharmacologist. *Eur J Intern Med* 26(6):399–406.

Hansen LB, Fernald D, Akaya-Guerra R, Westfall JM, West D, Pace W. 2006. Pharmacy clarification of prescriptions ordered in primary care: A report from the Applied Strategies for Improving Patient Safety (ASIPS) collaborative. *J Am Board Fam Med* 19:24–30.

Hatton J, Chandra R, Lucius D, Ciuchta E. 2018. Patient satisfaction of pharmacist-provided care via clinical video teleconferencing. *J Pharm Pract* 31(5):429–433.

Houle SKD, Chuck AW, McAlister FA, Tsuyuki RT. 2012. Effect of a pharmacist-managed hypertension program on health system costs: An evaluation of the Study of Cardiovascular Risk Intervention by Pharmacists—Hypertension (SCRIP-HTN). *Pharmacotherapy* 32: 527–537.

Hume M. 1999. Changing hospital culture, systems reduces drug errors. *Exec Solut Healthc Manag* 2:1,4–9.

Johnson ST, Brown GC, Shea KM, 2002. Reengineering a pharmacist intervention program. *Am J Health Syst Pharm* 59:916–917.

Joint Commission on Accreditation of Healthcare Organizations. 2018. *Benefits of Joint Commission Accreditation.* Available at https://www.jointcommission.org/benefits_of_joint_commission_accreditation/. Accessed April 12, 2019.

Joint Commission on Accreditation of Healthcare Organizations. 2019a. *History of the Joint Commission.* Available at https://www.jointcommission.org/about_us/history.aspx. Accessed January 24, 2019.

Joint Commission on Accreditation of Healthcare Organizations. 2019b. *Facts about the Joint Commission on Healthcare Organizations.* Available at https://www.jointcommission.org/facts_about_the_joint_commission/. Accessed January 24, 2019.

Joint Commission on Accreditation of Healthcare Organizations. 2019c. *2019 Hospital National Patient Safety Goals.* Available at https://www.jointcommission.org/assets/1/6/2019_HAP_NPSGs_final2.pdf. Accessed January 24, 2019.

Jokanovic N, Tan EC, Sudhakaran S, et al. 2017. Pharmacist-led medication review in community settings: An overview of systematic reviews. *Res Social Adm Pharm* 13(4):661–685.

Knight D, Pearce CL, Smith KG, et al. 1999. Top management team diversity, group process, and strategic consensus. *Strateg Manag J* 20(5):445–465.

Kohn L. 2000. To err is human: An interview with the Institute of Medicine's Linda Kohn. *Jt Comm J Qual Improv* 26:227–234.

Kozma CM, Reeder CE, Schultz RM. 1993. Economic, clinical and humanistic outcomes: A planning model for pharmacoeconomic research. *Clin Ther* 15:1121–1132.

Law AV, Okamoto MP, Brock K. 2009. Ready, willing, and able to provide MTM services? A survey of community pharmacists in the USA. *Res Social Adm Pharm* 5(4):376–381.

Lazarus IR, Butler K. 2001. The promise of six sigma, part 1. *Manag Healthc Exec* 10:22–26.

Lazarus IR, Stamps B. 2002. The promise of six sigma, part 2. *Manag Healthc Exec* 12:27–30.

Leape LL, Kabcenell A, Berwick DM, et al. 1998a. Change concepts for reducing adverse drug events. In *Reducing Adverse Drug Events: Breakthrough Series Guide.* Boston, MA: Institute for Healthcare Improvement, p. 49.

Leape LL, Kabcenell A, Berwick DM, et al. 1998b. Achieving breakthrough improvement in reducing adverse drug events. In *Reducing Adverse Drug Events: Breakthrough Series Guide.* Boston, MA: Institute for Healthcare Improvement, p. 79.

Leape LL, Kabcenell A, Berwick DM, et al. 1998c. A step-by-step guide to reducing adverse drug events. In *Reducing Adverse Drug Events: Breakthrough Series Guide.* Boston, MA: Institute for Healthcare Improvement, p. 13.

Leape LL. 1994. Error in medicine. *JAMA* 272:1851–1857.

Leapfrog. 2019a. *Our History. The Leapfrog Group.* Available at http://www.leapfroggroup.org/about/history. Accessed January 25, 2019.

Leapfrog. 2019b. *Welcome to the 2019 Leapfrog ASC Survey.* Available at http://www.leapfroggroup.org/ASC. Accessed January 25, 2019.

Lohr KE. 1990a. Health, health care, and quality of care. In *Medicare: A Strategy for Quality Assurance.* Washington, DC: National Academy Press, p. 19.

Lohr KE. 1990b. Concepts of assessing, assuring, and improving quality. In *Medicare: A Strategy for Quality Assurance.* Washington, DC: National Academy Press, p. 45.

Mainz J. 2003. Defining and classifying clinical indicators for quality improvement. *Int J Qual Health Care.* 15(6):523–530.

Marwick C. 1997. NCQA: Quality through evaluation. National Committee for Quality Assurance. *JAMA* 278(19):1555–1556.

McAdam-Marx C, Dahal A, Jennings B, Singhal M, Gunning K. 2015. The effect of a diabetes collaborative care management program on clinical and economic outcomes in patients with type 2 diabetes. *J Manag Care Spec Pharm* 21:452–468.

Milosavljevic A, Aspden T, Harrison J. 2018. Community pharmacist-led interventions and their impact on patients' medication adherence and other health outcomes: A systematic review. *Int J Pharm Pract* 26(5):387–397.

Mishra A, Krishna GS, Alla S, et al. 2017. Impact of pharmacist–psychiatrist collaborative patient education on medication adherence and quality of life (QOL) of bipolar affective disorder (BPAD) patients. *Front Pharmacol* 8:722.

Moczygemba LR, Barner JC, Lawson KA, et al. 2011. Impact of telephone medication therapy management on medication and health-related problems, medication adherence, and medicare part D drug costs:

A 6-month follow up. *Am J Geriatr Pharmacother* 9:328–338.

Mohammed MA, Moles RJ, Chen TF. 2016. Impact of pharmaceutical care interventions on health-related quality-of-life outcomes: A systematic review and meta-analysis. *Ann Pharmacother* 50(10): 862–881.

Moore LD, Smith MG. 2018. Positive impact of technician-driven MTM program on performance measures. *J Pharm Pract* [Epub ahead of print].

Morgado MP, Morgado SR, Mendes LC, Pereira LJ, Castelo-Branco M. 2011. Pharmacist interventions to enhance blood pressure control and adherence to antihypertensive therapy: Review and meta-analysis. *Am J Health Syst Pharm* 68(3): 241–253.

Morriss FH, Abramowitz PW, Nelson SP, et al. 2009. Effectiveness of a barcode medication administration system in reducing preventable adverse drug events in a neonatal intensive care unit: A prospective cohort study. *J Pediatrics* 154(3):363–368.

Murphy PZ, Sands C, Ford F. 2016. Effectiveness of a pharmacist-led cardiovascular risk reduction clinic in rural Perry County, Alabama. *Int J Chronic Dis* 2016; doi: 10.1155/2016/4304761.

Murray MD, Young J, Hoke S, et al. 2007. Pharmacist intervention to improve medication adherence in heart failure: A randomized trial. *Ann Int Med* 146(10):714–725.

Nagel DC. 1988. Human error in aviation operations. In Nagel DC (ed.) *Human Factors in Aviation*. New York, NY: Academic Press, p. 263.

National Association of Boards of Pharmacy (NABP). 2014. *CPPA Community Pharmacy Practice Accreditation Program Now Accepting Applications*. Available at https://www.nabp.net/news/cppa-community-pharmacy-practice-accreditation-program-now-accepting-applications. Accessed July 17, 2015.

National Center for Patient Safety (NCPS). 2011b. *NCPS Triage Cards for Root Cause Analysis*. Available at www.patientsafety.gov/CogAids/Triage/index.html#page=page-1. Accessed June 13, 2011.

National Committee for Quality Assurance (NCQA). 2019a. *NCQA About NCQA – Overview*. Available at https://www.ncqa.org/about-ncqa/. Accessed January 23, 2019.

National Committee for Quality Assurance (NCQA). 2019b. *Report Cards*. Available at https://www.ncqa.org/report-cards/. Accessed January 24, 2019.

National Committee for Quality Assurance (NCQA). 2019c. *HEDIS & Performance Measurement*. Available at https://www.ncqa.org/hedis/. Accessed January 24, 2019.

National Committee for Quality Assurance (NCQA). 2019d. 2019 *Summary Table of Measures, Product Lines, and Changes*. Available at https://www.ncqa.org/wp-content/uploads/2018/08/20190000_HEDIS_Measures_SummaryofChanges.pdf. Accessed January 24, 2019.

National Coordination Council for Medication Error Reporting. 2007. *Recommendations for Regulators and Standard Setters to Prevent Medication Errors Associated with the Label, Labeling, and Packaging of Pharmaceutical (Drug) Products and Related Devices*. Available at https://www.nccmerp.org/recommendations-regulators-and-standards-setters-prevent-medication-errors-associated-label. Accessed April 12, 2019.

National Coordination Council for Medication Error Reporting. 2015. *Recommendations to Enhance Accuracy of Dispensing Medications*. Available at https://www.nccmerp.org/recommendations-enhance-accuracy-dispensing-medications. Accessed April 12, 2019.

National Guideline Clearinghouse (NGC). 2000. *Evidence-Based Clinical Practice Guidelines. Agency for Healthcare Research and Quality*. Available at https://www.qualitymeasures.ahrq.gov/. Accessed March 19, 2019.

Ni W, Colayco D, Hashimoto J, et al. 2018. Budget impact analysis of a pharmacist-provided transition of care program. *J Manag Care Spec Pharm* 24(2):90–96.

Nolan TW. 2000. System changes to improve patient safety. *BMJ* 320:771–773.

O'Malley C. 1997. Quality measurement for health systems: Accreditation and report cards. *Am J Health Syst Pharm* 54:1528–1535.

Obreli-Neto PR, Marusic S, Guidoni CM, et al. 2015. Economic evaluation of a pharmaceutical care program for elderly diabetic and hypertensive patients in primary health care: A 36-month randomized controlled clinical trial. *J Manag Care Spec Pharm* 21:66 75.

Ovretveit J. 1992. *Health Service Quality*. Oxford, England: Blackwell Scientific.

Ovretveit J. 2001. Quality evaluation and indicator comparison in health care. *Int J Health Plan Manag* 16:229–241.

Park KS. 1997. Human error. In Salvendy G (ed.) *Handbook of Human Factors and Ergonomics*. New York, NY: Wiley-Interscience, p. 150.

Pellegrin KL, Krenk L, Oakes SJ, et al. 2017. Reductions in medication-related hospitalizations in older adults with medication management by hospital and community pharmacists: A quasi-experimental study. *J Am Geriatr Society* 65(1):212–219.

Pharmacy Quality Alliance (PQA). 2019a. *The PQA Story.* Available at https://www.pqaalliance.org/our-story. Accessed January 25, 2019.

Pharmacy Quality Alliance (PQA). 2019b. *PQA Measures.* Available at https://www.pqaalliance.org/pqa-measures. Accessed January 25, 2019.

Pinto S, Simon A, Osundina F, Jordan M, Ching D. 2018. Study to measure the impact of pharmacists and pharmacy services (STOMPP) on medication non-adherence: Medication adherence and clinical outcomes. *Inov Pharm* 9(1):11.

Poon EG, Cina JL, Churchill WW, et al. 2005. Effect of bar-code technology on the incidence of medication dispensing errors and potential adverse drug events in a hospital pharmacy. *AMIA Annu Symp Proc* 2005:1085.

Pringle JL., Boyer A, Conklin MH, McCullough JW, Aldridge A. 2014. The Pennsylvania project: Pharmacist intervention improved medication adherence and reduced health care costs. *Health Aff* 33(8):1444–1452.

Merriam-Webster Dictionary. 2019a. *Quality.* Available at https://www.merriam-webster.com/dictionary/quality. Accessed January 25, 2019.

Merriam-Webster. 2019b. *Quality Control.* Available at https://www.merriam-webster.com/dictionary/quality%20control. Accessed January 25, 2019.

Merriam-Webster. 2019c. *Quality Assurance.* Available at https://www.merriam-webster.com/dictionary/quality%20assurance. Accessed January 25, 2019.

Quality Care Pharmacy Program. 2015. *Quality Care Pharmacy Program.* Available at http://www.qcpp.com/about-qcpp/what-is-qcpp. Accessed July 17, 2015.

Rasmussen J, Pejtersen AM, Goodstein LP. 1994. *Cognitive Systems Engineering.* New York, NY: Wiley.

Rogers B. 1997. Preventing medication errors. *Healthplan* 38:27–31, 34.

Sakthong P, Sangthonganotai T. 2018. A randomized controlled trial of the impact of pharmacist-led patient-centered pharmaceutical care on patients' medicine therapy-related quality of life. *Res Social Adm Pharm* 14(4):332–339.

San-Juan-Rodriguez A, Newman TV, et al. 2018. Impact of community pharmacist-provided preventive services on clinical, utilization, and economic outcomes: An umbrella review. *Prev Med* 115:145–155.

Santschi V, Chiolero A, Paradis G, Colosimo AL, Burnand B. 2012. Pharmacist interventions to improve cardiovascular disease risk factors in diabetes: A systematic review and meta-analysis of randomized controlled trials. *Diabetes Care* 35(12):2706–2717.

Schuessler TJ, Ruisinger JF, Hare SE, Prohaska ES, Melton BL. 2016. Patient satisfaction with pharmacist-led chronic disease state management programs. *J Pharm Pract* 29(5):484–489.

Shane R, Gouveia WA. 2000. Developing a strategic plan for quality in pharmacy practice. *Am J Health-Syst Pharm* 57:470–474.

Sheridan TB. 1988. The system perspective. In Nagel DC (ed.) *Human Factors in Aviation.* New York, NY: Academic Press, p. 27.

Shortell SM, Bennett CL, Byck GR. 1998. Assessing the impact of continuous quality improvement on clinical practice: What it will take to accelerate progress. *Milbank Q* 76:510, 593–624.

Shortell SM, O'Brien JL, Hughes EF, et al. 1994. Assessing the progress of TQM in U.S. hospitals: Findings from two studies. *Q Lett Healthcare Lead* 6:14–17.

Skinner JS, Poe B, Hopper R, Boyer A, Wilkins CH. 2015. Assessing the effectiveness of pharmacist-directed medication therapy management in improving diabetes outcomes in patients with poorly controlled diabetes. *Diabetes Educ* 41:459–465.

Stanton-Robinson C, Al-Jumaili AA, Jackson A, Catney C, Veach S, Witry MJ. 2018. Evaluation of community pharmacist-provided telephone interventions to improve adherence to hypertension and diabetes medications. *J Am Pharm Assoc* 58(4S):S120–S124.

Theising KM, Fritschle TL, Scholfield AM, Hicks EL, Schymik ML. 2015. Implementation and clinical outcomes of an employer-sponsored, pharmacist-provided medication therapy management program. *Pharmacotherapy* 35(11):e159–e163.

van Bokhoven MA, Kok G, Vander Weijden T. 2003. Designing a quality improvement intervention: A systematic approach. *Qual Saf Health Care* 12:215–220.

van Boven JFM, Stuurman-Bieze AGG, Hiddink EG, Postma MJ, Vegter S. 2014. Medication monitoring and optimization: A targeted pharmacist program for effective and cost-effective improvement of chronic therapy adherence. *J Manag Care Pharm* 20:786–792.

von Bertalanffy L. 1968. *General Systems Theory: Foundations, Development, Application.* New York, NY: George Braziller.

Van Eikenhorst L, Taxis K, van Dijk L, de Gier H. 2017. Pharmacist-led self-management interventions to improve diabetes outcomes. A systematic literature review and meta-analysis. *Front Pharmacol* 8:891.

Warholak-Juarez T, Rupp MT, Salazar TA, Foster S. 2000. Effect of patient information on the quality of pharmacists' drug use review decisions. *J Am Pharm Assoc* 40:500–508.

Weinstein MC, Fineberg HV. 1980. *Clinical Decision Analysis*. Philadelphia, PA: Saunders.

Wooldridge AR, Carayon P, Hundt AS, Hoonakker PL. 2017. SEIPS-based process modeling in primary care. *Appl Ergon* 60:240–254.

Zarbo RJ, Tuthill JM, D'Angelo R, et al. 2009. The Henry Ford production system reduction of surgical pathology in-process misidentification defects by bar code–specified work process standardization. *Am J Clin Pathol* 131(4):468–477.

■ APPENDIX 10A. CQI CYCLE CHECKLIST

Cycle Background

Focus description

Should describe practice setting, the portion of the medication use process where the focus occurs, and baseline data (if possible).

Focus importance

State why the focus is important.

Literature review

Relate the focus to the literature.

Goal

Global and specific goals should be clearly stated and relate to the focus described in background.

Cycle Methods

Intervention

Describe and justify the intervention made (if any) for this cycle.

Processes and outcomes measured

Describe and justify the processes and outcomes measured (should relate to goal).

Data collection procedures

Measurement methods should be clearly described and appropriate.

Data analysis

Planned statistical analysis should be clearly described and appropriate.

Cycle Measurement

Cycle results

Sample description

Type and size of sample should be clearly described.

Results presented

Results should be reported for each stated goal. Result presentation should include graphs and/or charts.

Cycle Conclusions and Recommendations

Conclusions

Describe the conclusions your team came to after examining the data.

Implications

Describe why these results are important and what actions need to take place.

Recommendations

Recommendations for additional CQI cycles in this area.

■ APPENDIX 10B. CQI PLANNING WORKSHEETS FOR A RESEARCH PROJECT

Research Planning Worksheet 1

Date of meeting: _____

Name and contact information of each team member present:

1. _____   4. _____
2. _____   5. _____
3. _____   6. _____

Introduction

1. Brainstorm possible areas of study (list here). _____
_____

2. Rank and select an area of focus from the list above.
3. Provide a detailed description of the area chosen for study.

Area or project: _____
Setting: _____
_____

Portion of the medication use process involved: _____
Baseline data (if available): _____
4. State why the proposed project is important.
_____
_____
_____

5. Relate the proposed project to the literature.
_____
_____

6. State the global goal of the project [*Hint*: Some options may include (1) discovery, (2) frequency estimation, and (3) measure of a change or a combination.] *Note:* Goal should relate to project stated in 3 above.
_____
_____

7. State the specific goal(s) of the project.
_____
_____

Methods

8. List possible interventions (some options may include reduce reliance on memory, simplify, standardize, use constraints or forcing functions, use protocols of checklists, improve access to information, decrease reliance on vigilance, reduce handoffs, differentiate, or automate).
_____
_____

9. Select best intervention to accomplish goals (listed in 7 above).

_____

_____

10. List process and/or outcome measures necessary to determine if goals were met.

_____

_____

11. Determine what data are already being collected and what measures exist.

_____

_____

12. Plan data collection methods [_Hint_: May choose from (1) inspection points, (2) focus groups, (3) monitoring for markers, (4) chart review, (5) observation, and (6) spontaneous report.]

_____

_____

13. Plan statistical analysis. Make sure you will collect all information needed.

_____

_____

14. Break the project into steps and detail practical considerations.

Step	Who	What	Where	When	How

15. Sketch preliminary timeline for project.

Timeline										
	Week									
Step	1	2	3	4	5	6	7	8	9	10

16. List challenges to be addressed before the next meeting.

_____

_____

_____

17. Assign a responsible party to address each challenge listed above.

Challenge	Person Responsible	Due Date
1.		
2.		
3.		

18. Set date for next team meeting. _____

Research Planning Worksheet 2

Date of meeting: _____

Name and contact information of each team member present:

1. _____   4. _____
2. _____   5. _____
3. _____   6. _____

Introduction/Methods Revision

1. Review materials from last meeting.
2. Review progress made.
3. Indicate plan changes, if needed.

_____

_____

_____

4. Add additional steps and detail practical considerations, if needed:

Step	Who	What	Where	When	How

5. Discuss challenges solved during this report period.

Challenge	How It Was Solved	Lesson Learned

6. List challenges to be addressed before the next meeting.

1. _____
2. _____
3. _____
4. _____

7. Assign a responsible party to address each challenge listed above.

Challenge	Person Responsible	Due Date
1.		
2.		
3.		
4.		
5.		
6.		
7.		

8. Update the timeline for project.

Timeline											
	Week										
Step	1	2	3	4	5	6	7	8	9	10	

9. Set date for next team meeting._____

_____

_____

Note: This worksheet can be used for several team meetings. Proceed to Worksheet 3 when data are collected.

Research Planning Worksheet 3

Date of meeting: _____

Name and contact information of each team member present:

1. _____   4. _____
2. _____   5. _____
3. _____   6. _____

Measurement

1. Just do it!

Results

2. Analyze data.
3. Describe sample type and size.

4. Describe a result for each specific goal.

Conclusions and Recommendations

5. Describe conclusions the group reached after examining the results.

6. Why are these results important, and what actions need to take place?

7. What are the team's recommendations for this project?

8. What are the team's recommendations for the next project?

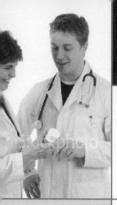

11

RISK MANAGEMENT IN CONTEMPORARY PHARMACY PRACTICE

Gregory L. Alston and Steve Boone

About the Authors: Dr. Alston is an Associate Dean and professor at Savannah Campus, South University School of Pharmacy. He has over 30 years of experience in community pharmacy management, both as a chain-pharmacy administrator and an independent pharmacy owner. He earned a Doctor of Pharmacy (PharmD) degree from the University of the Pacific and has published three best-selling management books, *The Bosshole Effect – Managing People Simplified*, *The Ten Things A New Manager Must Get Right From the Start*, and *Own Your Value: The Real Future of Pharmacy Practice*. His passion lies in teaching the next generation of pharmacists how to create value for the stakeholders they serve.

Steve Boone has over 30 years' experience in the insurance industry and is currently the pharmacy insurance practice leader at Heffernan Insurance Brokers of Chesterfield, Missouri. The Heffernan Brokerage works with a range of insurance carriers to provide customized coverage to pharmacists across the country. Steve has presented pharmacy insurance webinars to pharmacist audiences throughout the United States and is endorsed by Pharmacy Development Service, Inc., as a pharmacy insurance expert. Currently Steve is working with Intuitive Captive Solutions in the design, structuring, and formation of an 831(b) micro captive pharmacy insurance company that will be another tool for pharmacy owners to better insure their businesses.

■ LEARNING OBJECTIVES

After completing this chapter, readers should be able to

1. Describe the role of risk management in pharmacy practice.
2. Identify critical components that constitute pure risk.
3. Describe the criteria for determining an insurable risk.
4. Discuss how risk management techniques can be used to manage emerging risks that may pose a threat to community pharmacy practice.

5. Describe how increased reliance on information technology and automation may exacerbate certain risks.
6. Describe the factors that affect performance risk of an information technology system used in pharmacies.
7. Characterize the risk of loss associated with the use of information technology in pharmacy operations.

■ SCENARIO

Bill Halsey, PharmD, has spent the past 2 years since graduating from pharmacy school working as a staff pharmacist for a well-respected community pharmacy to refine his skills as a clinically oriented community pharmacist. Bill's dream is to someday return to his hometown and purchase the pharmacy that had inspired him to pursue this career. That day seemed to arise even sooner than Bill expected when he learned that Mr. Simmons, the long-time owner of Corner Drug in his hometown, had suffered a minor heart attack. Mr. Simmons would like to sell Corner Drug and move to a retirement village. Bill quickly scheduled a trip back home to visit with Mr. Simmons and inspect the pharmacy to see what it might be worth. He also evaluated the current state of the pharmacy for providing specialized services in diabetes and geriatrics. Bill was somewhat surprised to see that the pharmacy was essentially in the same condition that it was when he worked there during high school. Mr. Simmons had always enjoyed chatting with his customers, so the pharmacy counter was very small with wide openings on both sides so that he and his employees could easily move in and out of the pharmacy department to interact with customers. The desk where the clerk took care of the insurance claims paperwork and charge accounts was in the corner of the customer waiting area. The computer appeared to be somewhat ancient, and Mr. Simmons joked that the high school students he hired as clerks often had to help him when the computer would start "acting up." Bill was understandably concerned. The delivery car could best be described as a "beater." He had been serving as the Health Insurance Portability and Accountability Act (HIPAA)

compliance officer for his current pharmacy and was wondering what, if any, security and privacy measures were in place at Corner Drug. Bill also remembered Mr. Simmons lecturing him on his philosophy of the unnecessary reliance on insurance and wondered how well the pharmacy was protected from harm or loss or liability. Mr. Simmons always told him, "Your customers will never sue you if they love and respect you, so treat them well." Bill was beginning to question himself as to what may lie in store for him if he bought Corner Drug, as he now contemplated several emerging unresolved issues that could threaten the ability of the pharmacy to exist and prosper.

■ CHAPTER QUESTIONS

1. What is the primary difference between a speculative risk and a pure risk for an individual?
2. What are the common risk threats that pharmacies share with any type of retail business?
3. Is it possible for a community pharmacy to avoid all risks? If not, how should risk be handled?
4. How might HIPAA privacy rules affect a pharmacy's liability insurance coverage and costs?
5. What are the four areas of risk that arise when pharmacies increase their reliance on information technology and automation?
6. What are the increased risks brought about by the interaction of information technology with the safety and health hazards this technology poses to employees in the workplace?
7. Which six factors characterize the operational risk associated with information technology and automation in pharmacies?

■ INTRODUCTION

An element of risk exists in every human activity. One can become injured in an automobile accident on the way to work, become ill from food poisoning eating at a favorite restaurant, or lose thousands in retirement savings when the value of a company's stock declines significantly owing to an unexpected product recall. Pharmacists who own or operate pharmacies always must deal with the risk of business declines or even failure. There are always threats from the economy and the competition, as well as the potential for damage caused by a tornado, fire, flood, or hurricane. Indeed, a degree of risk is inherent in performing a most common task in almost any pharmacy—that of dispensing a patient's prescription. The changing health care environment requires pharmacists to critically examine risks in all aspects of their practice, especially as they look to take on more patient-oriented roles.

Historically, the primary risk exposure for pharmacists was related to traditional business risks (i.e., fire, theft, etc.), coupled with negligence related to medication errors. Modern pharmacy practice must also consider new risks related to the use of technology and electronic data transmission, patient counseling and drug utilization review requirements, and protected private health information. As the practice of pharmacy continues to evolve, so do the risks associated with the changing environment and scope of pharmacy practice. Pharmacists must be aware of the inherent and evolving risks of delivering health care goods and services and develop risk management strategies to deal with the risks. This chapter will review the concept of risk management and then focus on the new and developing risks associated with modern pharmacy practice in a technology-based environment.

■ DEFINITION OF RISKS

Risks are associated with negative outcomes. A *risk* is anything that threatens the ability of a person or organization to accomplish its mission. To fully understand risk in one's life or business venture, one must realize that there are several factors related to defining a risk as a threat. A risk may best be described as some *degree of probability* that *exposure* to a *hazard* will lead to a *negative outcome or consequence*, such as loss, damage, injury, or death (Ropeik & Gray, 2002). Exposures to some risks are a part of daily life. You could have an auto accident on any given day. For a risk to be a threat, there must be some statistical chance (probability) that a negative event will occur. One may or may not be exposed to a risk that may diminish or eliminate the risk as a real threat. You cannot drown if you are not near water. You cannot suffer an adverse reaction from a drug you have never consumed. To be a risk, it also must constitute a hazard (hence the sports phrase "No harm, no foul"). The severity or consequences also must be negative to be a risk. A drug may have a small probability of anaphylactic shock, but anaphylactic shock may result in death. A new computer virus could destroy all the patient files and records stored in the pharmacy computer system.

From an insurance perspective, there are two basic types of risks: speculative risks and pure risks. A *speculative risk* involves a chance of gain or benefit as well as a chance of loss. Speculative risks are not insurable. Gambling is the prototypical speculative risk. When the $1 scratch-off lottery ticket you just bought didn't win the instant $1000, you knew you had a very good chance of losing your dollar. The individual decides on the amount of risk he or she is willing to assume, including how much money to gamble and at what odds. Choosing to purchase shares of a mutual fund or common stock as an investment also involves speculative risk. Based on an investor's choices and a great number of other factors, his or her investment portfolio can experience substantial gains or suffer significant losses. Operating a pharmacy also involves speculative risk, in that there is no guarantee of success or failure. The number of independent community pharmacies in the United States declined from 31,879 in 1990 (U.S. Department of Health and Human Services [DHHS], 2000) to about 22,000 stores in 2018 (National Community Pharmacists

Association, 2018). In general, small-business owner-ship is inherently a risky venture. Data from the U.S. Bureau of Labor Statistics (2016) has found that only 56% of businesses launched in 2014 survived at least 5 years.

Pure risk involves a risk in which there is only the opportunity of sustaining a loss; there is no oppor-tunity for gain. Pure risks are considered accidental, unanticipated, or unavoidable. Illness, death, fire, flood, and most accidents involve pure risk. Insurance is a product designed to assist people in managing their exposure to these unanticipated or accidental risks. Individuals and businesses can purchase insur-ance for risks involving health, death, and damage to home and business property. Damage to a place of business from fire or a tornado could cause cata-strophic loss with little chance of gain for the owner and is therefore an insurable pure risk. The identifica-tion and management of pure risks are essential for a business to manage potential threats to its mission.

CRITERIA FOR INSURABLE RISKS

For a pure risk to be insurable, it must meet certain requirements (Schafermeyer, 2007):

- The loss must be measurable in dollar figures, easy to measure, and result in a substantial loss.
- The loss must have a defined time and place.
- The loss must be accidental for the insured. There should be no prospect of gain or profit for the individual.
- The probability of the event occurring in a popula-tion can be accurately calculated. There must be a sufficiently large number of homogeneous individ-uals with similar risks to make losses predictable.
- The insured must have an insurable interest. Com-pensation cannot be awarded to those not actually suffering the loss.
- The insurance premium must be available at a rea-sonable cost. One would not want to pay an insur-ance premium greater than the value of the item insured.

DEVELOPING A RISK MANAGEMENT STRATEGY

What strategies should pharmacists pursue to identify and minimize their risk exposure? A risk management process should be developed to analyze and identify strategies to manage risk threats. A risk management strategy should be designed to protect the vital assets of a pharmacy through coping with uncertainty. This process involves not only identifying risks but also assessing their threat potential and making decisions on managing those risks. Recall the definition of risk in this process—that some type of probability exists that exposure to some type of hazard will lead to a negative outcome or consequence.

THE RISK MANAGEMENT PROCESS

There are five steps that organizations should follow when developing a risk management process.

1. *Establish the context.* What are the goals of the risk management process? What are potential vulner-abilities of the business? Do employees or patients risk injuries? How might the reputation of the pharmacy suffer if a patient was injured owing to a medication error, or if a patient's health condition was inadvertently made public by an employee? Could costly claims be avoided by not providing certain goods or services?

2. *Identify and analyze risks.* Pharmacy managers should start by analyzing each dimension of their operation. Some examples of risks faced by phar-macies include the activities inherent in their busi-ness (i.e., filling prescriptions, counseling patients, and providing professional services). Other risks faced by pharmacies include making deliveries; maintaining the building, sidewalks, and parking lot; preparing sterile products; maintaining a com-puter system; and protecting patient health infor-mation. Problems in any of these could result in substantial losses for the pharmacy.

3. *Evaluate and prioritize the risks.* Pharmacy managers must prioritize their risks because every risk cannot be addressed at one time. Some risks are fairly common yet are not associated with a high degree of loss (e.g., prescription insurance claim rejections and shoplifting). Other risks are much less common yet are associated with substantial losses (e.g., catastrophic damage from a fire, flood, or storm, or harm to a patient associated with a medication error). Pharmacies should prioritize managing risks that have the greatest potential to result in substantial losses for their business.

4. *Select an appropriate risk management strategy and implement the technique.* Pharmacy managers must determine which risks could (and should) be avoided. Policies and procedures should be developed for appropriate risk prevention measures. Additional insurance policies or add-on riders should be secured as necessary. *Riders* are supplemental policies that provide additional coverage for something not covered in the original policy at some additional charge. There may be a ceiling or maximum amount the original policy will cover to replace personal property or equipment that may not provide adequate cost replacement for an asset(s). Thought should go into the level of deductibles to appropriately balance risk sharing issues and risk transfer issues (see "Techniques to Manage Risks" below). These strategies and the evaluation of which risks to avoid versus those that should be managed should be discussed with consultants or advisors (e.g., attorney, accountant, etc.) of the business operation.

5. *Monitor decisions and update the risk management program.* Pharmacy managers should monitor and update their risk management strategies to meet new challenges, threats, and opportunities. For example, when a pharmacy decides to offer immunizations to their patients, it not only creates new patient care and business opportunities but it also exposes itself to additional risks (e.g., patients could experience an anaphylactic reaction to the immunization, patients could receive an inappropriate or incorrect immunization, and pharmacy employees could be exposed to pathogens). Once these new risks are identified, managers must create new strategies for their management.

■ TECHNIQUES TO MANAGE RISKS

Although risk is inherent to some degree in all our activities, there are different types of risks that require different techniques to manage. Each risk should be evaluated individually as to which technique(s) would be the most appropriate for that given risk.

1. *Risk avoidance.* Although avoiding risks may sound like a logical approach, it is often impractical for many risks in a business environment. For example, most pharmacies cannot (and would not want to) avoid dispensing prescriptions despite the inherent risks involved in the process. However, there may be situations where not offering a specific good or service with an unreasonable risk may be the most prudent action. Many pharmacies choose simply not to perform sterile compounding services rather than incur the expense and risks associated with the preparation of these products.

2. *Risk prevention/modification.* Pharmacy managers may not be able to eliminate a risk, but they can take steps to minimize the likelihood of its occurrence. All pharmacies take steps to avoid medication errors. This commonly involves the development of policies and procedures to prevent errors and improve patient safety (see Chapters 10 and 12).

3. *Risk absorption/retention.* Pharmacies often choose to retain or absorb some risks. Pharmacies commonly accept losses owing to shrinkage (i.e., shoplifting, employee theft, and unsalable products), usually by losing profits or passing on higher prices to consumers. A deductible on an insurance policy is absorption of risk. Some may choose to pay higher deductibles when losses occur in exchange for lower insurance premiums.

4. *Risk sharing or transfer.* Another technique to manage risk is to share or transfer the risk to another

party. Insurance companies commonly share or transfer the risks inherent in paying for health care for their beneficiaries by entering capitated agreements with providers, paying them a set amount per member per month, regardless of how much or how little their beneficiaries need health services. Another method to share or transfer risk is to purchase reinsurance (insurance for insurance companies). Health care providers can also purchase insurance to share or transfer the risks involved in providing care to patients whose costs may exceed the income provided in the capitated contract.

On an individual level, one can avoid some unnecessary risks (i.e., someone may never go swimming to avoid the risk of drowning), but from a business perspective, this strategy is impractical. One may choose to absorb certain risks if the cost of insurance is very high and the potential loss is small. Foregoing automobile collision insurance on a vehicle of minimal value would be an example (while retaining legally required liability insurance). Risk prevention is an important component of effective risk management strategies and is generally used in tandem with risk transfer. On the most basic level, risk prevention includes the use of smoke alarms, security systems, and theft detection. In addition, for a business such as a pharmacy, employee training programs, education, and established policies and procedures are essential to deal with such risks as prevention of medication errors. With the possible exception of risk avoidance, most instances of conducting risk management will use some combination of each of the techniques of risk prevention, risk absorption, and risk sharing.

■ BASIC INSURANCE CONCEPTS

A pharmacy, like any other business entity, needs to protect itself, its employees, and its customers from physical and financial harm. No matter how careful a pharmacy is about preventing risks, it is practically impossible to eliminate accidents, such as when a customer or employee slips on the pharmacy's floor.

At the same time, insuring for these risks does not eliminate the need for pharmacies to take effective risk prevention measures. Indeed, insurers commonly require that pharmacies have risk prevention measures in place to keep insurance policies in good standing for these risks or to reduce premiums. For instance, insurance for fire damage generally requires a sprinkler system or smoke detectors or alarms.

Common Insurance Terms

Insurance companies often use language that may be confusing to individuals not in the insurance industry. Pharmacy managers should have an understanding of the following terms commonly used in insurance policies (Insurance Information Institute, 2015):

- *Coverage.* The scope (extent) of protection provided under an insurance contract.
- *Coinsurance.* A provision that requires the insured party to share (absorb) some of the costs of covered services or losses on a fixed percentage basis. For example, this may require the insured to pay 20% of the replacement costs.
- *Deductible.* The amount (a fixed amount specified in dollars) of an insured loss to be paid (or absorbed) by the policyholder. Deductibles may range from several hundred to several thousand dollars. For automobile collision insurance, $500 deductibles are common.
- *Disability insurance.* A type of health insurance that provides monthly income to the policyholder if he or she becomes unable to work because of an illness or accident.
- *Insured.* The party covered by the insurance contract or persons entitled to benefits under the terms of the policy (e.g., family members may be covered under the employee's employer-sponsored health insurance plan).
- *Liability.* Individual responsibility for causing injury to another person or damage to another's property through negligence.
- *Negligence.* The failure to use reasonable care. The failure to do something a reasonably prudent person would do in similar circumstances.

- *Peril.* Insurance terminology for risk, possible cause of injury, or event causing damage or loss.
- *Policy.* A written contract for insurance between an insurance company and the insured party.
- *Rider.* Term used to describe a document that amends or changes the original policy.
- *Umbrella liability.* A form of insurance protection in excess of the amount covered by other liability insurance policies. It also protects the insured in situations not covered by the usual liability policies.
- *Worker's compensation.* A policy that pays benefits to an employee (or his or her family) for job-related injury or death.

Types of Insurance for a Pharmacy

Depending on the needs of the individual pharmacy, several different types of insurance policies may be required to provide adequate risk protection for the business. The geographic location, type of practice, and services offered will influence the types of insurance needed. The risk management process is a continuous process, and periodic evaluations are necessary to address new or emerging risk threats to the pharmacy. Emerging threats discussed later in this chapter exemplify how recent changes in health care practices and technology create new and different risk threats to the pharmacy.

Property Insurance

This is one of the most common types of insurance for protecting the property and physical assets of any business entity. These policies generally cover losses owing to fire or lightning and theft and the costs of removing property to protect it from further harm. Property that should be insured includes buildings (leased or owned), equipment, supplies, fixtures, inventory, money, accounts receivable records, computers and other data storage devices, vehicles, and intangible assets (e.g., goodwill and the value of a trade secret). Additional coverage can be purchased for specific "extended perils" such as windstorms, hail, floods, explosions, riots, or other specific events. A pharmacy manager should know exactly what is covered in his or her basic property insurance policy to determine if additional coverage is warranted owing to geographic location or local circumstances.

Liability Insurance (also known as Casualty Insurance)

Liability insurance protects a business entity against claims when it is sued for damages or injuries caused by the negligence of the business or its employees. Liability insurance generally covers bodily injury, property damage, personal injury (including libel and interference with privacy), and advertising injury. Advertising injury may occur when advertising activities cause loss to another person through slander, defamation, libel, violation of privacy, or misuse of a copyright or trademark (Rupp, 2002). The legal expenses involved in a negligence suit (i.e., investigation, settlement, or trial) also should be covered by the policy. In today's litigious society, liability insurance is essential for any business entity, including pharmacies. Even fraudulent lawsuits brought by plaintiffs with little hope of success will result in expenses necessary for the pharmacy to defend itself. When a pharmacy is found to be negligent (such as in a medication error), a single judgment could result in a claim into the millions of dollars, resulting in financial ruin for an uninsured pharmacy. Liability insurance does not protect against nonperformance of a contract, wrongful termination of employees, sexual harassment, or race or gender lawsuits.

Business Owner's Policy

Insurance companies commonly bundle property and liability coverage together in the same policy for small-business owners. This policy allows for broader coverage, generally with less expensive premiums, than if property and liability insurance were purchased separately. Small businesses must meet certain criteria to qualify for these policies, such as having fewer than 100 employees and revenues not exceeding set amounts. These policies generally do not include professional liability coverage, worker's compensation, or employee health insurance. These must be purchased separately.

Individual Professional Liability Insurance

Pharmacists frequently purchase individual professional liability insurance policies in addition to what their business or employer may provide. This policy protects the individual against claims emanating from actual or alleged errors or omissions, including negligence, in the course of professional duties or activities. Individual policies are purchased because the business policy limits may not be high enough, and they will not cover the pharmacist outside that workplace. In addition, an organization's policies are designed to protect the organization, such as a pharmacy or hospital. An employer-paid legal defense team may choose to defend a lawsuit by claiming that the employee violated a company policy thereby absolving the company of any liability. If this were to occur the entire liability for the claim could fall on the individual pharmacist. Individual professional liability insurance policies commonly provide coverage of up to $1 million to $2 million per incident. The costs of these policies are generally low (often less than $250 per year). Many pharmacists choose to purchase their own professional liability insurance, regardless of the coverage they may be provided by their employer.

Key Person Insurance

This is insurance designed to protect a business entity from financial loss if key individuals (very likely the owner or partners) were to die or experience a disability. For instance, if the pharmacist-owner were to die suddenly or become disabled, this policy would pay to find and train a replacement or replace profits the company may have earned if the person had not died.

Umbrella or Excess Liability

It is possible that a lawsuit filed against a pharmacy could exceed the limits of the primary liability protection. For instance, a pharmacy's base liability policy may provide a maximum of $300,000 of coverage, but the pharmacy experiences a lawsuit in which the settlement or judgment reaches $1 million. The umbrella policy would cover the difference between the base liability limits and the judgment amount. An umbrella policy is activated only when the limits of the underlying base policy have been exceeded and exhausted. Umbrella liability policies can add substantial coverage for a relatively small additional cost.

Worker's Compensation

This statutory insurance covers medical expenses, disability income, and death benefits to dependents of an employee whose accident, illness, or death is job related. Businesses are required to provide a safe working environment for their employees. Failure to provide a safe environment makes an employer liable for harm to their employees and may result in damage claim lawsuits from their employees. Worker's compensation can be a costly expense for some types of business in which the risk of injury to the worker is high, such as construction. Examples of injuries related to a pharmacy would be those owing to falls, overexertion, or repetitive motion, such as using a computer keyboard. Coverage rates depend highly on individual state laws and the type of work employees are engaged in.

Disability Insurance

Disability insurance provides income for an employee and his or her family in the event something happens that prevents the employee from working. Many employers provide disability insurance to their employees as part of their standard benefit package. Employees may also purchase additional disability insurance coverage. Short-term disability insurance (6 months or less) provides income replacement for employees who are temporarily unable to work. Employees commonly use their short-term disability benefit when taking a medical leave of absence or after the birth or adoption of a child. Long-term disability insurance replaces an employee's salary if he or she is unable to work for long periods (6 months or more) or if an employee becomes permanently disabled.

Independent Pharmacy Insurance

There are a number of insurance companies that specialize in providing insurance coverage to pharmacies. It is a good idea for pharmacy owners to meet with representatives from these companies to discuss their specific insurance needs and compare policy offerings. Pharmacies may also purchase additional coverage for the specialty services they may offer. Examples include policies for home medical equipment, consultant pharmacist services, and professional liability insurance for pharmacists. As previously mentioned, it is generally a good idea for pharmacists to purchase individual professional liability insurance for more comprehensive protection.

■ EMERGING RISKS ASSOCIATED WITH MODERN PHARMACY PRACTICE

The health care industry, including pharmacy, is one of today's most dynamic environments. Health care is a technology-rich environment, with pharmacy often leading the way in technological innovations and advancement. For example, pharmacies now commonly use robotics to assist in the prescription-filling process. They have long used computers in the transmission of third-party prescription claims and to share information between pharmacies. Today, prescriptions are increasingly transmitted electronically from the physician to the pharmacy, a process known as *electronic prescribing* (or *e-prescribing*). Although advances in technology may offer many benefits in terms of patient safety and cost reductions, pharmacies need to incorporate these new technologies into their risk management processes. Employees need to be trained to become aware of new patient privacy regulations and requirements. Pharmacists may need to check and verify not only prescription dispensing activities by technicians but also computer input and data review. Ignoring or not understanding the impact of new professional requirements or technologies can place the pharmacy at risk. The Omnibus Budget Reconciliation Act of 1990 (OBRA 90) and the HIPAA are examples of significant changes in pharmacy practice, which present risk factors the pharmacy must consider in risk management.

OBRA 90

The OBRA is enacted by Congress to establish the budget for all the nation's governmental agencies. Generally an OBRA has little to do specifically with pharmacy. However, the OBRA passed by Congress in 1990 (OBRA 90) had implications for pharmaceutical costs and state Medicaid pharmacy programs. In general, OBRA 90 specified what was expected of pharmacists in providing drug therapy to Medicaid patients. By 1993, pharmacists providing medications to state Medicaid recipients were required to provide prospective drug use review (Pro-DUR), patient counseling, and maintain proper patient records. Most states quickly amended their state pharmacy practice acts to require that all patients receive this level of pharmacy services. Although patients had the option to refuse counseling, pharmacists now had the legal responsibility to provide information to their patients. While most pharmacists welcomed the legal acknowledgment of the professional responsibilities of modern pharmacy practice, OBRA 90 and the resulting changes in state pharmacy practice acts required that pharmacies reassess their risk exposure. Historically, pharmacists and pharmacy liability exposure had been limited to errors (negligence) when a prescription was filled incorrectly. A policy known as the *learned intermediary doctrine* traditionally held that pharmacists had no duty to warn patients against potential adverse reactions or other problems associated with a properly filled prescription. The duty to warn resided with the prescribing physician. Despite the pharmacist's developing role, courts that recognize expanded legal liability for pharmacists remain in the minority but case law is emerging that defines a pharmacist's duty as to: "endeavor to *minimize the risks of harm* to [the patient] and others which a reasonably careful and prudent pharmacist would foresee" (Roybal, 2018). While three-fourths of all claims against pharmacists are still related to dispensing the wrong drug or strength, drug review claims against pharmacists (i.e., checking for interactions, allergies, and other problems), which virtually did not exist before 1991, now account for 8% of all claims (O'Donnell & Vogenberg, 2014).

HIPAA of 1996

The HIPAA, which set standards for the privacy of individually identifiable health information, was signed into law in 1996 and went into effect in 2003. The Department of Health and Human Services (DHHS) was required by Congress to promulgate the privacy standards and to set security standards for patient health information (U.S. Department of Health and Human Services [DHHS], 2003). An individual's health information is referred to as *protected health information* (PHI) and is subject to the HIPAA privacy and security rules.

Pharmacies are affected by these rules in two ways. Pharmacies, by definition, deal with PHI (e.g., a prescription itself is PHI). HIPAA protects all "individually identifiable health information" held or transmitted by a covered entity or its business associate in any form or media, whether electronic, paper, or oral (U.S. Department of Health & Human Services [DHHS], 2003). This covered information includes demographic data, including the individual's physical or mental health (past, present, or future); the health care provided to the individual; and payment information and common identifiers (e.g., name, address, birth date, and Social Security Number) that can be used to identify the individual. Pharmacies must have numerous policies and procedures in place to be in compliance with the HIPPA mandates. These include conducting risk assessments, appointing security and privacy officers to ensure compliance, and implementing policies and procedures to detect and prevent security violations.

There are a host of issues involving HIPAA that can place a pharmacy at risk. These include procedures for handling PHI in the event of fire, theft, system malfunctions, and disaster situations. Even such seemingly benign events such as sticky-note reminders regarding customer requests in the pharmacy area or a technician verbally inquiring at the counter if the Zoloft® for Mr. Jones prescription that came in the morning wholesaler shipment are likely HIPAA violations. Risk exposure involving PHI goes beyond violations of federal law. It can include personal injury claims (nonbodily injury) or claims that involve libel, slander, or the unauthorized release of confidential records. The release of a patient's PHI constitutes the unauthorized release of confidential records.

Information Technology–Related Risks

The health care sector in general and pharmacies specifically have become increasingly dependent on information technology (see Chapter 9). Almost all aspects of goods, services, and activities provided or conducted by pharmacies have become interlinked with information technology. Many pharmacies have invested heavily in information technology systems not only to dispense prescriptions and maintain patient records but also to digitize their financial and accounting systems, enterprise resource planning, human resources, and almost every other element of pharmacy operations. Information technology has benefited pharmacy in many ways. However, pharmacy's increased dependence on information technology has brought about a relatively new and increasingly important risk known as *information technology–related risk* (ITRR), often referred to as *digital risk*. Indeed, hardly a day passes without the report of some business losing confidential client information or having its computer network compromised by unauthorized intruders.

In addition to the usual ITRR that any business must confront, pharmacies possess patient health, prescription, and financial data that can be an attractive target to unauthorized individuals wishing to gain access to those data. Therefore, risks owing to the implementation of and dependence on information technology potentially can offset the benefits derived if the implementation and management of information technology are not given sufficient attention. The ITRR incurred by pharmacies can be grouped into several areas:

Strategic Risk

Strategic risk is the first and foremost risk confronted by pharmacies implementing information technology. To make any information technology project successful in the long run, pharmacies must assess the compatibility of the technology with their mission and goals (see Chapter 6). Businesses must make choices between investing in information technology and other types of resources to achieve their overall goals and objectives. Although the purpose of most information technology is to achieve efficiencies and competitive advantages, there are always risks that the organization would have been better off by pursuing other options. The costs of these risks are known as *opportunity costs*. Such risks can even result in failure to meet a pharmacy's goals and objectives and potentially can put the pharmacy at risk for significant financial loss.

In pharmacies, failures of this sort can be numerous and wide-ranging. For example, a new information technology system may not interface with automated dispensing robotics or the automated telephone call management systems, causing a customer service disruption. Or the anticipated workflow improvements may actually make the workflow process more tedious and cumbersome. It is difficult to evaluate the function and effectiveness of technology for your business without actually embedding the software in to the process and seeing how it works. Companies can waste time, energy, and money on technology that doesn't produce the promised results.

Organizational behavior problems can arise when integrating information technology into pharmacy practice. These often occur when stakeholders (i.e., employees and patients who interact with these systems) are not provided appropriate training before or after information technology implementation. The intended outcomes of information technology integration into pharmacy operations can occur only if there is good communication, commitment, cooperation, and coordination among all the stakeholders. Pharmacy managers incur risks associated with the acquisition and implementation of information technology resources when there is denial of the potential adverse events that can occur in the future. Pharmacy managers must "think outside the box" and consider each and every bad situation that can arise from the implementation and increased dependence on information technology.

Performance Risk

Performance risk is the degree of uncertainty inherent in the procurement and application of information technology solutions that may keep the system from meeting its technical specifications or from being suitable for its intended use and the consequences (Browning, 1999). The most important aspects of performance—those contributing most to performance risk—will vary with the needs and desires of the pharmacy.

Performance risk arises from product complexity. Product complexity involves the number of components, functions, and interfaces in the pharmacy information system. There are several factors that contribute to product complexity:

1. *System Requirements*. Specifications required by a pharmacy in its information technology are directly related to the degree of product complexity and performance risk. These challenges result from the various individual tasks pharmacies require of their information technology and the desire to integrate these tasks into a single piece of technology. Pharmacy information systems must handle a multitude of complex and interrelated elements, such as prescription entry, claim processing, prescription pricing, inventory, and financial management (see Chapter 9). These interrelationships make it difficult to balance optimal performance in all these areas and achieve the ultimate design goal of the system (i.e., enhanced operational efficiency and patient safety). For example, the information system must work to adjudicate third-party prescription claims and at the same time check therapeutic substitution or drug–drug interaction for a particular patient. Another area of concern to pharmacies is data storage. Pharmacy information systems have become a huge repository of PHI for patients. The need to prevent unauthorized third-party access to sensitive patient data increases the chances of data becoming corrupted or lost due to improper maintenance, inadequate replication (backup), and complex encryption and decryption processes. Therefore, there is a tradeoff between data privacy and longevity data storage.

2. *Modularity*. The ability of important components to function independent of the main application is preferable for information technology systems operated by pharmacies. The system should be decomposable into subsystems that make the product less complex. This provides room for individual component upgrades instead of redesigning the whole system when specifications change in certain areas such as claim processing.

Operational Risk

Operational risk generally is defined as risk of loss resulting from inadequate or failed internal processes, people and systems, or external events (Bank for International Settlements, 2015). Information technology operational risks in today's digitized pharmacy are characterized by six event factors:

1. *Internal fraud* is an act committed by at least one internal party (typically an employee) that leads to data theft and/or loss. Information technology creates a tempting environment for employees to create fraud not only because the payoff from such activities can be high but also because the risk of detection is minimal.

    An *intranet* can help a pharmacy operate more efficiently by allowing information to be shared and communicated quickly and reliably. However, having a large number of users increases the intranet's vulnerability to internal threats. Intranet applications and their content may be exposed to a far greater audience than just those authorized users of the intranet. A pharmacy intranet can become more vulnerable as the user base becomes larger and more complex. Pharmacy intranet users commonly include employees, wholesalers, vendors, business partners, and other associated parties such as pharmacy students. Coincidentally, pathways from outside the intranet to the network can become less effective as the gateways needed to protect the organizational assets (mostly data) grow in scope and size. Finally, the degree of protection offered by firewalls can diminish as more and more exceptions to otherwise tight controls to the pharmacy's intranet are granted.

2. *External fraud* is an act committed by a third party that leads to data theft, data loss, and function disruption. People with technology skills can access (hack) the computer systems of pharmacies to steal or manipulate patient information for financial or nonfinancial reasons. For example, Target experienced a serious credit card security breach in December of 2013. This data breach cost the company over $160 million dollars by the end of 2014 (Target Stores, 2014). One can only imagine the problems that could arise if patient data contained in a pharmacy's database were to be exposed, stolen, or manipulated. A 2018 survey by Hiscox Insurance reported that more than 47% of small businesses reported at least one cyberattack in 2017 and 44% of businesses that were attacked had multiple attacks (Hiscox, 2018).

    In general, threats from external users can be classified into one of the two groups: information attack and business-functions attack. *Information attack* can lead to Web site defacement, financial data theft, denial of service, and network performance degradation. *Business-function attack* may cause disruption of online refill requests, physician e-prescribing, and inventory management and interference with automated schedule actions. One of the most vulnerable areas of information technology for pharmacies is Web servers for Internet applications (e.g., pharmacy Web sites where patients can go to place refill orders or make other purchases). Web servers that have not been configured specifically to the pharmacy's needs (i.e., default configuration, insufficient input validation, poor encryption, improper cleaning of temporary files, and poor management of user sessions) are susceptible to serious attacks that may compromise these applications.

    Another important tool of pharmacy automation is the barcode, which can be used to increase patient safety, facilitate inventory management, deliver checked prescriptions to patients, and refill automated stock cabinets. However, barcodes can be bypassed and are increasingly easy to exploit. To duplicate a barcode, one needs only the font of the barcode, a scanner, and the right software program. Exploitation of the barcode system can place a pharmacy at great risk in maintaining the security of its supply system as the risk of counterfeit drugs becomes increasingly common. To help control this risk threat, radiofrequency identification (RFID) chips have been developed to help maintain the security of the drug supply system.

3. *Cyber security* The Food and Drug Administration has become increasingly concerned about the potential for electronic medical devices to cause harm. The 2018 draft guidance for the management of cyber security in medical devices states, "The need for effective cybersecurity to ensure medical device functionality and safety has become more important with the increasing use of wireless, Internet- and network-connected devices, portable media (e.g. USB or CD), and the frequent electronic exchange of medical device-related health information. In addition, cybersecurity threats to the healthcare sector have become more frequent, more severe, and more clinically impactful. Cybersecurity incidents have rendered medical devices and hospital networks inoperable, disrupting the delivery of patient care across healthcare facilities in the US and globally. Such cyberattacks and exploits can delay diagnoses and/or treatment and may lead to patient harm," (Food and Drug Administration, 2018).

4. *Digital veil* is the term applied when the use of computer and automated machinery to execute business-related tasks creates a unique state of mind among the employees, resulting in complacency and blind trust in automation. This results in a mental disengagement with the work process, as if existing under a veil of digitization.

In July 2013, a 16-year-old patient was given a dose of Septra DS 39 times greater than the correct dose. This patient experienced seizures and required emergency treatment and intensive care before he stabilized and could return home. The error originated because the hospital's management software required the physician to convert the correct dose for this patient to a mg/kg equivalent. The physician entered 160 mg thinking she was ordering one Septra DS tablet. However, the software converted the dose to 160 mg/kg for a 40 kg child resulting in the child receiving 39 tablets. The original error was compounded when the verifying pharmacist rushed through the screen alerts, the medication was dispensed from an automatic robotic dispensing device, and the nurse who gave the doses relied on the barcode scanning system to verify the dosing. In this case a manual dispensing process would have likely caught this gross dispensing error, but trust in the computers eventually allowed each player to rationalize their actions based on a misplaced trust that the computer was correct (Wachter, 2015).

Similar circumstances can occur in today's highly automated pharmacy. Employees can be become complacent, and the outcomes to both patient and pharmacy safety and security can be catastrophic.

5. *The human automation tradeoff* becomes more prominent as pharmacies become more dependent on automation. Years of experience and situational factors cannot be incorporated into software, which makes it less capable than humans to deal with emergency situations. Machines do not have the problem-solving capabilities that humans do have for responding to new types of situations or threats.

6. *System failures* can occur in a multitude of ways once a pharmacy business is automated. System failures can have disastrous consequences. The use of sophisticated and intertwined Web services such as Internet refill request and processing, insurance processing, and inventory management create an overlay data level network that ties multiple business functions together. If one function crashes, its failure potentially creates a cascading effect, causing other Web services to fail as well. In addition, an attack against a single node supporting a purchase transaction in a supply chain could corrupt databases at several pharmacies, interfere with logistics and third-party shipping organizations, and create errors in financial reports and inventory management. The damage may not be localized to

the node that was attacked initially. The damage could extend across a business network, spanning companies.

The examples of system failures just cited are general and can happen in any automated business. However, some system failures are unique to pharmacies because of time and regulation constraints. Automated dispensing devices have become increasingly common to enhance pharmacy efficiency and improve patient safety. Although the implementation of automated dispensing reduces personnel time for medication administration and improves billing efficiency, reductions in medication errors have not been uniformly realized. A systematic review of prescription errors suggests that error rates for "wrong drug" and "wrong dose" in an automated computerized physician order entry system still run from 6% to 77% of orders (Korb-Savoldelli et al., 2018).

The authors assert that the more reliable the technological system is, the less skilled workers become in responding to eventual system breakdowns. Finally, the desire to avert human error by practitioners can lead to automation-induced errors and unanticipated forms of failure that can be impossible to plan for.

Psychosocial Risk

Psychosocial risk involves the moral and legal issues related to the interaction of information technology and the safety and health hazards that technology poses to employees in the workplace (Burton, 2006). Pharmacies with an increased risk of these conditions also risk higher worker's compensation costs, absenteeism, short- and long-term disability, and decreased productivity. Repetitive process driven businesses, such as pharmacies, may seem like a safe work environment but actually may have hazardous work conditions. Repetitive-motion injuries are common among pharmacists and technicians. The Centers for Disease Control and Prevention issued a report in 2018 which made the following conclusions, "Pharmacists and the pharmacy technician were exposed to work-related factors such as repetitive and forceful

movements, awkward wrist and shoulder postures, and contact stress such as opening or closing bottle caps that put them at risk for musculoskeletal disorders including de Quervain tenosynovitis, carpal or radial tunnel syndrome, and/or upper extremity tendinitis" (CDC, 2018).

Electronic Health Records and E-Prescribing

Electronic health records (EHR) and e-prescribing are becoming the standard of care, and bear special discussion. By April 2014, 70% of physicians were prescribing using an EHR. Between 2009 and 2014, 48 states experienced an increase in utilization by at least 50 percentage points (Gabriel & Swain, 2014). There is no doubt that a large part of the increased acceptance of e-prescribing and EHR can be attributed to federal incentive programs, specifically the Medicare Improvements for Patients and Providers Act (MIPPA) and the Medicare or Medicaid Electronic Health Records Incentive Programs (EHR Incentive Programs) (Grossman et al., 2011). The purpose of increased use of EHR and e-prescribing is to attain increased patient safety and increased efficiency (cost savings). However, with the increased reliance on information technology, there is an increased concern for the security of PHI and the need for risk management concern. In fact, in a report by the U.S. Department of Health and Human Services Office of Inspector General, there were serious concerns regarding information technology security controls for health information technology (HIT). The report noted that while there were application controls, information technology controls were deficient. The specific information technology controls cited included encrypting data stored on mobile devices, requiring two-factor authentication when remotely accessing HIT, and patching operating systems of computer systems that process and store EHR (U.S. Department of Health & Human Services [DHHS], 2011).

With the increased concerns regarding HIT, pharmacies must be concerned regarding the exposed risks of this increasingly adopted form of technological communication. In reality, it would serve the pharmacy well to have an information security consultant assess the pharmacy's information technology systems for potential risks.

RISK PARADIGM

Risk can be defined either as a negative outcome (e.g., lung cancer is a risk among smokers) or the cause for any negative outcome (e.g., smoking is a health risk). When there are several causes for a single outcome or several outcomes from a single cause, the qualitative assessment of risk becomes complicated. The *quantitative* approach in defining risk does not divide the events into causes and outcomes explicitly, rather, a probability is assigned to each possible relationship whose development is undesirable. The impact of the previously discussed four categories of risk associated with integration of information technology in pharmacies can be viewed as probability events (which are also risks) because they happen at a discrete time and have impact on financial and nonfinancial aspects of pharmacies, as described in Table 11-1.

The *qualitative* explanation for risk provides a better understanding of risk in terms of both cause and outcome. However, the identification of causes and predictions of outcomes is better rather than identifying the outcomes and predicting the causes to minimize the risk because the failure rate of information systems projects is high and is an ever-changing field bringing new and advanced solutions almost every year.

REVISITING THE SCENARIO

Bill Halsey clearly saw a huge task in front of him if he was to purchase Corner Drug. He started making a list of all the issues and risks he would have to address. Not only would he need to update most of the fixtures in the store, but he also foresaw problems with the current layout of the pharmacy department from a security standpoint. He would have to purchase a new computer system and install other information technology and then consider the security issues related to this new technology. Two local physicians were interested in having Bill monitor drug therapy for all their geriatric patients. Bill knew that he also would have to develop a training program for the store's employees to meet HIPAA requirements and for counseling and monitoring documentation. One of his first tasks would be to develop a risk management program to assess current and future risk threats and to ascertain which techniques would have to be employed to address the risks. Bill breathed a sigh of relief that his current employer had included him in meetings with his insurance agent and that

Cause/Effect	Financial Risk	Reputation Risk	Privacy Risk	Human Capital Risk
Strategic risk	Budget constraint; low or no return			Skill shortage; key personnel loss
Performance risk	Low or no return; patient injury	Loss of customers/ trading partners		
Operational risk	Data theft/loss; patient injury	Loss of customers/ trading partners	Data theft	
Psychosocial risk	Productivity loss; increased health benefits			

Table 11-1. Pharmacy Risk Paradigm

he had become well versed in insurance terminology and planning. He would have a big job in front of him and a lot of additional learning to do, but Bill thought he was prepared to know where to start and what needed to be done.

■ CONCLUSION

Just as with human beings in our daily lives, business entities such as pharmacies face risks that may threaten their financial health or ability to exist. Risk management is the process of identifying risks and developing strategies to manage or eliminate negative outcomes for the business. Risk management programs are an important component of business management. Risk management techniques include not only the use of insurance to transfer risk but also implementing strategies to minimize the likelihood of hazards occurring. Pharmacists need to be aware of these potential threats and seek assistance from their professional business consultants and experienced colleagues to develop and maintain appropriate risk management programs. Advice from experienced professionals may be crucial because most pharmacists have little training or experience in these areas.

The use of advanced information technology in pharmacies continues to rise. Managers must be continually vigilant in safeguarding not only the pharmacy's own assets but also patient data from individuals both within and outside the pharmacy. As pharmacies grow more reliant on information technology and attacks on pharmacy systems grow more frequent and sophisticated, the successful pharmacy manager must manage the various risks brought about by this technology.

■ QUESTIONS FOR FURTHER DISCUSSION

1. Why is a risk management program an important component of a progressive patient-oriented pharmacy practice?
2. Many pharmacists have argued and fought for expanded roles in patient-oriented medication therapy management. These newer roles obviously increase the risk exposure of the pharmacists and the pharmacy. Therefore, should they be avoided?
3. A local physician has approached you about the possibility of establishing a paperless e-prescribing system with your pharmacy. What are the risks involved, and how can you minimize those risks?
4. You have decided to establish a Web site that can be used by your patients to order both over-the-counter medications and prescription refills. Would you also like to incorporate inventory management? What are the specific patient security risks? What are the pharmacy data security risks? Are other strategic, operational, performance, and psychosocial risks involved?

■ ACKNOWLEDGMENTS

The authors would like to acknowledge the contributions of Dr. Kevin Farmer and Dr. Donald Harrison in their preparation of this chapter for the third edition.

REFERENCES

Bank for International Settlements. 2015. *Operational Risk.* Available at https://www.bis.org/publ/bcbs195.pdf. Accessed January 15, 2019.

Browning T. 1999. *Sources of Performance Risk in Complex System Development.* Available at http://sbuweb.tcu.edu/tbrowning/Publications/Browning%20(1999)—INCOSE%20Perf%20Risk%20Drivers.pdf. Accessed March 3, 2019.

Bureau of Labor Statistics. 2016. *Table 7. Survival of Private Sector Establishments by Opening Year.* Available at https://www.bls.gov/bdm/entrepreneurship/entrepreneurship.htm. Accessed January 15, 2019.

Burton J. 2006. *Psychosocial Risk Management: What Every Business Manager Should Know!* Available at www.iapa.ca/pdf/2006_hwp_psychosocial_risk.pdf. Accessed March 3, 2019.

CDC. 2018. *Ergonomic Evaluation of Pharmacy Tasks March 2018.* Available at https://stacks.cdc.gov/view/cdc/53113. Accessed January 16, 2019.

Food and Drug Administration. 2018. *FDA Content of Premarket Submissions for the Management of Cybersecurity in Medical Devices; Draft Guidance for Industry and Food and Drug Administration Staff.* Available at https://www.fda.gov/downloads/MedicalDevices/DeviceRegulationandGuidance/GuidanceDocuments/UCM623529.pdf. Accessed January 16, 2019.

Gabriel M, Swain M. 2014. E-Prescribing trends in the United States. Available at: http://www.healthit.gov/sites/default/files/oncdatabriefe-prescribingincreases2014.pdf. Accessed March 3, 2019.

Grossman JM, Boukus ER, Cross DA, Cohen GR. 2011. *Physician Practices, E-Prescribing and Accessing Information to Improve Prescribing Decisions.* Washington, DC: Center for Studying Health System Change.

Hiscox. 2018. *Hiscox Small Business Cyber Risk Report.* Available at https://www.hiscox.com/how-to-develop-strong-small-business-cyber-security-strategy. Accessed January 15, 2019.

Insurance Information Institute. 2015. *Glossary of Insurance Terms.* Available at http://www2.iii.org/glossary/. Accessed September 11, 2015.

Korb-Savoldelli V, Boussadi A, Durieux P, Sabatier B. 2018. Prevalence of computerized physician order entry systems-related medication prescription errors: A systematic review. *Int J Med Inform* 111:112–122.

National Community Pharmacists Association Website. 2018. *About NCPA.* Available at https://www.ncpanet.org/home/ncpa's-mission. Accessed January 15, 2019.

O'Donnell J, Vogenberg FR. 2014. Legal risk management opportunities, pharmacy practice, and P&T Committees. Part 1: Deconstructing dispensing errors. *Pharm Ther* 39(8):559.

Roybal PM. 2018. Of remand and responsibility: Oakey v. may maple pharmacy and the pharmacist's professional standard of care in New Mexico. *N M Law Rev* 48(3):491.

Ropeik D, Gray G. 2002. *Risk: A Practical Guide for Deciding What's Really Dangerous in the World Around You.* Boston, MA: Houghton Mifflin.

Rupp RV. 2002. *Rupp's Insurance & Risk Management Glossary.* Chatsworth, CA: NILS Publishing.

Schafermeyer KW. 2007. Private health insurance. In McCarthy RL, Schafermeyer KW (eds.) *Health Care Delivery: A Primer for Pharmacists,* 4th ed. Boston, MA: Jones and Bartlett.

Target Stores. 2014. *Annual Report.* Available at https://corporate.target.com/_media/TargetCorp/annualreports/2014/pdf/Target-2014-Annual-Report.pdf?ext=.pdf. Accessed March 3, 2019.

U.S. Department of Health and Human Services (DHHS). 2000. *The Pharmacist Workforce: A Study of the Supply and Demand for Pharmacists.* Rockville, MD: Health Resources and Services Administration.

U.S. Department of Health & Human Services (DHHS). 2003. *OCR Privacy Brief: Summary of the HIPAA Privacy Rule.* Available at http://www.hhs.gov/ocr/privacy/hipaa/understanding/summary/. Accessed March 3, 2019.

U.S. Department of Health and Human Services (DHHS). 2011. *OIG Audit of Information Technology Security Included in Health Information Technology Standards (A-18-09-30160). Washington, DC.* Available at https://oig.hhs.gov/oas/reports/other/180930160.pdf. Accessed March 3, 2019.

Wachter R. 2015. *How Medical Tech Gave a Patient a Massive Overdose.* Available at https://medium.com/backchannel/how-technology-led-a-hospital-to-give-a-patient-38-times-his-dosage-ded7b3688558. Accessed April 12, 2019.

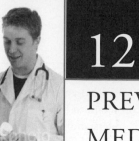

12

PREVENTING AND MANAGING MEDICATION ERRORS: THE PHARMACIST'S ROLE

Matthew Grissinger and Michael Cohen

About the Authors: Matthew Grissinger, RPh, FISMP, FASCP is the Director of Error Reporting Programs at the Institute for Safe Medication Practices (ISMP). He works with health care practitioners and institutions to provide education about medication errors and their prevention and review medication errors that have been voluntarily submitted by practitioners to a national ISMP Medication Errors Reporting Program (ISMP MERP). He has published numerous articles in the pharmacy literature, including regular columns in Pharmacy and Therapeutics (*P&T*) and the Pennsylvania Patient Safety Authority's (PSA) *Patient Safety Advisory* and is a journal reviewer for several publications including the Joint Commission Journal on Quality and Patient Safety, Pharmacoepidemiology and Drug Safety, and Annals of Internal Medicine. He is a chapter contributor to a textbook published by McGraw-Hill entitled *Pharmacy Management: Essentials for All Practice Settings, Remington and Medication Errors.*

Mr. Grissinger serves as the Chair for the National Coordinating Council for Medication Error Reporting and Prevention (NCC MERP) and serves on the National Quality Form (NQF) Common Formats Expert Panel, the Editorial Board for P&T, the Faculty Advisory Board for the Pharmacy Learning Network (PLN), and the Publications Advisory Board for Davis's *Drug Guide for Nurses*. He also served on the United States Pharmacopeia's (USP) Safe Medication Use Expert Committee from 2005 to 2010, the Food and Drug Administration (FDA) Proprietary Name Review Concept Paper workshop panel in 2008, FDA Naming, Labeling, and Packaging Practices to Minimize Medication Errors workshop panel in 2010, and the Joint Commission Home Care Compounding Pharmacy Technical Advisory Panel in 2013.

Michael R. Cohen, RPh, MS, ScD (hon.), DPS (hon.) is founder and president of The Institute for Safe Medication Practices. Dr. Cohen's passion for medication safety began in 1974 when he was involved in a serious adverse event with insulin in the hospital where he was employed. He immediately saw the value in sharing his story with other hospital pharmacists to prevent the same error from occurring. Dr. Cohen founded ISMP in 1994 and launched the first of five ISMP Medication Safety Alert! publications in 1997. The newsletters along with Safety Alerts now reach over a million health professionals in the United States as well as regulatory authorities and others in over 30 foreign countries.

Dr. Cohen is active in many patient safety initiatives including coeditor of the ISMP consumer website, Chairperson of the International Medication Safety Network, former member of the US FDA Drug Safety and Risk Management Advisory Committee (DSaRM) and the Nonprescription Drugs Advisory Committee (NDAC) and is currently a consultant to FDA.

Among his many recognitions for his advocacy, contribution, and understanding of medication safety, Dr. Cohen has received the John M. Eisenberg Patient Safety and Quality Award from the National Quality Forum and the Joint Commission and the Harvey A. K. Whitney Award from the American Society of Health-System Pharmacists. In 2006, he was recognized as a MacArthur Fellow by the John D. and Catherine T. MacArthur Foundation.

■ LEARNING OBJECTIVES

After completing this chapter, readers should be able to

1. Discuss the role of the pharmacist in preventing and detecting medication errors.
2. Define latent and active failures and the role each plays when a medication error occurs. Define the types of medication errors that can occur during the ordering and dispensing process.
3. List some commonly used drugs that can result in medication error-related deaths.
4. Describe what changes are needed at the risk management level to better address medication safety issues, including the use of failure mode and effects analysis (FMEA) to reduce the potential for errors.
5. Identify specific problems in our approach to error prevention and what needs to be changed to ensure patient safety.
6. Describe a variety of methods that can be used to identify risk and provide meaningful data on the relative safety of a facility's medication use process.
7. Select high-leverage error-reduction strategies based on sound safety principles.

■ SCENARIO

This scenario is based on a true story that demonstrates the multiple breakdowns that can occur during the medication use process.

An infant was born to a mother with a prior history of syphilis. Despite having incomplete patient information about the mother's past treatment for syphilis and the current health status of both the mother and the child, *a decision was made to treat the infant for congenital syphilis*. After phone consultation with infectious disease specialists and the health department, an order was written for one dose of "benzathine penicillin G 150,000 units IM."

The physicians, nurses, and pharmacists were unfamiliar with the treatment of congenital syphilis and had limited knowledge about this medication. The pharmacist consulted *Drug Facts and Comparisons* to determine the usual dose of penicillin G benzathine for an infant. However, *she misread the dose as 500,000 units/kg*, a typical adult dose, instead of 50,000 units/kg for an infant. Consequently, the pharmacist also *incorrectly read and prepared the order as 1,500,000 units, a 10-fold overdose*. Owing to the lack of a consistent pharmacy procedure for independent double checking, *the error was not detected*. The pharmacy *dispensed the 10-fold overdose in a plastic bag containing two full syringes of Permapen®*

(the brand name of penicillin G benzathine) 1.2 million units/2 mL each, with green stickers on the plungers to "note dosage strength." A pharmacy label on the bag indicated that 2.5 mL of medication was to be administered intramuscularly to equal a dose of 1,500,000 units. After glancing at the medication sent from the pharmacy, the infant's primary care nurse expressed concern to her colleagues about the number of injections required to give the infant the medication (since a maximum of 0.5 mL per intramuscular injection allowed in infants, the dose would require five injections).

Anxious to prevent unnecessary pain to the infant, the two nurses *decided to investigate the possibility of administering the medication intravenously instead of intramuscularly*. The monograph on penicillin G did not specifically mention penicillin G benzathine; instead, it noted the treatment for congenital syphilis with aqueous crystalline penicillin G slow intravenous push or penicillin G procaine intramuscularly. Nowhere in the two-page monograph was penicillin G *benzathine* mentioned, and no specific warnings regarding "IM use only" for penicillin G procaine and penicillin G benzathine were present. Unfamiliar with the various forms of penicillin G, a nurse practitioner *believed that "benzathine" was a brand name for penicillin G* and concluded that the drug could be administered safely intravenously. While preparing for drug administration, *neither nurse noticed the 10-fold overdose and nor noticed that the syringe was labeled by the manufacturer, "IM use only."* The nurses *began to administer the first syringe of Permapen as a slow intravenous push*. After approximately 1.8 mL was administered, the infant became unresponsive, and resuscitation efforts were unsuccessful (ISMP, 1998).

The three nurses involved in this case were indicted for criminally negligent homicide in the death of the baby. Over 50 different system failures allowed this error to occur, go undetected, and ultimately, reach a healthy newborn child, causing his death. Had even just one of these failures not occurred, either the accident would not have happened, or the error would have been detected and corrected before reaching the infant.

■ CHAPTER QUESTIONS

1. At what stages of the medication use process do medication errors occur?
2. What types of contributing factors lead to medication errors during the ordering process?
3. What procedures should be followed when taking a verbal order?
4. What steps should be followed during the prescription-filling process to prevent medication errors?
5. What three important factors play a role in any patient interface?
6. Which types of patients are at risk for nonadherence?

■ INTRODUCTION

Patient safety has been a major concern since the November 1999 release of the Institute of Medicine's (IOM) report *To Err Is Human*. Health care practitioners may have been surprised to learn from this report that errors involving prescription medications kill up to 7000 Americans a year (Kohn et al., 1999). The IOM released a report in 2006 entitled *Preventing Medication Errors* and indicated that medication errors are among the most common medical errors, harming at least 1.5 million people every year. The reports concluded that 400,000 preventable drug-related injuries occur each year in hospitals. Another 800,000 occur in long-term care settings, and roughly 530,000 occur just among Medicare recipients in outpatient clinics. Assuming conservatively, an annual incidence of 400,000 in-hospital preventable adverse drug events (ADEs) yields an annual cost of $3.5 billion in 2006. The report noted that these are likely underestimates because the data excluded errors of omission such as the failure to prescribe medications for which there is an evidence base for the ability to reduce morbidity and mortality (Aspden et al., 2006).

With this increased attention to medication errors, concern has intensified in both the public and health care sectors. Research demonstrates that injuries resulting from medication errors generally are not the fault of individual health care professionals, but rather represent failures in a complex health care system. Medication error prevention starts with recognizing that errors are multifactorial and are faults of the system as a whole rather than results of the acts or omissions of the people in the system. Even when an error can be traced directly to a specific individual (e.g., the pharmacist dispensing or nurse administering the wrong medication), further investigation often determines that a number of factors, such as poor order communication between the physician and pharmacist, dangerous storage practices in pharmacies, and lookalike labeling, may have played a role in the error. Protecting patients from inappropriate administration of medications has become an important focus for pharmacists and technicians, including those in ambulatory, acute care, long-term care, home care, and managed-care settings.

Pharmacists and technicians play a pivotal role in assuring medication safety. In a study performed in community pharmacies, an overall dispensing accuracy rate for prescription medications was reported to be 98.3% (Allan et al., 2003). Although most of these errors probably have minimal clinical relevance and do not affect patients adversely, many experts believe that medication error rates may be higher in the outpatient setting because errors may not always be evident to the health professionals who work there. For example, medication errors can occur when a patient purchases over-the-counter (OTC) medications without speaking with the pharmacist about any potential interactions with his or her prescription medications, or if patients fail to verify the appropriate dose of the OTC medication.

This chapter focuses on system enhancements and the checks and balances needed to proactively prevent medication errors as pharmacists and technicians prepare, dispense, and monitor the effects of medications in all practice settings. In addition, focus is placed on the importance of determining latent failures that contribute to medication errors by developing effective reporting programs to discover how latent failures occur and how they can be prevented.

■ BACKGROUND

Many organizations take an ineffective approach to preventing medication errors. Investigations tend to focus on the *front end* or *active end* of the error (e.g., the frontline practitioner, such as the pharmacist dispensing the medication). When an error occurs, human nature tends to assign blame to someone or something. In addition, health care practitioners work in an environment where they strive for perfection. Individuals involved in the commission of an error may be considered inattentive, incompetent, lazy, and uncaring. They are often subject to punitive action such as disciplinary action, public or private reprimands, remedial education, suspensions, or termination. As a result, the practitioner develops feelings of inadequacy, denial, and embarrassment.

Effective approaches, on the other hand, consider factors that contribute to medication errors that occur at the organizational level, known as the *latent end* or *blunt end* of an error. Latent failures are weaknesses in organizational structure, such as faulty information management or ineffective personnel training, that may have resulted from decisions made by upper management (Reason, 1990). Latent failures can also stem from incomplete patient information, such as missing allergy or diagnosis information, unclear communication of a drug order, lack of an independent double check before dispensing, lack of computer warnings, ambiguous drug references, drug storage issues, and look-alike/sound-alike medications. These latent failures are properties of the medication-use system. To prevent medications errors, we must change and improve the processes in the medication-use system and not rely on changing people and their behaviors.

ISMP has identified 10 key elements that have the greatest influence on the medication-use system. System-based causes of medication errors can be directly traced to weaknesses or failures in these key elements:

- Patient information
- Drug information
- Communication of drug information

- Drug packaging, labeling, and nomenclature
- Drug device acquisition and use
- Drug storage, stock, and distribution
- Environmental factors
- Staff competency and education
- Patient education
- Quality processes and risk management (Cohen, 2007)

By themselves, latent failures are often subtle and may not cause problems directly. The potential consequences are often hidden, becoming apparent only when they occur in a certain sequence and combine with the active failures of an individual.

Medication use is a complex process that consists of subprocesses such as the ordering, preparing, dispensing, administration, and the provision of patient education. Because failed communication of medication orders is at the heart of many errors, pharmacists must be aware of the types of breakdowns that can occur during the ordering process that can lead to medication errors.

■ ORDERING MEDICATIONS

Physicians or their designees—pharmacists, nurse practitioners, physician assistants, and nurses—initiate the drug dispensing and administration process through a medication order or prescription. Computerized prescriber order entry (CPOE) and electronic prescribing (e-prescribing) systems, each with clinical decision-support tools, have been implemented in many health care settings.

"True" electronic prescribing, or "e-prescribing," exchanges prescriptions directly between a prescriber's computer system and a pharmacy's computer system. When fully implemented, e-prescribing can improve medication safety. In fact, the Southeast Michigan e-prescribing Initiative (SEMI), a broad coalition involving General Motors, Ford Motor Company, Chrysler, the United Auto Workers, Blue Cross Blue Shield of Michigan, Health Alliance Plan, Henry Ford Medical Group, Medco Health Solutions, and CVS Caremark Corporation, recently reported promising

results from an evaluation of e-prescriptions (SEMI, 2012). Their analysis, conducted in December 2011 on a sample of 23 million prescriptions written by SEMI physicians since the program began, found the following:

- A severe or moderate drug-to-drug interaction alert was sent to physicians for more than 6.2 million prescriptions, resulting in 1.8 million (or 28%) of those prescriptions being changed or cancelled by the prescribing doctor;
- Physicians received nearly 923,000 medication allergy alerts, resulting in more than 250,000 (or 27%) of those prescriptions being changed or cancelled by the prescribing doctor;
- 8.2 million lists of dispensed prescription histories were downloaded by physicians; and
- When a formulary alert was presented, physicians changed the prescription to comply with formulary requirements 28% of the time.

The use of e-prescribing continues to grow. According to SureScripts, operators of the Pharmacy Health Information Exchange that facilitates the electronic transmission of prescription information, 13.7 billion prescriptions were electronically prescribed in 2017, representing a 26% increase from the previous year , including 4.8 million e-prescriptions daily (SureScripts, 2017).

Electronically generated prescriptions, including those faxed or hand delivered to pharmacies, may solve legibility issues; however, they have introduced a number of other types of errors. ISMP has received reports in which prescribers have included a second set of directions that conflict with the pre-programmed label (i.e., sig) for a medication (see Figure. 12-1).

Rx	HYTRIN
Sig:	5 MG PO HS
Dispense:	180 Tablet (s)
Directions:	2 HS

Figure 12-1. Prescription that includes a second set of directions that conflict with the pre-programmed "sig" for a medication.

Often these pre-programmed directions are selected from a drop-down list, and the prescriber does not know how to change or delete them. Also, prescribers may not be aware of the increased risk of error that conflicting directions create. For example, a community pharmacy received an e-prescription for the anticonvulsant gabapentin with "1 tablet PO TID" in the sig field but "i po bid × 7 days, then i po tid thereafter" in the notes field. A second report indicated that an e-prescription for MIRALAX™ (polyethylene glycol 3350) powder, an osmotic laxative, was sent by the prescriber with the directions "1 tablet(s) PO BID." Clearly this was an inappropriate sig for a powder, so the pharmacist looked at the notes field at the bottom of the e-prescription and found the correct directions. A third report described an e-prescription for ONE TOUCH™ ULTRA blood glucose test strips which was transmitted with a sig of "lnVt" while the notes field contained "use as directed up to 10 times daily" (ISMP, 2011).

ISMP has also received reports that some electronically generated prescriptions have misspelled drug names, missing container size information, and pre-programmed sigs that contain error-prone abbreviations. The prescription in Figure 12-2, although legible, includes trailing zeros, uses error-prone abbreviations, and has conflicting directions.

Another reported concern with e-prescribing is the lack of communication with changes in orders. For example, a near miss occurred in a small clinic pharmacy where three e-prescriptions were received for a patient from the same doctor. These included doxycycline 100 mg BID for 7 days, moxifloxacin 400 mg once daily for 30 days, and prednisone 20 mg BID for 7 days. The patient was also taking sotalol 120 mg BID to control an arrhythmia. All the prescriptions

were entered by a pharmacy technician and reviewed by a pharmacist, at which point the computer system flagged a drug interaction between sotalol and moxifloxacin. The prescriber was then contacted by the pharmacist. He stated he sent the prescription electronically but immediately realized the drug interaction and discontinued moxifloxacin in the computer system on his end. He incorrectly assumed that this would send a message to the pharmacy as well; however, that did not happen (ISMP, 2009).

A number of vendors offer e-prescribing systems. However, the structure and design of the prescriptions these systems generate are not standardized. Vendors should collaboratively work with practitioners to standardize the structure of electronically generated prescriptions. Error-prone abbreviations and dose designations should be removed from these systems, and users should avoid using them in free-text fields (ISMP, 2007). Pharmacists should communicate and share copies of error-prone electronically generated prescriptions with prescribers and software vendors to illustrate the issues these prescriptions can create.

Illegible Handwriting

Although there continues to be an upward trend in the use of e-prescriptions, illegible, ambiguous, or incomplete handwritten prescriptions or medication orders still contribute to many errors made by nurses, pharmacists, pharmacy technicians, and other health care workers. To minimize the chance of misinterpretation due to illegibly handwritten orders, encourage physicians with poor handwriting to print prescriptions and medication orders in block letters. In the institutional setting, have physicians review orders with the nursing staff before leaving the patient care area. More importantly, ask physicians to include the purpose of the medication as part of the prescription or medication order to help readers distinguish drug names when handwriting legibility is less than ideal. Pre-printed orders, dictation, and direct order entry into the computer by physicians are other solutions for poor handwriting. Pre-printed orders should be reviewed at least annually to make sure the information is up-to-date.

Rx	Clonazepam
Sig:	1(1.0 MG) PO QHS × 30 days
Special Instructions:	take 0.5 mg q am and 1.0 mg po qhs
Directions:	60

Figure 12-2. Prescription that includes trailing zeros, error-prone abbreviations, and has conflicting directions.

Because even skilled individuals can misread good handwriting, a system of independent double checks for order/prescription transcription should be in place in which several individuals interpret and transcribe an order. In the pharmacy, pharmacists and technicians have a number of opportunities to check the order, including a double check against labels, printouts, and the drug containers. A technician often screens the order and sometimes enters it into the computer. After data entry, a label is printed, and a pharmacist should interpret the original order/prescription and verify the technician's computer entry by comparing it with the label. Later, the order and label can be read again by technicians and pharmacists as doses are prepared and dispensed. In the outpatient setting, this system should include a final check when providing counseling to the patient. In no case should pharmacy technicians interpret orders on their own because this process does not offer enough checks to prevent an error. In addition, orders must not be filled only from computer-generated labels. Rather, the original order should accompany the label to serve as another check.

Look-Alike Drug Names

While there may be fewer handwritten orders due to the increased use of prescriber order entry systems, medications with names that are spelled similarly can be easily misread for one another. Pharmacists and technicians must be alert to this problem and should never guess about a prescriber's intent.

Study the handwriting in Figures 12-3 and 12-4. These are actual examples of handwritten orders in

Figure 12-3. Order for Vantin 200 mg misread as Vasotec 20 mg.

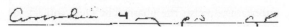

Figure 12-4. Order for Avandia 4 mg misread as Coumadin 4 mg.

both the inpatient and outpatient settings, each of which led to medication errors. The problem was not uncertainty. On the contrary, each order was misread from the start. No consideration was ever given to the alternative drug because in each case, the pharmacy staff members thought they were reading the order correctly.

When pharmacists and technicians interpret prescriptions and medication orders, newly marketed drugs are a particular problem. Staff members are not as familiar with names of the drugs, and they tend to misinterpret them as older drugs. It is important that up-to-date education on all new medications is provided to the pharmacy staff, including any potential for error that may exist with these new products. In the outpatient setting, physicians can write both the generic and trade names legibly on the prescription, and they can add the intended purpose of the medication to further alert pharmacy staff to the correct medication name. Many medications have look-alike names, but very few name pairs that are spelled similarly are used for similar purposes.

Sound-Alike Names

Drug orders communicated orally, by phone or in person, are often misheard, misunderstood, misinterpreted, or transcribed incorrectly. Pyridoxine and pralidoxime sound alike, as do clonidine and Klonopin®, alprazolam and lorazepam, Flomax® and Volmax®, and hundreds of other name pairs. Each of these drugs has been confused for the other, resulting in patients receiving incorrect medications. In many cases, serious injuries have occurred because of misinterpreted verbal orders. This is a good reason for health care facilities such as hospitals and long-term care facilities to establish policies that prohibit verbal requests for medication without pharmacy review of a hard copy of the order. Sound-alike drug names present many of the same problems as look-alikes. Obviously, when uncertainties exist, the pharmacist must contact the prescriber for clarification.

To decrease the opportunity for misunderstanding, health care facilities and community pharmacies should discourage verbal orders. The Joint Commission, a national accrediting agency for health care organizations, requires in its standards that accredited organizations improve the effectiveness of communication among caregivers by implementing a process for taking verbal or telephone orders that mandates that a verbal order to be transcribed and then "read back" completely by the person receiving the order (The Joint Commission [TJC], 2015).

Greater use of computerized order entry among hospital areas, medical offices, pharmacies, and nursing units has improved the communication of medication orders. When verbal communication is unavoidable, strict adherence to these procedures can minimize errors:

- In acute care settings, spoken orders should be limited to true emergencies or circumstances in which the prescriber is physically unable to write or electronically transmit orders (e.g., the prescriber is working in a sterile field).
- Prohibit spoken orders for selected high-alert medications (e.g., chemotherapy, IV insulin for neonates) because of their complexity and potential for serious errors.
- Verbal orders should be taken only by authorized personnel.
- If possible, a second person should listen while the prescription is being given.
- The order should be written down and then read back (i.e., the "write down, read back" method), repeating exactly what has been ordered, sometimes spelling the drug name for verification and the strength by using a digit-by-digit technique for the dose (1–5, not 15).
- Obtain the prescriber's phone number in case it is necessary for follow-up questions.
- The prescribed agent must make sense for the patient's clinical situation (Cohen, 2007a).

To prevent sound-alike and look-alike errors, physicians must be encouraged to include complete directions, strengths, route of administration, and indication (purpose) for use. With this information, pharmacists and other skilled health care professionals can judge whether the drug ordered makes sense for the patient in the context in which it is written. For example, knowing that the patient has a diagnosis of diabetes would be important in determining that Avandia® is intended by the medication order in Figure 12-4. Diagnostic procedures along with orders could also provide important information. This is why it is important for pharmacists to verify all orders processed by technicians. When in doubt, technicians should check with the pharmacist, who can contact the prescriber for clarification if the intent is not completely clear.

Abbreviations to Avoid

Certain abbreviations are easily misinterpreted. Discouraging the use of dangerous abbreviations can reduce communication errors. Although many health care facilities have lists of abbreviations that are approved for use by professional staff, it would be far safer if each facility also develops a list of abbreviations that should never be used.

The ISMP has developed a list that contains several easily misinterpreted abbreviations from actual medication errors, some of which resulted in patient harm (ISMP, 2018). These abbreviations should never be used in medication orders (both written and electronic), on pharmacy labels, in newsletters, or in other communications that originate in a pharmacy or pharmacy computer systems. Examples of some of the most problematic abbreviations used to communicate orders include the following:

- *The abbreviation* U *for units.* Errors have occurred when the letter *U* was mistaken for the numerals 0, 4, 6, and 7, and even cc, resulting in disastrous drug overdoses of insulin, heparin, penicillin, and other medications whose doses sometimes are expressed in units. For example, an order written as "Humalog 6U" has been misinterpreted as "60 units" (see Figure. 12-5).
- *Q for "every," as well as other abbreviations with this letter (QD, QID, and QOD; or qd, qid, and qod).* QD

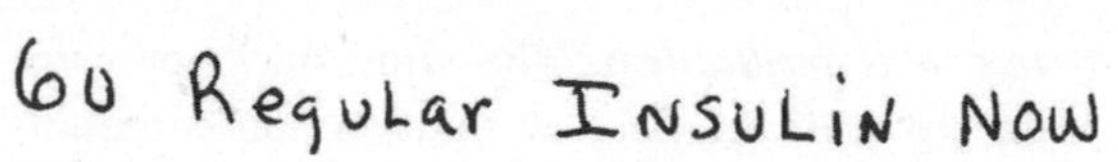

6U Regular Insulin Now

Figure 12-5. Misinterpretation of 6 units (U) of Humalog insulin for 60 units.

for "daily" can result in four-fold overdosages if seen as QID (q.i.d.) for "four times daily," or subtherapeutic doses if seen as QOD for "every other day." Errors associated with QD and QOD have been reported to the Pennsylvania PSA (PSA, 2005). In one case, an order for Zithromax® (azithromycin) 500 mg written as QD was misinterpreted as QID. In another report, an order was written for digoxin 0.125 mg po QOD (every other day), but the medication was given QD (every day).

- *D/C.* It has been written to mean either "discontinue" or "discharge," sometimes resulting in premature stoppage of a patient's medications. In Figure 12-6, the "d/c" order was incorrectly interpreted as "discontinuation" of an antibiotic that the patient had never even received. In reality, the "d/c" is really "OK," meaning that the drug was approved for use by the infectious disease physician.

Drug names also should not be abbreviated. Abbreviating drug names have led to frequent medication errors, including the following:

- *Magnesium sulfate (MgSO₄ or simply Mg) and morphine sulfate (MSO₄ or simply MS).* In one example, a prescriber used an abbreviation for $MgSO_4$ and wrote "$MgSO_4$ 2g IV × 1 dose" for a 45-year-old female patient. However, the unit clerk and nurse misinterpreted the order as MSO_4 "2 mg IV × 1 dose." The patient received a 2-mg dose of MSO_4. Contributing to this error was the fact that the patient was having pain, so morphine seemed reasonable (PSA, 2005).

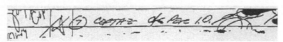

Figure 12-6. Ceftazidime "OK" per ID misread as ceftazidime "d/c" per ID.

- *MTX.* This means "methotrexate" to some health professionals, but others understand it as "mitoxantrone."
- *AZT.* This has been misunderstood as "azathioprine" (Imuran®) when "zidovudine" (Retrovir®) was intended. In one case, this misinterpretation led to a patient with AIDS receiving azathioprine, an immunosuppressant, instead of the intended antiretroviral agent. The patient's immune system worsened, and he developed an overwhelming infection.
- *HCT and HCTZ.* Orders for "HCTZ50 mg" (hydrochlorothiazide) can be mistaken for "HCT 250 mg" (hydrocortisone).

Ambiguous Orders

Errors can result when ambiguous orders are interpreted in a manner other than what the prescriber intended. Proper expression of doses is vital in a drug order. Pharmacists should be able to recognize improper expressions of doses and their potential for error. When the order is not clear, the pharmacist must contact the prescriber for clarification. Pharmacists and technicians should avoid using dangerous expressions of doses as they process orders, type labels, and communicate with others. The following examples include several improperly expressed orders that were reported to the ISMP:

- *Zeros and decimal points.* When listing drug doses on labels or in other communications, never follow a whole number with a decimal and a zero. For example, "Coumadin 1.0 mg" is a very dangerous way to express this dose. If the decimal point were not seen, the dose would be misinterpreted as "10 mg," and a 10-fold overdose would result. The same could happen when "Dilaudid 1.0 mg" is written. The proper way to express these orders would be "Coumadin 1 mg" and "Dilaudid 1 mg."
- *Leading zeros.* Always place a leading zero before a decimal point when the dose is smaller than 1. For example, "Vincristine .4 mg" was seen as "Vincristine 4 mg" due to a poor impression of the decimal, as is common on faxes or copies of orders. Avoid using

decimal expressions when recognizable alternatives exist because whole numbers are easier to work with. For example, "Digoxin 0.125 mg" is acceptable, but "Digoxin 125 mcg" is a better alternative. So too would be to indicate a dose as "500 mg" instead of "0.5 g."

- *Tablet strengths.* Orders specifying both strength and number of tablets are confusing when more than one tablet strength exists. For example, "Metoprolol 1/2 (one-half) tablet 25 mg once daily" appears clear enough. However, when you realize that this product is available in both 25- and 50-mg tablets, the ambiguity of this order becomes apparent. What is the intended dose, 25 or 12.5 mg? Orders are clearer if the dose is specified regardless of the strengths available (e.g., "Metoprolol 12.5 mg once daily"). For doses that require several tablets or capsules, the pharmacy label should note the exact number of dosage units needed. For example, the label on an 800-mg dose of Asacol® (mesalamine), which is available only in 400-mg tablets, should read "2 × 400-mg tablets = 800 mg." For a 6.25-mg dose of captopril, which is available in 12.5-mg tablets, the label should read one-half (1/2) × 12.5-mg tablet = 6.25 mg." Fractions should be displayed in fraction format and not as 1 slash 2 (1/2) (ISMP, 2011). The same type of notation should be used on electronic medication administration records (eMARs) for nurses.

- *Liquid dosage forms.* Expressing the dose for liquid dosage forms in only milliliters or teaspoonfuls is dangerous. For example, acetaminophen elixir is available in many strengths, including 80, 120, and 160 mg per 5 mL. If the prescriber wrote "5 mL," the intended number of milligrams would be unclear. However, an order of "80 mg" states the appropriate dose. The amount of drug by metric weight, as well as the volume, should always be included on the pharmacy label (e.g., "Acetaminophen elixir 80 mg/5 mL"). Further, the patient dose should also be included. For a 320-mg dose, the label should read, "320 mg = 20 mL." The same holds true for unit dose and bulk labels.

- *Injectable medications.* The same rules apply for injectable drugs. Because solution concentrations can vary, list the metric weight of the dose, or the metric weight and volume of the dose, but never the volume alone. An example of this type of error occurred at a hospital where hepatitis B vaccines were being administered. A pre-printed physician's order form was used to prescribe the vaccine, listing only the volume to be given. When the clinic switched to another brand of vaccine, containing a different concentration of vaccine, the same pre-printed forms continued to be used. This resulted in the underdosing of hundreds of children until the error was discovered. This could have been avoided had the amount of vaccine been prescribed in micrograms rather than just the volume in milliliters.

- *Variable amounts.* A drug dose should never be ordered solely by number of tablets, capsules, ampules, or vials because the amounts contained in these dosage forms vary. Drug doses should be ordered with proper unit expression (e.g., "20 mEq potassium chloride").

- *Spacing.* Overdoses have been reported because a lowercase "l" (el) was the final letter in a drug name and was misread as the number 1. In one case, an order for 300 mg Tegretol® (carbamazepine) twice daily appeared as "Tegretol 300 mg bid" and was misinterpreted as "1300 mg bid" (see Figure 12-7). In another case, a nurse misread an order for 2 mg Amaryl® (glimepiride) as 12 mg because there was insufficient space between the last letter in the

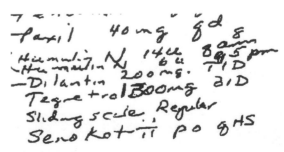

Figure 12-7. Order for Tegretol misread as 1300 mg instead of 300 mg.

drug name and the numerical dose. In addition, when labels are printed, make sure that there is a space after the drug name, the dose, and the unit of measurement.

■ PREPARING AND DISPENSING MEDICATIONS

An important safety enhancement for preventing dispensing errors is the development of a system of redundant checks from the time the original prescription is ordered in the physician's office or on the nursing unit to receipt in the pharmacy and through dispensing and administration. The more independent "looks" an order receives (while efficient workflow is maintained), the better. Health professionals can review orders at several checkpoints and thereby maximize the chances of errors being discovered.

Steps in Prescription Filling

It is important that all health care professionals, including prescribers, nurses, and pharmacy personnel, work together when filling prescriptions so that the lines of communication are kept open if questions should arise. It is also important that pharmacy personnel understand the processes involved in the communication of orders in their particular practice setting so that breakdowns can be addressed, and improvements can be made to improve both efficiency and safety.

Outpatient/Community Pharmacy

1. The prescriber sees the patient; performs an assessment; determines the appropriate medication, dose, route, and frequency; and writes the order or communicates the order electronically to the pharmacy.
2. A direct copy of the order is transported by the patient, faxed/scanned to the pharmacy, or the prescriber's computer entry system (e-prescribing) to the pharmacy order entry system.
3. The pharmacist or pharmacy technician reads the order and enters it in the pharmacy computer system.

   a. If the technician finds a duplicate order, incorrect dose, drug allergy, or other problem, it is documented and called to the attention of the pharmacist during prospective drug utilization review (DUR).

4. A pharmacist reviews the prescriber's or pharmacy technician's computer entry, compares it with the original prescription, and performs a DUR of the prescription with respect to the need for the drug, allergies or other contraindications, proper dose, and proper route of administration.
5. A label and/or medication profile is printed. It is important that a copy of the original prescription or medication order continues to accompany the label or medication profile is available to review once the order is filled. Orders should never be filled solely on the basis of what appears on the label or medication profile because the computer entry may have been in error.
6. To choose an item for dispensing, a technician reviews both the label and the medication order for possible discrepancies.
7. A pharmacist checks the technician's work, reviewing the label against the medication order and the dose that has been prepared. The drug is labeled and dispensed.
8. The pharmacist uses the patient counseling session to further assess that the correct medication is being dispensed and that the patient has a condition treatable with the product being provided.

   a. Pharmacists should not simply ask patients if they have any questions about their medication but confirm their understanding of the medication and its proper use by using open-ended questions.

   b. Patients should be educated about the common adverse effects of medications they are taking and understand what clinical signs to watch for and report to health professionals.

   c. If patients or caregivers are provided with an administration device, such as an oral syringe or inhaler, pharmacists must ensure that the patient or caregiver understands how to use the device properly by using the show-and-tell technique.

d. For refills and medications patients have received in the past, pharmacists should ask questions about how the medication is working and whether or not the patient is experiencing any problems with the medication. Adherence should also be assessed. If the patient is taking too much medication or is not taking the drug as frequently as prescribed, the pharmacist should speak with the patient to determine the reasons for and address the variation. Finally, patients should be encouraged to ask the pharmacist about any changes in the appearance of the product.

e. At the point-of-sale, have the patient review the pharmacy labels and contents of each prescription container to check that the medication is correct—even if this requires opening the bag. This simple step alone can cut the risk in half of patients taking home a correctly filled prescription intended for another patient (ISMP, 2015).

Hospital Pharmacy

1. The prescriber sees the patient; performs an assessment; determines the appropriate medication(s), dose(s), route(s), and frequency(ies); and writes orders or communicates the orders electronically to the pharmacy.

2. The pharmacist reads the order and verifies it in the pharmacy computer system. If the technician finds a duplicate order, incorrect dose, drug allergy, or other problem, it is documented and called to the attention of the pharmacist during prospective DUR.

3. A pharmacist reviews the prescriber's or pharmacy technician's computer entry, compares it with the original prescription (handwritten or electronic), and performs a DUR of the prescription with respect to the need for the drug, allergies or other contraindications, proper dose, and proper route of administration.

4. The pharmacy label is printed. A copy of the medication order(s) continues to accompany the label while the order is filled. Orders should never be filled solely on the basis of what appears on the label because the computer entry may have been in error.

5. To choose an item for dispensing, a technician reviews both the label and the medication order for possible discrepancies and obtains the product from its storage area.

6. A pharmacist checks the technician's work, reviewing the label against the medication order and the dose that has been prepared. The drug is labeled and dispensed.

7. The medications are delivered to the patient's care area. Medications are stored in a variety of areas that include individual patient cassettes/bins or automated dispensing cabinets (ADCs).

8. The nurse obtains the drug and compares the medication and pharmacy label against the copy of the physician's order, as well as the MAR/eMAR.

9. The nurse administers the dose, giving the drug's name, explaining the drug's purpose and potential adverse effects, and answering questions and concerns raised by the patient.

Selecting Medications

The importance of reading the product label while selecting medications and filling prescriptions cannot be overemphasized. Too often the wrong drug, strength, or concentration is dispensed. Such errors often stem from failure to read the label thoroughly. During drug preparation and dispensing, the label should be read three times:

1. When the product is selected,
2. When the medication is prepared, and
3. When either the partially used medication is disposed of (or restored to stock) or product preparation is complete.

Selecting the correct item from the shelf, drawer, or bin can be complicated by many factors. Similar labeling and packaging, as well as look-alike names, are common traps that lead to medication errors (see Figures 12-8 and 12-9). Restocking errors are common and can lead to repeated medication errors before being detected.

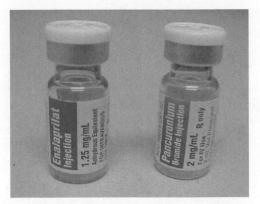

Figure 12-8. Similar packaging might lead to medication errors.

ADCs are computerized drug storage devices or cabinets that allow medications to be stored and dispensed near the point of care, while controlling and tracking drug distribution. They are now used in the majority of hospitals and have become more prevalent in the outpatient setting. Many health care organizations have moved beyond storing only narcotics and floor stock in ADCs and are using ADCs as their primary method of drug storage and delivery in patient care areas (ISMP, 2019). The use of ADCs as the predominant distribution model in the hospital setting has increased from 22% in 2002 to 70% in 2017, whereas a centralized manual dose distribution

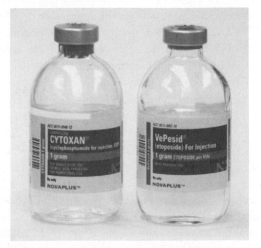

Figure 12-9. Another example of packaging that might lead to medication error.

model has continued to decrease over the last 15 years (Schneider, 2018). This change in the pharmacy distribution model has had broad implications for pharmacist, pharmacy technician, and nurse workflow and safety.

ADCs offer a variety of benefits to the organization and the user. They provide nurses with near total access of medications needed in patient care areas. This has decreased the delivery turnaround time from the pharmacy to the patient care unit for new medications ordered. ADCs also ensure greater control of the charge capture of medications, support security measures, and potentially reduce the number of medication errors. Expanded ADC software can provide additional clinician support aimed at enhancing patient safety, including linking ADC and pharmacy management system (profiled system) to allow pharmacist review of new medication orders, machine-readable bar codes for restocking and selection of medications, integration into automated refilling systems, drug safety alerts and decision support when selecting medications from the cabinets, and the capacity to link with telepharmacy operations for after-hour drug verification and distribution (Grissinger et al., 2007).

ADCs create several situations that can result in errors. While these machines are routinely restocked, the wrong drug still can be placed into the wrong bin during this process. Devices that have multiple medications in each drawer have an open matrix configuration and/or that do not require pharmacist review of orders before access have drawbacks that are identical to the flaws in traditional floor-stock systems:

- The pharmacy can replenish the system with an incorrect medication.
- The nurse can retrieve either the wrong item or additional items to use for other patients.
- For ADCs without profiling capabilities, the lack of pharmacist double checking and screening orders before a nurse withdraws a medication from the cabinet allows prescribing errors, wrong dosages, incorrect routes of administration, and other clinical errors to occur.

ISMP held a national ADC forum to create interdisciplinary guidelines for the safe use of ADCs. During the forum, attendees reviewed a list of core elements believed to significantly influence the safe use of ADCs and developed process recommendations for each element (ISMP, 2019). Those core elements include the following:

- Provide Ideal Environmental Conditions for the Use of ADCs
- Ensure ADC System Security
- Provide Profiled ADCs and Monitor System Overrides
- Select and Maintain Appropriate ADC Configuration and Functionality
- Select and Maintain Optimal ADC Inventory
- Implement Safe ADC Stocking and Return Processes
- Display Important Patient and Drug Information
- Develop Procedures for Accurate ADC Withdrawal and Transfer to the Bedside for Administration
- Provide Staff Education and Competency Validation

The term *confirmation bias* is used to describe the phenomenon that when choosing an item, people see what they are looking for, and once they think they have found it, they stop looking any further. Often health professionals choose a medication container based on a mental picture of the item. Staff members may be looking for some characteristic of the drug label, the shape and size or color of the container, or the location of the item on a shelf, in a drawer, or in a storage bin instead of reading the name of the drug itself. Consequently, they may fail to realize that they have the wrong item in hand.

A number of approaches can be used to minimize the possibility of such errors in the pharmacy, care areas, and in automated dispensing machines. Physically separating drugs with look-alike labels and packaging reduces the potential for error. Some pharmacies also separate drugs with similar names and overlapping strengths, especially those labeled and packaged by the same manufacturer. For example, chlorpromazine 100-mg tablets and chlorpropamide

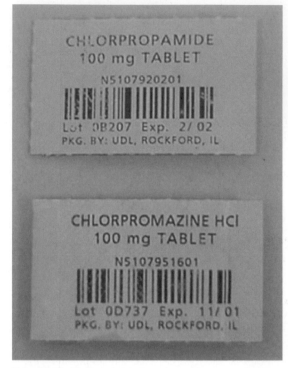

Figure 12-10. Similarity in labeling of two different medications.

100-mg tablets, both from the same unit-dose packager (see Figure 12-10), might pose a problem. So might tramadol 50 mg and trazodone 50 mg or metformin 500 mg and metronidazole 500 mg. Another strategy would be to change the appearance of look-alike product names on computer screens, pharmacy shelf labels and bins, and pharmacy product labels by highlighting, through boldface, color, or the use of "tall man" letters, the parts of the names that are different (e.g., hydrOXYzine and hydrALAzine). In fact, the FDA Office of Generic Drugs requested that the manufacturers of 16 look-alike name-pair drug products voluntarily revise the appearance of their established names to minimize medication errors resulting from look-alike confusion. Manufacturers were encouraged to differentiate their established names visually with the use of "tall man" letters. Examples of established names involved include chlorproMAZINE and chlorproPAMIDE, vinBLASTINE and vinCRISTINE, and NICARdipine and NIFEdipine.

In institutional and community pharmacies with several staff members, everyone should have input in deciding how and where drugs are available, how doses are prepared, who is responsible for preparing them, the appearance of the storage containers, and how they are labeled. In addition, staff members should be encouraged to use a technique known as *failure mode and effects analysis* to examine the use of new products to determine points of potential failures and their effects *before any error actually happens* (see Chapter 10). In this regard, FMEA differs from *root-cause analysis* (RCA). RCA is a reactive process, employed after an error occurs, to identify its underlying causes. In contrast, FMEA is a proactive process used to carefully and systematically evaluate vulnerable areas or processes. FMEA can be employed before the purchase and implementation of new products to identify potential failure modes so that steps can be taken to avoid errors before they occur (ISMP, 2011a, 2019b). Procedures to ensure safe medication use must be written, and the importance of adhering to the guidelines must be shared by all involved pharmacy, medical, and nursing personnel.

Selecting Auxiliary Labels

To help prevent errors and improve patient outcomes, pharmacists and technicians should judiciously apply auxiliary labels in certain circumstances, especially in the community setting. For example, amoxicillin oral suspension is available in dropper bottles for pediatric use. When the suspension is used for an ear infection, some parents have been known to place the suspension in the child's ear rather than to give it properly (orally). An auxiliary label, "For oral use only," would help to prevent this administration error. However, this practice can be unsafe if auxiliary labels are relied upon in lieu of direct patient education and/or the patient is unable to understand the warning. The application of an auxiliary label should not be done in lieu of speaking with the patient. A study that appeared in the *American Journal of Health-System Pharmacy* showed that there is a high level of misunderstanding of auxiliary labels among adults with low literacy, defined as a reading level at or below the

sixth-grade level (Wolf et al., 2006). The rate of correct interpretation of these labels ranged from 0% to 78.7%. With the exception of the label "Take with food," less than half of all patients were able to provide adequate interpretations of the warning labels' messages. In fact, no one was able to correctly interpret the label, "Do not take dairy products, antacids, or iron preparations within 1 hour of this medication." Studies also have shown that a combination of a verbal description of a warning along with visual symbols improves the overall comprehension of the warning (Lesch, 2003).

■ STERILE ADMIXTURE PREPARATION

In preparing fluids for injectable administration, the potential for grave errors is increased for several reasons. First, patients are often sicker when they need intravenous drugs, so the medications used have more dramatic effects on the body's function and physiology. Further, most injectable solutions are clear, colorless, water-based fluids that look alike, regardless of what drug and how much of it are actually in the fluid.

A five-hospital observational study on the accuracy of preparing small- and large-volume injectables, chemotherapy solutions, and parenteral nutrition (PN) showed a mean error rate of 9%, meaning almost 1 in 10 products was prepared incorrectly and then dispensed (Flynn et al., 1997). Error rates for complex solutions, such as PN, were especially high—37% for manual preparation and 22% for preparations that were partly automated. More recently, a 2009 State of Pharmacy Compounding Survey showed that 30% of hospitals have experienced a patient event involving a compounding error in the past 5 years (Pharmacy Purchasing & Products, 2009). In 2006, an infant received a lethal dose of zinc stemming from an error that occurred during the order entry and compounding of a total parenteral nutrition (TPN) solution. TPN was prescribed for a preterm infant born at 26 weeks gestation. On the day of the event, the physician's TPN order included directions to add zinc in a concentration of 330 µg/100 mL. Because the automated compounder used for TPN required entry of zinc in a µg/kg dose, the pharmacist converted the µg/mL dose to a µg/kg dose. She performed this calculation correctly, but accidentally entered the zinc dose in the pharmacy computer in mg, not µg. This resulted in a final concentration of 330 mg/100 mL—a 1,000-fold overdose (ISMP, 2007).

Based on this information, the ISMP held a national invitational Sterile Preparation Compounding Safety Summit where participants identified best practices that applied to the preparation of the following items (ISMP, 2016):

1. Simple compounded sterile preparations (CSPs) (those with one or two ingredients, such as patient controlled analgesia infusions, single electrolyte infusions, bolus doses, or maintenance IV infusions with no more than two ingredients),
2. Complex CSPs (those with greater than two ingredients, such as PN, cardioplegia solutions, or dialysis solutions),
3. Pediatric and neonatal preparations, and
4. Chemotherapy.

These guidelines consisted of 13 consensus statements that range from a focus on policies and procedures for compounding sterile preparations to compounding to staff management.

In the sterile admixture preparation setting, dosage miscalculations and measurement errors must be minimized by systems designed with procedures that require independent double checks by two staff members. In many pharmacies, independent double checks are required for all calculations or measurements, whereas others may require it only for calculations falling in special categories, such as dosage calculations for admixture compounding for any child under age 12, critical care drug infusions requiring a dose in micrograms per kilogram per minute, insulin infusions, chemotherapy, and patient-controlled analgesia. Calculators and computer programs may improve accuracy, but they do not eliminate the need for a second person to review the calculations and solution concentrations used.

Another important way to minimize calculation errors is to avoid the need for calculations in the first place. This can be accomplished by using the unit-dose system exclusively as follows:

- Using commercially available unit-dose systems such as premixed critical care parenteral products.
- Standardizing doses and concentrations, especially of critical care drugs such as heparin, insulin, dobutamine, dopamine, and morphine.

Similar steps can be taken in community pharmacies that provide sterile admixtures to physician offices, home care programs and patients, long-term care facilities, and other clients.

The use of standard dosage charts on nursing units in institutions and standard formulations in the pharmacy minimizes the possibility of error and makes calculations much easier. For example, in critical care units, physicians need to order only the amount of drug they want infused and list any titration parameters. No one has to perform any calculations because dosage charts can be readily available for choosing appropriate flow rates by patient weight (in kilograms) and dose ordered.

Standard concentrations for frequently prepared formulations should be readily accessible for reference in the admixture preparation area of the pharmacy. All calculations must be double-checked and documented by the pharmacist. Diluents as well as active drugs must be checked before they are added to the base solution. (Proxy methods of verification of ingredients, such as the syringe pull-back method of verification, should never be used.) The stock container of each additive with its accompanying syringe should be lined up in the order it appears on the container label to facilitate the checking procedure. When compounding TPN solutions, at least three verification processes should occur in the pharmacy after initial order entry of TPN; before manually injecting additives into the TPN; and once the TPN has been compounded. Each verification should require a pharmacist to compare the actual prescriber's order to the printed labels, and the printed labels to the additives and final product, as appropriate. Verification of manual additives should include inspection of the actual vials and syringes that contain the additives. The final verification of the compounded TPN should include a comprehensive review of the TPN order, the label on the product, and the work label.

In many hospitals and home infusion pharmacies, automated compounding equipment is being used for admixing both large- and small-volume parenterals. While automated equipment improves the accuracy of compounding parenterals, accidents can occur when solutions are placed in the wrong additive channel. These can result in serious medication errors. Therefore, it is important that the pharmacy have an ongoing quality assurance program for the use of automated compounding equipment. This program should include double checks and documentation of solution placement within the compounder, final weighing or refractometer testing of the solution to ensure that proper concentrations have been compounded, and ongoing sampling of electrolyte concentrations. Pharmacists who prepare special parenteral solutions in batches (e.g., TPN base solutions or cardioplegic solutions) should have additional quality assurance procedures in place, including sterility testing and quarantine until confirmation.

■ PATIENT COUNSELING AND EDUCATION

The patient is the last individual involved in the medication use process. The pharmacist–patient interface can play a significant role in catching medication errors before they occur. Unfortunately, many health care organizations do not take advantage of this key interaction. Three important factors play a role in any patient interface and often determine the outcome of error-prevention efforts. These include direct patient education, health care literacy, and patient adherence.

Community pharmacies in the United States filled over 4 billion prescriptions in 2017 (StateHealthFacts, 2017). This increase in prescription volume often results in a decrease in the amount of time available for direct pharmacist involvement in patient education.

A 1999 study involving community pharmacies in eight states revealed that 87% of all patients received written information with their prescriptions. However, only 35% of pharmacists made any reference to the written leaflet, and only 8% actually reviewed it with the patient (Svarstad, 2000). A follow-up study by Svarstad showed that about 63% of the shoppers were given oral drug information and that counseling practices varied significantly according to the intensity of a state's counseling regulation, with frequency of any information provision climbing from 40% to 94% as states' counseling regulations increased in intensity (Svarstad, 2004). Contributing to this gap in patient education is the failure to provide patients with understandable written instructions.

The second factor is patient literacy, which includes general literacy levels and health care literacy. Many people have difficulty understanding their illness or disease, proper management of disease, and their role in maintaining their health. Whether limited by knowledge, socioeconomic factors, emotional or clinical state, or cultural background, patients' level of health literacy (i.e., the ability to read, understand, and act on health care information) is often much lower than many health care providers appreciate. Examples of patients who have had difficulty reading and understanding medication directions are plentiful. For example, an elderly patient could not tell the difference between his bottle of Coumadin® (warfarin) and Celebrex® (celecoxib). A mother, who after reading the label on a bottle of acetaminophen, could not accurately state her child's dose. And a teenager who misunderstood directions for contraceptive jelly and ate it on toast every morning to prevent pregnancy.

According to a report published by the American Medical Association Ad Hoc Committee on Health Literacy, more than 40% of patients with chronic illnesses are functionally illiterate, and almost a quarter of all adult Americans read at or below a fifth-grade level. Unfortunately, medical information leaflets typically are written at or above a tenth-grade reading level. Further contributing to the dilemma is the fact that an estimated three-quarters of patients throw out the medication leaflet stapled to the prescription bag without reading it, and only one-half of all patients take their medications as directed (American Medical Association, 1999).

One reason for this lack of understanding may be that people who have difficulty reading or understanding health information are too embarrassed or ashamed to acknowledge their deficits. Instead, they are hesitant to ask questions of their health professionals and often pretend to understand instructions. In addition, low literacy is not obvious. Researchers have reported poor reading skills in some of the most poised and articulate patients (ISMP, 2011a).

Adherence is the third patient-related factor contributing to medication errors. One study found a 76% difference between medications patients actually are taking when compared with those recorded in their charts as prescribed. Two factors that contribute to this high rate of discrepancy include confusion that may accompany advancing age and the increase in the number of prescribed medications (Bedell et al., 2000). Another study demonstrated that patient nonadherence played a role in 33% of hospital admissions (McDonnell et al., 2002). Additional studies have showed that between 21% and 41% of patients do not understand their diagnosis, treatment, or follow-up (Waisman, 2003; Zavala, 2011), 20% are aware of their lack of understanding (Engel, 2009), between 12% and 20% do not fill their prescription, and 40% do not adhere with their recommended prescription regimen (Hohl, 2009). A major factor in patient nonadherence is poor understanding of instructions (Watt, 2005), which in turn is often due to inadequate physician-patient communication and/or pharmacist-patient communication (Clark, 2005; Thomas, 1996).

Nonadherence may be exhibited by patients in many ways, such as not having a prescription filled initially or refilled, dose omissions, taking the wrong dose, stopping a medication without physician's advice, taking a medication incorrectly or at the wrong time, taking someone else's medication, and financial inability to purchase their medications. Patients at risk for being nonadherent include those taking more than one drug, those with a chronic condition who are on complex drug regimens that may result in bothersome side effects, those who take a drug more than once daily, and those who have a condition that produces no overt symptoms or physical impairment such as hypertension or diabetes (National Council on Patient Information and Education [NCPIE], 2007). In addition, older adults are more at risk owing to factors such as decrease in mental acuity and increased confusion, lack of family or caregiver support, decreased coordination and dexterity, and impaired vision (Lombardi & Kennicutt, 2001). Pharmacy managers must consider these factors in developing and providing patient education tools or methodologies.

A New Model of Accountability

Despite a growing awareness of the system-based causes of errors, many in health care are still struggling to come to terms with the role of individual accountability. Even when we seem to understand the system-based causes of errors, it's still hard to let individuals "off the hook." We ask, "How can we hold individuals accountable for their actions without punishment?" Some have suggested that a nonpunitive approach to error reduction leads to increased carelessness as people learn that they will not be punished for their mistakes. However, another perspective is that staff awareness of safety issues, as well as their enthusiasm for changing systems and practices associated with errors, actually grows in a nonpunitive system. A nonpunitive, system-based approach to error reduction does not diminish accountability; it redefines it and directs it in a more productive manner by focusing on the most manageable component of the error: the medication-use system itself.

Typically when an error happens, only those individuals at the "sharp end" of an error (e.g., pharmacists and pharmacy technicians) are held accountable. But, we must shift from this thinking and realize that accountability must be shared among all health care stakeholders. In the new patient safety model, each individual becomes accountable, not for zero errors (which is an unrealistic and unattainable expectation for any human), but for making patient safety a part of every aspect of their job. In addition, all become accountable for identifying safety problems, implementing system-based solutions, and inspiring and embracing a culture of safety.

Because we are not capable of practicing without making errors, health care practitioners should be held accountable for speaking out about patient safety issues, voluntarily reporting potential and actual errors as well as hazardous situations, and sharing personal knowledge of what went wrong when an error occurs. Also, practitioners must be empowered to ask for help when needed, consistently provide patient education, and be willing to change their practices to enhance safety.

In an effort to make health care safer, many health care organizations are attempting to adopt the characteristics of high-reliability organizations (HROs) that have achieved impressive safety records despite operating in unforgiving environments (ISMP, 2014). Several examples of HROs include nuclear power plants, air traffic control systems, naval aircraft carriers, and wildland firefighting crews. HROs consistently navigate through complex, dynamic, and time-pressured conditions in a nearly error-free manner. Research suggests that HROs achieve their exceptional performance through a collective behavioral capacity and culture of safety to detect and correct errors and adapt to unexpected events despite a changing environment. At the core of HROs is a set of principles that enable organizations to focus attention on evolving problems and to address those problems before they escalate. These principles, termed mindfulness, directly impact reliability in a manner different than strategies traditionally employed by health care organizations. This state of mindfulness embodies five cognitive processes that capture the essence of HROs: (1) preoccupation with failure, (2) reluctance to simplify interpretation, (3) sensitivity to operations, (4) commitment to resilience, and (5) deference to expertise.

Management should be held equally accountable for making a safe and rewarding culture for practitioners to openly discuss errors and patient safety issues. They must hold regular safety briefings with staff to learn about improvement needs, discuss strategic plans, and identify new potential sources of error. When practitioners recommend error-prevention strategies, leaders must support them and provide necessary resources within a reasonable timeframe to implement system enhancements to improve efficiency and safety. Leaders should be held accountable for understanding and addressing barriers to safe practice such as distractions and unsafe workloads. Leaders should incorporate patient safety as a value in the organization's mission and engage the community and staff in proactive continuous quality improvement (CQI) efforts, including an annual self-assessment of patient safety. All health care personnel should be held accountable for working together as a team, not as autonomous individuals. Finally, leaders and staff alike need to review and share safety literature frequently and offer visible support to their colleagues who have been involved in errors.

This model of shared accountability spreads far beyond the walls of individual health care settings to encompass licensing, regulatory, and accrediting bodies; institutions that educate and train students and health care professionals; professional associations; governments and public policy makers; the pharmaceutical industry; medical device and technology vendors; and even the public at large. These often-overlooked participants share equal accountability for doing their part to make medication use safer. For example, licensing, regulatory, and accrediting bodies should be held accountable for adopting standards related to error reduction recommendations that arise from expert analysis of adverse events and scientific research. Educators should seek out patient safety information and use it in curriculum design. Professional organizations should support local and national reporting systems and disseminate important patient safety information to their members. Companies that produce medical devices, pharmaceutical products, health care computers and software, and other health-related products should be held accountable for pre- and post-market evaluation, continuous improvement in the design of devices and products as well as labels and packages. Purchasers of health care should provide incentives and rewards for patient safety initiatives. And all health care professionals, including pharmacists, should encourage the public to ask questions and stay informed about their care and ways to avoid errors.

The system-based model of accountability requires that all who interact with the health care system help to define its weaknesses and find ways to make it stronger. Organizational leaders and other stakeholders who simply hold the workforce accountable when an error happens are inappropriately delegating their own responsibility for patient safety. Managers must stop blaming and punishing those closest to an error, and instead accept a model of shared accountability to collectively translate our sincere concern for patient safety into effective system-based error solutions. Implementing such solutions and inspiring and embracing a culture of change to reach the goal of safety may not be easy, but is certainly necessary.

Effective Risk-Reduction Strategies

Selecting the best error-prevention strategies is not an easy task. Often, the most effective action is not obvious, and the best error prevention tools to use in each situation are not clear, even when system-based causes have been identified. In addition, pharmacists should focus their efforts on medications that may lead to harm if involved in an error. Although most medications have a wide margin of safety, a few drugs have a high risk of causing patient injury or death if they are misused. Special precautions are needed to reduce the risk of error with these "high-alert" medications. Errors with these drugs may not be more common than with other medications, but their consequences can be more devastating (ISMP, 2008).

Listed below are examples of error-prevention strategies for creating lasting system changes for safe medication use (see Table 12-1). Those listed first are considered to be "high leverage" strategies, such as constraints and forcing functions, are more powerful because they focus on changes to the system in which individuals operate. As the list descends, strategies that target system changes but rely in some part

Table 12-1. Medication Error Reduction Strategies

Error-Reduction Strategy	Power (leverage)
Fail-safes and constraints	*High*
Forcing functions	
Automation and computerization	
Standardization	
Redundancies	
Reminders and checklists	
Rules and policies	
Education and information	
Suggestions to be more careful or vigilant	*Low*

Reproduced with permission from Institute for Safe Medication Practices (ISMP): Root Cause Analysis Workbook for Community/Ambulatory Pharmacy, 2006.

on human vigilance and memory, considered to be "low leverage" strategies, such as education and information, are presented. Strategies toward the end are familiar and often easy to implement, but rely entirely on human vigilance (ISMP, 1999, 2006).

- Fail-safes and constraints are among the most powerful and effective error-prevention strategies. They involve true system changes in the design of products or how individuals interact within the system. In the hospital setting, one example includes removing concentrated potassium chloride for injection from all patient care areas. In this situation, a nurse could not accidentally administer this medication because it would not be available to select from stock. Another acute care example includes eliminating nursing access to the pharmacy when it is closed by establishing a carefully selected night time formulary and dispensing cabinet. At a community pharmacy where the pharmacy computer system is integrated with the cash register, a fail-safe would prevent the clerk from "ringing up" the prescription unless final verification by a pharmacist was noted in the system.

- Forcing functions are procedures that create a "hard stop" during a process to help ensure that important information is provided before proceeding; often referred to as a "lock and key" design. Examples outside of health care would include the inability to drive your car unless you first place your foot on the brake before shifting the car into "drive." For example, a pharmacy order entry system that requires a weight to be entered for each patient receiving an order for a weight-based medication (e.g., heparin, enoxaparin) before it is processed, or a bar code scanning system that does not allow final verification of a product without a positive match between the selected product and the profiled medication.

- Automation and computerization of medication-use processes and tasks can lessen human fallibility by limiting reliance solely on vigilance or memory. Examples include use of electronic prescribing software that includes clinical decision support; pharmacy computer systems that can receive prescriptions sent electronically from a prescriber's hand-held device or computer and thus eliminate transcriptions and misinterpretations; robotic prescription preparation and dispensing technology; and computer systems that provide accurate warnings related to allergies, significant drug interactions, and excessive doses.

- Standardization creates a uniform model to adhere to when performing various functions and it tends to reduce the complexity and variation of a specific process. For example, standardized processes could be created to guide the pharmacist's final verification of a medication or to enhance the safety of giving or receiving a telephoned medication order. Prescriber use of carefully designed pre-printed prescription blanks or standardized order forms that contain commonly used protocols (e.g., steroid tapers, insulin regimens, and weight-based heparin) or frequently prescribed medications can reduce problems with confusing or missing instructions and illegible handwriting. On its own, standardization relies on human vigilance to ensure that a process is followed; therefore, it is less effective than the strategies mentioned previously.

- Redundancies incorporate duplicate steps or add another individual to a process to force additional checks in the system. Involving two individuals in a process reduces the likelihood that both will make the same error with the same medication for the same patient. However, the potential for error still exists since the redundant step may be omitted or ignored. Examples of redundancies include use of both brand and generic names when communicating medication information or requiring independent double checks of high-alert medications before dispensing. Patient counseling is often an underutilized redundancy that can detect many errors.

- Reminders and checklists help make important information readily available. For example, using auxiliary labels to distinguish products; building look- and sound-alike alerts into order entry systems; and using preprinted prescription blanks that include prompts for important information (e.g., medication indication, allergies, patient's birth date).

- Rules and policies are useful and necessary in organizations. Effective rules and policies should guide staff toward an intended positive outcome. However, some may add unnecessary complexity and may be met with resistance, even rightfully so, especially when implemented in response to an error. Because their use relies on memory, they should be used as a foundation to support more effective strategies that target system issues.

- Education and information are important tactics when combined with other strategies that strengthen the medication-use system. But, the effectiveness of these tactics relies totally on an individual's ability to remember what has been presented. Thus, on their own, they offer little leverage to prevent errors.

While each tool mentioned above can play an important role in error prevention, beware of those that, on the surface, seem to provide the easiest and fastest solution. While strategies at the bottom of the list may be used initially, we must realize that they will not be effective for long-lasting error prevention when used alone. In order to do a better job at preventing errors, detecting errors or mitigating harm to patients, we need to employ a variety of strategies that focus on the medication-use system issues and address human factors issues for those who work within that system. Since people cannot be expected to compensate for weak systems, managers should routinely evaluate the error-prevention strategies being used in their organizations. Consider if there are more powerful strategies that could be implemented to enhance medication safety.

Risk Identification Methods

All medication dispensing procedures should be examined regularly, both proactively and retrospectively, and the potential problems as well as causes of system breakdowns must be discovered so that prevention measures can be designed. Pharmacy staff needs to communicate clearly to managers what it takes to do the job correctly in terms of personnel, training programs, facilities design, equipment, drug procedures and supplies, computer systems, and quality assurance programs. In addition, reducing medication errors requires using a number of effective risk identification methods including a nonpunitive environment and a voluntary medication error reporting system.

Self-assessments can help organizations assess the safety of medication practices throughout the facility, identify opportunities for improvement, and possibly compare their experiences with the aggregate experiences of demographically similar hospitals (ISMP, 2019b). One key consideration when undergoing this type of process is the establishment of an interdisciplinary team that should consist of representatives from all aspects of an organization, ranging from leadership (CEO, CMO, and nurse executives), directors of pharmacy as well as frontline staff, including nursing, pharmacists, and physicians.

It is also important for pharmacy staff not only to focus on their own internal errors but also to look at other pharmacies' errors and methods of prevention and to learn from them. Organizations such as the ISMP, TJC, and many others provide ongoing features to facilitate these reviews in publications such as *Hospital Pharmacy, Pharmacy Today, Pharmacy Practice News,* and *Pharmacy and Therapeutics* or newsletters that report on current medication safety issues and offer recommendations for changes.

The direct observation technique, in which a trained observer accompanies the person giving medications and witnesses the preparation and administration of each dose, was developed by Barker and McConnell (1962). The observer writes down in detail what the subject does when preparing and administering the drug (Barker et al., 2002). The notes are then compared with the prescriber's orders. An error is counted if the subject did not carry out the order accurately. The error rate is the percentage of doses administered in error, and the accuracy rate is the percentage of doses accurately administered. This method has many advantages. For example, it is not affected by lack of awareness of errors, lack of willingness to report errors, faulty memory, poor communication skills, or selective perception of the subject observed. Its reliability has been established through replication over many years. A large quantity of data can be accumulated at a rate 24 times that of chart review and 456 times that of incident reports. It can detect more errors and more types of error per unit of time than other methods, and it can identify clues about the causes so that future errors can be prevented (Cohen, 2007b).

A retrospective, voluntary, confidential reporting program provides pharmacists and pharmacy technicians with the opportunity to tell the complete story without fear of retribution. The depth of information contained in these stories is critical to understanding the error. This information is critical to identification of system deficiencies that can be corrected to prevent future errors. However, successful and sustained improvement of error-prone processes cannot occur if there is little information available about factors that contribute to an error.

Many organizational factors inhibit the reporting of medication errors. Examples include inconsistent definitions of a medication error within an organization, a punitive approach to medication errors, failure to improve the medication system or address reported problems reported by staff, lack of feedback to staff, over-concern with medication error rates when reporting of an error may increase a facilities "error rate," complex reporting processes, a perception that reporting is a low priority, and concern for personal liability. A voluntary program encourages practitioners to report hazardous situations and errors that have the potential to cause serious patient harm. A confidential reporting system where everyone understands that errors will not be linked to performance appraisals is critical. Many pharmacy organizations have regular meetings where medication errors are addressed. The results of these meetings are often not shared with the front-line staff, therefore giving the impression that "nothing is being done" when errors are reported. In addition, busy practitioners tend to avoid reporting errors owing to the cumbersome nature of their organizations' reporting forms and processes. It is important to make error reporting easy, reward error reporting, and provide timely feedback to show what is being done to address problems. Consistently applying a nonpunitive approach to errors is important. If even one person is disciplined for an error, mistakes will be hidden. Employees should not be evaluated based on errors or lack of making mistakes but on positive measures that evaluate an employee's overall contribution to the organization. Armed with these tools, pharmacists can become aware of the deficiencies in their organizations and make performance-improvement changes. Without them, pharmacies can only address errors when they surface rather than at the root cause.

To be successful, medication error-reduction efforts must result in system improvements that are identified through a four-pronged analysis of errors. The first two prongs, both reactive in nature, include analysis of organization-specific errors that have caused some degree of patient harm and analysis of aggregate medication error data (e.g., trends by drugs or location of drugs involved in errors). Equally important, the other two prongs, both proactive in nature, include analysis of "close calls" (errors that have the potential to cause patient harm) and analysis of errors that have occurred in other organizations. Each prong contains valuable information about

weaknesses in the system that, collectively, can lead to effective error-reduction strategies. Yet many organizations focus primarily on the first two prongs of error analysis and action. Most often proactive efforts are not given high priority. As a result, organizations may be busy "fighting fires" rather than preventing them. A "close call" should be clear evidence that a tragic event could occur. Unfortunately, too often this wakeup call is not heard. Little attention is focused on thorough analysis of errors that, fortunately, do not cause actual patient harm, especially if organizations identify errors that require analysis by a severity rating that is based on actual patient outcome. For example, a serious overdose detected before administration may not be given the same priority and analysis as a similar error that actually reached and possibly harmed the patient. Worse, some organizations fail to use errors that have occurred elsewhere as a road map for improvement in their own organization. Staff will be more comfortable discussing a serious external error than one that has occurred within its own organization. Because blame is not an issue, defensive posturing and other obstacles to effective discussion will not be present. Staff can identify possible system-based causes of the error more easily and the likelihood of a similar error in their facility and make suggestions for improvement. As improvements are made, enthusiasm builds for identifying, reporting, and analyzing errors that are actually occurring within the organization. In the end, discussion about external errors leads to more effective analysis of internal errors.

Multidisciplinary educational programs should be developed for health care personnel about medication error prevention. Because many errors happen when procedures are not followed, this is one area on which to focus through newsletters, discussions during staff meetings, and in-service training.

Finally, organizations should report medication errors externally so that the lessons learned from these events can be shared with others to prevent future occurrences in their facilities. In 1999, the IOM issued a landmark report entitled, *"To Err is Human: Building a Safer Health System"* that highlighted critical areas of research and activities needed to improve

The National Medication Errors Reporting Program (ISMP MERP)

Operated by the Institute for Safe Medication Practices, a federally certified Patient Safety Organization and an FDA MEDWATCH partner

Do not provide any identifiable health information, including names of practitioners, patients, healthcare facilities, or dates of birth.

Date and time of event: _____

Please describe the error. Include description/sequence of events, type of staff involved, and work environment (e.g., code situation, change of shift, no 24-hour pharmacy, floor stock). If more space is needed, please attach a separate page.

_____
_____
_____

Did the error reach the patient?　　☐ Yes　　☐ No

Was the incorrect medication, dose, or dosage form administered to or taken by the patient?　☐ Yes　　☐ No

Circle the appropriate Error Outcome Category (select one—see back for details):　A　B　C　D　E　F　G　H　I

Describe the direct result of the error on the patient (e.g., death, type of harm, additional patient monitoring). _____

Indicate the possible error cause(s) and contributing factor(s) (e.g., abbreviation, similar names, distractions). _____
_____

Indicate the location of the error (e.g., hospital, community pharmacy, clinic, nursing home, patient's home). _____

What type of staff or healthcare practitioner made the initial error? _____

Indicate if other practitioner(s) were also involved in the error (type of staff perpetuating error). _____

What type of staff or healthcare practitioner discovered the error or recognized the potential for error? _____

How was the error (or potential for error) discovered/intercepted? _____

If available, provide patient age, gender, diagnosis. Do not provide any patient identifiers. _____

Please complete the following for the product(s) involved. (If more space is needed for additional products, please attach a separate page.)

	Product #1	Product #2
Brand/Product Name (If Applicable)	_____	_____
Generic Name	_____	_____
Manufacturer	_____	_____
Labeler	_____	_____
Dosage Form	_____	_____
Strength/Concentration	_____	_____
Type and Size of Container	_____	_____

Reports are most useful when relevant materials such as product label, copy of prescription/order, etc., can be reviewed.

Can these materials be provided? ☐ Yes　　☐ No　　Please specify: _____

Suggest any recommendations to prevent recurrence of this error, or describe policies or procedures you instituted or plan to institute to prevent future similar errors. _____
_____

(___) _____　　　(___) _____

Name and Title/Profession　　　　　　　　Telephone Number　　　Fax Number

Facility/Address and Zip　　　　　　　　　　　　　　E-mail

Address/Zip (where correspondence should be sent)

Please check the box that applies:　☐ Consumer　　☐ Licensed Healthcare Practitioner　　☐ Student/Technician

Copies of reports, without any identifying information, will be sent to third parties such as the manufacturer/labeler and to the Food and Drug Administration (FDA). You have the option of including your name on these copies.

ISMP may release my identity to these third parties as follows (check boxes that apply):

☐ FDA　　☐ The manufacturer and/or labeler as listed above　　☐ Anonymous to all third parties

Signature　　　　　　　　　　　　　　　　Date

©ISMP 2012

Submit via the web at: **www.ismp.org/merp**　　　Email: **merp@ismp.org**

Mail: ISMP, 200 Lakeside Dr., Ste. 200, Horsham, PA 19044　　Phone: 800-Fail-Saf(e) (800-324-5723)　　Fax: 215-914-1492

Figure 12-11. ©The Institute for Safe Medication Practices. All rights reserved.

the safety and quality of health care delivery. One critical area of the IOM report addressed the reporting and analysis of data on adverse events.

The IOM report and its findings spotlighted a serious need to capture information that would help to improve quality and reduce harm to patients. Addressing this need, Congress passed The Patient Safety and Quality Improvement Act of 2005 (Patient Safety Act). To implement the Patient Safety Act, the Department of Health and Human Services issued the Patient Safety and Quality Improvement final rule. The Patient Safety Act and the Patient Safety Rule authorize the creation of Patient Safety Organizations (PSOs) to improve quality and safety through the collection and analysis of data on patient events (Agency for Healthcare Research and Quality [AHRQ], 2011).

PSOs are organizations that share the goal of improving the quality and safety of health care delivery. Organizations that are eligible to become PSOs include public or private entities, for-profit or not-for-profit entities, provider entities such as hospital chains, and other entities that establish special components to serve as PSOs. By providing both privilege and confidentiality, PSOs create a secure environment where clinicians and health care organizations can collect, aggregate, and analyze data, thereby improving quality by identifying and reducing the risks and hazards associated with patient care. ISMP is certified as a PSO by the AHRQ, which offers the highest level of legal protection and confidentiality for medication error reporting and analysis.

Reporting errors to organizations like ISMP can also inform pharmaceutical companies of labeling and packaging problems. Many pharmaceutical companies have responded to suggestions made by technicians and pharmacists. Health professionals can report all of the aforementioned close calls and actual medication errors by using the ISMP Medication Error Reporting Program (ISMP MERP, 2015). Reports are forwarded to the individual pharmaceutical company and the FDA, and ISMP provides follow-up when appropriate. Call 1-800-FAILSAFE, visit ISMP's website at www.ismp.org, or complete an ISMP MERP report (see Figure 12-11).

■ CONCLUSION

Pharmacists play a key role in the drug use process throughout any health care organization. Pharmacists and other members of the pharmacy department should lead a multidisciplinary effort to examine where errors arise in this process. Pharmacy department administrators should encourage their staff to collaborate in designing quality assurance programs to obtain information that helps to establish priorities and make changes. Programs can be established to monitor the accuracy of order entry into computers in the pharmacy. Quality assurance efforts that include a review of medication error reports help to develop a better understanding of the kinds of systemic or behavioral defects being experienced so that necessary corrections can be identified. The medication error problem will never be eliminated completely,

■ QUESTIONS FOR FURTHER DISCUSSION

1. Have you witnessed or been involved in a medication error, and what actions did you take to prevent any future errors?
2. Have you counseled a patient whom you know did not understand his or her doctor's instructions? What steps did you take to ensure that the patient thoroughly knew his or her medication, directions, and indication for use?
3. Will you include medication error-prevention strategies in the orientation process for new employees and ongoing education for pharmacy staff?
4. Do you think that you will be involved in reporting medication errors both internally within your organization and externally to reporting agencies such as the ISMP or the FDA? Do you think this will make a difference in your pharmacy practice setting?

but pharmacy managers, working together with their staffs and other health care providers, can use their expertise to address issues of safety and thus ensure best outcomes in the safest environment possible.

REFERENCES

Agency for Healthcare Research and Quality (AHRQ). 2011. Patient Safety Organizations. Available at http://www.pso.ahrq.gov/about. Accessed September 15, 2015.

Allan EL, Barker KN, Carnahan BJ. 2003. National observational study of prescription dispensing accuracy and safety in 50 pharmacies. *J Am Pharm Assoc* 43:191–200.

American Medical Association (AMA), Ad Hoc Committee on Health Literacy for the Council on Scientific Affairs. 1999. Health literacy: Report of the Council on Scientific Affairs. *JAMA* 281:552–557.

Aspden P, Wolcott JA, Bootman L, Cronenwett LR (eds.). 2006. *Preventing Medication Errors: Quality Chasm Series*. Washington, DC: The National Academies Press.

Barker KN, Flynn EA, Pepper GA. 2002. Observation method of detecting medication errors. *Am J Health Syst Pharm* 59(23):2314–2316.

Barker KN, McConnell WE. 1962. The problems of detecting medication errors in hospitals. *Am J Hosp Pharm* 19:360–369.

Bedell SE, Jabbour S, Goldberg R, Glaser H, Gobble S, Young-Xu Y, et al. 2000. Discrepancies in the use of medications: Their extent and predictors in an outpatient practice. *Arch Intern Med* 160:2129–2134.

Clark C, Friedman SM, Shi K, Arenovich T, Monzon J, Culligan C. 2005. Emergency department discharge instructions comprehension and compliance study. *Can J Emerg Med* 7:5–11.

Cohen MR (ed.). 2007. *Medication Errors*, 2nd ed. Washington, DC: American Pharmacists Association, p. 56.

Cohen MR (ed.). 2007a. *Medication Errors*, 2nd ed. Washington, DC: American Pharmacists Association, pp. 192–193.

Cohen MR (ed.). 2007b. *Medication Errors*, 2nd ed. Washington, DC: American Pharmacists Association, p. 27.

Engel KG, Heislier M, Smith DM, Robinson CH, Forman JH, Ubel PA. 2009. Patient comprehension

of emergency department care and instructions: are patients aware of when they do not understand? *Ann Emerg Med* 53:454–461.

Flynn EA, Pearson RE, Barker KN. 1997. Observational study of accuracy in compounding IV admixtures at five hospitals. *Amer J Health-System Pharm* 54:904–912.

Grissinger M, Cohen H, Vaida AJ. 2007. Using technology to prevent medication errors. In Cohen M (ed.). *Medication Errors*, 2nd ed. Washington, DC: American Pharmacists Association, pp. 413.

Henry J, StateHealthFacts. Kaiser Family Foundation. 2017. Total number of retail prescription drugs filled at pharmacies, 2017. Available at http://kff.org/other/state-indicator/total-retail-rx-drugs/. Accessed February 14, 2019.

Hohl CM, Abu-Laban RB, Brubacher JR. 2009. Adherence to emergency department discharge prescriptions. *Can J Emerg Med* 11(2):131–138.

Institute for Safe Medication Practices (ISMP). 1998. *ISMP Medication Safety Alert!* Washington, DC: ISMP, p. 3.

ISMP. 1999. Medication error prevention "toolbox." *ISMP Medication Safety Alert* 4(11):1.ISMP. 2006. Selecting the best error-prevention "tools" for the job. Community/Ambulatory Care Edition. *ISMP Medication Safety Alert* 5(2):1–2.

ISMP. 2007. Electronically-generated prescriptions: An Rx for E-rror? Community/Ambulatory Care Edition. *ISMP Medication Safety Alert* 6(12):1–2.

ISMP. 2007. Fatal 1,000-fold overdoses can occur, particularly to neonates, by transposing mcg and mg. *ISMP Medication Safety Alert* 12(18):1–2.

ISMP. 2008. ISMP's List of High-Alert Medications. Available at http://www.ismp.org/Tools/highalertmedications.pdf. Accessed September 15, 2015.

ISMP. 2009. A cautionary note for ambulatory e-Rx users! Community/Ambulatory Care Edition. *ISMP Medication Safety Alert* 8(8):1–2.

ISMP. 2011. E-prescribing issues. Community/Ambulatory Care Edition. *ISMP Medication Safety Alert* 10(3):1–2.

ISMP. 2011a. Principles of designing a medication label for oral solids for patient specific, inpatient use. Available at http://www.ismp.org/Tools/guidelines/labelFormats/. Accessed September 15, 2015.

ISMP. 2015. Open the bag to catch errors at the point-of-sale. ISMP Medication Safety Alert! *Community/Ambulatory Care* 14(7): 1–3.

ISMP. 2016. ISMP Guidelines for Safe Preparation of Compounded Sterile Preparations. Available at https://www.ismp.org/sites/default/files/attachments/2017-11/Guidelines%20for%20Safe%20Preparation%20of%20Compounded%20Sterile%20Preperations_%20revised%202016.pdf. Accessed February 18, 2019.

ISMP. 2018. ISMP's List of Error-Prone Abbreviations, Symbols, and Dose Designations. Available at http://www.ismp.org/Tools/errorproneabbreviations.pdf. Accessed April 15, 2019.

ISMP. 2019. Guidelines for the Safe Use of Automated Dispensing Cabinets. Available at https://www.ismp.org/resources/guidelines-safe-use-automated-dispensing-cabinets. Accessed April 22, 2019.

ISMP. 2019b. Medication Safety Self Assessment® for high-alert medications. Available at https://www.ismp.org/self-assessments. Accessed February 15, 2019.

ISMP. 2014. Safety Requires a State of Mindfulness. *ISMP Medication Safety Alert!* 19(15):1–3. Available at https://www.ismp.org/resources/safety-requires-state-mindfulness. Accessed February 13, 2019.

Kohn LT, Corrigan JM, Donaldson MS, (eds.). 1999. To Err Is Human: Building a Safer Health System, Institute of Medicine Report, November 29. Available at https://iom.nationalacademies.org/Reports/1999/To-Err-is-Human-Building-A-Safer-Health-System.aspx/. Accessed September 15, 2015.

Lesch MF. 2003. Comprehension and memory for warning symbols: Age-related differences and impact of training. *J Safety Res* 34:495–505.

Lombardi TP, Kennicutt JD. 2002. Promotion of a safe medication environment: Focus on the elderly and residents of long-term care facilities. Available at https://www.medscape.com/viewarticle/421217. Accessed April 15, 2019.

McDonnell PJ, Jacobs MR, McDonnell PJ. 2002. Hospital admissions resulting from preventable adverse drug reactions. *Pharmacotherapy* 36:1331–1336.

National Council on Patient Information and Education. 2007. Enhancing Prescription Medicine Adherence: A National Action Plan 2007. Available at http://www.bemedwise.org/docs/enhancingprescriptionmedicine-adherence.pdf.html. Accessed February 14, 2019.

National Medication Errors Reporting Program (ISMP MERP). 2015. Institute for Safe Medication Practices. Available at www.ismp.org/merp. Accessed September 15, 2015.

Pennsylvania Patient Safety Authority. 2005. Abbreviations: A shortcut to medication errors. *PA-PSRS Patient Safety Advisory* 2(1):19–21.

Pharmacy Purchasing & Products. 2009. State of pharmacy compounding 2009: survey findings. *Pharmacy Purchasing & Products* 6(4):4–20.

Reason J. 1990. The contribution of latent human failures to the breakdown of complex systems. *Philos Trans R Soc Lond B Biol Sci* 327:475–484.

Schneider PJ, Pedersen CA, Scheckelhoff DJ. 2018. ASHP national survey of pharmacy practice in hospital settings: dispensing and administration. *Am J Health Syst Pharm* 75(16):1203–1226.

Southeast Michigan e-prescribing Initiative (SEMI). 2012. Southeastern Michigan ePrescribing Initiative Reports SE Michigan E-Prescribing Initiative Kicks Off Seventh Year, Enrollment Up 33%. Press release on 29 Mar 2012. Available at http://detroit.cbslocal.com/2012/03/29/se-michigan-e-prescribing-initiative-kicks-off-seventh-year-enrollment-up-33/. Accessed April 15, 2019.

SureScripts, LLC. 2017. National Progress Report. Available at https://surescripts.com/docs/default-source/national-progress-reports/2151_npr_2017_finalB.pdf. Accessed August 7, 2019.

Svarstad B. 2000. *FDA-Commissioned Research, University of Wisconsin–Madison.* Presented February 2000, Rockville, MD, and June 2000, Kuopio, FL.

Svarstad BL, Bultman DC, Mount JK. 2004. Patient counseling provided in community pharmacist: effects of state regulation, pharmacist age, and busyness. *J Am Pharm Assoc* 44(1):22–29.

The Joint Commission (TJC). 2015. Standard PC.02.01.03. In *Comprehensive Accreditation Manual for Hospitals.* Oakbrook Terrace, IL: Joint Commission Resources; 2015 Han.

Thomas EJ, Burstin HJR, O'Neil AC, Orav EJ, Brennan TA. 1996. Patient noncompliance with medical advice after the emergency department visit. *Ann Emerg Med* 27(1):49–55.

Waisman Y, Siegal N, Chemo M. 2003. Do parents understand emergency department discharge instructions? A survey analysis. *Isr Med Assoc J* 5:567–570.

Watt D, Wentzler W, Brannan G. 2005. Patient expectations of emergency department care: phase I – a focus group study. *Can J Emerg Med* 7:12–16.

Wolf MS, Davis TC, Tilson HH, Bass PF 3rd, Parker RM. 2006. Misunderstanding of prescription drug warning labels among patients with low literacy. *Am J Health Syst Pharm* 63:1048–1055.

Zavala S, Shaffer C. 2011. Do patients understand discharge instructions? *J Emerg Nurs* 37(2):138–140.

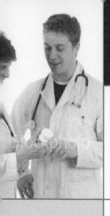

13

COMPLIANCE WITH REGULATIONS AND REGULATORY BODIES

Jennifer L. Adams

About the Author: Dr. Jennifer Adams is a graduate of Boise State University, Idaho State University, and George Washington University. She serves as the Associate Dean for Academic Affairs at the Idaho State University College of Pharmacy providing oversight for the PharmD curriculum, experiential education, interprofessional education, and assessment. Dr. Adams teaches pharmacy law to third-year student pharmacists, oversees the professional development course series, and co-curricular activities for the college. Her previous experience includes working in hospital and community pharmacy settings and in association management at the American Pharmacists Association (APhA) and the American Association of Colleges of Pharmacy (AACP). She has received national awards in recognition of her leadership skills.

■ LEARNING OBJECTIVES

After completing this chapter, readers should be able to

1. Describe the reasons for the evolution of pharmacy and drug regulation that have created the current legal environment for pharmacy practice organizations.
2. Summarize and explain the basic provisions of major pharmacy practice and drug laws discussed in this chapter.
3. Describe the manager's role in monitoring a pharmacy's compliance with applicable laws and professional standards.
4. Explain the role of the manager in developing and maintaining appropriate policies that help prevent violations of the law in order to manage organizational risk.
5. Analyze practice-based situations where laws and/or professional standards may have been violated; in these analyses, the reader will consider the implications (statutory, regulatory, and civil) of a manager's actions in resolving problems that these situations present and then propose appropriate courses of action for the manager.

■ SCENARIO

Few examples of how much trust is put in the hands of a pharmacist and the extent to which that trust can be betrayed come close to the story of Robert Courtney, a former pharmacist from Kansas City. During the 9 years leading up to his arrest in August 2001, Courtney secretly diluted the chemotherapy drugs of over 4200 cancer patients to increase the profits of his home infusion pharmacy business. Courtney broke the law while betraying the trust of his patients and damaging the reputation of his profession.

Patients place their trust in pharmacists to do and know things that they themselves do not understand. State and federal laws provide additional layers of protection to shield the public from dangerous and/or contaminated drugs and from dangerous and/or dishonest professionals. But as with any protective system, it can be breached. Consider how Courtney accomplished his deception.

Courtney began by diluting chemotherapy drugs for patients who were near death. He started out by diluting the drugs only a bit, thinking no one would notice. Later, he became more bold and diluted medications to the point that only a trace of the prescribed dose remained. He started out cheating "just a little" and then slid down a slippery slope until he was convicted of his crimes and sentenced to 30 years in prison. As stated in a newspaper feature about his case:

> "The path to hell leads one step at a time," says Mike Ketchmark, the brash but persistent attorney who successfully litigated a $2.2 billion civil judgment against Courtney. "I think he started from the gray market and realized you could make a whole bunch of money. Then he'd get orders in from people who were on their deathbed, and he'd slice a little bit. Then he realizes he can just continue to cut it, and no one's going to notice. It's a felony once you engage in the gray market; you're then breaking down the barrier of a person's inhibition. You don't go from being John-Boy to Charles Manson overnight" (Draper, 2003).

Although the Courtney case is an extreme example of just how far someone can go in betraying their professional duties and in breaking the law, it is important to understand that Courtney's transgressions started out small and were almost undetectable. Then his moral compass drifted further, and greed became his guide. His patients no longer mattered to him. Their trust in him was betrayed. Laws were broken. Courtney's crimes provide a hideous but poignant example of just how vulnerable patients are and exactly why there are pharmacy and drug laws in the United States to protect them.

■ CHAPTER QUESTIONS

1. Do you think that statutes and regulations are necessary to protect the public from dangerous drugs and/or incompetent pharmacists? Why or why not?
2. What areas of pharmacy regulation do you find excessive and overly restrictive? Justify your contention based on evidence and/or personal experience.
3. What areas of pharmacy practice and pharmacy operations can you identify that you think need to be regulated more closely? Justify your contention based on evidence and/or personal experience.
4. How have standards and legal requirements for pharmacists evolved to the point where we see them today?
5. What is the significance of the current state of pharmacy and drug regulation for pharmacy managers?

■ INTRODUCTION

The purpose of this chapter is not to present a study guide for pharmacy law, an area to which entire texts have been devoted (Abood, 2012). Instead, its purpose is to provide an orientation to the professional and operational implications of food and drug law, pharmacy law, and professional regulation for pharmacy managers. This orientation should encourage pharmacy managers to think seriously about how the legal and regulatory environment that is external to a pharmacy practice organization can exert substantial influences on both the organization and its members. This encouragement includes a strong recommendation to know, understand, and follow applicable laws and professional standards in the operation of a pharmacy.

■ STANDARDS FOR PHARMACISTS' PROFESSIONAL PERFORMANCE AND THEIR IMPORTANCE TO A MANAGER

Webster's Dictionary defines a *standard* as "something established by authority, custom, or general consent as a model or example" and states that *standard* "applies to any definite rule, principle, or measure established by authority (standards of behavior)" (Webster's Online Dictionary, 2019). From a contemporary managerial perspective, standards of conduct for a pharmacist and for the operation of a pharmacy are derived both from laws and from professional standards or values. Standards for professional conduct and the operation of a pharmacy, whether stated formally in statutes and regulations or presented in professional codes of ethics, are important for managers to understand and apply. Violations of these standards can affect the licensure status of a pharmacy practice site and/or its pharmacists, may result in litigation if a patient is harmed subsequent to a violation, and in the most serious cases can result in criminal prosecution. Both criminal prosecution and civil liability resulted in the case of Robert Courtney, the pharmacist discussed in the scenario. Courtney was sentenced to 30 years in prison, fined $25,000, and ordered to pay $10.4 million in restitution to the patients and families affected. These penalties were in addition to the civil judgment of $2.2 billion (Stafford, 2002).

What are Standards and What are Their Origins?

Before there were laws in the United States for regulating the behavior of professionals, there were standards and codes of ethics established by professional guilds and associations. These codes of ethics stated in a formal way the type and level of professional performance that a guild or association expected from its members. These expectations were derived from the kinds of expert services that society needed from members of that profession. The professional standards in codes of ethics helped to align the highest standards of a profession with society's expectations. Knowing that professionals worthy of their title and status should adhere to their profession's standards, society came to expect no less. Yet, there was and continues to be an inherent tension between the desire of professions to self-regulate and the often justified cynicism of members of the public who fear that self-regulation can lead to lax oversight and endanger the public. The result is that we see not only professional standards and codes of ethics that emanate from professional associations (e.g., the APhA Code of Ethics and Oath of a Pharmacist) but also federal and state statutes and regulations designed to protect the public from dangerous products and practitioners.

Bledstein (1976) discussed the evolution of the relationship between professionals and those whom they serve and noted that in mid-Victorian America, there seemed to be a prevailing sense of insecurity among some members of the population. Professionals in places such as the courtroom, classroom, and hospital were regarded as experts and trusted by public citizens. People who were seeking to expand their cultural horizons looked to professionals even for such things as recommendations concerning what should be considered appropriate reading material (Bledstein, 1976). The trust in the professional came at a time in the history of American culture long before the existence of the commercial aspects of professional–client relationships sometimes seen today (May, 1988).

Why Laws Governing Drugs and Professional Conduct Became Necessary

Despite such lofty expressions of the duties owed to society by those who served them, maximization of profits (rather than adherence to the highest standards) sometimes was the goal of those selling "medicinal" products. Philip J. Hilts (2003) describes the evolution of drug regulation in the United States beginning in the late 19th century through the end of the 20th century. During the late 19th century and well into the middle 20th century, laws governing the content and quality of medicinal products provided, by today's standards, little or no protection to an unknowledgeable and unsuspecting public. Members of a relatively uninformed society were left to their own devices in making decisions for the purchase and use of medications. Subsequently, it took the occurrence of sentinel events, such as the Elixir Sulfanilamide tragedy of 1937 and the thalidomide disaster of 1962, to raise consumer ire and prompt government action aimed at protecting the public from dangerous drug products.

The evolution of the pharmacy profession in the United States from colonial times to the present is rather astounding. During this time, pharmacy made the transition from an unlicensed occupation that in many ways resembled a trade to its current status requiring a professional doctorate (PharmD) degree to become eligible for licensure. At first, scant formal education and long periods of apprenticeship were required to attain full status as a pharmacist. During this period, the American Pharmaceutical Association (now the APhA) was established in 1852. Contemporaneously, the more classic definitions of professions and professionals applied. Professionals were expected to be ethical and honest in their dealings with the public, and the pharmacy profession was largely self-regulating, with sanctions from within its ranks as the only punishment for violation of the profession's standards.

■ HISTORICAL OVERVIEW OF LEGAL DEVELOPMENTS IN THE REGULATION OF DRUGS, PHARMACIES, AND PHARMACISTS

This section examines some of the more pivotal pieces of legislation enacted during the last century and discusses how they have evolved to provide pharmacy with the current legal and regulatory environment for the regulation of drugs, pharmacists, and pharmacies.

Regulation of Food and Drug Safety: Standards for Foods and Drugs Sold at Retail

The authority to regulate foods and drugs sold in interstate commerce is given to the federal government by the commerce clause of the US Constitution (US Constitution, Article I, Sec. 8, Clause 3). Until the beginning of the 20th century, the only federal law regulating drugs in the United States was the Drug Importation Act of 1848, which empowered the US Customs Service to prevent the importation of adulterated (i.e., contaminated) drugs from other countries (FDA, 2018). Beginning in the early 20th century, a series of highly publicized dramatic events provided the impetus for changes and improvements in the regulation of food, drug, and cosmetic safety.

Pure Food and Drug Act of 1906

The Pure Food and Drug Act of 1906 (59th Congress, Session I, Chap. 3915, pp. 768–772) was prompted by increased interest in the popular press concerning food safety that culminated in the publication of Upton Sinclair's exposé, *The Jungle,* a book that highlighted filthy and unsanitary conditions in meat packing plants. As stated in the 1906 act, the purpose of the new law was "for preventing the manufacture, sale, or transportation of adulterated or misbranded or poisonous or deleterious foods, drugs, medicines, and liquors, and for regulating traffic therein." In essence, this law required that foods and drugs be hygienic and accurately labeled. Before this law was enacted, there was a lack of standards and "traveling medicine shows," "patent medicines," and other unregulated products and activities were rampant. Products such as Lydia Pinkham's Vegetable Compound were nothing more than alcohol, whereas "soothing syrups" marketed as remedies for teething babies contained undisclosed and varying amounts of opium (Hilts, 2003).

The Food, Drug, and Cosmetic Act of 1938 and Amendments

Passage of the Food, Drug, and Cosmetic Act of 1938 was preceded by the Elixir Sulfanilamide tragedy of 1937. The 1906 act required drugs to be pure and labeled accurately but contained no requirement that drugs be safe. As one of the first effective oral anti-microbial drugs, sulfanilamide was very popular with physicians and was used widely to treat streptococcal infections. Bitter in taste, it was not easy to administer to children. Therefore, with some difficulty, the manufacturer developed a liquid dosage form called *elixir sulfanilamide*. Sulfanilamide powder is not soluble in either water or alcohol. Chemists at the manufacturer settled on ethylene glycol—the same chemical used today as an automobile antifreeze/coolant. This sweet-tasting chemical is highly toxic, causing painful kidney failure and death within a few days of ingestion.

In 1937, no safety testing was required prior to marketing a drug product, and no premarketing safety tests were performed on elixir sulfanilamide. Two hundred and forty gallons were shipped to physicians and pharmacies all over the country, and 107 children died after using the product. Despite the extreme danger that this product represented to the public, the only legal basis the Food and Drug Administration (FDA) had for removing it from the market was that the product label stated "elixir," whereas technically it was not an elixir because it contained no alcohol and therefore was misbranded. The danger of allowing drug products to enter the market without safety testing became obvious, and the public demanded that something be done. The result was the requirement for premarketing safety testing in the Food, Drug, and Cosmetic Act of 1938.

The 1938 act was strengthened subsequently by amendments. The 1951, Durham–Humphrey Amendments created separate categories for prescription-only and over-the-counter (OTC) drugs. Prior to passage of these amendments, there was no legal prohibition against selling drugs without a prescription. These 1951 amendments transformed pharmacy in ways likely unintended by their sponsors (Representative Carl Durham and Senator Hubert Humphrey were both pharmacists). There was a synergy between these amendments and the increased availability of finished-dosage forms in the post-World War II pharmaceutical industry boom that transformed the professional activities of neighborhood pharmacists. This transition from compounding and selling drugs at retail to "lick, stick, count, and pour" occurred simultaneously with the creation of the prescription-only market niche—a niche that only pharmacists were allowed to fill.

Next, the early 1960s saw another tragedy related to an unsafe drug product. Thalidomide was a drug marketed in Europe as a tranquilizer and used extensively to treat morning sickness in pregnant women. Although the manufacturer was eager to market this product in the United States, the efforts of FDA pharmacologist and reviewer Dr. Frances Kelsey prevented thalidomide from reaching the US market. At the time, an FDA reviewer had 60 days either to approve or reject a new drug application (NDA) from a manufacturer. However, an FDA reviewer could request further information from the manufacturer and restart the 60-day clock—a tactic that Dr. Kelsey employed several times because she was satisfied with neither the quantity nor quality of the data she had received about thalidomide's safety.

Tragedy in the United States was averted by Dr. Kelsey's efforts. Her refusal to approve the thalidomide NDA without further proof of safety occurred just as news from Europe revealed that thalidomide was responsible for a birth defect that caused infants to be born with flipper-like limbs. This near miss in the United States led to passage of the 1962 Kefauver–Harris Amendments to the 1938 act. These amendments established requirements that testing for *both* safety and proof of drug efficacy had to be conducted in well-controlled clinical trials before an NDA could be approved and a drug allowed to reach the market (Bren, 2001).

Establishment of State Pharmacy Practice Acts and State Boards of Pharmacy

Prior to 1870, when Rhode Island became the first in the nation to enact a state pharmacy practice act, regulation of the pharmacy profession was accomplished sporadically—generally at the local level or through the regulation of the medical profession (Green, 1979). States subsequently enacted their own pharmacy practice acts over the next several decades. The establishment of state pharmacy practice acts and the state boards of pharmacy created by these acts represent a legally binding codification of society's expectations of professional performance and a delineation of legal consequences for violation of these standards. The regulation of professional behavior by the states is pursuant to the police powers granted to the individual states by the US Constitution. The establishment of state statutes and regulations governing the practice of pharmacy and operation of a pharmacy business not only provided a new layer of safety for the public but also created a real barrier to entry into the pharmacy profession. This was a significant step in increasing both the professionalism of pharmacy and the expectations that society had of pharmacists. Prior to establishment of such standards and legal requirements, practically anyone could operate a business and call it a pharmacy.

Currently, all states have some form of a pharmacy practice act (a state statute) and state board of pharmacy regulations. These laws establish legally binding standards for the conduct of pharmacists and ancillary personnel, as well as standards for the physical facilities licensed as pharmacies. In comparison to other health professions, pharmacy has the largest percentage of state rules and regulations, making pharmacy the most regulated health profession. These regulations place restrictions on the health services and the circumstances around those services a pharmacist is allowed to perform which can compromise professional pharmacy practice standards (Adams, 2018). Most health professions are regulated based on a "standard of care" that is set by the profession. The term "standard of care" as it relates to medical regulation generally refers to "that which a minimally competent physician in the same field would do under similar circumstances" (Moore, 2011). Pharmacy regulation, on the other hand, has many state laws that are so specific as to delineate the types of hinges a pharmacy must use on the door and the exact square footage required for the pharmacy space (Cacciatore, 1997). The highly regulated approach used in pharmacy sets a "standard of care" that is created by state boards of pharmacy and state legislatures, rather than the approach used by other health professions where the profession itself

sets the standard of care and the court systems defer to a standard set by expert testimony from within the profession to determine if a health professional has been negligent. This poses a problem for both the profession of pharmacy and the court systems in that pharmacists are held to a limited standard of care that is dictated by a state legislature rather than the profession itself. As of 2018, only one state, Idaho, has attempted to regulate their pharmacists based on a standard of care set by the profession of pharmacy (Idaho, 2018). It is important for pharmacy managers to understand this conundrum and to be aware of the applicable statutes and regulations in the state(s) where they oversee pharmacy practice.

These state statutes and regulations are not to be taken lightly. Violations can result in penalties ranging anywhere from reprimands and fines to the loss of licensure to practice the profession or maintain operation of a given pharmacy facility. Practicing pharmacy without a license is a violation of criminal law, so it is important for pharmacy managers to have a clear understanding of their responsibilities under these statutes and regulations and to communicate these responsibilities clearly to nonpharmacist management personnel involved in operation of the pharmacy. For example, consider the situation where a pharmacy is located within a larger store that is open when the pharmacy department is closed. If the nonpharmacist store manager decides to open the pharmacy to get someone's medication during hours when the store is open but the pharmacy department is closed (and, of course, there is no pharmacist on duty), this would violate the pharmacy practice act and board of pharmacy regulations in any state. A managing pharmacist has to make clear to nonpharmacist managers what they are not allowed to do under the law. Further, a pharmacist who allows such illegal practices also has committed a violation and may be subject to both sanctions from the board of pharmacy as well as criminal prosecution.

The Pharmacist-in-Charge Role of Pharmacy Manager

As of March 2019, 48 states and the District of Columbia require that each pharmacy has a Pharmacist-in-Charge (PIC). Maryland and Idaho are the two states that do not have a PIC designation. In general, the role of a PIC is to oversee all operations and activities in the pharmacy and must ensure proper policies, procedures, and adherence to state laws by all pharmacy staff. Often the pharmacy manager assumes the role of PIC in addition to their managerial duties. The assumption of this role is a great task for an individual to assume, as no one person can always be in a pharmacy during the hours of operation to oversee every task or action.

From a legal perspective, there is potential personal liability for the pharmacy manager PIC to be responsible for every action in the pharmacy whether or not they were involved in the actions. For example, if one of the staff pharmacists fails to renew their license on time, the PIC may be held responsible by a state board of pharmacy for not reminding the staff pharmacist and ensuring their license is current. For those who manage chain pharmacies, where some pharmacy operations are overseen at the corporate level, the PIC may be responsible for activities that happen at the corporate level. For example, if a state law requires that data for controlled substance dispensing be reported to a prescription drug monitoring program (PDMP) every 24 hours, and a glitch in the system causes this not to happen in the appropriate time frame, the PIC for every pharmacy in that chain affected in that state may be held personally responsible by the board of pharmacy in that state. Pharmacy managers should not take this responsibility lightly as it has potential for significant personal liability.

■ FEDERAL LAW AND THE CONDUCT OF PHARMACISTS

Omnibus Budget Reconciliation Act of 1990

Until the passage of the Omnibus Budget Reconciliation Act of 1990 (OBRA 1990; Public Law 101–508), federal law in the pharmacy arena had been concerned primarily with drug product safety, with the courts generally recognizing clerical accuracy, as it relates to patient safety, as the standard for the pharmacist's duty of care. OBRA 90, while not explicitly usurping the police powers of the states, required that to be eligible for federal matching dollars, states participating in the Medicaid program would have to establish standards for:

- *Maintaining proper patient records.* Pharmacies must make reasonable efforts to obtain, record, and maintain at least the following patient information: patient name, address, telephone number; age and gender; individual history (where significant), including disease state or states, known allergies and/or drug reactions, and a comprehensive list of medications and relevant devices; and the pharmacist's comments about the patient's drug therapy.
- *Prospective drug use review (pro-DUR).* Prior to dispensing a prescription, a pharmacist must conduct an evaluation of a patient's medication record to detect potential therapy problems, such as therapeutic duplication, drug–disease contraindications, drug–drug reactions (including serious interactions with OTC medications), incorrect drug dosage or duration of drug treatment, drug–allergy interactions, and evidence of clinical abuse/misuse.
- *Patient counseling.* A dispensing pharmacist must offer to counsel regarding matters that are, in the pharmacist's professional judgment, significant, which include but are not limited to name and description of the mediation, route of administration, dose, dosage form, and duration of therapy. In addition, such standards require pharmacists to discuss special precautions and directions, common severe side effects or interactions, therapeutic contraindications that may be encountered (including how to avoid them and what to do if they occur), proper storage, techniques for self-monitoring of drug therapy, what to do if a dose is missed, and refill information.

Not wanting to establish two separate legal standards of care—one for Medicaid patients and another for non-Medicaid patients—states generally adopted standards to meet the OBRA 90 criteria while extending the standards to benefit all pharmacy patients, not just Medicaid patients (Catizone et al., 1993). Implications for pharmacy management include how the manager decides to structure employee duties and the organization of work in the pharmacy. It is the managing pharmacist's duty to maintain compliance with applicable state and/or federal laws by ensuring that requirements for pro-DUR and patient counseling are followed. From a management perspective, this means organizing work in the pharmacy and staffing the pharmacy to facilitate performance of these legal duties. Individual states may have their own requirements that may be stricter—but not more lenient—than federal law.

Health Insurance Portability and Accountability Act of 1996

This statute and its rules establish, for the first time, federal standards for protecting the privacy and security of patients' protected health information (PHI). These standards include, but are not limited to, how patient PHI must be stored, under what conditions it may be released, and to whom. This law has sweeping implications for pharmacies and pharmacists alike. The Health Insurance Portability and Accountability Act (HIPAA) privacy rules are designed to strike a balance between maintaining the flow of patients' health information among persons and entities providing health care to patients while simultaneously maintaining privacy for individuals. Essentially, this combination of statute and implementing regulations increases privacy and security for private information by establishing a "need to know" basis for who may have access to someone's PHI and to what extent they may have that access. Further, it establishes requirements for security of storage and for transmission of PHI by anyone who has access to the information. The purpose of this chapter does not include an exhaustive summary and explanation of this landmark legislation; numerous resources have been devoted to the subject.[1] The rules implementing this federal statute became effective as of April 14, 2003. Suffice it to say that pharmacy managers are responsible for making

sure that their staff and policies and procedures are in compliance with HIPAA.

From a pharmacy manager's perspective, it is essential to understand that HIPAA establishes transaction standards, security standards, and privacy standards for PHI. Transaction standards and security standards are concerned primarily with how data are handled and transmitted. In the day-to-day operation of pharmacy, a manager needs to understand and comply with the requirements for privacy standards.

A pharmacy manager should know the answers to the following questions regarding these privacy standards:

1. *Who is covered by the privacy rule?* The privacy rule considers health plans, health care providers, and health care clearinghouses as covered entities (Centers for Medicare and Medicaid Services, 2019). This definition includes pharmacies.

2. *What information is protected?* According to the Department of Health and Human Services Office of Civil Rights, The Privacy Rule protects all *individually identifiable health information* held or transmitted by a covered entity or its business associate, in any form or media, whether electronic, paper, or oral. The Privacy Rule calls this information PHI. Further, the Privacy Rule states that *individually identifiable health information* is information, including demographic data, which relates to:
   • the individual's past, present, or future physical or mental health or condition,
   • the provision of health care to the individual, or
   • the past, present, or future payment for the provision of health care to the individual, and that identifies the individual or for which there is a reasonable basis to believe can be used to identify the individual. Individually identifiable health information includes many common identifiers (e.g., name, address, birth date, Social Security Number) (US Department of Health and Human Services (DHHS), 2003).

3. *What must the covered entity do to protect information?* Every covered entity must have an individual designated as the facility's "privacy officer"—a person who is charged with the responsibility

---

[1]See (1) *HIPAA Privacy Standards: A Compliance Manual for Pharmacists.* National Association of Chain Drug Stores, Inc., and Mintz, Levin, Cohn, Ferris, Glovsky, and Popeo, P.C. 2003; and (2) Fitzgerald WJ. 2003. *The NCPA HIPAA Compliance Handbook for Community Pharmacy.* Alexandria, VA: National Community Pharmacists Association.

of keeping the site in compliance with HIPAA. Essentially, a covered entity may not release or disclose PHI except as allowed under the privacy rule. The following subsections summarize briefly what a pharmacy manager (a person who also may be the privacy officer) must be aware of.

Employee Training

Employees of a pharmacy should be trained in HIPAA rules and procedures as a condition of employment. Newly hired personnel should receive training before being allowed to work with PHI. This training should be documented as having been completed and repeated, if necessary, for employees who do not perform up to the standard. At a minimum, the training should include making clear to employees: (1) how, to whom, to what extent, and under what circumstances PHI may be released and (2) that PHI should not be included in casual conversations with others—even in conversations with other health care providers if they are not involved in the patient's care. Also, employee access to PHI should be restricted to what is necessary in the performance of their duties.

Notice of Privacy Practices

Under the HIPAA privacy rule, all covered entities are required to provide patients with a "notice of privacy practices." The covered entity must provide this notice to all patients, and it should be written in understandable language. The privacy officer, most likely the pharmacy manager, is responsible for documenting patient signatures acknowledging receipt of the notice and documenting the reasons for any patient refusals of the notice or any patient refusal to sign in acknowledgment of having received the notice. The covered entity must maintain records of these documents for 6 years. Again, the importance of maintaining well-organized and easily retrievable records cannot be overemphasized.

Business Associates

The HIPAA privacy rule definition of a business associate and requirements regarding business associates are as follows:

"*Business Associate Defined.* In general, a business associate is a person or organization, other than a member of a covered entity's workforce, that performs certain functions or activities on behalf of, or provides certain services to, a covered entity that involve the use or disclosure of individually identifiable health information. Business associate functions or activities on behalf of a covered entity include claims processing, data analysis, utilization review, and billing. Business associate services to a covered entity are limited to legal, actuarial, accounting, consulting, data aggregation, management, administrative, accreditation, or financial services. However, persons or organizations are not considered business associates if their functions or services do not involve the use or disclosure of PHI, and where any access to PHI by such persons would be incidental, if at all. A covered entity can be the business associate of another covered entity. (DHHS, 2003)."

"*Business Associate Contract.* When a covered entity uses a contractor or other nonworkforce member to perform "business associate" services or activities, the Rule requires that the covered entity includes certain protections for the information in a business associate agreement (in certain circumstances, governmental entities may use alternative means to achieve the same protections). In the business associate contract, a covered entity must impose specified written safeguards on the individually identifiable health information used or disclosed by its business associates. Moreover, a covered entity may not contractually authorize its business associate to make any use or disclosure of PHI that would violate the Rule. (DHHS, 2003)."

In general, a pharmacy manager and/or privacy officer (in consultation with legal counsel) should tailor the pharmacy's relationships with business associates via the business associate contract. The overarching goals in an appropriately constructed business associate contract are to minimize the business associate's exposure to PHI while clearly establishing what uses of the PHI are permitted by the business associate. The privacy officer should have a clear idea of what business associates plan to do with any PHI they obtain and should make sure that any subcontractors have similar agreements. The privacy officer should monitor the business associate for any violations of the contract. In fact, the contract should stipulate that it is the responsibility of the business associate to report unauthorized disclosures of PHI. Finally, the privacy officer is responsible for the disposition of any PHI released to the business associate and should make sure that after it has been used by the business associate, PHI is either returned, held securely, or destroyed.

Patient Authorization Required for Release of PHI

A pharmacy, as a covered entity, needs to obtain a patient's written authorization for any disclosure or use of PHI that is not for treatment, payment, or health care operations. This authorization cannot be used as a precondition for benefits eligibility, payment, or treatment. The authorization document must be written in plain and specific language, and it may allow use and disclosure of PHI by the covered entity. An example of a disclosure of PHI that would require a written authorization by a patient is disclosure of such information to a drug manufacturer for marketing purposes. All authorizations must specify what information may be disclosed and must identify the person(s) disclosing and receiving the information, must specify an expiration date for the authorization document, and must state that a patient has the right to revoke the authorization in writing. Patient authorization for the release of PHI is not required for circumstances where a pharmacist reports spousal abuse or child neglect, becomes involved in legitimate law enforcement situations (including compliance with workers' compensation laws), is avoiding a threat to health or safety, or is reporting an adverse drug reaction to the FDA Medwatch program.

Circumstances Where PHI may Be Released Without Explicit Patient Authorization

PHI may be released without explicit patient authorization under certain circumstances defined in the law and rules. These circumstances (with examples) include treatment (e.g., when a pharmacist discusses a patient's condition with the patient's physician), payment (e.g., when a claim for payment is submitted to a third-party payer), regular health care operations (e.g., the transfer of PHI among departments within a hospital), and when the information has been "deidentified."

PHI is considered to be "deidentified" when the following data elements have been removed:

- Patient's name, social security number, and telephone and/or fax numbers
- Patient's town, street address, and/or ZIP code (state of residence need not be removed)
- Any dates of service (except year)
- Medical record number, health plan number, account number, and/or prescription number
- Any vehicle identifiers (e.g., license plate number), medical device identifiers and/or serial numbers, patient's website URL, computer IP address, and/or email address
- Biometric identifiers (e.g., DNA, fingerprints, voice recording, body description, retinal scan, etc.), photographic images (identifiable)
- Any other unique characteristic or code

Remember, though, that "deidentification" of information is not necessary between covered entities involved in a patient's care. "Deidentification" is also not necessary between a covered entity and a business associate with which the covered entity has a business associate contract.

The HIPAA statute and rules have created considerable confusion for pharmacy managers who have wondered about how these changes may affect normal operations in their pharmacies. Questions arise regarding situations such as when a neighbor is picking up a prescription for a patient. (*Note:* HIPAA rules allow the pharmacist to release a prescription to a patient's neighbor and counsel that neighbor as the patient's *agent*.) In response to these sorts of questions, the U.S. Department of Health and Human Services (DHHS) website has a search function that finds answers to many common questions about a wide variety of health care practice situations (U.S. DHHS, 2017).

An Amendment to the Social Security Act Enacted as Part of HIPAA

When HIPAA was passed, a small but significant amendment to the Social Security Act [Section 1128A(a)(5)] was included. This amendment prohibits offering inducements (i.e., remuneration) for Medicare or Medicaid recipients to utilize the services of any particular provider. This provision is enforced by the Office of Inspector General (OIG) within the U.S. DHHS. The OIG interpretation of the amendment permits "Medicare or Medicaid providers to offer beneficiaries inexpensive gifts (other than cash or cash equivalents) or services without violating the statute. For enforcement purposes, inexpensive gifts or services are those that have a retail value of no more than $10 individually, or no more than $50 in the aggregate annually per patient" (U.S. DHHS, 2002).

When a pharmacist manager works in a setting with a nonpharmacist manager (e.g., a large community pharmacy or a pharmacy department in a discount or grocery store), the nonpharmacist may not be aware of this prohibition, and may want to include Medicare and Medicaid recipients in coupon offerings or discounts in the store, but outside of the pharmacy department, to keep the recipients' business. This situation provides a difficult, but absolutely necessary opportunity for the pharmacist to educate the nonpharmacist manager regarding compliance with federal law. Failure to comply with this provision can result in serious legal and financial consequences—"… a person who offers or transfers to a Medicare or Medicaid beneficiary any remuneration that the person knows or should know is likely to influence the beneficiary's selection of a particular provider, practitioner, or supplier of Medicare or Medicaid payable items or services may be liable for civil money penalties (CMPs) of up to $10,000 for each wrongful act" (U.S. DHHS, 2002). So, as difficult and cumbersome as it may seem, a pharmacy engaged in offering small "gifts" to Medicare and Medicaid beneficiaries must limit individual gifts to a monetary value of $10 or less and must limit the annual total to $50 for each beneficiary. Actions that would likely be in violation of this statute include providing in-store gift cards or coupons that can be spent in the store just like cash as incentives to utilize a given pharmacy's services. For example, it is not difficult to imagine that someone who receives a $15 store coupon every time they get a Medicare/Medicaid prescription filled might be more likely to find ways to increase their prescription drug utilization.

Prescription Drug Marketing Act

Pharmacy managers must also comply with federal laws regulating other economic issues in pharmacy. The Prescription Drug Marketing Act of 1987 (PDMA) represents one area where some pharmacists have encountered considerable legal problems, resulting in large fines and/or prison sentences (Associated Press, 2000; Eiserer, 1999). In brief, the PDMA prohibits the diversion of prescription drug samples into the retail market sector. Pharmacies may not have in their stock any prescription drug samples, and pharmacies may not possess or sell any prescription drug samples. Further, the PDMA restricts the annual distribution of prescription drugs by pharmacies to other pharmacies to no more than 5% of the annual dollar value of prescription drug sales for the distributing pharmacy (e.g., one pharmacy providing prescription drugs to another pharmacy that has run out of stock of an item). Pharmacy managers must ensure compliance with the PDMA or be prepared to face stiff penalties. In a Nebraska case, a pharmacist violated the PDMA by colluding with a pharmaceutical manufacturer's sales representative to divert and profit from the sale of drug samples. In 1999, the pharmacist pled guilty to illegally selling prescription drug samples over a 15-year period (Eiserer, 1999). In 2000, the pharmacist was sentenced to 18 months in prison and ordered to pay nearly $147,000 in fines and restitution (Associated Press, 2000).

State Prescription Drug Monitoring Programs

Prescription opioid abuse has become a national issue in the United States, with the DHHS declaring a public health emergency in 2017 (U.S. DHHS, 2019). According to the National Institute on Drug Abuse, in 2017, more than 70,200 Americans died from drug overdoses, more than double the deaths just 10 years prior (National Institute on Drug Abuse, 2019). To curb the epidemic, all states require a PDMP. The state of Missouri has not yet passed regulations detailing the use of their program, but all other states have implemented a PDMP. These PDMPs collect information on controlled substances and "drugs of concern" dispensed within the state and maintain an electronic database of the information. The agencies that administer and house these programs vary from state to state as do "drugs of concern." The National Council for Prescription Drug Programs tracks the variation across states and provides information about the frequency and format of information reporting, as well as other "drugs of concern" reported that are not controlled substances in all states. Two common drugs tracked by states are gabapentin, a GABA analog with potential for misuse and naloxone, an opioid antagonist (National Council for Prescription Drug Programs, 2019).

Information collected by PDMPs is then distributed to individuals authorized by state law to receive such information for their professional purposes. Individuals authorized to access PDMP data vary from state to state, but usually include prescribers and pharmacists. For example, in a state with a PDMP where both prescribers and pharmacists are allowed to access PDMP data, each is able to check if their patient is obtaining prescriptions for controlled substances from other prescribers and/or other pharmacies. This sharing of information can help to deter abuse and diversion of controlled substances while identifying patients who may need to be directed to drug abuse treatment programs. Also, in cases of criminal prosecution for drug diversion via falsified prescription documents, data from prescription monitoring programs would be discoverable and could be used as evidence by prosecutors. The effectiveness of PDMPs has been studied in many different ways and have found decreases in opioid prescriptions, overdose deaths, and total morphine milligram equivalents (a value assigned to indicate relative potency of an opioid) since the implementation of PDMPs (Ponnapalli, 2018). However, PDMPs are only effective if they are used by prescribers and pharmacies (Ponnapalli, 2018).

A PDMP is a useful tool for pharmacy staff to use to maintain compliance with federal- and state-controlled substance statutes and regulations. Pharmacy managers should ensure that pharmacists practicing at their site take advantage of this resource. Failure to do so could result in board of pharmacy actions against the license of a pharmacist who did not use the PDMP tool to ascertain whether or not prescriptions for controlled substances and "drugs of concern" were valid prior to dispensing.

Civil Law and Liability Concerns

When a pharmacist or pharmacy organization is sued, the issue of negligence becomes the key to what the outcome of the lawsuit will be. Negligence theory revolves around either the failure to do something that a reasonable and prudent person *would* do or doing something that a reasonable and prudent person *would not* do. In this case, the person is the pharmacist. The pharmacist's role has changed over time because of the evolving nature of pharmacy practice (e.g., OBRA 90 ushered in the requirement to offer patient counseling). Case law also changes pharmacy practice standards. Case law is based on precedents established by the outcomes of civil cases. For example, if the result of a lawsuit establishes that a pharmacist had a duty to warn a patient about certain dangers of a drug that was dispensed, then a new standard of behavior for pharmacists is established through case law, not by statute or regulation.

The thought of being sued for something one has done while practicing, or the thought of a pharmacy manager being sued for the actions of his or her staff, is not at all pleasant. The first thing someone might think of is, "How can I prevent that from happening to me?" This question opens the door to a field of management called *risk management* that deals with how to reduce and manage exposure to risk (see Chapter 11). Sound practice site design, consistent adherence to applicable law, and a well-organized workflow system designed to detect errors before they reach the patient are all essential to minimizing exposure to risk. As with all laws governing the activities of pharmacists, managers are encouraged to become familiar with these important provisions.

HOW DO LEGAL STANDARDS AFFECT WHAT AN ORGANIZATION SHOULD AND/OR NEEDS TO DO?

It is important for managers to understand that statutory and regulatory standards create an environmental context for an organization, a factor critical in determining whether or not the organization prospers and grows. The manager is a person embedded within an organization that is, in turn, embedded within the environment—an environment that is constantly changing. For pharmacists and pharmacies, statutes and regulations represent society's codification of standards beyond its normative expectations—beyond the sanctions implicit in not meeting the expectations of professional peers. Statutes and regulations also provide for enforcement by way of penalties if they are violated. Regulations are standards that are derived from statutes and have legal enforcement mechanisms (i.e., potential penalties) attached to them. For example, a state's pharmacy practice act creates a board of pharmacy and empowers that board to establish rules and/or regulations to interpret and implement the practice act. Board of pharmacy regulations carry the full force of the law and establish penalties anywhere from warnings, fines, and on to suspension and/or revocation of pharmacist's or pharmacy's licensure.

Performance Improvement versus Meeting Minimum Performance Standards

To avoid legal sanctions for practitioners and/or the pharmacy, the manager can take steps to prevent or avoid substandard practices that could lead to penalties. How should a manager approach such a task? One way some organizations approach making sure they meet minimum legal standards is by developing programs to foster performance improvement. Meeting minimum performance standards is

compliance with the bare minimum legal requirement, whereas performance improvement goes beyond this and can provide additional protection in the risk prevention and risk management arenas. If a pharmacy and its pharmacists aim to establish standards for the performance of the organization that exceed the legal minimum, it is much less likely that performance quality will result in violations of the law or in performance so poor that it results in a civil lawsuit. For example, a pharmacist manager may decide to establish a policy that every patient visiting the pharmacy will receive a personal offer of counseling from a licensed pharmacist, even where state law may allow pharmacy interns or other pharmacy staff to perform this function. Further, if a lawsuit is filed against the pharmacy, it can work in a pharmacy's favor if the pharmacy has in place standards of care and policies and procedures that exceed the legal minimum and afford better protection for patients. Also, with such systems in place, it is much less likely that a pharmacy will encounter legal difficulties of either kind. Establishment of a patient-centered practice environment and philosophy while knowing and obeying all applicable laws is essential to avoiding legal problems in either the civil or criminal realm.

Quality measurement of pharmacy professional services by groups such as the Pharmacy Quality Alliance (PQA, see http://www.pqaalliance.org/) develops measures beyond minimal legal requirements for medication safety, appropriateness, and adherence that pharmacies can use to evaluate themselves. Other groups (including third-party payers) are currently developing standards to evaluate the quality of a pharmacy practice site and professional services—standards that will be used to determine eligibility to participate in provider networks and levels of payment for pharmacist services (see Chapter 10).

FUTURE CONSIDERATIONS

While it may be difficult to predict the future, early trends in the pharmacy practice and legal landscape may allow pharmacy managers to consider what may impact their future pharmacy practice and the business of pharmacy.

Pharmacists' Patient Care Process

A growing body of evidence demonstrates that when pharmacists are fully deployed as part of the health care team, patient outcomes improve and total health care costs are reduced (Giberson, 2011). In 2014, national pharmacy associations presented the Pharmacists' Patient Care Process (PPCP), a consensus-based document to establish a consistent, stepwise approach for the array of pharmacist-delivered services available in any pharmacy practice setting (Joint Commission of Pharmacy Practitioners [JCPP], 2014). The process consists of five steps: (1) collect; (2) assess; (3) plan; (4) implement; and (5) follow-up. The entire process is based on patient-centered care, close collaboration with the patient's broader health care team, and robust documentation of services provided (JCPP, 2014).

The PPCP has been embraced within the profession, Doctor of Pharmacy curricula, and is gaining traction from public health agencies (Accreditation Council for Pharmacy Education, 2016; Bonner, 2015; Centers for Disease Control and Prevention, 2016). State "scope of practice" laws and regulations establish what pharmacists are legally authorized to perform in practice and as pharmacists integrate the PPCP into practice, there may be legal barriers that impede patient care and prevent pharmacists from fully performing steps in the process. This may drive change in pharmacist scope of practice laws and regulations to allow pharmacists to practice at the top of their education and training, rather than limiting them by the scope of practice allowed by their pharmacist license.

Pharmacists as Prescribers

Currently, nearly all states allow pharmacist prescribing in some fashion. The authority to prescribe exists along a continuum where the authority is either dependent (delegated through a collaborative practice agreement) or independent (authority comes directly from the state, no delegation required) authority (Adams, 2016). Collaborative prescribing is most restrictive when a patient-specific collaborative practice agreement is required and least restrictive when a population-specific collaborative practice agreement is allowed. Independent prescribing is most restrictive when authorized via a state-wide protocol and least restrictive when allowed independently with few (category specific) to no restrictions (Adams, 2016).

Most states allow for more than one type of prescribing, some collaborative, and some independent prescribing; however, the majority of independent prescribing is medication, or medication category specific and generally addresses a public health issue (e.g., naloxone or opioid antagonists, epinephrine auto-injectors, hormonal contraceptives). The state that has the most pharmacy-friendly laws related to pharmacist prescribing, Idaho, allows pharmacists to independently prescribe for any condition that: (1) does not require a new diagnosis; (2) is minor and generally self-limiting; (3) has a test that is used to guide diagnosis or clinical decision-making and are waived under the federal clinical laboratory improvement amendments of 1988; or (4) in the professional judgment of the pharmacist, threaten the health or safety of the patient should the prescription not be immediately dispensed. In this context, pharmacists in Idaho are prohibited from independently prescribing controlled substances, compounded drugs, or biological products. If all states reached this level of pharmacist autonomy in prescribing, pharmacy practice and the business of pharmacy, particularly in the community and ambulatory settings, will look different than it does today.

■ CONCLUSION

This chapter concludes with the following case examples for discussion of laws pertinent to the operation of a pharmacy. These cases are presented as starting points for discussion and analysis of practice-based situations a pharmacy manager is likely to encounter. Pharmacy and drug law, as well as civil law, all present managers with criteria on which to fashion their own management style in operating a pharmacy. Law, while quite explicit in its language, can often be silent on some issues and thus open to interpretation and the exercise of professional judgment. Student pharmacists reading this chapter are encouraged to work together in analyzing the situations presented here and to come up with their own plausible solutions to the problems presented.

■ QUESTIONS FOR FURTHER DISCUSSION

Case Examples for Discussion of Laws Pertinent to Operating a Pharmacy

Case 29.1: Why Won't the Pharmacist Just Refill My Prescription?

A FEDERAL DRUG LAW: THE CONTROLLED SUBSTANCES ACT OF 1970 Maureen Smith, RPh, the Pharmacist Manager of ABC Drugs Community Pharmacy, encounters the following situation within 10 minutes of arriving at the pharmacy on a Tuesday morning. She finds herself dealing with a complaint from a patient, Mr. Jones, about one of the staff pharmacists. Yesterday evening, Monday, at about 8:30 PM, Mr. Jones came to the pharmacy and presented an empty prescription vial to the pharmacist on duty and asked for a refill of his acetaminophen with codeine no. 3 tablets. Acetaminophen no. 3 is a schedule III controlled substance, and the federal Controlled Substances Act limits prescriptions for such medications to a maximum of five refills within 6 months of the time they are issued. Mr. Jones had not seen the prescribing physician in about 7 months and was now experiencing pain unrelated to the reason for his visit 7 months ago. However, the label on his vial stated that he had three refills remaining, and he wanted one right away.

Sally Howard, PharmD, the pharmacist who was on duty Monday evening, explained to Mr. Jones that she would need further authorization from Mr. Jones' prescriber because the prescription had been written over 6 months ago and was now no longer valid for refilling. Sally tried to reach Mr. Jones's doctor to

obtain authorization but was unsuccessful in reaching the prescriber before the pharmacy closed at 9:00 PM. Therefore, she informed Mr. Jones that the pharmacy would not be able to refill the prescription until it could reach the prescriber. Mr. Jones became angry when he heard this and remains very angry as he tells Maureen about the situation.

DISCUSSION QUESTIONS

1. What are the essential legal issues involved?
2. How should the pharmacy manager handle this situation?
3. How might another manager deal with the problem presented by this difficult patient?

Case 29.2: The Grandmother Who Did Not Need an Easy-Open Prescription Vial

A FEDERAL CONSUMER PROTECTION LAW: THE POISON PREVENTION PACKAGING ACT The (federal) Poison Prevention Packaging Act requires that prescription medications (with very few exceptions, such as sublingual nitroglycerin tablets) be dispensed in child-resistant containers. Mrs. Mabel Brown, a 79-year-old great grandmother to 2-year-old Barbara Brown, is a longstanding patient at the community pharmacy where you are the manager. You have just been informed by Mrs. Brown's great granddaughter's pediatrician that little Barbara was treated at the local hospital emergency room yesterday evening. It seems that while Barbara and her parents were visiting Mabel at her house, Barbara climbed up on the kitchen counter and grabbed Mabel's prescription vial containing propranolol 80-mg long-acting capsules. Little Barbara had only been out of her mother's sight for about 2 minutes when her mother walked into the kitchen and found Barbara sitting on the kitchen counter munching away on Mabel's medicine. Although she became a bit lethargic, luckily she did not have enough time to consume a dangerous quantity and was treated and released.

After speaking with the pediatrician, you do some checking in Mabel's patient record, and you discover that all her medications have been dispensed in non-child-resistant containers (i.e., "easy open" flip-top containers). On further investigation, you discover that there is no request on file where Mabel or her physician actually asked for easy-open containers. While discussing this with your pharmacy staff, you learn that everyone just assumed that a 79-year-old patient would want the non-child-resistant containers but that no one had ever asked her if she wanted them.

Discussion Questions

1. How would the pharmacy manager need to articulate and address the issues presented by this situation?
2. What are the key issues, and how should a pharmacy manager handle them with pharmacy staff?
3. What recommendations for change, if any, would be appropriate to assist the pharmacy in refining the pharmacy's policies and procedures?
4. What additional civil liability issues arise from situations like this one?

Case 29.3: The Super-technician

A state practice act/board of pharmacy provision Trudy Hamilton, PharmD, is a licensed pharmacist and is currently the manager of a hospital pharmacy department. In the state where Dr. Hamilton is licensed, nonpharmacist personnel are prohibited by both statute (the state pharmacy practice act) and state board of pharmacy regulation from engaging in activities defined as the practice of pharmacy. The specific activities that fall within the definition of the practice of pharmacy are limited to being personally performed by licensed pharmacists only. Such activities include counseling patients about their medications and responding to drug information requests from other health care professionals (e.g., physicians and nurses).

Robert Allen recently earned his certification as a certified pharmacy technician (CPhT) and has been working as a technician in the pharmacy department for the past 3 years. Robert is rightly proud of his accomplishment and recently has expressed interest in applying for admission to pharmacy school. Today, Dr. Hamilton received a phone call from Ann Brown, DO, an attending physician at her institution. Dr. Brown was noticeably angry. Yesterday, Dr. Brown called the pharmacy with a drug-interaction question about a drug that is new to the hospital's formulary (i.e., the list of drugs that the hospital pharmacy regularly keeps in stock). She was told by the "pharmacist" who answered the phone that the pharmacy department's computer system showed no interactions. Today, Dr. Brown's patient experienced a severe interaction between the new drug and a medication that the patient was already taking.

At a recent continuing-education seminar, Dr. Hamilton and her staff pharmacists learned of the potential for a significant interaction between the two medications in question. She was puzzled as to why one of the pharmacists would have told a physician that there are no drug interaction problems with the new drug. Dr. Hamilton and the staff pharmacists are aware that the hospital information technology department has not yet updated the pharmacy department computer system to include this interaction. As she concludes her conversation with Dr. Brown, she promises to find out what happened and take corrective action.

In Dr. Hamilton's investigation, she discovers that technician Robert Allen in fact took the phone call and answered Dr. Brown's question. Dr. Hamilton calls a meeting of the pharmacists to discuss how to prevent such problems from occurring in the future. During the meeting, she discovers that a few of the staff pharmacists have, on occasion, observed Robert stepping outside his technician role because he was trying to be helpful. They tell her that they have attempted to correct his behavior but have had little success. This is the first time Dr. Hamilton has heard of the problem.

Discussion Questions

1. How should Dr. Hamilton address this situation?
2. Are there problems with the way the department is functioning as a unit?
3. Is this situation simply a "personnel" issue confined to Robert's behavior?
4. Are there other issues or combinations of issues that should be addressed?

Case 29.4: A Recently Hired Pharmacist and the Nonpharmacist Store Manager

FEDERAL STATUTES (SOCIAL SECURITY ACT AND HIPAA) Pauline Rodgers, PharmD, recently started working as a staff pharmacist at Big Box Stores, Inc. right after she passed her board examinations and became licensed as a pharmacist. The pharmacy manager, Len Roberts, RPh, has been working for Big Box for about 20 years and has a fairly cordial relationship with Don Smith, the store manager. Mr. Smith, a business school graduate, is very "pro" pharmacy and wants to do all he can to help the pharmacy department increase its business through various marketing promotions. After working at the store for a few weeks, Pauline notices that Len makes a practice of giving in-store coupons to patients who are Medicare and Medicaid beneficiaries. These coupons, each worth $10, can be used to purchase groceries, DVDs, clothing, and so on. Realizing that she will soon likely encounter a situation where a Medicare or Medicaid beneficiary will expect to receive a coupon from her, Pauline asks Len what recordkeeping system is in use for tracking the total annual value of coupons given to each beneficiary. Len responds with a puzzled look on his face and asks: "Why would we do that? Mr. Smith wants us to keep handing out these coupons to increase our business. When it comes to running the business, I do what Mr. Smith wants and I don't ask questions."

DISCUSSION QUESTIONS

1. How should Pauline respond to Len?
2. What do you think are the important legal and managerial issues here?
3. How should Pauline respond to a request for a coupon from a Medicaid beneficiary?
4. Describe how you would handle this situation if you were Pauline.

Case 29.5: The Poorly Written Prescription and the Hurried Pharmacist

CIVIL LIABILITY (TORT LAW) Stuart Johnson, RPh, is manager of Johnson's Apothecary, a community pharmacy. When he arrived at the pharmacy today, there was a frantic voicemail message left for him in the middle of the night while the pharmacy was closed. It seems that a staff pharmacist, Dave, made a dispensing error yesterday, and Suzie Jones, a 3-year-old child, was taken unconscious by ambulance to the local community hospital emergency room at 2:00 AM. Suzie and her family had just moved to town about 2 weeks ago, and yesterday was their first visit to Johnson's Apothecary.

In the process of both calling the hospital and interviewing Dave, the staff pharmacist, Stuart learns the following: somehow Dave misinterpreted a poorly written prescription that was supposed to be for glycerin suppositories (Directions: "Use as directed") as a prescription for Glynase 5-mg tablets (a drug used to treat diabetes in adults). As a result of this error, Suzie's blood sugar dropped to dangerously low levels, and she is now in a coma. Dave was very busy when the error occurred and did not determine that the patient, Susan Jones, was in fact a 3-year-old child. He also did not speak to Suzie's mother, who brought in the prescription. Because he was very busy, he quickly checked a pharmacy technician's work and let her dispense the prescription to Mrs. Jones, an uninsured cash-paying customer. The sad truth is that the doctor had not even intended this written note to be a prescription (glycerin suppositories are available without a prescription); it just looked like one because it was on one of the doctor's prescription blanks.

DISCUSSION QUESTIONS

1. From this case, describe violations of both state and federal law and the tort law implications (i.e., potential for being sued).
2. What is the manager's role in determining what happened internally that was out of conformance with standards, with external regulatory bodies, and with professional performance standards beyond the letter of the law?
3. How can all these be brought to bear on the pharmacy?
4. How should Stuart as the manager respond when the local TV station and newspaper want interviews?

REFERENCES

Abood RR. 2012. *Pharmacy Practice and the Law*, 7th ed. Boston, MA: Jones and Bartlett.

Accreditation Council for Pharmacy Education (ACPE). Standards 2016. Available at https://www.acpe-accredit.org/pdf/Standards2016FINAL.pdf. Accessed March 17, 2019.

Adams AJ. 2018. Transitioning pharmacy to "standard of care" regulation: Analyzing how pharmacy regulates relative to medicine and nursing. *Res Social Admin Pharm* [Epub ahead of print].

Adams AJ, Weaver KK. 2016. The continuum of pharmacist prescriptive authority. *Ann Pharmacother* 50(9):778–784.

Associated Press. 2000. *Drug Representative, Pharmacist Sentenced*. Omaha World-Herald, February 12, 2000, p. 16.

Bledstein BJ. 1976. *The Culture of Professionalism*. New York, NY: Norton, p. 78.

Bonner L. Pharmacists' patient care process gains traction. Pharmacy Today. June 26, 2015. Available at http://www.pharmacist.com/pharmacists-patient-care-process-gains-traction. Accessed March 17, 2019.

Bren L. 2001. Frances Oldham Kelsey: FDA medical reviewer leaves her mark on history. *FDA Consum* 35(2):24–29.

Cacciatore GG. 1997. The overregulation of pharmacy practice. *Pharmacotherapy* 17(2):395–396.

Catizone CA, Teplitz J, Clark BE (eds.). 1993. *NABP Survey of Pharmacy Law*. Park Ridge, IL: National Association of Boards of Pharmacy.

Centers for Disease Control and Prevention (CDC). 2016. Using the pharmacists' patient care process to manage high blood pressure: A resource guide for pharmacists. CDC. Atlanta, GA. Available at https://www.cdc.gov/dhdsp/pubs/docs/pharmacist-resource-guide.pdf. Accessed March 17, 2019.

Centers for Medicare and Medicaid Services. 2019. Are you a covered entity? Available at https://www.cms.gov/regulations-and-guidance/administrative-simplification/hipaa-aca/areyouacoveredentity.html. Accessed March 25, 2019.

Draper R. 2003. The Toxic Pharmacist. *New York Times Magazine*, June 8, 2003, A83.

Eiserer T. 1999. 2 Plead Guilty in Fraudulent Drug Sale Case. Omaha World-Herald, October 9, 1999, p. 34.

Giberson S, Yoder S, Lee MP. Improving Patient and Health System Outcomes through Advanced Pharmacy Practice. A Report to the U.S. Surgeon General. Office of the Chief Pharmacist. U.S. Public Health Service. Dec 2011.

Green MW. 1979. *Epilogue, Prologue. In From the Past Comes the Future—The First 75 Years of the National Association of Boards of Pharmacy*. Chicago: National Association of Boards of Pharmacy.

H.R. 5835—101st Congress: Omnibus Budget Reconciliation Act of 1990. Available at: https://www.govtrack.us/congress/bills/101/hr5835; Accessed August 8, 2019.

Hilts PJ. 2003. *Protecting America's Health: The FDA, Business and One Hundred Years of Regulation*. New York, NY: Knopf.

Idaho Board of Pharmacy. 2018, *Idaho Pharmacy Laws*. Available at https://bop.idaho.gov/code_rules/2018-07-02_2018_IDBOP_LawBook.pdf. Accessed February 20, 2019.

Joint Commission of Pharmacy Practitioners. Pharmacists' Patient Care Process. May 29, 2014. Available at https://www.pharmacist.com/sites/default/files/files/PatientCareProcess.pdf. Accessed March 17, 2019.

May WF. 1988. Code and covenant or philanthropy and contract: Hastings Center report 1975. In Callahan JC (ed.) *Ethical Issues in Professional Life*. New York, NY: Oxford University Press, p. 93.

Moffett P, Moore G. 2011. The standard of care: Legal history and definitions: the bad and good news. *West J Emerg Med* 12(1):109–112.

National Council for Prescription Drug Programs. 2019. Implementation information for state prescription monitoring programs. Available at https://www.ncpdp.org/NCPDP/media/pdf/State_PMP_Tracking_Document.xlsx. Accessed April 12, 2019.

National Institute on Drug Abuse. 2019. Overdose death rates. Available at https://www.drugabuse.gov/related-topics/trends-statistics/overdose-death-rates. Accessed April 12, 2019.

Ponnapalli A, Grando A, Murcko A, Wertheim P. 2018. Systematic Literature Review of Prescription Drug Monitoring Programs. AMIA Annual Symposium Proceedings, pp. 1478–1487.

Stafford M. 2002. Ex-Pharmacist Gets 30 Years for Diluting Cancer Drugs. Omaha World Herald, December 5, 2002, p. 1.

U.S. Department of Health and Human Services. 2002. Office of Inspector General (OIG) Special Advisory Bulletin, Offering Gifts and Other Inducements to Beneficiaries. Available at https://oig.hhs.gov/fraud/docs/alertsandbulletins/sabgiftsandinducements.pdf. Accessed March 25, 2019.

U.S. Department of Health and Human Services. 2003. Office of Civil Rights (OCR) Privacy Brief: Summary of the HIPAA Privacy Rule. Available at https://www.hhs.gov/sites/default/files/privacysummary.pdf. Accessed March 25, 2019.

U.S. Department of Health and Human Services. 2017. HIPAA FAQs for professionals. Available at https://www.hhs.gov/hipaa/for-professionals/faq/index.html. Accessed March 25, 2019.

U.S. Department of Health and Human Services. 2019. What is the U.S. opioid epidemic? Available at https://www.hhs.gov/opioids/about-the-epidemic/index.html. Accessed April 2, 2019.

U.S. Food and Drug Administration (FDA). 2018. Milestones in U.S. food and drug law history. Available at https://www.fda.gov/aboutfda/history/forgshistory/evolvingpowers/ucm2007256.htm. Accessed March 25, 2019.

Webster's Online Dictionary. 2019. Available at http://www.merriam-webster.com/dictionary/standard. Accessed March 25, 2019.

SECTION III

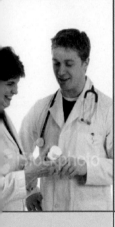

MANAGING PEOPLE

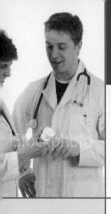

14

MANAGING YOURSELF FOR SUCCESS

Dana P. Hammer

About the Author: Dr. Hammer is the Faculty Lead for Student Professional Development at the University of Colorado Skaggs School of Pharmacy and Pharmaceutical Sciences. Prior to this appointment, she served as Director of the Teaching Certificate Program in Pharmacy Education, and Director of the Bracken Pharmacy Care Learning Center at the University of Washington. Dr. Hammer received a B.S. in pharmacy from Oregon State University, worked in hospital and community independent pharmacies, and then returned to school to earn M.S. and Ph.D. degrees in Pharmacy Practice with an emphasis in education from Purdue University School of Pharmacy. Her research involves assessment of students' educational outcomes, professional development, and interprofessional education. Dr. Hammer has served on the editorial boards of several pharmacy education, practice and research journals, and has won awards for teaching, innovations in teaching and education, and educational research. She practices her personal and time management skills balancing a faculty position, relief work in an independent pharmacy, and parenthood of two teenagers.

■ LEARNING OBJECTIVES

After completing this chapter, readers should be able to

1. Determine if they need to improve their personal and time management skills.
2. Critically analyze the choices they make in how they spend their time.
3. Describe common myths or pitfalls with regard to time management.
4. Take action to avoid time management pitfalls.
5. Discuss various theories and approaches to time management.
6. Apply concrete suggestions and steps to improve their personal and time management skills.
7. Explain how personal and time management techniques apply to pharmacy practice.
8. Recognize the relationships between personal and time management, stress, health, and career success.

■ SCENARIO

Revisit the Krista Connelly scenario from Chapter 2. It appears as though Krista is a somewhat successful "personal manager"—she seems to attend all her classes, prepares for classes ahead of time and reviews material with professors, holds down a part-time pharmacy job, and even is able to squeeze in routine home activities and downtime with friends and family. Unfortunately, Krista may not be taking very good care of herself with regard to diet, exercise, and sleep which can eventually be detrimental to her success, but she seems to have her act together for the most part. One question that remains after reading about Krista is when does she study? Perhaps she is one of the "genius" students who does not seem to have to study very much but is still able to achieve high grades. Consider a different scenario discussed further.

Tom Gupta is also a second-year pharmacy student. Tom describes himself as a busy pharmacy student, although he would not necessarily say that he is stressed out most of the time. Tom tries to get out of bed by 7 AM so that he can get to class by 8 AM, but he often oversleeps and misses his first class. He realizes that he should go to bed earlier, but it seems that the only time he can find to study or maybe watch some TV to unwind is between 10 PM and 2 AM Tom's normal day consists of attending classes, getting in an hour of basketball, and then heading to work at his pharmacy intern job at a local chain pharmacy. In between classes, he usually hangs out with friends, eats, or attends extracurricular activities and meetings. Tom finds it hard to try to get in any quality study time during the day and usually puts off studying for major exams or completing large assignments until the night before they are due. Because of this, he usually pulls all-nighters once every week or two. During midterm and finals weeks, he sometimes will stay up all night on several occasions. Tom averages B's and C's in school, although he got a D in pharmacology last year and had to repeat the course.

Tom usually works about 20 hours per week to help pay his tuition and other school-related expenses, as well as costs related to his cell phone, cable TV, and Internet subscriptions; car payment and insurance; rent; and other living expenses. He usually manages to have a little left over each month to buy music, go to movies, and go out on the town with friends, but he also maintains some credit-card debt from furniture and apartment supplies he bought when he started pharmacy school. The local chain that employs Tom as a pharmacy intern has an intern development program that helps interns to learn chain pharmacy management and administrative skills. At a recent employee annual review, Tom's preceptor shared his disappointment with Tom's tardiness to work, his inability to prioritize work tasks very well, and his lack of desire to want to improve or become engaged in management functions. Tom was discouraged with his preceptor's observations and is not sure what to do.

A third student is Ming-Lee Chan. In her first year of a PharmD program, she is experiencing overwhelm of pharmacy school. She has always done well in college courses, but the transition to the rigor of the PharmD curriculum, the realization of the competitive postgraduation market, learning an entirely different "culture" of her school's program, and developing new relationships has left her exhausted and feeling depressed and anxious. She is not even sure she wants to stay in the PharmD program, let alone go to class, study, and engage in other activities.

Do you have classmates like Krista, Tom, or Ming-Lee? Do their lives sound similar to yours? Read on to find out how to help yourself and others to maximize your potential and achieve your goals, while staying healthy and happy along the way. This chapter focuses on "personal management," with an emphasis on time management. After all, it is hard to manage a practice and its staff if you are not able to manage yourself!

■ CHAPTER QUESTIONS

1. How do I know if I need to manage myself and my time better?
2. What can I do to better manage myself and my time?

3. What are some resources I can use to help me better manage myself and my time?

4. What are some of the common pitfalls with regard to time management?

5. How does personal time management relate to time management in pharmacy practice?

6. How can time be better managed in pharmacy practice?

7. How do personal and time management relate to stress, health, and career success?

■ THE IMPORTANCE OF PERSONAL MANAGEMENT FOR SUCCESS IN SCHOOL AND YOUR CAREER

Life is hard! You worked hard to get into pharmacy school. Pharmacy school is hard. Placement into postgraduate residencies and jobs is more difficult, and students feel the pressure to be successful at "everything" in pharmacy school in order to be more competitive for these positions. Navigating the pharmacy school culture and managing relationships that come with it can be enriching but taxing. Add financial pressures and family and/or work responsibilities, and life before, during, and after pharmacy school can be downright stressful and overwhelming!

These stressors and others can make it difficult to maintain the mental, emotional, and physical health needed to be successful in school and beyond. Recent studies have shown high levels of stress and mental health concerns among undergraduate and graduate student populations (Henriques, 2014; Evans et al., 2018). For students unable to either remove or cope with these stressors in healthy ways, their chances to succeed, let alone become a good manager of a practice and its staff, are diminished.

Thankfully, college campuses have recognized this phenomenon and have placed increased emphases on mental health support, student wellness and resilience, and other related initiatives. There are local, regional, and national campaigns to inspire students to seek support when they feel overwhelmed with negative feelings, and to help overcome the stigma associated with "mental health."[1,2,3] These types of initiatives also encourage peers to seek support for loved ones of whom they have concern. Many college programs include training, workshops, and even courses to help students better cope with life's and situational stress.

The bottom line (and relevance of) this discussion is the importance of maintaining all aspects of your health in order to do well in school and in your career. While a full discussion of maintaining your overall health is beyond the scope of this chapter, you should take advantage of resources available to you from your school's or university's student services. There are also numerous resources available via internet and apps for your smartphone.[4,5,6] Your health serves as the foundation for "personal management;" it is also important, as a future (or current) manager, that you role model healthy behaviors for your staff. Their health and well-being are critical for their work productivity and success, as well as your collective practice and care for patients.

While multiple definitions of personal management exist, that which is most applicable to this discussion is "the personal skills, attitudes, and behaviors that drive one's potential for growth."[7] Personal

[1]Active Minds. Available at www.activeminds.org. Accessed Feb 25, 2019.

[2]JED Foundation. Available at www.jedfoundation.org. Accessed Feb 25, 2019.

[3]National Alliance on Mental Illness. Available at www.nami.org. Accessed Feb 25, 2019.

[4]American Association of Colleges of Pharmacy. Available at https://www.aacp.org/resource/wellness-and-resilience-pharmacy-education. Accessed February 25, 2019.

[5]Calm app. Available at www.calm.com. Accessed February 25, 2019.

[6]Omada Health Inc. Available at www.omadahealth.com. Accessed February 25, 2019.

[7]Conference Board of Canada. Available at https://www.conferenceboard.ca/edu/employability-skills.aspx?AspxAutoDetectCookieSupport=1. Accessed February 25, 2019.

management means making deliberate decisions and taking action to achieve your potential and your goals.

A large component of personal management, and reduction of stress, is time management. Using effective time management skills can help you succeed in school and in your career, as well as help you to be an effective pharmacy manager. People with poor time management skills are less likely to achieve their career goals due to a lack of ability to stay focused and organized. Read on to dig deeper into the magical and elusive concept of time, and how you can best use it as a critical component to your health and success.

■ TIME MANAGEMENT: A PRIMARY FACTOR OF PERSONAL MANAGEMENT

There are 24 hours in a day. Research tells us that for a person to be healthy, roughly 7 to 8 hours of that time should be used for sleeping. That leaves 16 to 17 hours to accomplish everything else we need and want to do in a day: go to school and/or work (usually 3 to 10 hours per day), study (rule of thumb for lecture courses is 2 hours outside class for every 1 hour in class, so let's say approximately 6 hours per day), prepare/acquire and eat food/beverage (approximately 1 to 2 hours per day), shower and get ready (0.5 to 1 hour per day), exercise (0.5 to 1 hour per day), routine maintenance (e.g., pay bills, pick up room, etc.— 1 hour per day), commute to/from school, home, and work (1 hour per day), participate in extra-curricular (1 hour per day), relax and have fun (0.5 to 1 hour per day), and spend time with family and/or friends (face-to-face, or via e-mail, phone, text or social media— 0.5 to 2 hours per day). Not all of us participate in all these activities each and every day, but if we did, we are looking at spending anywhere from 1 to 24 hours per day engaged in them. And this estimate does not even include time spent on unexpected events.

Time is one of the most valuable resources we have. Several philosophies have been iterated about time:

- The gift of your time is the most valuable gift you can give.

- If you want to know what people's *real* values are, look at how they spend their time and their money.
- Time is money.
- Time management is *not* about managing time; it is about managing yourself.

Many advances in technology and other areas are all about saving time. Think about computers, food processors, microwaves, and airplanes, for example. How about smartphones, wearables, and one-click purchase and shipping of items? All these inventions were created to make our lives easier and allow us to be more productive and spend the time we save through their use on other activities. It has been written, however, that we can never *save* time—we can only *spend* it—so we must make wise decisions about how we choose to spend our time (Ensman, 1991). Moreover, author Randy Milanovic writes, "When you study technology over a long enough time horizon, you notice an interesting trend: Even though each new development is in itself time-saving, people tend to be busier and busier, from one generation to the next" (Milanovic, 2014).

Time management and organizational skills are important both personally and professionally. You can likely recall a workshop or seminar related to time management during your pharmacy school orientation, or at least a mention of how important it is to be a good time manager to be successful in pharmacy school. Poor time management can lead to frustration, stress, and a failure to complete daily tasks or achieve personal and professional goals. We already know that frustration and stress can be physically detrimental. Poor time management can also cause others to lose respect for and faith in us—we may be considered less reliable and dependable, less likely to follow through on commitments, and less responsible. If others feel this way about us, we are less likely to be involved in committed relationships or receive promotions at work. Safety can also be compromised— personal safety, for example, if one is constantly late and so feels compelled consistently to drive over speed limits. Patient safety certainly can be compromised if pharmacists practice in a manner that is hurried, disorganized, and haphazard. These pharmacists may always be behind in their work, operate in "crisis-mode," contribute to errors, and lack good customer service. Conversely, good time management skills can lead to a higher quality of life for most people because they affect so many aspects of our lives, both personal and professional. The reasons to become a better time/self-manager are compelling and important—readers of this chapter should be motivated to improve their time management skills.

■ COMMON MYTHS/PITFALLS OF TIME MANAGEMENT

Myth/Pitfall #1 "I don't have time …"

How often do you hear this phrase or utter it yourself? The truth is that we *all* have 24 hours in every day to accomplish what we need and want to do, so saying that you don't have time is actually a lie. The difference is how we *choose* to spend our time. Thus, unless you are in prison or some kind of work camp where you do not make the decisions on how your day is spent, most of us consciously decide how to spend our time. It was your choice to apply to pharmacy school. It is your choice to go to class. It is your choice to study. It is your choice to get a part-time job. It is your choice to read this book. No one is forcing you to do these things. Granted, there may be significant consequences if you do *not* choose to do these things, but the bottom line is that you *choose* how to spend your time. The next time that you feel compelled to say, "I don't have time to—[fill in the blank]," rephrase it to, "I can't take the time to—[fill in the blank]." At least that way you will not be lying!

Myth/Pitfall #2 "I'm too busy …"

Once again, you *choose* how to spend your time. If you feel that you are too busy to maintain your personal health, achieve your personal and professional goals, or be as successful in all your tasks and responsibilities as you would like to be, then *change your schedule.* Do not take on as many tasks. Find your success limit and maintain it! Contrary to popular belief, the busier people are, the more productive they are, and the more they accomplish, to a certain extent. Think about the last time that you had a week without appointments or without deadlines. How much did you get done? Granted, you may have caught up on some needed rest and relaxation, but you may not have attended to many other items on your to-do list because you were in relaxation mode and were not feeling the subtle pressure of "something needs to be done." Deadlines creep up and cause stress when the realization occurs that you do not have as much time to meet that deadline as you would like. Although it was stated that busy people are more productive, it is not necessarily true to say that *all* busy people are productive. Many folks spend their time working on tasks and activities that could be better handled by others. They may not be able to prioritize their responsibilities very well or may be easily distracted or consistently interrupted. One of the most common distracters nowadays is over-involvement in social media. Yet, it is certainly true that some folks are just *too* busy. You know that your plate is too full when your health begins to fail, your personal relationships begin to fail, and you cannot follow through reliably with all your responsibilities. You begin to forget things. You miss meetings and deadlines. You may feel consistent stress, and guilt if you relax at all or "get off task." These are not healthy feelings and can escalate to the point of illness, exhaustion, and burnout. It is important to find that balance of where your health, happiness, and productivity are maximized; where you are in the stage of "eustress" (Figure 14-1).

Myth/Pitfall #3 "I need time to focus in order to …"

"… finish that assignment," "… . check that order," "… counsel that patient." While you may be more successful at any particular task when time and conditions are ideal, the reality is that this does not happen regularly in daily life. The ability to effectively shift focus from one task to another is an absolute necessity for any pharmacist or pharmacy student. This does *not* mean doing several things simultaneously—if that were the case, you would never get anything fully

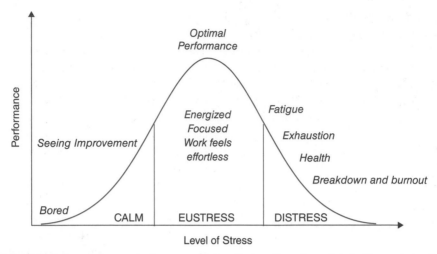

Figure 14-1. Relationship of stress to human performance. (Yerkes-Dodson Curve is reprinted with permission from Yerkes RM, Dodson JD (1908), The relation of strength of stimulus to rapidity of habit-formation. J. Comp. Neurol. Psychol., 18: 459–482. Copyright © 1908 The Wistar Institute of Anatomy and Biology.)

accomplished, and patient safety would certainly be compromised. Studies show that multitasking is not effective (Uncapher, 2017; Martín-Perpiñá, 2019). What it *does* mean, however, is that it is important that you have the ability to "switch gears" easily and maintain a sharp mind so that you can give your undivided attention for a few moments to the task at hand and then move on to the next task or back to the original task. Rarely will you have full days without any appointments or activities scheduled, or interruptions, so that you can spend large amounts of time on one or a few tasks.

Myth/Pitfall #5 "I'm a perfectionist … "

It is certainly important to do your best and to always "put your best foot forward," but as a pharmacy student or pharmacist with many demands on your time, it is critical that you discern which tasks must be perfect and which can be less than perfect. Dosing and preparation of chemotherapeutic agents, for example, should be as close to perfect as possible—it is crucially important that enough time be spent on these tasks to make sure that they are correct because people's lives are at stake. Revising a term paper five times for a three-credit course, however, does not have such severe consequences, and the time spent in the extra

three revisions could have been spent studying for an examination that is worth twice the number of points as the paper. There is also some evidence to support that higher levels of perfectionism are correlated with higher levels of stress and anxiety (Mandel, 2015; Damian, 2017). It is okay not to be perfect all the time, unless, of course, the consequence of *not* being perfect is severe. In other words, sometimes we have to "choose our battles" in order to win the time management war. And don't let yourself get caught up in "analysis to paralysis."

■ HOW TO "DO" TIME MANAGEMENT

Of the many resources on time management, care has been taken to distill the most pertinent themes that would apply to busy pharmacy students and practitioners. The most commonly suggested strategies involved in practicing better time management are:

- Recognize the need for improvement.
- Conduct an honest analysis of how you currently use your time.
- Establish your "mission" and set goals.

- Get organized (sort through tasks, create a master list, schedule tasks, use a system).
- Take action.
- Review, revise, and modify.

These themes are described more fully further in text, along with a variety of helpful tips from many different sources.

Recognize the Need for Improvement

Almost all literature that describes successful behavioral change programs (think 12-step programs, smoking cessation, weight loss, and others) start at the same point: the recognition that one's behavior needs to change or that a person desires to change his or her behavior. Hopefully, you have decided already that your personal and time management skills could use some improvement. If you have not decided this, then the chances of your being able to improve are much less. If you are in this latter category, then the next section may just convince you that you could benefit from changing some of your current habits.

Conduct an Honest Self-Reflection or Analysis of How You Currently Use Your Time

Conducting a thorough review of how you currently spend your typical day or week can be very helpful in determining how to best proceed with improving your time management. Asking yourself some key questions can also help to identify problem areas and how you should best plan your time based on your personal preferences and style (Table 14-1). There are many electronic, as well as paper, resources used to conduct a time analysis, such as Rescue Time,[8] Toggl,[9] and TimeLogger,[10] just to name a few. You can also use an electronic or paper calendar to keep a short-term

[8]RescueTime. Available at www.rescuetime.com. Accessed on February 25, 2019.

[9]Toggl. Available at www.toggl.com. Accessed on February 25, 2019.

[10]Timelogger. Available at www.timeloggerapp.com. Accessed on February 25, 2019.

time journal, and document how you spend your time in blocks of 15 minutes. The most accurate way to do this would be to keep your calendar with you at all times; document an activity and the time you spent on it each time you change activities. Do this for an entire week, and *be honest,* for example, 75 minutes surfing the Internet/social media for fun, 15-minute day-dreaming, 30-minute power nap, and so on. After a week, analyze those areas where you think your time could have been better spent and evaluate factors that could have contributed to wasting time. For example, Tom Worrall, ambulatory care clinical pharmacy specialist for the Ralph H. Johnson Veterans' Affairs Medical Center in Charleston, South Carolina, explained that as a student he chose to study in the city library instead of the school's library so that he could get more done. "What takes 4 hours at the student center can take 2 hours at the city library because of fewer distractions" (English, 2003).

Woodhull (1997) suggests that identifying your time management style will help you to better know how to use your unscheduled time, or "white spaces." She states that workaholics often have no white spaces in their schedules, which is unhealthy. She describes the four basic types of time managers:

- "*Leaders*, above all, value getting the job done and moving forward … . Their communication style is direct and succinct. Their motto is 'be brief and be gone.' Say what you have to say in 10 words or less. They are experts at making quick decisions" (Woodhull, 1997, p. 43).
- "*Analytics* value getting tasks done with precision and accuracy. They pay a lot of attention to detail. Their style is systematic. They use facts, logic, and structure. When communicating with them, make sure you tie new ideas to old concepts and make sure you provide a thorough explanation" (Woodhull, 1997, p. 45).
- "*Relaters* believe that getting along with others is the most important thing. Nourishing the primary relationships in their life is of utmost importance to them. They dislike making decisions that affect others. Sometimes they feel overburdened by all the

Table 14-1. General and Specific Questions to Help Analyze One's Time	
General Questions	**General Questions**
1. What went right today (with regard to spending your time wisely)? What went wrong? Why?	1. What am I doing that does not really need to be done?
2. What time did I start my top-priority task (assuming that you have identified your top-priority task)? Why? Could I have started earlier in the day?	2. What am I doing that could be done by someone else?
3. What patterns and habits are apparent from my time log?	3. What am I doing that could be done more efficiently?
4. Did I spend the first hour of my (work) day doing important work?	4. What do I do that wastes others' time?
5. What was the most productive part of my day? Why?	5. If I do not have time to do it right, do I have time to do it wrong?
6. What was the least productive part of my day? Why?	**Specific questions to ask for each activity**
7. Who or what caused most interruptions (or what kept you from staying on task)?	1. Why am I doing this?
8. How might I eliminate or reduce the three biggest time wasters?	2. What is the goal?
9. How much of my time was spent on high-value activity and how much on low-value tasks?	3. Why will I succeed?
10. Which activities could I spend less time on and still obtain acceptable results?	4. Is what I am doing at this minute moving me toward my objective?
11. Which activities needed more time today?	5. What will happen if I choose not to do it?
12. Which activities could have been delegated? To whom?	

Data from Douglass and Douglass, 1993; Bond, 1996.

things they have agreed to do for others" (Woodhull, 1997, p. 45).

- *Entertainers.* "Once considered too offbeat for the normal world of work, these types are now the ones who generate new ideas that are keeping companies alive. Unlike the other three types, entertainers do not like having a precise, predictable schedule. Instead, they enjoy a great deal of variety and flexibility" (Woodhull, 1997, p. 46).

If you are unsure of which type of time manager you are, Woodhull (1997, p. 47) offers a quiz you can take to find out. She advocates, however, that better time managers incorporate features of each style in order to be more flexible and adaptable to a variety of situations.

Now that you have thoroughly analyzed your time management style, preferences, and current use of time, you are ready to move on to the next step of becoming an improved time manager.

Establish Your "Mission" and Set Goals

While this step and the diagnostics just described are not necessarily critical to becoming a better time manager, completing them should increase your likelihood for success in becoming a better self-manager. Setting short- and long-term personal and professional goals *is* critical to help determine priorities and stay focused. Covey (1989) and Douglass and Douglass (1993) each advocate writing your personal mission statement; from this, all your goals and priorities should flow. According to Covey, a personal mission statement is "the most effective way I know to begin with the end in mind" (Covey, 1989, p. 106). Your personal mission statement, or philosophy or creed, "focuses on what you want to be (character) and to do (contributions and achievements) and on the values and principles upon which being and doing are based" (Covey, 1989, p. 106). Covey provides several examples of people's mission statements and guidance on how to write such statements. Douglass and Douglass describe a personal mission statement as focusing "directly on your roles, relationships, and responsibilities ... where you really figure out who you are and why you are here ... carefully consider your relationships with [a higher power, significant other, loved ones], friends, community, employers, and self. What kind of a person do you really want to be? What should the sum total of your life add up to? Write out your rough ideas, then edit and refine them" (Douglass and Douglass, 1993, p. 179).

Once you have thought through these deeper questions, it is much easier to identify long- and short-term goals and priorities. Douglass and Douglass (1993, pp. 16–17) describe how to write SMART (specific, measurable, achievable, realistic, and timed) goals. Incidentally, these are the same considerations in writing goals used in strategic and business planning, as well (see Chapters 6 and 7):

1. *Goals should be specific.* The more specific a goal, the more direction it provides, and the easier it is to measure progress. For example, you may have a goal of studying more, which is stated very broadly. However, if you were to say, "I will increase my study time by 1 hour every day or at least 6 hours a week," this goal is more specific and clearly defined.
2. *Goals should be measurable.* Similar to the preceding comments, it is easier to determine if you are making progress toward your goal if you can quantify the specifics in your goal. The preceding example would be easy to quantify if you were keeping track of how your time is spent each day.
3. *Goals should be achievable.* "Goals should make you stretch and grow," but they should not be set so high that they are unachievable. For example, a person may want to be a famous singer, but if that person has no previous musical training or talent, this goal could be unachievable. Goals "should be set at a level at which you are both able and willing to work. In general, your motivation increases as you set your goals higher." If a goal is set too high, however, so that steps and time to achieve it seem daunting, then you are more likely to fail. Think about trying to lose fifty pounds in 12 months vs. 5 pounds in 2 months.
4. *Goals should be realistic.* Closely related to achievability, goals should be realistic—take into account available time, resources, and skills. The preceding examples illustrate this case well.
5. *Goals should be timed.* You are much more likely to achieve a goal if it has a target date by which it should be accomplished. Assigning target dates for accomplishing goals increases motivation, commitment, and action. Goals without time schedules quickly become daydreams under the pressure of daily affairs. For each step along the way, you should set a realistic target date that can, and should, be adjusted if conditions change.

Douglass and Douglass go onto to describe three additional recommendations to help you achieve your goals: (1) *Goals should be compatible*—because if they are not, working to achieve one goal may prevent you from accomplishing another; (2) *goals should be your own*—otherwise, your motivation to achieve them is much less—you should take ownership of at least *part* of the goal if it is not your own; and (3) *goals should be written*—writing helps to clarify goals and makes them more real—our commitment to goals improves if they are written and posted in a place where they can be seen regularly.

If you have a lot of goals, some people find it easier to focus on them if they categorize them into personal vs. professional and short- vs. long-term. It is important, however, to keep your goals posted somewhere, perhaps in multiple places, so that you will look at them regularly. The more often you are reminded of your goals, the more likely you are to continue working toward them. Morgenstern (2000, pp. 71–72) tells readers to classify their "big picture" goals into one of six categories: self, family, work, relationships (such as spouse and friends), finances, and community (such as making contributions and getting involved). She goes on to say that it is much easier to determine specific activities and then daily tasks that help to achieve each goal in each category. Often some daily tasks can be used to help achieve more than one goal, such as exercising with a good friend.

With regard to tackling one's goals, Woodhull (1997, p. 221) advocates using the Benjamin Franklin approach—do not try to accomplish all your goals in the same time frame, or you will become overwhelmed and discouraged (consider New Year's resolutions). Instead, work on one or two at a time. Franklin also believed that it took 21 days for a new behavior to take root and become a routine habit; he would carry a card in his pocket with his goal for at least 21 days to constantly remind him of it.

Get Organized (Sort Through Tasks, Create a Master List, Prioritize and Schedule Tasks, and Use a System)

You have now come to the meat of time management—*getting organized.* Organizing your life and keeping it that way are the absolute best ways to save time and feel good about how you use your time. There are several steps that many experts recommend when getting organized. First, you need to sort through what you already have. This refers to tangible items such as possessions, papers, e-mail messages, electronic documents, bills, and tasks that need to be accomplished. There are numerous resources to help people get their possessions organized. One need only think about closet-organizing companies and "storables" stores. A complete discussion of these is beyond the scope of this chapter. However, this section will provide you with some tips about organizing some of the other parts of your life that are more difficult: papers, e-mails/texts, electronic documents, and tasks that lie before us.

Sort Through Tasks
You probably have heard the statement "Handle each piece of paper once," or some people use the acronym

OHIO (Only Handle It Once). This is a very good rule of thumb that literally means that each time we get a new piece of mail or paper of some sort, we need to decide how we are going to use that piece of paper and do something with it—keep it, recycle it, or read it later. This implies that we need to set up a filing system that works for us. Also, it is not bad to have a "read it later" pile as long as you make sure that you *schedule some time* somewhere in your calendar to actually read through the pile. Perhaps this is a task that you could work on once a week. These same ideas apply to e-mail and text messages, and electronic documents. Most of us have some sort of computer file system set up on our hard drives or in the "cloud" that allows us to keep computer documents organized. Similar to handling paper, as you receive new e-mail/text messages or computer documents, you need to determine whether to file them, delete them, or respond to them later. Most e-mail programs allow users to create files in which to store e-mail messages in a place other than one's inbox. Just like paper, however, e-mails. Photos, videos, and other electronic files take up space on a server and/or hard drive that has limited capacity. With both paper and computer files, it is important to go through them periodically, at least once or twice a year, to clean them out and make sure that you are not running out of space.

Create a Master List
Organizing and prioritizing your tasks are often more difficult than organizing papers and e-mails. Many authors advocate creating a master list of all the tasks you need to do and then prioritizing and scheduling them. You can create your master list on your computer, on paper, on a calendar or with various apps, as long as it is on something that you can refer to regularly and easily. Some folks have more than one master list, such as a "work or school list" and a "home list." Whatever system works best for you, the main idea is to document *all* tasks that you need to complete at some time or another. This includes any new tasks that may come your way after reviewing your mail, e-mail, texts, assignment and exam trackers/notifications, and others. Make sure to cross off tasks

as you complete them, which adds to your sense of accomplishment!

Prioritize Tasks

Creating a master list is not too challenging as long as you remember to document everything. The more difficult task is determining how to approach the multitude of tasks on your list. Where do you start? Sometimes it can be overwhelming to think about if you have a variety of tasks that all seem very important. Thankfully, experts have helped us determine how best to prioritize tasks and responsibilities so that we can be most effective and satisfied. Three general approaches to prioritizing tasks are (1) the goal-achievement approach, (2) the deadline approach, and (3) the consequences approach. Using a combination of these three will be help you to prioritize the tasks in your life effectively.

Briefly, the goal-achievement approach advocates prioritizing tasks that you know will directly help you achieve your goals as most important. For example, if one of your goals is to achieve a grade-point average (GPA) of 3.5 or higher, then the task of studying at least 4 hours a day should be high on your priority list. As another example, if you are seeking a certain internship position, then completing the application and other tasks necessary to get hired should be high on your priority list. The deadline approach is relatively self-explanatory—when are your tasks due? Using the deadline approach to prioritize your tasks is easy when the deadlines have been set by others (think assignments, exams, birthdays, and others) as long as you allocate yourself enough time to complete the tasks. The deadline approach is not as effective, however, when certain tasks have no externally assigned deadlines and you have to set a deadline yourself. Regular exercise, for example, is easy to put off because it does not have a deadline (unless you are training for an athletic event). The deadline approach is also not very effective in helping you to achieve your goals. The consequence approach is somewhat related to the deadline approach and essentially asks the question, "What will happen if this task is not completed or not completed on time?" The more detrimental the consequences, the higher the priority of the task. For example, if the brakes on your car are beginning to fail, it is extremely important that you get them fixed right away, or the consequences could be fatal. On the other hand, if the penalty for turning in a late assignment is only a loss of 5 points out of 100, then completing that assignment on time may have a lesser priority than getting your brakes fixed.

Similar to these approaches is the "big rock" approach. You may have heard the story about the time management seminar speaker who was presenting to a class of business students one day.[11] He had a large glass jar and proceeded to fill it up with large rocks. He asked the class if the jar was full.

"Yes," the students responded.

He then took a bag of gravel and proceeded to add it to the jar and shake it down—the gravel filled up space among the large rocks in the jar. "Is the jar full?" he asked the class.

"Probably not," replied one student.

"Good!" the speaker responded. Then he added a bag of sand to the jar, which filled up any remaining space among the rocks. "Now?" he asked the class.

"No!" the students emphatically responded.

Then the speaker brought out a pitcher of water and proceeded to pour the entire amount into the jar without causing the jar to overflow. "What's the point of this illustration?" the speaker asked.

One student responded, "The point is, no matter how full your schedule is, if you try really hard, you can always fit some more things in it!"

"No," the speaker replied, "that's not the point. The truth this illustration teaches us is: If you don't put the big rocks in first, you'll never get them in at all." He goes on to explain that the big rocks in our lives are time spent with family and friends, taking

---

[11]Nash G. 2011. The Rock Parable. Available at http://www.psybersquare.com/work/parable.html. Accessed February 16, 2019. The story has also been described as filling up the jar last with beer instead of water, with the moral being, "no matter how full your life gets, there's always room for a beer."

care of ourselves, our faith, and time spent on other worthy causes. The sand and water are "fillers" in our lives, and although some quantity is important, if we fill up our jars with these activities first, then we will have no room left for the big rocks or gravel.

Lastly, you probably have observed that some of these approaches discussed delegating certain tasks. As you review your master list, especially the tasks that are of lesser priority and importance, ask yourself if any of those tasks could be done by someone else or if someone else could help you with them. Would it be appropriate to enlist the help of a significant other, a roommate, a friend, a family member, or another person to complete a task? This is a very important question to ask so that you can avoid getting bogged down in activities that detract from your higher-priority tasks.

Establishing priorities, both in your professional and personal lives, can have a significant impact on your overall time and stress management skills. By focusing on what is most important to achieving your personal goals and practice responsibilities, you should be able to have more time to focus on these activities and less stress in worrying about how you will be able to get everything done.

Schedule Tasks

This is not without its own set of challenges because it is often difficult to know how much time a particular task will take—especially if it is a task that you have not done before. It is best to take a conservative approach and allow yourself *more* time than you think you will need to complete a task. It is always better to under-commit and over-deliver (e.g., telling your boss that you will have a particular project done by a date later than you actually think it will take for you to complete and then turning the project in early *or* telling a patient that her prescription will be ready in 15 minutes when you are positive that it will only take 5 to 10 minutes) than to overcommit and under-deliver. Convince yourself of the phenomenon that "things always take longer than I think they will" to allow for unexpected interruptions and other unscheduled events. Then, when you finish a task early, you can reward yourself with a break or fun activity that you had not scheduled previously.

It is also important to break larger tasks into smaller ones with their own deadlines. If you are working on a semester-long research paper for a class, for example, you are much more likely to do a better job and save yourself a lot of stress if you set some deadlines for yourself to complete the paper:

Month 1: Complete literature search and reading about the topic; draft outline of paper.
Month 2: Complete rough draft of paper; turn in to instructor voluntarily for feedback.
Month 3: Revise first draft based on instructor's feedback; turn in final paper.

Breaking down large tasks also makes them seem less daunting and less overwhelming. Setting intermediate deadlines and sticking to them helps you not to procrastinate.

Lastly, it is important to schedule *all* tasks if not on paper or electronically, at least in your mind; otherwise, they will not get done. Some doctors make weekly appointments with *themselves* to make sure that they can squeeze in some personal time or downtime without being interrupted by another appointment. This is not to say that you need to be so rigid that you have every activity in your life entered into a master schedule, but at least allocating time for quadrant II activities is vital to make sure that they are accomplished (e.g., family time, working out, and personal time). It is also important to review your schedule and master list several times a week to make sure that you are prepared for tasks that are coming up. Some authors advocate doing this each night before going to bed. If that initiates insomnia, however, then save that task for mornings.

Use a System

You have the tasks on your master list prioritized and scheduled—but how are you going to keep track of all this? Many people have found that the busier they are and the more tasks they need to complete, the more they rely on some sort of planner system to stay organized. There are a wide variety of daily, weekly, monthly, and yearly planning systems available. While a comprehensive discussion of such systems is beyond the scope of this chapter, several useful approaches are described:

- *Paper Systems.* What, you ask? PAPER? Believe it or not, some people still prefer paper for certain types of documentation over electronic.

  Calendars. A simple portable calendar can be used to document scheduled tasks as well as a master or to-do list. If this system sounds appealing, make sure that the squares on the calendar are large enough so that you can legibly write down all your tasks and appointments. You also want to make sure that your master list can be attached easily to the calendar so that you can keep track of unscheduled tasks that need to be completed. The written calendar system has the advantage of allowing you to easily review daily tasks as well as others coming up in the week or month.

  Planner/organizer systems. You may have heard of the Franklin–Covey planner system or the Day Runner system or seen them in stores. These are just two examples of popular paper-based organizing systems that go beyond the traditional paper calendar. These systems help the user to prioritize and schedule tasks and to keep a detailed calendar, master to-do list, and address book. They allow the user to customize it so that you only include the types of pages you use most. They come with instructions on how to best use their systems in order to get the most out of them.

- *Computer programs and smartphone apps.* In this digital age, more and more people are opting for electronic systems. Many pharmacy students already use apps and other programs on their smartphones to store drug information references as well as keep a daily schedule, maintain contacts, and check e-mail/texts/social media. These systems have the ability to sound an alarm to alert you of an upcoming meeting or event. Another advantage is that many of the phone systems can be backed up to and synced with a computer system, or they exist in "the cloud" so that if either system crashes or is lost, you do not completely lose everything. One challenge of these systems, however, is that it is difficult to look at multiple pages easily. The master list may be kept in a different place than the daily schedule, and the weekly schedule may not show up in much detail. Many of the paper-based organizer programs are now available as computer programs or phone apps. The former works well for those who work on a primary computer most of the time, but if you are not able to download the information onto something that you can carry, such programs may not be as useful.

Take Action

You are ready! On paper, computer, or mobile device you are extremely organized and ready to hit the ground running. In order to help you be successful in accomplishing all your well-organized tasks, Douglass and Douglass (1993, pp. 22–23) feel that it is important to review some of the realities of human nature and how we normally spend our time—not all of which are bad. Some highlights from their 21-item list are noted in Table 14-2.

Table 14-2.	**Observations of Human Behavior for How We Spend Our Time**
• We do what we like to do before we do what we do not like to do.	• We tackle what we know how to do faster than we tackle what we do not know how to do.
• We do activities that we have resources for.	• We do things that are scheduled before we do nonscheduled things.
• We respond to the demands of others before we respond to demands from ourselves.	• We wait until a deadline approaches before we really get moving on projects.

Data from Douglass and Douglass, 1993.

Being aware of some of these patterns can better help you to avoid them and to stay on track in accomplishing your tasks. Always keep the big picture in mind—think of the goals that you want to achieve and how completing a task will help you do that. A great slogan for dieters who are having trouble with self-discipline is "Nothing tastes as good as healthy feels." Constant self-motivation is important when you are trying to change your behavior.

Morgenstern (2000, p. 195) says, "Plan your work, and then work your plan." She recommends three actions to help you stay focused and disciplined so that you can overcome bad habits and achieve more each day (p. 196):

1. Minimize interruptions (i.e., unexpected events) and their impact.
2. Conquer procrastination and chronic lateness.
3. Overcome perfectionism.

She goes on to provide helpful suggestions on how to do all these things because they sound much easier than they are (pp. 196–210). In the end, if you are able to "containerize" your activities, you will be able to get your to-dos done and move through your day "feeling energized, optimistic, and satisfied" (p. 195).

General Tips From the Experts

To make the most of your personal and time management, thereby increasing your chances to be healthy and achieve your goals, here is a recap of some strategies that are worth mentioning again:

• Take care of yourself. It is extremely difficult to be productive and successful if you subsist on unhealthy food, get less than 7 hours of sleep per night, or only exercise when you walk from your apartment to the bus stop.
• Most people do their best work in the morning, so tackle the tough projects at that time.
• Schedule meetings and less intensive activities in the afternoon.
• Check your e-mail, text, and phone messages only twice a day, once in the morning and once in the afternoon or evening.

• Cluster tasks and activities together when possible. For example, if you have a class or meeting in building A, what other tasks or activities can you accomplish that need to be done in or near building A before you trek across campus to building Z?
• Quantity does not equal quality.
• Busy does not equal productive.
• Working harder does not equal working smarter.
• Reward yourself. It gives you something to shoot for and look forward to. Besides, all work and no play is unhealthy and no fun!

Douglass and Douglass (1993, pp. 184–186) offer 39 tips for becoming a "top time master." They have even created a poster with these tips that they offer free to anyone who contacts one of the authors (contact information is included in their book). They describe it as "an excellent way to keep reminding yourself to develop good time management habits" (p. 186).

Review/Revise/Modify

Now that you are working on your plan in full swing, it is important to review periodically all the steps that you went through to determine if your system is working well. Are you accomplishing tasks and goals to your satisfaction? Are you feeling less stressed? Do you procrastinate less often? Have your preferences or your style changed in any way? Do you want to try out a new organizational system? Have your goals or priorities changed? What major changes have occurred in your life to modify your goals and priorities? When you ask yourself these questions, especially the first three, remember to cut yourself a little slack. Real change takes time, and old habits are hard to break. It is okay if you did not follow your plan to a tee. Celebrate your successes, learn from your failures, and keep striving to improve.

■ TIME MANAGEMENT IN PHARMACY PRACTICE

So how does all this information about personal and time management relate to pharmacy practice? As mentioned earlier, it is unlikely that a person who is unhealthy and disorganized at home will be healthy and organized in his or her work environment, and vice versa. The practice environment in which you work can affect your personal and time management abilities. If you have a position that is more administrative, project-based, or appointment-based, you will have more control over how your time is spent, allowing you to better use many of the skills described in this chapter. In many practice environments, however, we do not get to determine how we spend our time—the nature of the job involves responding to the demand of medication orders and questions from patients, health care providers, and others. Rarely do we have the luxury of planning our daily work activities. White (2007) offers several strategies that any pharmacist could use to improve work efficiency (Table 14-3).

Personal and time management in practice are based on two issues: how you organize and perform your work and space, i.e., factors of which you may have some control, and what the general workflow is like in your environment, i.e., of which you may not have as much control. If you do have some control in yours' and others' duties and how the workflow progresses, there are numerous recommendations about how to improve efficiency, patient safety, and work life. A full discussion of these is beyond the scope of this chapter, but a few specific recommendations are shared further in text.

Table 14-3.	General Strategies for Working More Efficiently
Determine the cost of your time	Prioritize your goals
Understand your responsibilities	Assign times for your tasks
Log your activities	Manage e-mail
Plan for productive time	Manage clutter
Avoid time-wasting behavior	Manage retrieval of information
Develop reminders	Employ other time savers, such as templates for regular reports

Data from White, 2007.

Karen Berger, PharmD, proposed "11 New Year's Resolutions to Improve Pharmacy Work Life," a few of which are pertinent to our discussion (Berger, 2017):

- *Set expectations to properly manage stress.* She gives an example of telling a patient to return 3 hours later than when she knows his prescription will be ready to fill, so that he won't be returning when the pharmacy opens (which is usually busy and more stressful).
- *Take accountability for unresolved issues.* She recalls an effective pharmacy manager who said that good pharmacists pick things up (notes, bottles, other clutter in the pharmacy) and ask, "What's this, and what do I need to do with it?" Doing so can improve patient care and work life for staff.
- *Set the tone, because attitude is contagious.* While this is relatively self-explanatory, she notes that it may not happen every day or in every situation but do your best to be positive. This might also be a time to practice "fake it til you make it."
- *Drink more water and eat healthy food.* She also recommends sitting down for 5 (at least!) minutes to eat, and take bathroom breaks. Prepare healthy snacks/lunch in the evenings that you can easily take to work the next day.

Mark Jacobs, pharmacist for Shopko Pharmacy in Beloit, Wisconsin, published his thoughts about making more time for patients in the pharmacy in the book *101 Ways to Improve Your Pharmacy Work-life* (as noted in Jacobs, 2002). Some of his suggestions related to managing the volume of phone calls to improve your professional satisfaction and ability to care for patients (a few of which apply specifically to outpatient and community practices):

1. *Make full use of pharmacy technicians and other support staff.* If you work with capable technicians, use them as fully as the law will allow. One example is never to answer the phone yourself unless it is a prescribers' line. Jacobs mentions that no other professionals (e.g., doctors, lawyers, etc.) answer their own phones (see Chapter 19).

2. *Respond to questions on the phone through your pharmacy technicians whenever possible.* This does not mean that you should avoid talking with patients on the phone at all possible costs, but by training your technicians to ask the caller the proper "triage" questions, you can avoid calls where the patient wants to talk to the pharmacist and then goes on to give you a prescription number to refill. Doctors most often respond to patients on the phone through their nurses.

3. *If a patient insists on speaking with a pharmacist, explain that the pharmacist is busy with another patient right now.* Jacobs advocates having the technician take down the patient's name and phone number and the reason for the call so that the pharmacist can prepare for the call prior to calling back, which also saves time.

4. *Find out when and where would be the best time to call the patient back.* Jacobs states that this will help "condition" patients to realize that you are a busy health care professional and that you may not always be available on-demand. In addition, if they really need help right now, they may be willing to ask the technician.

5. *Gracefully exit the conversation after 2 minutes* "by explaining to the patient that you have time for one more question. They will either ask it or thank you for your time."

6. *Have the technician take down all the information for prescription transfers* (depending on what the law will allow). At the very least, the technician can pull up the prescription on the computer or pull the hard copy before handing the phone to the pharmacist.

For some patients and phone calls, it may not be appropriate to adhere to all these suggestions, but these tips could help a busy pharmacist to better manage time each day. Other efficiencies that many practices are implementing include a variety of dispensing technologies and robotics, automated refill phone lines, interactive websites, and revisions to technicians' and pharmacists' responsibilities so that technicians perform most technical duties and pharmacists can concentrate on medication therapy management activities, as well as engaging in patient and provider education. All these suggestions can be implemented relatively easily so as to better manage time in the pharmacy. Jeff Rochon, PharmD, Chief Executive Officer of the Washington State Pharmacists Association, reminds us that above all, we must make time to communicate with patients and other health care providers (Rochon, 2003).

■ STRESS AS A PRIMARY CONSEQUENCE OF POOR PERSONAL AND TIME MANAGEMENT

Recall the conversations earlier in the chapter about health and wellness in student populations, and how stress levels can be classified as calm, eustress, or distress (Figure 14-1). In the postgraduate working world, conversations about stress are equally important. There are calls for health care systems to consider the work life of their employees to reduce job dissatisfaction and burnout of health care providers (Bodenheimer and Sinsky, 2014). Stress among health care providers has been shown to lead to lower patient satisfaction, reduced health outcomes, a possible increase in costs (Reid et al., 2010), and even suicide (Center et al., 2003). Personal factors can also play a part in stress at work, such as family; friends; health; and spirit/self (Byrne, 2005). The issue of balance, in all aspects of one's life, is the crux of this chapter. Effective use of personal and time management strategies should help to reduce the probability that a person will feel overly stressed.

Stress can be very high for pharmacy students. Earlier-year (P1-P2) students reported higher stress levels than later-year (P3-P4) students (Votta and Benau, 2013), and 3-year accelerated programs students reported higher stress levels than traditional 4-year program students (Frick et al., 2011). Another study indicated that stress among pharmacy students was partially related to "excessive study load" (Dutta, 2001). Votta and Benau found that coursework, lack of sleep, finances, and grades were reported as the top stressors by pharmacy students (Votta and Benau, 2014). Similarly, Marshall and colleagues reported that the top five triggers of stress for a group of pharmacy students were (Marshall et al., 2008):

1. Family and relationships,
2. Examinations and tests,
3. Monday morning examinations,
4. Outside of class assignments,
5. Financial concerns.

Certainly, lack of sleep and grades might be able to be improved with better time management skills. Other research on consequences of pharmacists' job stress could be informative for students (Table 14-4). It is logical to conclude that what is considered "job stress" for pharmacists could be "school stress" for students or a combination of work and school. Thus, if students feel stressed about school and perhaps their internship, they likely might suffer similar consequences as pharmacists: dissatisfaction with their PharmD program or internship, lower commitment to completing one's degree program or even pharmacy as a career, quitting school or the internship or both, and the potential for substance abuse and burnout.

Thankfully, coworker social support, or the material and emotional support received from one's coworkers, has been shown to buffer the impact of job stress on job dissatisfaction for a number of health professionals, including pharmacy technicians (Desselle and Holmes, 2007). For students, this applies to coworkers and classmates. It is presumed that most pharmacy students probably have a network of friends in their academic class experiencing the same "stress" (at least related to the PharmD program), so a natural buffer exists. How one copes with stress also makes a difference; problem-focused coping strategies, where one attempts to tackle the problems at hand, are most effective in reducing the impact of job stress on job dissatisfaction (Gupchup and Worley-Louis, 2005). Implementing time management strategies could be an example of a problem-focused coping strategy and could certainly help to reduce stress related to excessive study load. Emotion-based coping strategies, such as distancing oneself from the problem or trying to avoid the problem, are unsuccessful (Gupchup and Worley-Louis, 2005). Other strategies to combat stress include meditation and relaxation (e.g., yoga and massage), biofeedback, and physical exercise (Gupchup and Worley-Louis, 2005). Wick and Zanni (2002) suggest a number of strategies for pharmacists, such as:

- Keep a journal and assess your automatic emotional reactions. Ask others for feedback and try to identify new patterns.
- Keep things in perspective. Laugh often and laugh hard.
- Try to connect with people compassionately.
- Recognize that you are not perfect or superhuman.
- Focus on the positive; count your blessings.
- Recognize situations that are beyond your control; act accordingly.
- Identify your successful stress-reducing strategies and avoid stress triggers.
- Manage your environment as well as you can.
- Pay attention to diet, sleep, and exercise.
- Adopt a pet.

Marshall et al. reported that the top five coping strategies pharmacy students used to cope with stress were:

1. Exercising (running and working out),
2. Time with family and friends,

Table 14-4.	Consequences of Job Stress for Pharmacists

- Job dissatisfaction
- Lower commitment to one's organization
- Job turnover (leaving one's job)
- Lower commitment to pharmacy as a career
- Substance abuse potential
- Burnout

Data from Gupchup and Worley, 2005.

3. Napping/sleeping,

4. Watching TV, and

5. Drinking alcohol.

The study prompted investigators to help students use healthy coping strategies vs. those that can have negative consequences.

REVISITING THE SCENARIOS

This chapter has presented a lot of tips and ideas that Krista, Tom, and Ming-Lee may heed so that they can improve their personal and time management skills. Krista likely needs to build in time to take care of herself. Tom may have a routine, but he definitely does not have a system. At the very least, Tom must ask himself some important questions and establish some goals and priorities. He may also consider the use of a master list and implement the use of technology to help him focus on the tasks at hand. We certainly would not want to see him lose his job or have to resign from the school of pharmacy. Ming-Lee will hopefully connect as soon as possible with an advisor or student services for support and strategies during this difficult time. If she doesn't, maybe one of her friends will do so on her behalf. Her situation could easily continue to decline if she does not get some help.

CONCLUSION

The goal of this chapter was to raise awareness about the importance of personal and time management to achieve one's goals while being happy and healthy during pharmacy school and practice. Readers should have come away with concrete strategies and resources about how to improve their skills so that they can achieve their full potential. Remember, time management is not about managing time, it's about managing yourself—and all of us can use some improvement so that we can be more effective in all that we do.

■ QUESTIONS FOR FURTHER DISCUSSION

1. After applying the techniques described in this chapter, are you better able to accomplish your goals?

2. Are you healthier? Why or why not?

3. Are you happier? Why or why not?

4. How can you help others to learn and employ these skills?

5. How can these skills help you as a practitioner?

6. What kinds of personal and time management techniques can you employ in your practice to help improve the process of health care delivery?

7. In addition to time management, what strategies would you employ to reduce your stress level?

REFERENCES

Berger K. 2017. 11 New Year's Resolutions to Improve Pharmacy Work Life. *Pharm Times*. Available at https://www.pharmacytimes.com/contributor/karen-berger/2017/12/11-new-years-resolutions-to-make-pharmacy-work-life-better. Accessed February 25, 2019.

Bodenheimer T, Sinsky C. 2014. From triple to quadruple aim: Care of the patient requires care of the provider. *Ann Fam Med* 12:573–576.

Byrne U. 2005. Work-life balance: Why are we talking about it at all? *Bus Info Rev* 22(1):53–59.

Center C, Davis M, Detre T, et al. 2003. Confronting depression and suicide in physicians: A consensus statement. *JAMA* 289(23):3161–3166.

Covey SR. 1989. *The 7 Habits of Highly Effective People: Restoring the Character Ethic*. New York: Simon & Schuster.

Damian LE, Negru-Subtirica O, Stoeber J, Băban A. 2017. Perfectionistic concerns predict increases in adolescents' anxiety symptoms: A three-wave longitudinal study. *Anx Stress Cop* 30(5):551.

Desselle SP, Holmes ER. 2007. Structural model of certified pharmacy technicians' job satisfaction. *J Am Pharm Assoc* 47:58–72.

Douglass ME, Douglass DN. 1993. *Manage Your Time and Your Work Yourself: The Updated Edition*. New York: AMACOM.

Dutta AP. 2001. Measuring and understanding stress in pharmacy students. Published dissertation, Virginia Commonwealth University.

English T. 2003. Yes, you can find the time: Experts present time management for dummies. *Pharm Stud* 33:16.

Ensman RG. 1991. Time test: How well do you manage time? *Consultant Pharmacist* 6:61.

Evans TM, Bira L, Gastelum JB, Weiss LT, Vanderford NL. 2018. Evidence for a mental health crisis in graduate students. *Nat Biotech* 3(36):282–284.

Frick LJ, Frick JL, Coffman RE, Dey S. 2011. Student stress in a three-year doctor of pharmacy program using a mastery learning educational model. *Am J Pharm Educ* 75(4):Article 64.

Gupchup GV, Worley-Louis MM. 2005. Understanding and managing stress among pharmacists. In Desselle S, Zgarrick D (eds.) *Pharmacy Management*. New York: McGraw-Hill, pp. 52–62.

Henriques G. 2014. College Mental Health Crisis, *Psych Today*. Feb 15. Available at https://www.psychology-today.com/us/blog/theory-knowledge/201402/the-college-student-mental-health-crisis. Accessed March 6, 2019.

Jacobs M. 2002. Time management in the pharmacy: Efficient use of your time will leave more time for your patients. *Wash Pharm*. Autumn:17.

Mandel T, Dunkley DM, Moroz M. 2015. Self-critical perfectionism and depressive and anxious symptoms over 4 years: The mediating role of daily stress reactivity. *J Couns Psych* 62(4):703–717.

Marshall LL, Allison A, Nykamp D, Lanke S. 2008. Perceived stress and quality of life among doctor of pharmacy students. *Am J Pharm Educ* 72:137.

Martín-Perpiñá MM, Viñas Poch F, Malo Cerrato S. 2019. Media multitasking impact in homework, executive function and academic performance in Spanish adolescents. Psicothema 31(1):81–87.

Milanovic R. 2014. 7 Time Management Tips for the Digital Age. *Soc Media Today*. March 13. Available at http://www.socialmediatoday.com/content/7-time-management-tips-digital-age. Accessed March 6, 2019.

Morgenstern J. 2000. *Time Management from the Inside Out: The Foolproof System for Taking Control of Your Schedule—and Your Life*. New York: Holt, Available at http://www.bridgewaypartners.com/WhoWeAre/Principals/MarilynPaulPhD.aspx. Accessed March 6, 2019.

Reid RJ, Coleman K, Johnson EA, et al. 2010. The Group Health medical home at year two: cost savings, higher patient satisfaction, and less burnout for providers. *Health Aff* (Millwood) 29(5):835–843.

Rochon J. 2003. Developing relationships is an essential aspect of your practice. *Wash Pharm*. Summer:9.

Uncapher MR, Lin L, Rosen LD, et al. 2017. Media multitasking and cognitive, psychological, neural, and learning differences. *Pediatrics* 140(Suppl 2): S62–S66.

Votta RJ, Benau EM. 2013. Predictors of stress among doctor of pharmacy students: Results of a nationwide survey. *Curr Pharm Teach Learn* 5(5):365–372.

Votta RJ, Benau EM. 2014. Sources of stress for pharmacy students in a nationwide sample. *Curr Pharm Teach Learn* 6(5):675–681.

White SJ. 2007. Working efficiently. *Am J Health Syst Pharm* 64:1587.

Wick JY, Zanni GR. 2002. Stress in the pharmacy: Changing the experience. *J Am Pharm Assoc* 42(1): 16–20.

Woodhull AV. 1997. *The New Time Manager*. Brookfield, VT: Gower.

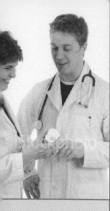

15

NEGOTIATION SKILLS

Mitch Barnett and Eric Fromhart

About the authors: Mitch Barnett is an associate professor with Touro University College of Pharmacy in California and an adjunct (clinical) associate professor with the University of Iowa College of Pharmacy. Dr. Barnett received his BS degree in pharmacy, MS in pharmacy administration, and PharmD from the University of Iowa. He has published numerous articles and is a frequent reviewer and served on the editorial boards for several peer-reviewed journals. Dr. Barnett's research focuses on using pharmacy claims data to adjust for comorbidity and severity of illness, the implementation of pharmacy guidelines in practice, and the measurement of pharmacy faculty workload and stress. He maintains an active full-time practice at Ryan Pharmacy, an independent community pharmacy located in rural Iowa.

Eric Fromhart is CEO of Secure340B, a company he founded to bridge the gap between independent pharmacies and health care providers participating in the 340B Drug Pricing Program. He has served as guest speaker at national conferences and delivers many workshops on pricing and on contracting with third-party payers throughout the country. Eric is an expert in 340B contracting and negotiations.

■ LEARNING OBJECTIVES

After completing this chapter, readers should be able to

1. Identify different types of negotiation styles.
2. Describe the attributes of a positional-driven negotiation.
3. Describe the attributes and proper usage of a principled-driven negotiation.
4. Differentiate between positional- versus principle-driven negotiation approaches.
5. Discuss the use of motivational interviewing (MI) in the context of negotiating, and provide examples of its use.
6. Identify the steps involved in MI, i.e., Desire, Ability, Reasoning, Need, Commitment, Activation, and Taking Steps (DARN CAT).

■ SCENARIO

Gary Rosen, PharmD, has been practicing pharmacy in a variety of settings since graduating from pharmacy school several years ago. Owning an independent pharmacy has been a dream of Gary's since entering pharmacy school. Gary and his family decide to move to a small town and purchase the town's sole independent community pharmacy, Taylors Drug Store. The pharmacy has served patients in town for 30 years, has a reputation as a pillar in the community, and maintains a good working relationship with the local hospital and its providers. However, over the years, Taylors Drug Store has been impacted by many changes in the health care environment, specifically in the pharmacy industry: pharmacy benefits manager (PBM) involvement, reimbursement cuts, chain pharmacy expansion, regulations, competition, fluctuating drug prices, specialty pharmacy, discounts, and chargeback or rebate (e.g., direct and indirect remuneration [DIR] fees). Faced with adapting to these changes, Gary has begun looking at alternative, creative methods to remain competitive, sustain profitability, and continue serving the community as a pharmacy owner. Gary quickly realizes that nearly all of the potential opportunities will require him to explore new agreements (or significantly expand existing ones) to be successful as the new owner. Gary is worried that he may lack the proper skills or tools necessary to negotiate effectively, but believes he likely has some time before having to worry about a high stakes negotiation.

Shortly after the purchase of the pharmacy, Gary is approached by the local Critical Access Hospital to participate as a contract pharmacy in their 340B program. The hospital, referred to as the "Covered Entity," operates a small primary care clinic in town as well. Prescribers affiliated with the hospital and/or primary care clinic (i.e., the Covered Entity) write 35% of Taylor's drug store prescriptions and represent a great deal of the store's business and revenue. The 340B program requires manufacturers, in order to be reimbursed by Medicaid and Medicare, to offer deep discounts on outpatient prescription drugs to "Covered Entities" that qualify. These Covered Entity facilities generally operate in underserved areas and rural communities such as the one served by Gary's drug store.

In lieu of investing in and operating in-house retail pharmacies to procure and dispense discounted medications, Covered Entities usually outsource the opportunity to local retail pharmacies by establishing contracts to fill and dispense 340B drugs to their patient population. Through this arrangement, the retail pharmacy collects reimbursements and copays from a patient and/or their insurance and the Covered Entity re-supplies the pharmacy with inventory purchased at the discounted 340B price. Uninsured patients are able to access prescription drugs at a savings, while patients with prescription coverage can also generate benefits to program participants (Covered Entity and participating pharmacies) as well. Based on the contract negotiated, the pharmacy remits a portion of the collected reimbursement back to the Covered Entity to pay the cost of the replenished inventory. Since the cost is deeply discounted, there are often significant "savings" or margins generated to Covered Entities between the amount due from the pharmacy and the 340B drug cost. This is commonly known as a "340B Contract Pharmacy" arrangement.

What began as a simple concept (340B Program) to offer discounted medications to those in need has grown more complex over time, as a new industry was born and opportunity has arisen. Each with their own unique set of challenges and realities, Covered Entities and pharmacies have much at stake when establishing 340B Contract Pharmacy arrangements. There are unique risks and benefits to both parties. The contract negotiation is the single-most critical component in determining the long-term success and sustainability of the partnership.

Gary is faced with the task of negotiating a successful contract with a major player and driver of his business. While there is an opportunity for Gary to increase his margins and to finance additional services for his patients, the potential also exists to accept a contract with less than favorable terms for his pharmacy. Gary believes the Covered Entity may have the upper hand in the negotiation and fears they may simply present a "take it or leave it" approach with little room for negotiation. At the same time, Gary fears a hard-nosed approach to negotiating the 340B contract may alienate the prescribers upon whom his business is dependent.

■ CHAPTER QUESTIONS

1. What are some of the common workplace situations and settings involving a pharmacist that might require a negotiation?
2. What are some of the consequences of approaching a negotiation from a positional style approach (an approach with a clear winner and loser)?
3. How might a principled centered style approach be used to uncover a solution that is not immediately apparent to either party at the beginning of the negotiation process?
4. How might a best alternative to a negotiated agreement, or BATNA, prevent you from entering into a poor agreement?
5. How might MI be useful to a pharmacist in successful negotiations with another client or stakeholder?

■ INTRODUCTION

John F. Kennedy Presidential Inaugural Address: "Let us never negotiate out of fear. But let us never fear to negotiate."

Negotiations take place routinely throughout pharmacy practice in every setting. These may include self-motivating a patient to be more adherent to a medication regimen, discussing the final details with a technician regarding her promotion, getting a prescriber to change an order to a less expensive or more appropriate medication, or getting a helpdesk representative from a PBM to grant a prior authorization or early refill override for a patient. All these examples involve some type of a negotiation on your part as a pharmacist.

Negotiations can occur over various length of time. In general, short-term negotiations leave less room to navigate, while long-term negotiations generally offer more opportunities. Both short-term and long-term negotiations may have low or high stakes, and may have near-term or far-reaching rewards or consequences. Many people will traditionally approach negotiations as a pyramid style discussion or arrangement; in other words, with a clear top-down hierarchy and a clear winner and loser. For example, imagine a parent with a fussy toddler or a substitute teacher thrown into a class of unruly middle school students. In these examples, there is clearly a pyramid style structure, and it is easy to identify the likely "winner" in these scenarios. They are steeped in tradition with a clear hierarchy of control and enforcement. Imagine, however, a relationship between a pharmacist and a patient or a relief pharmacist and the pharmacy's most trusted technician. There is not such an easily identifiable top-down structure with expected norms to which might be adhered. Additionally, you might envision the relationship between a large chain pharmacy and a large PBM or a large hospital pharmacy network and the largest employer in the region. There may be several individuals involved in a negotiation, and the same or different individuals involved in simultaneous or ongoing negotiations or multiple negotiations. There also may be representatives or other third parties brought in on the negotiations, e.g., government regulators, stakeholders or investors, legal counselors, and/or even the news media.

■ TRADITIONAL NEGOTIATING STYLES (HOW TO WIN ENEMIES AND ALIENATE PEOPLE)

Traditional negotiating styles can often be thought of in terms of a battle or sports competition, usually with a clear winner (party that is the victor) and loser (party that has been defeated). Negotiations may be drawn out over a long period of time, sometimes stretching out over a number of years. It may involve multiple parties, who may come and go or suddenly change roles in mid-negotiation. There may be little progress at times, where things seem to drag on or even come to a standstill, only to suddenly move quickly at the next stage. Feelings often run strong, and individuals may have passionate views, which only become stronger when the other party tries to change or discount those views. It is little wonder that most people fear and thus try to avoid negotiating. People are often left feeling worn down, have lingering doubts about being cheated, and are overall somewhat dissatisfied with the outcome (often the case with the process of buying a new car, even if you love the car, itself).

The academic study of negotiation can be traced backed to John Nash's 1950s articles in *Econometrica* on cooperative gaming theory (see the movie, "A Beautiful Mind"). In Nash's seminal articles, he argued that there is a solution or equilibrium (Nash equilibrium) for each finite game if each player has chosen a strategy, and no player can benefit by changing their strategy or choice if other players are forced to keep their strategy or choice unchanged (Nash, 1950, 1953). If Bill and Ted are playing the game, they are said to be in a Nash equilibrium if Bill is making the best decision he can, taking into account Ted's possible decisions. This solution operates under the assumption that neither can change his decision once it is revealed. Applied, Nash's theory of equilibrium predicts what will happen in a decision-making process, but requires that each player know the other players' decisions to maximize their own strategy. It involves a level of trust and cooperation for both players to "win." Such a game is often described in story format called the "deer hunt" or the "prisoner's dilemma."

In the deer hunt example, two players (hunters) each require the cooperation of the other hunter in order to succeed and capture a large prize (the deer). A hunter is able to capture a small prize (rabbit) by themselves, but a rabbit has much less meat and is therefore less desirable for a hunter than splitting a deer. If one player goes after a rabbit, then neither will get a deer, as doing so requires their mutual cooperation. If a hunter has chosen to go after the deer, hoping their partner will do the same, but the other party chooses instead to go after a rabbit,

the former will get neither and go hungry (no prize). In this example, the Nash equilibrium (greatest payout) would appear to be for both hunters to cooperate and go after the deer, assuming the meat yielded from half a deer is substantially more than a single rabbit. However, there are actually two valid Nash solutions here. One is that risk-averse hunters go after the rabbit (to have something to eat) and one in which they cooperate and go after the deer (have plenty to eat). If one hunter is going after the deer, they will often go to great lengths to communicate or let the other hunter know of their intentions to hunt the deer before the other hunter commits to their decision, thus yielding the most efficient outcome of both of them hunting the deer (and lots of meat). You can imagine endless scenarios where a researcher or investigator offers different prizes for cooperation or acting alone to study human behavior as opposed to sending people out hunting. What would you do if you were in such an experiment and the cooperation or large prize was $10,000 and the prize for acting alone was $10? Does your answer change if the cooperation prize is $100 and the prize for acting alone prize is $99? Does your answer change based on whether the other player is a trusted friend or a complete stranger?

Now imagine that two bank robbers are apprehended shortly after their big heist and are both being questioned in separate rooms away from each other. The interrogator offers each robber an opportunity to implicate the other, in exchange for a lighter sentence for themselves. If neither robber (prisoner) implicates the other, they are both likely to be found guilty, but each will serve only a single year in jail. However, if only one of the robbers implicates the other, the one being implicated will serve 3 years in jail, while the other robber (who was not implicated by his partner in crime) will be set free. If both robbers (prisoners) implicate each other, they will both have to serve 2 full years in jail each. In this situation, although it may not be clear at first, each robber's best option is to implicate the other when given the knowledge that the other robber is being offered the same chance to "defect." Thus, while the overall best outcome would be for both robbers to cooperate and not implicate each other, the individual robber's best option is to turn on their partner. The Nash equilibrium in the "Prisoner's Dilemma" is thus for both prisoners to defect, and for neither robber to cooperate and help the other by remaining silent. As highlighted above, Nash equilibrium solutions need not be efficient. Solutions also tend to become increasingly complicated with more players and may result in seemingly illogical solutions. An extension of Nash's game theory has also been applied to explain pharmacy contract negotiations between pharmacies and large PBMs or insurers (Brooks et al., 1999). In this study, the negotiating or bargaining power of independent versus chain pharmacies was modeled using actual reimbursement claims data. The results suggested that the negotiating power of the independent pharmacies is hampered when preventing (through anti-trust laws) their ability to communicate their intentions to each other. Such unintended or illogical equilibrium solutions in the health care marketplace are often the result of well-intended laws or policy decisions.

Table 15-1.	Types of Negotiation Philosophies in Positional and Principled Bargaining

- Win-Lose (Positional bargaining)
  - Authoritarian, competitive, little flexibility
- Lose-Win (Positional bargaining)
  - Appeasing, capitulate, "give-in" to maintain the relationship
- Lose-Lose (Positional bargaining)
  - Entrenched positions, won't agree at any cost, willing to accept a lose or a negative so other side doesn't win
  - May be vindictive and focused on getting even or extracting revenge
- Win-Win (Principled bargaining)
  - Cooperation, both parties committed to a larger goal or mutual benefit. Generally, the most sustainable long-term approach to keep both parties engaged.

Data from Fisher, 2011; Covey, 2004; Clay-Williams, 2018.

■ POSITIONAL VERSUS PRINCIPLED NEGOTIATION

With positional negotiations, the goal is winning, or a victory. Positions of one or both parties are bounded and often at opposing ends of a spectrum. The positional negotiating process generally starts (and ends) with entrenched positions. A party using the positional approach to negotiations will try to appeal to the other party's emotions (good or bad, soft or hard). In positional negotiations, a party tries to convince the other party that they are right, or that the other party has some obligation compelling them to accept their terms. In other words, a party using positional negotiation techniques tries to sway the other party to see their side or agree to their position. A hallmark of positional negotiations is the use of the "F" word—"Fair." A person using a positional style of negotiation may exclaim that a proposal is "unfair" for them, while a party trying to convince another of their position may state that they have a made a "fair" offer, or that the deal is "fair" and therefore needs to accepted. Different types of negotiation principles are listed and briefly described in Table 15-1.

The typical haggling process is often a product of positional negotiations, and a common outcome of positional negotiation is to "meet-in-the-middle" or "split-the-difference." Think of the typical marketplace transaction with a single buyer and seller where the price of the good is listed, but generally expected to be flexible. A more specific example is the listing price for a new car or the price of a house. With few exceptions, the listed price in these two examples can generally be thought of as the upward position of the seller, be it the real estate agency or the car dealer. The buyer then begins the haggling process by initially offering an amount less than the listed price. A common tactic is for the buyer to offer an initial amount approximately equal to the listed price minus the amount they are willing to pay, subtracted from the amount they are willing to pay. For example, if the listed price is $12,000 and the buyer is willing to pay

$10,000, the buyer may begin the haggling process with an offer of $8,000. In this example, if the seller is willing to sell for $10,000, there will likely be a predictable series of back and forth offers in increasingly smaller adjustments until the buyer and seller meet at a price very near $10,000. Note, that there can be some efficiencies inherent in this style of negotiation. Specifically, if both parties have a clear expectation that a haggling process will occur, an agreement may be reached relatively quickly with both sides having invested very little outside time or resources in the negotiating effort.

Alternatively, one party may ultimately "give in" to preserve the relationship in a positional bargaining situation. People in negotiations often incorrectly assume that if they "give in" this time, the other party will "owe" them the next time, or expect the other party to be more flexible the next time. Note, that in the real world this seldom happens. Rather, parties that are convinced they have won a positional negotiation will generally expect to win the next round of negotiations, because of a history of success or getting what they want.

With principled negotiation, the focus is on the problem, not the people or their positions. If numbers are used, they should be based on actual or objective data from real-world examples. Skilled negotiators communicate their interests and put the problem before the answer. They are willing to learn, invent, and invite options. They bear in mind that the other party in the negotiation is/are people with emotions, feelings, and opinions. The other party may have a cultural background different from yours, so you cannot assume that they share your values or interests. A key to this approach is communication with no predetermined position. The impetus here is not to convince the other party of your principles, but rather in finding solutions within both sides' principles. It employs the use of illustrations, not demands. It uses objective data and agreed upon standards. The principled negotiator must be willing to discover, reason, and be open to reason. They concentrate on merits and resist the temptation to attack or defend. They listen and try to understand the other side. They ask

questions in attempting to do so. They often discover other options where neither side has to compromise. They consider many ideas before agreeing on one. They create multiple solutions versus just single options. If the other party shares your goals and values, they are more likely to agree with your proposals. Likewise, the other party is more likely to agree and become motivated when they have had input in drafting the proposals and when the options seem reasonable and legitimate.

When the focus is in the problem at hand instead of the people involved, you are less likely to have emotions and egos driving the decisions, and parties are less likely to become entrenched into a predetermined position. The problem-versus-people focus can be illustrated with an example of two cooks and a single lemon. Imagine a television cooking show competition involving two chefs and a basket of ingredients, which they must share. Both chefs have a recipe calling for an entire lemon, but the basket contains a single lemon, and thus they must negotiate a solution—one not involving the use of sharp knives used as weapons to obtain the lemon! The chefs may likely negotiate a solution where each gets a portion of the lemon, perhaps half a lemon each. In other words, using a position-centered approach, each will gain a portion of what they want and agree to give in or lose a portion of want they want in the name of negotiation and fairness. To an outside observer or arbitrator, it may even seem reasonable to suggest one chef gets to cut the lemon while the other chef gets to choose which half they would like. Imagine though that the chefs first explain or discuss their reasons for wanting the lemon, or take a more principle-centered approach. Discussing their intent or recipes further, they discover that one recipe requires the juice from a whole lemon, while the other recipe requires the rind from an entire lemon. In this hypothetical example, there is a simple principle-centered solution where each chef could get what they wanted to complete their respective recipes without compromising their needs. Such principled-centered solutions, or collaborations, have also been described in health care and pharmacy settings as a useful management style to resolve interpersonal conflicts, versus compromising, directing, or avoiding conflict resolutions styles (Austin et al., 2010; Sportsman et al., 2002). Read more about conflict resolution in Chapter 3.

As mentioned previously, the hallmark of principle-centered negotiations is communication. It has even been said that the three most important aspects of principle-centered negotiation are communication, communication, and communication. There are of course entire books written on communication and the science and art of communication, so the approach taken in this chapter is brief. Standard advice for improved communication includes becoming a good or active listener with frequent feedback to the other party to indicate you understand what they are saying. Note that understanding and providing feedback to the other party does not have to entail agreeing with them, only an acknowledgment that you have heard and understand what they are trying to say. When communicating to the other party, give them an opportunity to ask questions or provide feedback and reflect on what you have said. Speak in terms of you, not them. For example, "I feel let down" will often be received by the other party in a more favorable light than "You let me down." Lastly, communicate with a purpose. While small talk can be great to get things going, do not let it interfere or become the sole focus of the communication. Sometimes a little silence can speak volumes, and those with little to say can speak the most.

In his negotiations with the Covered Entity, Gary has surmised that communication is going to be key. Gary discovers that previous work has shown that compromise and avoidance are frequently used styles for communication in a health care setting, in addition to competitive and accommodative styles of communication (Austin et al., 2009). Gary further learns that a collaborative style is likely the superior approach and decides to approach the negotiations with the Covered Entity as an opportunity for all parties to get the needed ingredients for a successful recipe.

Closely related to communication is the invitation or exploration of options. Brainstorming or roundtable type discussions can be a great forum to reprioritize the goals of the negotiation and explore or invent options before the list of final recommendations are narrowed down and a final decision is made. During the discussion, resist the temptation to label something "their problem" or an item "none of their concern." Rather, you should welcome critique and explore mutually beneficial ways to work together on all the issues at hand. Frequently, one party may have a simple solution to an issue or concern that may seem insurmountable to the other party. An example is the patient at the pharmacy who is unwilling to pay for their expensive prescription because they believe it may not work, and a prescriber who is unwilling to change the order to a less expensive alternative. How might a pharmacist approach this seemingly intractable situation after a discussion with both the patient and the prescriber? Perhaps the pharmacist in this situation offers to dispense a 3-day supply to the patient as a trial. In this simple example, the patient, prescriber, and pharmacist are all getting a likely benefit from the solution. Look to discover solutions that are low-cost and high benefit to each party. These are the solutions that have a high likelihood of being accepted and ultimately successful.

Regardless of the path to the solutions or possibilities, they should ideally be based on reliable objective data with mutually acceptable standards. Viewpoints and likes and dislikes are based in culture and are highly subjective. Data, however, should be relatively independent of the viewer's culture and free of opinion. It is also much easier to defend data as opposed to an opinion. Negotiations are less tense and move smoothly when objective criteria and standards of fairness are utilized, as no one side digs in to a predetermined side and appears weak if/when they move away from the position. You are encouraged to ask to the other party the theory behind a figure or how they arrived at those numbers. Mutually agreed upon standards should generate similar data regardless of the side generating the numbers. One should reason, and be open to reason but not yield to pressure. Your principles, not your positions should guide the negotiation.

If you or the other party cannot arrive at an agreement, strive for a recommendation in its place. A recommendation can also be useful if the party you are negotiating with is not the ultimate or final decision maker. In this instance, arriving at "I'm going to recommend to the board," or "I'm going to take to the directors my recommendation that we proceed with this solution," may be an acceptable ending point.

Much like the description found on the label on a bottle of a fine wine (or a lesser bottle trying to pass itself off as a bottle of fine wine), principle-centered negotiation involves being concrete, with notes of flexibility and a nod to creativity. It is well-grounded and intellectually satisfying; it is mature, structured, and well-balanced. It is likely to have a delightfully surprising but honest finish. The principle-centered negotiator must resist the desire to make a decision until all complexities and subtleties have played out.

■ BATNA (BEST ALTERNATIVE TO NEGOTIATED AGREEMENT)

It is a good idea to have a best alternative to a negotiated agreement (BATNA) with a principled negotiation style. The BATNA can be thought of as a reset option or "tripwire" which causes a pause or exit from the negotiation process. A BATNA should be driven by analyses, and is often much better than some arbitrary or predetermined bottom line. Additionally, consider the various facets of a BATNA. If you can use your BATNA to obtain extra time, hitting the tripwire may not mean the "end of the deal." If you have a predetermined and reasonable BATNA, you are more likely to feel empowered and confident heading into the negotiation process. The power in a negotiation comes from either or both parties being able to "walk away" from the table. You will have a clear idea of your "walk away" or exit point by having a carefully thought-out BATNA, which serves to protect you from accepting an outcome worse than rejecting all proposals and exiting the negotiations. Remember, the goal of negotiating is to arrive at an agreement better than your BATNA, or the best alternative you would have with no negotiations. While you are certainly not obligated to reveal or even discuss your BATNA with the other party, doing so may be in your best interest at times during the negotiation process. Examples may include when the other party has not carefully considered all the possible options available or when they appear to be stalling for time with no apparent intent on returning to negotiations. Divulging (all or a portion) of your BATNA may be useful in these instances to refocus and re-engage the other party in the process. Regardless of your decision of disclosure, your BATNA should be determined by exploring options and basing the predicted outcomes on actual data or objective measures. If you follow this guideline, you will not only be able to explain your BATNA to the other party (if you decide to reveal it) but also be able to defend it if necessary. Skilled negotiators know that if they cannot defend or explain their BATNA to themselves, it is unlikely the other party will accept it as fact, if disclosed. Negotiating without a defined BATNA is negotiating blindly and is ill-advised. If a proposed agreement is better than your BATNA, you should generally accept it or continue trying to negotiate a more favorable proposal. If negotiations are closed, or the proposal cannot be improved, it should be rejected in favor of the BATNA. Note that a BATNA need not be rigid, and may change during the discussion if other options are uncovered during the negotiation process. Generally, the party with the best BATNA has an advantage during negotiations, so it may be useful to try and determine the other party's BATNA.

As such, steps in the principle-centered negotiation process are summarized and briefly explained in Table 15-2.

Referring back the chapter scenario, Gary has learned about and read up on having a BATNA. He had previously conducted a cost-of-dispensing analysis that took into account all of his costs, but also the costs from losing customers who might shop for additional nonprescription items. He has identified what are somewhat "typical" of contracts between Covered Entities and pharmacies. Gary has also

Table 15-2.	Four Aspects to Principle-Centered Style Negotiation

People. Separate the people (negotiators) from the problem or issue at hand

Interests. Focus on (mutual) interests, not the positions

Options. Invent and invite multiple options, particularly ones with mutual gains before making a decision or coming to an agreement

Criteria. Insist that the result (final outcome) be based on an objective standards or criteria. Ideally one that can be replicated by both sides using data

Adapted from Fisher, 2011.

talked with other health practitioners and administrators from various hospitals and has gained a much finer appreciation for what Critical Access Hospital and its patients have to gain and lose by contracting with Taylors pharmacy. He will enter the negotiation process with data, empathy for other players in the negotiation, and with a BATNA from his perspective.

■ NEGOTIATE AS IF YOUR LIFE DEPENDED ON IT

Principle-driven negotiation can help you get to the table. Now what? In Voss and Raz's best-selling book, "*Never Split the Difference*," he provides some insight gleaned from a decades-long career as a hostage negotiator for the FBI. In essence, he asks what one would do when actually entrenched in a high-stake negotiation situation. Voss and Raz stress to try to negotiate face-to-face, or over the web or phone as a second choice, since much communication is nonverbal. As mentioned above, communication is key, and it is paramount in effective communication to actively listen to the other party. Voss and Raz state that the three most important things in negotiating are Listening, Listening, and Listening. Use the listening process to uncover issues and be ready for surprises. An experienced negotiator will use her skill to reveal the surprises that are almost certain to exist in any negotiating situation.

Voss and Raz goes through the steps in how he tries to approach tense negotiations, including many that involve a life-or-death situation. These steps include using a calm, late-night "disc jockey (DJ) voice." A voice that is calm, strong, yet not overly aggressive can slow the cadence of conversation and diffuse anger. They then suggests to use a simple "I'm sorry," followed by a mirrored or reflective statement based on what the other party just stated or demanded, but posed in the form of a question. Finally, follow the mirroring statement with a few seconds of silence to allow the other party to hear what you are saying in their words. Repeat this process as needed. Imagine an upset or angry patient at the pharmacy who demands to have a prescription filled immediately. The pharmacy student, using a calm and soothing voice responds, "I am sorry, it seems like you are in a hurry. Do you need this prescription filled immediately?" This is followed by a few seconds of silence to allow the patient the chance to speak next. The patient in this situation is likely to rephrase their request, but in a calmer, less threatening manner or tone. "Yes, I would like the prescription filled as soon as you can, but I can see you are busy, so I realize I may have to wait a few minutes." The pharmacy student in this situation just used a common technique to quickly and calmly diffuse a tense situation as opposed to escalating it. Voss goes on to state that using tactful empathy has served him well as a high stakes FBI negotiator. He recommends repeating phrases back to the other party and using terms such as "It sounds like," "It seems like," and "It looks like" to defuse negative situations and rebalance power. This technique relabels the negative comments. It is important to remember that generally one is negotiating with people who want to be appreciated and understood.

With negotiating, being right is not as important as getting in the right mindset. Do not commit to assumptions; view them as hypotheses. Test scenarios during the listening process and solicit feedback from the other party. Remember, the goal with communication during a negotiation is not to conquer, or change someone's long-held views, but rather to uncover useful information. It is important to remember that all negotiations are defined by norms and the other party's environment. Be sensitive to others. People, almost universally, are more likely to comply or follow through if they feel like they have had a hand in the agreement and have been treated respectfully. Give others a chance to weigh in. People from many cultures have been shown to be risk averse. That is, they tend to stick with what is safe and known versus an unknown.

■ BEWARE THE YES; INSTEAD, LEARN TO START FROM NO

Voss and Raz state that most meaningful negotiations begin with a "No," which seems paradoxical. However, they succinctly argues that a "No" often begins the negotiation process (see Table 15-3). Nonetheless, he stresses not to take a "No" then simply leave the negotiation process. Rather, use it as an opening to ask for clarifications and identify opportunities. He further elaborates that "No" may mean many things, including: I'm not comfortable, I need some additional information, or I don't quite understand. Once you have some additional clarification or information, see if the other party is open to revisiting the topic. Voss and Raz also highlight that you should strive toward a "That's right" (which signals an understanding), and is often more powerful than "Yes." An early "Yes" may be noncommittal and used simply as a way to save time with another party that is planning to "weasel out" later. Do not negotiate to "Yes," negotiate from "No" and get to "How." Voss claims that "How" is really the key, and a yes without a how may be meaningless. Use terms like "how do we proceed?," "when do we meet again?," "what would you like me to do as a follow up?" as non-confrontational phrases to re-engage the other party and move to a "How." Remember, How only happens when the other party intends to act, after the agreement and following the Yes (see Table 15-4).

Table 15-3.	Voss' Recommendations for Approaching Tense Situations

Reassure. Use a calm, reassuring voice. Smile and people will generally smile back—this technique often works with the inflection or tone in your voice. Be mindful of your tone and use your voice as an opportunity to convey warmth and trust to the other party.

Mirror. Mirroring is the technique of repeating what someone has said, especially if said in an angry or demanding tone, in the form of a question. When mirrored, people will usually provide more information and elaborate what they just said in a less assertive tone.

Empathize. Try to instill a sense of understanding by conveying a sense of understanding or what the other person must be feeling. It is not necessarily agreeing with someone, only acknowledging that you understand them.

Employ labeling. Use phrases such as, "I understand" or "It seems like you…" to communicate a sense of empathy and understanding.

Slow down, use silence. When you slow a situation down, you have a chance to calm it down.

Data from Voss, 2016.

Table 15-4.	Useful Standby Phrases to Use During Negotiations

What about this issue is most important to you?

How can I help make this situation better for both of us?

How would you like me to proceed, what do you need from me in terms of next step(s)?

Can you think of some ways we can solve this problem?

What are we trying to accomplish here, what is the objective?

How I am supposed to do that?

Data from Voss, 2016.

Don't be afraid to use "No" tactfully. A "No" can be used as a tool to intentionally slow the negotiation process and seek additional time. A "No" may also allow real issues to be brought up. People generally do not like to say no. Voss and Raz suggest that when dealing with a party you are trying to move forward, try asking if they have given up on the project, rather than whether or not they still interested. "Have you given up on this project?" will generally illicit a quicker and more favorable response than "would you like to continue with this project or agreement." Finally, there are times when a "No" may be better than a bad deal. Think of a couple who are planning an evening on the town to celebrate a special occasion. If the wife wishes that her husband wear his black suit, while he prefers to wear his blue suit, a "No" by either party may prevent a mismatched blue coat-black pants scenario as a compromise.

Negotiation Types

Voss and Raz distill negotiators into three main types: analytical, accommodator, and assertive. Being able to recognize which of these types or styles you are, as well as which type you are dealing with, can be helpful to you as a negotiator. Analytical types tend to be methodical and diligent. They tend to move "slowly" as long as they are working in a systematic manner. They like to be thought of as minimizing errors and mistakes. Voss and Raz note that analytical types tend to work alone and rarely deviate from a schedule or task. They are detail-oriented and can come across as cool or even cold, but are generally thought of as being fair, if firm. They hate surprises and do not like to be unprepared. Do not expect immediate answers or decisions from them. They will often want to go back and reanalyze any new pieces of information or counter offer. The next type of negotiating style is the accommodator. The most important thing to these types of negotiators is building the relationship. They are generally most happy when they are doing the communication and will generally error on the side of keeping their counterpart happy. Voss and Raz note that these types are often easy to talk to and get along with, although they tend to be somewhat poor time managers. Another potential downside to accommodators is that sometimes agree to things, even when they cannot deliver, just to be agreeable. The final type is the assertive negotiator. The assertive type insists that time is money and wants to get things done or accomplished even if they are not perfect or the best solution. The assertive type is very aware of their output or accomplishments and love winning above all else. They tend to be very direct and candid. If they make a concession, they will expect something in return. If you make a concession, they may be oblivious to it; they focus on their own goals and not yours. The assertive type prefers to tell and not ask. Appreciate that the three types generally view time as a resource differently as well as silence. Finally, never assume that your counterpart thinks like you—especially if they are a different type.

Remember, regardless the type of negotiator, your counterpart likely has constituents who will hold them accountable for a bad agreement. Be mindful of this and be respectful and reasonable. Try to treat others involved in the negotiation process as you would like to be treated, ideally honestly and fairly at all times.

Dirty Tricks

A discussion of negotiation skills would be remiss if it were not to mention some of the "dirty tricks" that a dishonest or high-pressure negotiator might employ. These tricks are presented here so as to make them recognizable by the user when undertaken by another party. These should not be thought of as acceptable styles or options for negotiating in good faith, but rather red flags, that when identified, should give you caution or pause in continuing the negotiation process with the other party.

Good cop, bad cop. This is a common tag-team or buddy approach in negotiating where one side will bring in at least two people. One person will present a very stern or unpleasant offer using a very dire or hardened approach. The job of the other person on the team is to be very affable and present what appears to be a much more agreeable or pleasant option. Presented with this situation, most people will naturally feel an affiliation to the more friendly party and may readily accept the more agreeable option with little thought or consideration. Be wary of anyone claiming to be on "your side" or offering to help you out when they clearly should have an allegiance to another party. The buddy approach can also be used to wear down, or tire out the other party in the negotiation process. Think of the couple at the car dealership who are paraded through a seemingly endless series of offices before being allowed to finish the final paperwork. A good rule of thumb is to try and have an approximately equal number of people representing all sides of an important negotiation and to plan for scheduled breaks.

Deliberate deception or lying. Probably the hardest tactic to defend against in negotiations is one where one side knowingly presents "made up" or erroneous data to make a point or influence another party's decision. Here is where you want to do your due diligence. Rather than having to accept another party's numbers or analyses as fact, rely on your own homework for guidance.

Ridiculous offers. Extreme or ridiculous offers or even escalating offers or demands are common in negotiations played out in a public arena or forum. Prime examples include peace negotiations or labor employment talks. Be aware that such negotiators may be trying to strengthen their position or may be trying to manipulate the negotiation process by anonymously leaking information to a third party or the public.

Ambiguous authority. Beware the party who negotiates a final agreement with you, only to have to then take it to their boss or board for final approval. Find out who has the authority to negotiate what at the start of the negotiation process. This will prevent you from having what you think is a good faith agreement being used against you as a ceiling for a second round of negotiations.

Psychological warfare and personal attacks or threats. Avoid the temptation to return the personal attacks or threats with like comments. When negotiations are taking place in front of others, remember that the other party may be making demands more for show than for good faith bargaining efforts. If you see this happening, try to refocus the negotiations on the problem. You can question the tactic, but should not question the integrity of a person.

Beware the deadline imposed by the other party. Informal or arbitrary deadlines are often used by unscrupulous negotiators to give a since of urgency to a negation. Realize that many deadlines are informal, and even formal deadlines can often be extended when it is in the interest of both parties. Eventually you will enter into a negotiation with someone using one of the above "dirty tricks"— if you have not already encountered such a situation. One defense against the above tactics is to refocus the negotiations on the issue at hand and away from the people involved. If possible, try to engage the other party in a principle-centered style negotiation. It is likely easier and more beneficial to reform the issue at hand rather than the people doing the negotiating. Good natured humor and suggesting a break can also be useful to defuse tense or unconformable situations. Being prepared is another good strategy; it is harder to be taken advantage of when you are well prepared and have studied the issues. It is always easier to define a well thought out principle than a deceitful tactic. Above all else, do not fall prey or allow yourself to be pressured into a bad agreement just because the other party has resorted to using one or more of these tactics. There is no shame in walking away from a shady or deceitful proposition.

Gary has encountered dirty tricks with negotiations in the past and has also heard from other pharmacy owners that while many insurers and other clients operate in good faith, some have resorted to dirty tricks. Gary has prepared accordingly by having data and making sure that he will be negotiating up front with the right person(s)—preferably on a one-to-one basis in person. Gary has further investigated the actual deadlines required for the contracts and requests that any discussions remain confidential until after a potential agreement is signed.

■ MOTIVATIONAL INTERVIEWING AS A NEGOTIATING TOOL

MI, or as some refer to it, motivational conversation, is a style of evidence-based change management that is often useful in negotiations. Use of MI has been shown in research to help resolve ambivalent attitudes and improve the success of initiatives and acceptance of new ideas (Grimolizzi-Jensen, 2018), including salary negotiations (Berman and Gottlieb, 2019). The hallmark of MI is to strengthen the other party's motivation or commitment to a new idea or option. Imagine a situation where the other person or party bluntly states, "I'm not willing to agree to any part of that offer—end of story." There exists a continuum of communication styles one might choose to respond to this statement. This spectrum or continuum as described by Miller and Rollnick in their book, *Motivational Interviewing, Helping People Change*, ranges from a directing type of style (command, decide, order) to a guiding type of style (assist, encourage, support), on to a following type of style (comprehend, listen, understand). MI lives in the middle ground (guiding style), in between directing and following. Miller and Rollnick highlight the importance of resisting the "righting reflux," or the urge to argue with the other party; in this example by methodically listing out all the reasons why they "should" accept your offer (directing). You can likely recall examples similar to this in your own life; often what happens is the other party's resolve actually becomes stronger. Simply listing out the logical reasons for an idea is unlikely to change their position or behavior. In fact, directing, by stating the reasons for accepting your offer may have the opposite of its intended effect. A person put in this situation is likely to begin listing reasons why they are against your offer. Hearing the reasons stated aloud by themselves, the other party only becomes more hardened in their original position and their argument becomes reinforced.

It is important to understand the other party as part of the negotiation. The reason why most people are unwilling to be told what to do is that they want to make their own choices and be in control. The issue is often not the actual offer or message, but an issue of motivation. Resistance to change (or the desire to sustain current behavior) and the motivation to agree is like an adjustable knob. How do you turn the knob away from resistance or sustain toward motivation to agree? If people are approached as a partner instead of lecturing to them, you can help uncover their motivation to agree and thus empower them to act. Most patients have heard the reasons to quit smoking or lose weight in the past, from providers, family members, the media, and friends. Hearing them again from a pharmacist is likely to induce feelings of guilt, failure, discouragement, and even anger. Likewise, a patient may have already been told the reasons to take a medication. The goal in MI becomes to move the ambivalence dial toward making a change or agreement and away from sustaining or from resistance. In MI, ambivalence should not be viewed as a negative, but rather a necessary step to motivation. MI helps refine the issue or idea at hand by having the other party clarify it. As they do this, they also will identify the steps necessary to act or affect change and bring to light how to make the agreement possible. The pharmacist's role as a facilitator of MI with a patient may be thought of as analogous to a more experienced mentor with a more novice mentee. The learning process is something that should be done together, not something that is done for them or without them. There may be times when a patient requires clear direction and you need to play a more instructor type of role, and times when a patient needs to lead, and you simply are required to follow or watch—even if they fail to some extent. However, overall MI between a pharmacist and a patient will be most successful when you serve in a guiding and facilitating role for your patient.

Miller and Rollnick suggest a technique they describe as OARS, or Open-ended questions, Affirmative responses or affirmation, Reflection or reflective responses, and Summary to engage the ambivalence process. Miller and Rollnick offer that the OARS approach should begin with an open-ended question, e.g., asking the party about their goals or ambitions.

With a patient, you may ask if they can think of any reasons they may want to take the prescribed medication. The question should be followed by careful listening on your part, containing an appropriate amount of empathy to help build support and rapport. Although not contained as part of the OARS acronym, listening is probably the single most important skill in MI. The open-ended question and careful listening process should next be followed by a reflective response identifying the discrepancies between the other party's goals and their current status or situation. The reflective response should not disseminate any value or judgment. The reflective statement should also not impart any roadblocks, but should instead move the conversation forward and give the other party a chance to speak. It is also important that the affirmative response remains, positive, "You did really well despite all the challenges!" sounds much more encouraging to a patient than "I'm disappointed that you didn't do better." It is important that the other party "own" their motivation to make a decision or plan to move forward. Remember that ambivalence is not only normal, but it is good and indicates a reluctant party may be weighing options and moving from resistance to motivation or change talk on the ambivalence dial. Be careful not to push too hard, accept a certain amount of resistance, and embrace the opportunity to identify ways to help the other party achieve their goals. Realize the OARS process will likely go through many cycles or iterations during the encounter.

MI at its core is very different from a more traditional client centered type of interaction. In fact, it is not so much "interviewing," per se, as it is listening and providing reflection to empower the other party to act on making a decision on their own accord. It should be a reassuring, positive exchange empowering both parties to realize their best chances for a favorable outcome. People are more likely to act, and act favorably, if they feel they have a stake and can take ownership of an evolving idea. Imagine a patient in your pharmacy being told what they must do, e.g., "You need to take this medication despite your concerns about the adverse effects" versus being part of the decision process, e.g., "How do you feel about giving the medication a try?"

DARN-CAT

A useful guide to enlist MI into a discussion or a negotiation process is DARN CAT. The first, DARN, can be considered prep talk to assess readiness. The second, CAT, can be considered action or actual forms of agreement talk. DARN, in MI, represents the first four initial steps, namely Desire, Ability, Reasoning and Need, respectively. Desire-related queries often contain words like want or wish. Simply asking, "What does our organization want to accomplish in the long run," or "If you had a wish list, what item(s) would be at the top?" may be sufficient to open a dialogue with a reluctant party. Ability refers to the person's or organization's ability to accomplish something, sometimes in hypothetical terms. An example may be asking, "What ideas do you have for accomplishing…" or "If given the resources, how confident are you that you could…." Reasons correspond to linking rationales for enacting an agreement to someone's ability. Note, no commitment is required at this point, only a reason. Often, a person will have already been cued to reasons during affirmative reflections if you are properly using OARS. The final piece of the prep talk is the need. Need language focuses on what needs to happen in order to act and provides some sense of timeliness or even urgency, but not panic. Asking a person how important something is, or asking them to rate the importance on a scale, say from 1 to 10, and then asking them to reflect on why their rating is not higher (or lower), may provide some stimulation here to move in the right direction toward need talk. It should be noted that wrong questions abound in the DARN realm. Examples of wrong things to ask include, "Why haven't you thought about this before," or "Why can't you just do that?" Remember, try not to judge; instead, try to relate and express support. As highlighted previously, open-ended questions (OARS) are key.

The next set of steps in MI is CAT, or Commitment, Activation and Taking steps—items more directly related to action and taking steps, now that another party is motivated or prepared to agree. Often, with proper guiding utilizing MI, a person will suggest a course of action and be somewhat sure that they are able to accomplish what they have decided to do. The next steps should focus on implementation or the mobilization of the agreement. To say that one wants to agree or act is not the same as saying one will. Consider the difference between, "I would like to," "I will" or "I should, but…" each has a very different meaning. Commitment language is different from anything in prep talk and often involves use of words such as "I promise" or "We are willing to…"—in other words, they imply the person is not only ready to act, but will. The second part of commitment language is activation. Activation is indicated by words or phrases such as "We are ready" or "Let's get started." In other words, the other party is prepared to act. The final component of activation is taking steps. This final step may not be realized in an initial meeting, or even the first follow-up meeting. It is important to note that not all motivational interview sessions will move smoothly through a DARN-CAT scenario, or in a sequential flow. As such, OARS and DARN-CAT serve as a guide. Asking thoughtful questions and listening, affirmative reflective questions and summaries, followed by an assessment of the other party's desire, ability, reasons, and needs will often link seamlessly to initiate talk of commitment, activation, and taking steps toward an agreement or negotiation. Remember, with MI you are leading people to a decision or agreement, not forcing them into it.

■ REVISITING THE SCENARIO

Gary, new owner of Taylors Drug Store, researched 340B extensively. He reached out to colleagues and industry experts to gather information about program specifics and the impacts on independent pharmacies, both good and bad. Despite an added level of operational attention required and possible cash flow burdens, Gary's conclusion was that 340B, when structured correctly could be a fantastic opportunity for his pharmacy to increase margins. More importantly, Gary felt it could create a formal relationship with the hospital to compliment his pharmacy's patient services with medication access, adherence, and clinical services, layering in a mutual financial incentive for both parties. Gary informed the hospital administration that they would like to move forward.

Use of Positional Negotiation

Hospital administration sends a contract template to Gary to review. "Standard" program structure and rates are already input. Administration expresses to Gary that the contract is "fair," based on comparisons to existing contracts with a major chain pharmacy in town and advice from their consultant, and is therefore non-negotiable. Gary requests a telephone meeting to discuss the contract with the hospital.

To begin the meeting, Gary reiterates the desire to work collaboratively with the hospital to enhance patient care and mutual economics knowing that all will build a healthier community. With regard to the contract initially provided, Gary expresses concern that structure and rates are not feasible in order to proceed with signing. Gary counter offers a rate that he believes will work for Taylor's Drug, a rate that is simply a 15% higher number than that proposed by the hospital. The hospital stands firm on their original offer adding that the 340B program was intended to allow Covered Entities to expand scarce federal resources to continue serving underserved patient populations and that the funds generated will allow them to purchase a new MRI machine and hire two new specialists, a podiatrist and a cardiologist. Gary, as a businessman and health care provider in the community, understands that to continue seeing patients and generate prescriptions the hospital must remain solvent. Gary, in order to preserve his existing relationship with the hospital, reluctantly agrees to accommodate the administrator and accepts the hospital's proposal. As a compromise, Gary asks that the parties reconvene in 90 days to review the program and adjust the contract if need be. The contract is executed and the program begins. The hospital sees a tremendous increase in savings while Gary consistently experiences cash flow issues and views his participation in the 340B program and ultimately his relationship with hospital passively, at times negatively.

Result: The hospital employed a positional negotiation technique that required little effort and led to an easy, timely negotiation process where they stated their position, thus leaving the decision in the hands of Gary on whether or not to accept. They appealed to Gary's emotional connection with the community and his patients to assert their position. Gary was left feeling slighted and that he somehow "lost" the negotiation. Continued hassle and aggravation experienced from the program leads Gary and his staff feeling resentful toward the hospital and their primary care providers, ultimately jeopardizing the sustainability of the program and the relationship as a whole.

Use of Principled Negotiation

Hospital administration sends a contract template to Gary to review. "Standard" program structure and rates are already input. Gary runs a model to project the economic impact of the contract provided using past claim data from his pharmacy system. The goal is to determine their current economics and how the 340B rates compare in order to weigh the financial benefits, if any, of contracting. Through his analysis, Gary discovers two things:

1. Based on the volume of prescriptions filled from Covered Entity hospital and clinic prescribers, the potential financial benefit to the hospital is considerable; signing a contract with his pharmacy will produce a significant new revenue stream that does not currently exist.
2. Compared with his current financial analysis, the proposed 340B rate will result in a "break-even" for his pharmacy, thus giving him no real financial incentive to participate.

Utilizing their contract, Gary formulates a structure and rate that he believes will be advantageous for his business at the same time maintaining viability for the hospital. Gary's proposed rate takes into account all things they both consider to be impactful on their operations by participating in the 340B program. Additionally, Gary calculates a "floor" rate that will be the point in the negotiation at which the contract will simply not make sense from a business standpoint. Gary requests an in-person meeting with a representative or two from the hospital to discuss.

To begin the meeting, Gary reiterates the desire to work collaboratively with the hospital to enhance patient care and mutual economics knowing that all will build a healthier community. With regards to the contract initially provided, Gary expresses that the proposed structure and rates are not feasible. Gary takes the opportunity to explain in detail the impact 340B will have on his business along with specific data-driven information to support his position. Gary offers to share his results with the hospital and invites questions.

- Existing pharmacy economics (margin without 340B is equal)
- Wholesaler purchasing and rebate impact
- DIR fees
- Inventory management and control
- Cash flow
- Time, resources, work-flow

This is a necessary step regardless of the outcome of the negotiation to ensure that Gary's counterpart, the hospital, understands his side of the situation, as the hospital has their own perspectives, challenges, and issues on their side. Rather than simply saying "no," Gary suggests an alternative structure and rate that will satisfy the pharmacy's needs economically and will account for the various challenges faced with program participation. While not what the hospital had originally proposed or assumed going into the negotiation, they are able to corroborate information with their industry experts, colleagues, and other data sources to see that this proposal will be beneficial and meet their needs, as well. However, hospital administration still believes the rate that Gary is requesting is too high and that to remain compliant with program regulations, counter with a slightly lower rate for the pharmacy to consider. The counter is still above the pharmacy's "floor," and Gary discerns that it is worth contracting and building a stronger relationship with the hospital than to stand firm on their initial proposal. Thus he agrees, the contract is revised and executed, and the program begins. Both the pharmacy and the hospital see significant increases in savings and are now in discussions to begin a bedside delivery program to enhance medication adherence upon hospital discharge.

Result: Gary used a principled method centered on the patient and community benefit that would result from a hospital and pharmacy partnership rather than their needs alone. While each's needs were critically important, they understood that they would not arrive at an agreement if the focus was on position rather than outcome. Gary used analytical data, which strengthened his argument for a different structure and rate proposal. Gary also displayed creativity in looking at alternatives to alleviate challenges brought upon by the program. Gary was able to illustrate to the hospital's administration that despite his proposed contract changes, all parties would still benefit greatly. Using analytics, Gary knew his flexibility and had determined a predetermined "floor" (BATNA) and was prepared to accept a counteroffer quickly and avoid further time and effort spent negotiating. Both parties were comfortable with the contract because the data that was provided were real, and the concrete reasons given as the basis of the proposal. The result of the successful negotiation achieved the goal of enhancing clinical care to the community and to patients by expanding the existing positive relationship between the hospital and the Taylors Pharmacy to collaborate on more patient-centric initiatives.

■ CONCLUSION

Learning to negotiate is a lifelong skill that will serve you well in many facets of your professional career. However, just like learning to play a musical instrument, learning to negotiate requires practice. Simply reading a book about playing a musical instrument will not make you a good musician. It may make you a better musician if you already play one and continue to practice the instrument. The same can be said of negotiating. Reading about negotiating sets you off on the right path. It provides you with advice on how to practice to become a better negotiator. Try to treat others fairly and based on principles, even if they are not doing the same. While negotiating theory can be reduced to a simple mathematical equation or model, people sometimes behave irrationally or at least

■ QUESTIONS FOR FURTHER DISCUSSION

1. Think about a recent higher stakes negotiation in which you were involved but did not use a principle-centered approach to negotiating. Now imagine you had utilized a principle-centered approach in the negotiations. How might the process have differed?
2. Thinking about the same above negotiation, how might the outcome have differed?
3. Why is an analytical or data-driven approach often the most useful to determine a BATNA?
4. Imagine you are applying for your first job as a pharmacist. It is a full-time position that requires 5 weekdays of staffing and some limited evenings and weekends on-call. You are very interested in the position, but wish to work 4 days a week so that you can continue working on a graduate degree part-time. Outline a hypothetical conversation you might have using MI and the OARS framework to bring up the idea of a 4-day workweek with the pharmacist in charge of hiring. You should have a brief statement or point for each of the four components in OARS.

differently than how we might hope or predict. Do not be afraid to walk away; no deal is better than a bad deal, and it is important to remember that there is no risk in being well-prepared to enter a negotiation.

REFERENCES

Austin Z, Gregory PA, Martin C. 2009. A conflict management scale for pharmacy. *Am J Pharm Educ* 73:122.

Austin Z, Gregory PAM, Martin JC. 2010. Pharmacists' management of conflict in community practice. *Res Soc Admin Pharm* 6:39–48.

Berman RA, Gottlieb AS. 2019. Job negotiations in academic medicine: Building a competency-based roadmap for residents and fellows. *J Gen Intern Med* 34:146–149.

Brooks JM, Doucette W, Sorofman B. 1999. Factors affecting bargaining outcomes between pharmacies and insurers. *Health Serv Res* 34(1 Pt 2):439–451.

Grimolizzi-Jensen, Conrado J. 2018. Organizational change: Effect of motivational interviewing on readiness to change. *Journal of Change Management* 18:54–69.

Miller WR, Rollnick S. 2013. *Motivational Interviewing: Helping People Change*, 3rd ed. New York, NY: Guilford Press.

Nash JF. 1950. The bargaining problem. *Econometrica* 28:155–162.

Nash JF. 1953. Two-person cooperative games. *Econometrica* 31:129–140.

Sportsman S, Hamilton P. 2002. Conflict management styles in the health professions. *J Prof Nursing* 23:157–166.

Voss C, Raz T. 2016. *Never Split the Difference: Negotiating as If Your Life Depended on It*. New York, NY: Harper Business.

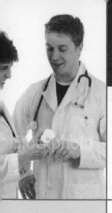

16

ORGANIZATIONAL STRUCTURE AND BEHAVIOR

Caroline A. Gaither

About the Author: Dr. Gaither is Senior Associate Dean, Professional Education Division and professor at the University of Minnesota College of Pharmacy. She received a BS in pharmacy from the University of Toledo and an MS and PhD in pharmacy administration from Purdue University. Her teaching interests include career and professional development, work-related attitudes and behaviors, interpersonal communication, and social and behavioral aspects of pharmacy practice. Her research interests include understanding and improving the work life of pharmacists, specifically focusing on individual-level (organizational and professional commitment, job satisfaction, job stress, role conflict, turnover, and gender and race/ethnicity effects) and organizational-level (culture and empowerment) factors, and the role of the pharmacist in addressing health disparities.

■ LEARNING OBJECTIVES

After completing this chapter, readers should be able to:

1. Discuss the field of organizational behavior and its development over time.
2. Describe the basic components of traditional and newer organization forms.
3. Compare and contrast different elements of formal and informal organizational structure.
4. Understand the role of teams in organizations and how to build effective ones.
5. Discuss the basic incompatibilities between organizational and professional models of structure.
6. Identify influences on pharmacists' job satisfaction, organizational commitment, job stress, job turnover intention, organizational identification and well-being, and how that affects organizational behavior and performance.
7. Describe the role of emotions, emotional labor, and emotional intelligence in organizational behavior.
8. Describe different leadership theories and how they can be applied to pharmacy practice.

■ SCENARIO

Joe Smart, a newly hired pharmacy intern, just completed his first week at the ambulatory pharmacy at State University Health System. Having worked previously in an independent community pharmacy, Sam's Pharmacy, he wanted to get some hospital experience before graduation. Now he is not so sure. He really liked working with the customers that came into Sam's Pharmacy, but frequently he and the pharmacist who worked there were so busy that neither had much time to do anything other than dispense prescriptions. His first week at the ambulatory pharmacy was also quite busy. There were many more people working here than at Sam's. He was overwhelmed by it all. During orientation, he received a copy of the policy and procedure manual that detailed the health system's mission and organizational chart. He was very impressed with all this but could not figure out why it was important to know about the rest of the organization. He was going to be a pharmacist and, as such, was only interested in things that pertained to the pharmacy. Also, he could not understand why the pharmacy staff was so uptight. At his old job, Sam, the owner, would always notice if an employee was distressed or unhappy about something. Sam had an "open door" policy and was always ready to talk. He really felt like part of the team. Joe only saw his new boss, the Director of the ambulatory pharmacy, once, and that was at orientation. The pharmacists he worked with were very concerned with showing him the tasks he needed to complete and not much else. Joe began to wonder if this was what it would be like to work for a large health system. He also heard the staff talking about a change in their electronic record system and that the health-system they worked for might be bought by a larger, for-profit company. He remembered that in his management class, the professor talked about working for large organizations, but he did not pay much attention. Joe thought that it was the responsibility of the manager to make sure that things ran smoothly and that he did not need to be concerned with details unrelated to patients' drug therapy. Anyway, he was new and thought that maybe he should give the place more time. In the back of his mind, however, he had this nagging feeling that things could be better, but he just did not know how to get there.

■ CHAPTER QUESTIONS

1. What is organizational behavior, and how has it developed over time?
2. Why do pharmacists need to understand how an organization works?
3. What is some basic terminology used to describe organizations?
4. What is the typical organizational structure among common employers of pharmacists? How do newer organizational structures differ from more traditional ones?
5. What factors should be taken into consideration when designing the most appropriate organizational structure?
6. What are the various types of teams found in organizations and how can they be structured for maximum effectiveness?
7. How does a professional work within a bureaucratic organization?
8. What are some of the typical organizational attitudes and behaviors of pharmacists?
9. What are some factors that lead to the focus on employee well-being?
10. What are some ways in which a leader is different from a manager?
11. What types of leaders do pharmacy organizations need?

■ WHAT IS ORGANIZATIONAL BEHAVIOR?

An *organization* can be defined as a group of individuals who work together and coordinate their actions to achieve a wide variety of goals (George & Jones, 2012). Organizations can be very small in number of personnel (fewer than three) or very large (>5,000). Personnel can include staff (e.g., ward clerk, cashier, technician, pharmacist, nurse, or physician) and management and administrators (e.g., owner, president, vice president, manager, director, or supervisor). Both staff and administrators are important to the overall functioning of any organization. It is not enough for pharmacists to understand only the technical and professional aspects of their job (e.g., dispensing, monitoring, and counseling); they must also understand how the organizations for which they work function and how the people within them work. This is something that Joe Smart has yet to figure out on his own. An examination of certain tenets in the field of organizational behavior will provide valuable insight into this area.

Organizational behavior is the systematic and scientific analysis of individuals, groups, and organizations; its purpose is to understand, predict, and affect human behavior to improve the performance of individuals, which ultimately affects the functioning and success of the organizations in which they work (Tosi et al., 1994). To be effective, managers must be able to understand why people in their organizations behave in certain ways. They must also be able to explain decisions and seek information from colleagues and employees even if turns out to be negative (Dragoni, et al., 2014). The study of organizational behavior provides guidelines that help managers understand and appreciate the many forces that affect behavior (George & Jones, 2012). This allows them to take corrective action if problems arise. Managers also must be able to predict how employees will react to new technologies and changes in the marketplace (e.g., implementation of robotics in a pharmacy department or moving from a drug-product orientation to a people orientation). Organizations exert control over their employees through rewards or sanctions to encourage fulfillment of organizational goals and objectives. Most have experienced working for an organization at some point in their lives, and it is important to understand and reflect on these experiences and how they shape one in both positive and negative ways.

Organizational behavior draws on a number of different behavioral science disciplines. Psychology, sociology, social psychology, anthropology, and political science all provide insights into how best to organize work (Robbins & Judge, 2018). Psychology allows one to understand individual behavior and focuses on such aspects as motivation, job satisfaction, attitude measurement, emotion, training, job stress, and work design. Sociology contributes by helping to understand how individuals fulfill their roles within a larger system through organizational structures, behavioral norms, and bureaucracies. Social psychology focuses on the influence of individuals on one another and helps to understand communication patterns, organizational and attitude change, and group functioning. Anthropology provides understanding of the environment in which the organization functions. Political science provides insight into organizational politics and informal organizational structures that greatly influence the functioning of an organization.

Understanding the functioning of organizations was not so important when the profession of pharmacy began. As noted in Chapter 1, most pharmacists started out as apprentices of apothecaries, from whom they learned the practice of pharmacy, and then went on to become practitioners who owned their own pharmacies and trained other apprentices. As the roles of the pharmacist have changed over time, so has their training and places of employment. Currently, a doctor of pharmacy degree requires 6 years or more of formal education. Unlike in the past, today most employers of pharmacists are large organizations. These organizations can be chain pharmacies (several stores under one owner or publicly traded on the stock market); integrated health systems that incorporate inpatient and outpatient pharmacies, ambulatory care clinics, and managed-care and mail-order operations; and even pharmaceutical manufacturers.

Other professions are following a similar trend, wherein their practitioners are transitioning from employers to employees. Very few graduates of medical or law school operate independent practices immediately after graduation (Carlin, 2011; Muhlestein & Smith, 2016). Many physicians are salaried employees of managed-care organizations, integrated health systems, or group practices. With the current emphasis on cost, quality, and outcomes of care, many health providers are members of a new health care entity, accountable care organizations, which reward lower spending and higher quality (Song & Lee, 2013). Ownership of an independent community pharmacy or a private medical practice is still a viable employment option for many, but they too will operate in an increasingly complex environment. Declining reimbursements and changes in payment schemes will continue to have deep impacts on the health care industry and the professionals who work in them (Borkowski, 2016). Changes in delivery approaches, implementation of electronic health records and publicly reported quality metrics have all affected clinician well-being (Dyrbye et al., 2017). Understanding how organizations function will enhance health professionals' employment experiences and increase their chances for a rewarding professional career.

Why is this shift from independent practitioner to salaried employee so important? This shift may appear to be in conflict with one of the hallmarks of a professional occupation—autonomy. "The major distinction between a profession and an occupation lies in legitimate organized autonomy—a profession is distinct from other occupations in that it has been given the right to control its work. Professions are deliberately granted autonomy including the exclusive right to determine who can do the work and how it should be done" (Freidson, 1970). Given that pharmacy and medicine are professional occupations, the status of practitioners as employees could result in conflict between the professional and the employing organization. In many cases, professionals' primary allegiance is to their work or patients and not to their employer. These practitioners also share a desire to exert at least some control over their work environments. If this desire is not met, job dissatisfaction, stress, and burnout can result (Gaither et al., 2015; Gregory & Menser, 2015; Jepsen & O'Neill, 2013; Kuiper et al., 2011). Even as an intern, Joe Smart is questioning the autonomy afforded the pharmacists at State University Health System. His initial frustration, however, may be compounded by a lack of knowledge of how operations and communication channels differ in a large organization compared with a much smaller one.

This chapter will help you gain a greater understanding of how organizations function by introducing basic organizational behavior principles, describing the structure of organizations, discussing the roles of employees within organizations, examining specific pharmacist organizational behaviors, and elaborating on the concept of leadership.

■ ORGANIZATIONAL PRINCIPLES

Chapter 6 discussed strategic planning and the development of mission statements and organizational goals and objectives. To understand an organization requires knowledge of its purpose or reason for being. Organizations do not function in isolation. They are created to meet some need in the external environment. As shown in Figure 16-1, at the center of any organization is a set of values that form the reason for existence, the philosophy, and the purpose of the organization (Jones, 1981). Articulations of these values are often represented as the goals of the organization. Some organizations will lose focus if the goals they set are at odds with the core values of the organization. To make the goals of the organization a reality, a structure must be put in place to make the organization operational. Typically, the structure includes such concepts as reporting relationships, communication patterns, decision-making procedures, responsibility/accountability, norms, and reward structures.

Structure produces the climate, or the psychological atmosphere of the organization (Jones, 1981). The climate of an organization consists of such factors as the amount of trust, the levels of morale, and the support employees experience (Gibb, 1978). Organizational climate is often confused with organizational culture (Schein & Schein, 2017). *Organizational culture* is defined as the system of shared meaning held by members that distinguish one organization from another (Robbins & Judge, 2018). *Culture* refers to the understandings and beliefs regarding how "things are done around here" (Schein & Schein, 2017). Once the culture is in place, practices within the

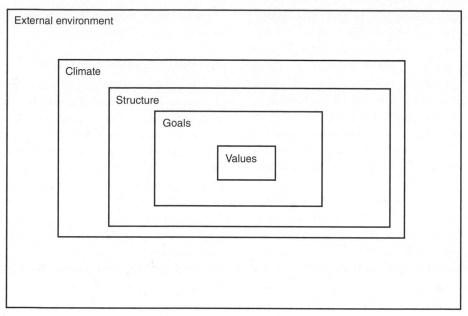

Figure 16-1. The organization.

organization act to maintain it by exposing employees to a set of similar experiences (Harrison & Carroll, 1991). The very specific and methodical training that Joe Smart is receiving is somewhat a reflection of the organization's culture.

Culture is not only influenced by the company's reason for existence and structure but also organizational ethics and the nature of the relationship a company establishes with its employees (George & Jones, 2012). Organizational ethics are the moral values, beliefs, and rules that establish the appropriate way for the members to deal with each other and those outside the organization. These ethics are influenced by the society in which the organization resides, the professional ethics that similarly trained people bring to an organization, and the personal moral values of employees, especially the founder. The company's hiring, promotion, and layoff practices and its pay shape the relationship an organization establishes with employees and benefits policies. These policies and procedures all influence whether or not an employee will be motivated to buy into a company's norms and values (Sagie & Elizar, 1996).

Organizational culture affects climate. A strong culture is characterized by the organization's core values being both intensely held and widely accepted (Korba et al., 2012). A weak culture is characterized by just the opposite—vagueness, ambiguity, and inconsistency. A strong culture will have a greater effect on the climate than a weak one because the high degree of sharedness and intensity creates an internal climate of high behavioral control (Robbins & Judge, 2018). Subcultures can develop to reflect common problems, goals, and experiences that members of a team, department, or other unit share (Daft, 2016). Problems in the climate can be traced back to problems in the organization's culture and structure. When improvements in the climate are needed, some managers may only monitor employees' overall job satisfaction and stress levels. While it is important to do this, managers should also determine if there are problems with communication patterns, reward structures, and decision-making procedures within the organization and focus on problem solving in these areas. Has the organization stayed true to its values? If not, the shared meaning that employees hold with management will be confused. Managers are essential in creating the culture, which influences interactions among coworkers and relationships with patients (Jacobs et al., 2011). An unhealthy climate can hinder employee productivity and ultimately affect the overall effectiveness of the organization.

Organizations exist in an environment that is constantly in flux. This is particularly the case in health care. Organizations that employ health professionals and the health professionals themselves must be flexible enough to cope with the unexpected (Jones, 1981). Leaders and managers of these organizations must assess the core values of the organization regularly to determine if they are being challenged or if they need revision (Dye, 2017). Assessing an organization's culture will assist in determining how

the organization is responding to both its internal and external environments.

Assessing Organizational Culture

A wide range of tools exist to assess organizational culture, including techniques ranging from observation, informal interviews, and attending meetings to the administration of carefully developed survey instruments. These instruments are designed to measure and compare the key cultural characteristics of a single organization or a number of different organizations. An example of such an instrument is the *competing values framework* (Figure 16-2) developed by Quinn and Rohrbaugh (1983; Quinn, 1988). Depending on the degree of flexibility or control in the structure of the organization and a focus on either

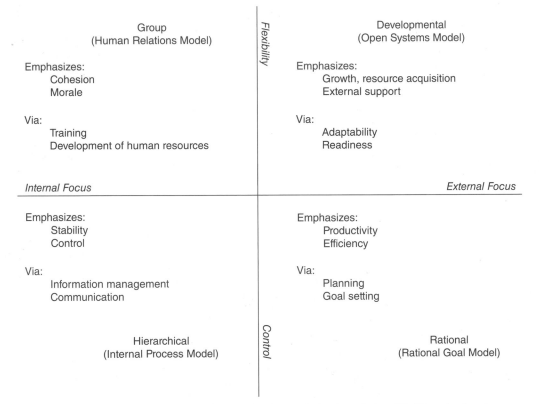

Figure 16-2. The competing values framework. (Adapted with permission from Quinn RE: Beyond rational management: mastering the paradoxes and competing demands of high performance. San Francisco: Jossey-Bass; 1988.)

the internal dynamics or external environment, four types of cultures are derived: hierarchical (i.e., internal focus, high control), group (i.e., internal focus, low control), rational (i.e., external focus, high control), and developmental (i.e., external focus, low control). Early research suggested that an overemphasis on any of the cultures could result in a dysfunctional organization (Quinn, 1988); therefore, organizations need to embrace some elements of each culture. A more recent meta-analysis suggested that organizations scoring higher on all four cultures are more successful in promoting positive employee attitudes and operational and financial performance (Hartnell et al., 2011). The most effective organizations embrace the dimensions that are most important and relevant to their goals and values (Jacobs et al., 2013).

To determine the type of organizational culture, employees are given an instrument that contains brief statements in which they are asked to rate out of 100 points how closely their organization reflects these dimensions. Using this instrument, a study of health-system pharmacists indicated that the majority of study participants felt that their organization had a hierarchical organizational structure (Lane et al., 2010). When asked about the type of culture they desired in their organization, staff pharmacists (those whose work activities involved overseeing drug distribution) were more likely to indicate they desired a hierarchical culture, while clinical pharmacists (those whose work involves no drug distribution activities) and administrative pharmacists desired a group culture. These results are similar to studies of other health system employees (Mahl et al., 2015; Sasaki et al., 2017). Depending on the type of staff member responding, cultures were seen as either hierarchical or group. Hierarchical cultures rate lower on staff job satisfaction, working conditions, and stress recognition. Quality improvement scores are shown to vary by culture with those in group cultures obtaining higher scores (Mahl et al., 2015).

Another way to look at organizational culture is to examine the congruence between individual and organizational values (Sarros et al., 2005). The Organizational Culture Profile presents respondents with a list of 40 values and asks them to rate each on a scale from 1 (Not at all) to 5 (Very much) regarding the extent to which the value is held by your organization. Pharmacists rated "performance orientation" (high expectations, results oriented, highly organized) and "supportive" (shares information freely, collaborative, team-oriented) as values most exhibited by their organization (Rosenthal et al., 2016). Pharmacists who worked for organizations that held "social responsibility" and "competitiveness" as important cultural values were more likely provide advanced services at their pharmacies (Rosenthal et al., 2015).

Other studies have demonstrated important implications of culture on pharmacy, pharmacist, and patient outcomes. Clark and Mount (2006) demonstrated that certain types of pharmacies had more of a culture toward providing patient-centered care than others. Similarly, it has been suggested that corporatization of community pharmacies may affect pharmacists' professional autonomy, yet a mixed market (i.e., various types of ownership) may be required to maintain a comprehensive range of public health services that provide maximum benefit to all patients (Bush et al., 2009). Other reports have shared that even beyond type of ownership, the culture instilled in an organization may have implications for pharmacist job satisfaction and turnover (Seston et al., 2009), effectiveness of the implementation of new policies (Tan et al., 2005), building capacity and establishment of policies for new cognitive services to patients (Feletto, 2010), the quality of care provided by pharmacists to patients (Desselle & Skomo, 2010), and even the rate of medication incident reporting among pharmacies (Boyle et al., 2011). A review added patient safety and business performance to the list (Jacobs et al., 2011). The importance of organizational culture simply cannot be understated.

Organizational Structure

Organizational theorists suggest that the structure of an organization encompasses seven major aspects: differentiation (also known as *complexity*), formalization, centralization, division of labor, unity of command, span of control, and departmentalization (Robbins

& Judge, 2018). *Differentiation* refers to the degree to which units are dissimilar. *Formalization* refers to the degree to which jobs in the organization are standardized, and *centralization* refers to the extent to which decision-making is concentrated at a single point in the organization. *Division of labor* refers to the degree to which activities are divided into separate jobs. *Unity of command* preserves the concept of an unbroken line of authority. *Span of control* determines the number of levels and managers an organization creates. *Departmentalization* is the way in which jobs must be grouped so that common tasks can be coordinated. Differentiation can occur either horizontally, vertically, or spatially.

Horizontal Differentiation

Horizontal differentiation describes the degree of differentiation based on how many different types of either people or units are included in the organization. Do all the employees of the organization have the same training and education? This is definitely not the case in pharmacy. Many pharmacy organizations focus not only on providing pharmacy services but also on merchandizing nonpharmacy-related items. If all personnel had the same training, managing the organization would be easier because everyone would have a similar orientation. Since this is not the case in pharmacy, coordinating the work among people in the different units can be more difficult. Horizontal differentiation can also take the form of multiownership of a variety of related industries. A health system can own several other types of facilities.

Vertical Differentiation

Vertical differentiation refers to the depth of the organizational hierarchy. One key feature of an organization is the chain of command, or the number of levels between the owner or president of the organization and the staff. Vertical differentiation is typically represented by what is known as an *organizational chart*.

An organizational chart depicts the reporting relationships and the hierarchy of authority in an organization. An example of a typical organizational chart is given in Figure 16-3. Authority usually flows from top to bottom, with those at the bottom of the chart holding the least authority. *Authority* is the rights given to a certain position in an organization to give orders and the expectation that those orders are carried out. Along with these rights, the responsibility for making sure work is completed is accepted. The solid lines represent direct reporting relationships important to the overall objectives of the organization (line authority). Line-authority positions include vice presidents, directors, managers, supervisors, and staff. The dashed lines in the figure represent advisory positions that supplement and support the line-authority positions (staff authority). Examples of staff-authority positions include chief personnel officer or vice president of personnel, finance, legal, real estate, information systems, etc. The degree of staff authority varies with the size of the organization. The smaller the size, the fewer are the number of positions needed to support the line authority. Many independent community pharmacies started out this way. One person (the owner) was responsible for numerous activities. As pharmacies grew and expanded, owners hired individuals to supervise different areas or functions of the store. As owners branched out into running additional stores at various locations, more personnel were needed to run the day-to-day operations of the organization.

If an organization represents a for-profit company (i.e., portions or shares of the company are sold on the stock exchange), the top position in the organization belongs to the stockholders. Typically, stockholders do not have a say in day-to-day operations but are very concerned about the profitability of the company and will sell their stock if earnings are not up to par. If the company is a not-for-profit organization, the top level will not be stockholders but may represent a board of directors or trustees who oversee the entire operation. This group is also not involved in day-to-day operations but will meet periodically to either review or make important decisions regarding the entire company. The next level represents the chief executive officer (CEO) or president. If the organization is an independent community pharmacy, the owner will occupy the top

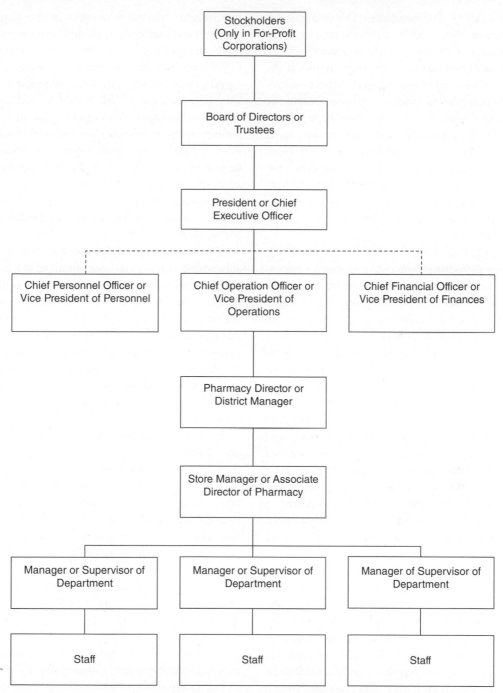

Figure 16-3. The organizational chart.

position in the organizational chart. Depending on the size of the company, a chief operations officer (COO) or the owner of the independent pharmacy will run the day-to-day operations of the organization. If the company is national or international, regional officers responsible for the operations in different areas of the country may assist this person. Under these officers are usually department directors or district managers. Departments in a health system can include nursing, medicine, quality assurance, managed care, long-term care, and so on. Each of these departments will have managers or supervisors who oversee staff who carry out the day-to-day responsibilities.

Spatial Differentiation

Spatial differentiation is the degree to which the location of an organization's units is in one place or spread across several locations. An independent community pharmacy may have only one location that has all operations in one place. A large health system or chain pharmacy operation can have multiple units spread across a city, state, or entire regions of the country. Spatial differentiation can also occur when different departments are located in different areas. A pharmaceutical manufacturer may have all its research and development departments in one city or state and the sales and marketing divisions in other areas of the country or the world. As organizations spatially differentiate, more coordination between these units is necessary. Spatial differentiation is also related to the amount of horizontal and vertical differentiation. The more complex the organization, the greater is the extent each of these will exist.

Formalization

Formalization can include the presence of rules (the degree to which the behavior of organizational members is subject to organizational control), procedural specifications (the extent to which organization members must follow organizationally defined techniques in dealing with situations they encounter), technical competence (the extent to which organizationally defined "universal" standards are used in the personnel selection and advancement process), and

impersonality (the extent to which both organization members and outsiders are treated without regard to individual qualities) (Hall, 1968). If a job is highly formalized, the employee has little discretion with regard to when and how the job is completed. Standardization grew out of beliefs held by early organizational behaviorists who suggested that in order to make work more efficient, error should be reduced (Taylor, 1911). One way to do this was to standardize procedures to reduce errors and increase efficiency. As noted in Figure 16-2, hierarchical and rational organizational cultures have high degrees of control usually through formalization and the standardization of procedures.

The degree of formalization can vary considerably within and between organizations (Robbins & Judge, 2018). Organizational charts depict different positions and/or units in an organization and formal lines of authority and decision-making. This is one type of formalization. Another type is related to performance of the work. Some pharmacies require all pharmacy personnel to punch a time clock at the beginning and ending of a shift; others do not have such a requirement. Positions that make up the organization can have very detailed job descriptions that inform employees what they can and cannot do, whereas other organizations are less formal and do not have written job descriptions. Or if they do, the descriptions are very vague. Individuals who are higher in the organization will have less formal job descriptions than those lower in the company. Some jobs also lend themselves to more or less formalization. The legal requirements of drug procurement and dispensing are highly formalized, but the individualized services that pharmaceutical care requires leave much discretion to the individual pharmacist.

Centralization

Centralization refers to the extent to which decision-making is concentrated at a single point in the organization. *Decision-making* and *authority* in this context refer to the rights inherent to the position that one holds in the organization. Usually the very top levels of management make most of the policy decisions in a centralized organization. More recently, the trend has been to decentralize decision-making and move it down in the organization to lower levels of management and/or even to staff-level employees. Problems with this approach arise when employees are responsible for achieving goals without the authority to make policies or gather the needed resources. Group and developmental organizational cultures have structures that allow for more flexibility in decision-making.

Centralization sometimes is confused with spatial differentiation. A hospital pharmacy that has satellite pharmacies located throughout the hospital is often referred to as being "decentralized." However, it is decentralized in location only if decision-making concerning the satellites still rests at one centralized point in the organization. Other organizational structure principles include division of labor, span of control, unity of command, and departmentalization.

Division of Labor

Division of labor divides work tasks into specific parts. This can be seen in pharmacy when there is a separation of pharmacists into those who only participate in dispensing functions and those who only participate in clinical functions. Even within clinical functions, pharmacists can specialize in a particular field (e.g., geriatrics, pediatrics, or disease states). This should result in more efficient use of the specialized skills of the individual (work specialization). A negative consequence of the division of labor is that the professional may become very narrow in his or her abilities, the job becomes routine, and job satisfaction is reduced. Some suggest that enlarging and reorganizing work functions rather than narrowing the scope of some jobs leads to greater productivity by using employees with interchangeable skills (Robbins & Judge, 2018). This can be seen in the health system setting, where pharmacists provide both traditional staffing functions on certain shifts and patient care (clinical) functions on others.

Unity of Command

Unity of command is the concept that an individual reports to only one supervisor, to whom he or she is responsible. As pharmacy organizations have tried to decentralize, employees may have more than one person to whom they are reporting. A structure that makes the most of this concept is called a *matrix organization*. A matrix organization integrates the activities of different specialists while maintaining specialized organizational departments (Tosi et al., 1994). Usually this takes the form of different specialists across several departments working in teams on specific projects. This translates into individuals having at least two supervisors. The structure works well when there is a need to coordinate a number of interdependent activities. It also works well where project work is the norm, and people are required to get together in interdisciplinary terms (La Monica, 1994).

Pharmaceutical manufacturers and cross-disciplinary teams in health systems (e.g., nurses, physicians, pharmacists, and social workers) are particularly well suited for this endeavor. This allows for diversity of ideas and for the best possible solution to emerge. On the negative side, there is little evidence that employees prefer reporting to more than one supervisor, and confusion, conflict, and ambiguity can develop as workers try to figure out who is responsible for what (George & Jones, 2012).

Span of Control

Span of control refers to how many people a manager effectively controls. In pharmacies, one can see a wide variation in the number of individuals a pharmacist supervises. One pharmacist can supervise only one or two technicians in the pharmacy (in some states, there are legal regulations in this area), or the pharmacist can manage the entire store, including non-pharmacy personnel. Recently, there has been a push to increase the span of control of managers owing to a number of drawbacks to small spans of control: they are expensive because they add layers of management, complicate vertical communication by slowing down decision-making, and discourage employee autonomy because of the close supervision by management. Managers can handle a wider span of control best when employees know their jobs inside and out (such as pharmacists) and can turn to colleagues when they have a question (Robbins & Judge, 2018). Some individuals find it quite discomforting to have some-one always looking over their shoulder, but others may prefer to have someone who can respond quickly to problems when they arise.

Departmentalization

Departmentalization refers to grouping individuals according to specific tasks. For example, persons responsible for purchasing, distributing, and managing drug products could constitute a department. One of the advantages of having departments is that the individuals in a department share a common vocabulary and training and expertise. This should increase efficiency and effectiveness of the unit. Given the increased complexities of health care and pharmacy in particular, some organizations are requiring that members work across departments so that a diversity of ideas and expertise is given to specific tasks. This team approach helps supplement the functioning of individual departments and allows for better communication between different areas.

Newer Approaches to Organizational Design

The idea that the best structure for an organization depends on the nature of the environment in which the organization operates is called the *contingency approach* to organizational design (Daft, 2016). In this approach, based on the work of Mintzberg (1983), there are five organizational forms: A *simple structure* is one in which a single person runs the entire organization. An independent community pharmacy would be an example of this structure. This type of organization is quite flexible and can respond to the environment quite quickly, but it is also quite risky because the success or failure of the business depends on one or two individuals. A *machine bureaucracy* is a highly complex formal environment with clear lines of authority. This type of organization is highly efficient in performing standardized tasks but may be dehumanizing and boring for employees. A chain or mail order pharmacy may be like this depending on the degree of structure and formalization that exists in the organization. On the other hand, a *professional bureaucracy* is one in which much of the day-to-day decision-making is vested in the professionals who carry out most of the work. In this type of structure, there are many rules and regulations that may inhibit creativity. An example of this type of structure would be found in a health-system pharmacy. The positive side of this structure is that it allows professionals to practice those skills for which they are best qualified. On the negative side, these professionals may become overly narrow, which may lead to errors and potential conflicts between employees as a result of not seeing the "big picture." A *divisional structure* is one that consists of a set of autonomous units coordinated by a central headquarter. In this design, divisional managers have a lot of control that allows upper level management to focus on the "big picture." A negative side of this structure is high duplication of effort. A college or school of pharmacy that is structured around the various disciplines of the pharmaceutical sciences is an example of this structure. A fifth structure is called an "adhocracy." An "adhocracy" is very informal in nature. There is very little formalization and centralization. Most of the work is done in teams. An example of this structure may be found in the research and development department of a pharmaceutical company. This type of design fosters innovation but can be highly inefficient and has the greatest potential for disruptive conflict.

One of the newest forms of organizational structure is the *boundaryless organization*. In this type of organization, the chains of command are eliminated, the spans of control are unlimited, and departments are replaced by empowered teams (Robbins & Judge, 2018). This type of organization is highly flexible and can respond quickly to the external environment. One form of the boundaryless organization is the virtual organization (George & Jones, 2012). A virtual (also called *modular* or *networked*) *organization* is one that has a small core of individuals, and major organizational functions are outsourced to others. Employees are linked to one another through computers, faxes, and video-conferencing and rarely see one another (Fulk & Desanctis, 1995). There are no departments in this type of organization, and all decisions are made centrally. An example of one aspect of this model in community pharmacy would be where all refill prescriptions are sent to a central location to be filled and then returned to the community pharmacy for distribution to patients or where technology is used to verify prescriptions while pharmacists are located at an off-site location.

One final organizational form that has emerged in recent years is the *leaner organization* (Robbins & Judge, 2018). A leaner organization is usually accomplished by downsizing. Downsizing refers to closing locations, reducing staff, or selling off business units that do not add value. This results in an intentional reduction in the size of the workforce. Due to the economic recession in 2009, many organizations, including pharmacies, downsized their staff (Schommer et al., 2009). This can cause stress and overload for employees who remain. Results from the 2014 National Pharmacist Workforce Survey suggest that reductions in staffing and hours available for pharmacists to work are still occurring (Gaither et al., 2015).

Organizational Teams

As previously mentioned, one of the newest forms of organizational structure involve the establishment of teams. Teams in health care are not new, as one can think of teams of clinicians working together to provide care to patients in the hospital or clinic setting. Teams can be thought of in terms of pharmacists and technicians working together at a community pharmacy on a particular shift. As health care becomes more specialized, there will be an increasing need for team structures to coordinate the work of individual specialists (Fried et al., 2012).

A *team* is defined as a small number of people who are committed to a common purpose, who possess complementary skills and who have agreed on specific performance goals for which team members hold themselves mutually accountable (Katzenbach & Smith, 1993). Teams differ from workgroups in that workgroups depend upon "individual bests" or the sum of individual performance for effectiveness. A team shares leadership roles and uses active problem-solving and open-ended discussions during meetings. Outputs are based on collective work products and

team performance is assessed using these outputs. Teams make decisions and then do the "real" work together (Katzenbach & Smith, 2005). Workgroups usually do not want to risk conflict and do not take collective action necessary to build a common purpose. Cohen and Bailey (1997) identified four types of teams: work teams, parallel teams, project teams, and management teams.

Work teams are continuing work units responsible for producing goods or providing services. They are usually directed by managers who make most of the decisions on what is done, how it is done, and who does it. An alternative form of the work team is the self-managing team that allows employees to decide how to carry out tasks, allocates work within the team, and makes decisions. The members of work teams are cross-trained in a variety of skills relevant to the tasks they perform.

Parallel teams draw members from different work units to perform functions that the regular organization is not equipped to perform well. These teams have limited authority and usually make recommendations to individuals higher up in the organizational hierarchy. A quality improvement team in a health system would be an example of a parallel team.

Project teams produce one-time outputs such as a new product or service. Project team members usually draw their members from different units so that specialized expertise can be applied to the project at hand. When the project is completed, the members either return to their functional unit or move on to the next project. A new drug development team that draws members from research and development, finance, marketing, and manufacturing would be an example of such a team.

Finally, *management teams* coordinate and provide direction to units under their authority. Management teams exist at the board of directors or trustee level, senior management level, or at the departmental level.

While many individuals enjoy the interactions and synergies that come from working on teams, there is probably no other aspect of organizational life that causes as much ambivalence and cynicism (Fried et al., 2012).

Many teams fail to provide the expected benefits and achieve far less than their potential because of coordination, communication, or motivation problems among group members (Franz, 2012). Interprofessional rivalries and status differences are often played out in teams causing anger, dissatisfaction, lower productivity, and a sense that individual knowledge and skills are being underutilized. True health care interprofessional teamwork is based on how well the members of the team collaborate and share power with one another (Barr & Dowding, 2016).

A meta-analysis of 298 studies found pharmacists to have positive effects on patient therapeutic and safety outcomes when participating in multidisciplinary teams that consist of physicians, nurses, and other health professionals (Chisholm-Burns et al., 2010). Another study found that shared team learning occurred more often in teams in which members felt that "they were all in this together" rather than ones in which members felt they had to get others "on board" (Bunniss & Kelly, 2008).

A study of pharmacists' identity development within multidisciplinary primary health care teams found that it takes time to begin to feel like a contributing member of a team (Pottie et al., 2009). Pharmacists needed mentors outside of the team to whom they could share ideas and ask advice. The progression to team member was not always linear and many felt there were days when progress was made and other days when steps back were taken. Pharmacists also began to see their profession through the "eyes" of doctors or nurses. They began to develop empathy for these perspectives rather than complaining about how the other health professionals do not understand their roles.

So how can effective team performance be built? Biech as cited in Gordon (2002) identified 10 characteristics of successful teams: (1) Clear goals—allows everyone to understand the function and purpose of the team; (2) defined roles—allows everyone to understand why they are on the team and enables them to form clear individual and team-based goals; (3) open and clear communication—is essential for team-building and is based on effective listening;

(4) effective decision-making—the team must be in agreement with the decisions that are reached through a consensus-building process; (5) balanced participation—ensures that all members are fully engaged; (6) valued diversity—the team must recognize each member's expertise and value variety of knowledge, skills, and abilities; (7) managed conflict—all team members feel safe to freely state their points of view without fear of reprisal; (8) positive atmosphere—requires a climate of trust be developed that requires team members to spend significant amount of time with each other; (9) cooperative relationships—team members need to recognize that they need one another's knowledge and skill to complete the given tasks; and (10) participative leadership—need to have leaders who are willing to share responsibility and recognition with the team. Borkowski (2016) added one more to this list: reflection and appreciative inquiry—teams need to allocate time for reflection and debriefing on the results of their actions and decisions so they can develop a vision of what they want to accomplish in the future and build on what worked best to reach their goals. A study of interprofessional practice confirmed these aspects of exemplar practice in primary care (Tubbesing & Chen, 2015).

Informal Organizational Structure

Alongside the formal organizational structure, an informal structure exists. The informal system has great influence in shaping individual behavior. Communication within the organization is one area that the informal structure affects. Formal communication patterns exist in the form of meetings, memos, and reports. Informal communication patterns ("the grapevine") can take the form of rumors, gossip, and speculation (George & Jones, 2012). The grapevine can be positive in that it allows formal communication to be translated into language that employees understand. In addition, it can provide feedback to the manager about pending problems in the organization. When employees feel frustrated at centralized decision-making and their level of input, the grapevine can be a useful source of information. Informal ways of influencing decision-making can also emerge through the formation of alliances and favoritism.

Organizational norms and accountability can be influenced by these informal means. *Norms* are explicit rules of conduct that govern such things as employee dress and punctuality in reporting for work. Informal norms can develop through peer-influence systems (e.g., if most pharmacists stay until all the prescription orders are processed, then someone who does not will be looked on unfavorably by peers). The *accountability* system considers ways to measure the achievement of organizational goals. This is usually accomplished through performance reviews (see Chapter 20).

Administrators and managers must monitor their treatment of employees continually to discern problems in the organization. Understanding and managing both the formal and informal structures of the organization are important for effective functioning and improved employee performance. Successful organizations have employees who provide performance beyond expectations (Robbins & Judge, 2018). This type of performance is described as organizational citizenship behaviors. Organizational citizenship behaviors are defined as behaviors which support the social and psychological atmosphere in which task performance takes place and are related to the culture and climate of the organization (Podsakoff et al., 2014). Their existence or lack of is manifested in a number of organizational behaviors (discussed later) and related to the degree to which professionals (such as pharmacists) are supported in bureaucratic organizations.

■ PROFESSIONALS IN BUREAUCRATIC ORGANIZATIONS

As noted previously, many organizations can be described as following the bureaucratic model of structure (characterized by control, hierarchy of authority, the presence of rules, and impersonality). While most pharmacists are employees of these organizations, they have been socialized through formal education and mentorship to value expertise, self-determination, and care to individual patients. This can be referred to as the *professional model*. Other aspects of this model include the use of professional associations as a major referent with regard to conduct and behavior, a sense of calling to the field (the dedication of the professional to work and the feeling that the practitioner would do the work even if few extrinsic rewards were available), and autonomy (the feeling that the practitioner ought to be able to make decisions without external pressures from clients, those who are not members of the profession, or the employer) (Hall, 1968).

In recent years, the professional value system of health care is challenged by escalating costs and the call for reform (Dye, 2017). Cost is particularly an issue for pharmacy because the cost of prescription drugs continues to escalate, and securing adequate payment for nondispensing services (e.g., drug therapy monitoring and evaluation) continues to be a struggle. One way in which health care organizations have responded to the need for change is to become more corporate or bureaucratic in values. The *corporate model* values the collective needs of its customers (not individual patients) both now and in the future and works to ensure institutional survival through measures of fiscal responsibility and operating efficiency (Stoeckle & Stanley, 1992). A professional values the care of individual patients and their present health needs, which leads to a focus on trust-building behaviors such as eliciting personal concerns and exercising technical competence. A professional responds to authority based on expertise, whereas the organization's authority is found in hierarchical positions. Allegiances of the professional outside the organization (professional associations) could conflict with organizational norms. The formalization and standardization found in organizations can stifle initiative and discourage creativity and risk taking. Although the occurrence of conflict depends on the degree to which the knowledge base of the professional leads to decisions that are inconsistent with those of management (Hall & Tolbert, 2009), there are some positive aspects to the organizational model. A highly developed division of labor and technical competence should be related to a high degree of professionalism because professionals are considered experts. Accountability and responsibility are important to the professional as well as to the corporation.

While important, the focus on technical competence, expertise, accountability, and responsibility has made it difficult for professionals to find meaning in their work (Cherniss, 1995; Dye, 2017). This focus encourages a critical, detached attitude toward the world that weakens the professional's ability to form a strong commitment to an ideology or a group. Frankl (1962) suggests that individuals can find meaning in activities done for the sake of a cause, a loved one, or a higher being. This research suggests that those individuals, who find meaning in their work, truly view their work as a "calling" to the field. These professionals are more likely to connect with clients, practice a set of ideals, and work in a community that shares and nurtures these ideals: a moral community.

How can pharmacy be infused with a greater sense of moral relevance? One might envision pharmacy and the health care system as a moral community rather than a service delivery system (Cherniss, 1995). Moral communities are those that share ethical concerns, value pluralism, and have a keen sense of social responsibility (Dharamsi, 2006). These communities are grounded in relationships with others (e.g., other pharmacists, health professionals, patients, and other stakeholders). The development of a moral community requires an interdisciplinary understanding of the moral and ethical situations that occur in the delivery of health care. Beginning a dialogue among these groups that address the multi-faceted challenges that arise within each group could open new ways of thinking, inquiry, and methods of addressing these challenges (Austin, 2007). Students and pharmacists need to articulate their value system and search for employers that allow them to express this value system. Research suggests that the day-to-day experiences pharmacists have with their employing organization can influence how they view the entire profession of pharmacy (Gaither & Mason, 1992).

Employers, who exhibit a commitment to professional ideals, align organizational structure and systems to support these ideals, and cultivate strong interpersonal relationships within the organization are ones to consider (Levinson et al., 2014). Organizations that allow pharmacists' expectations to be met find increased commitment to the organization (organizational commitment) (Gaither, 1999). Increased commitment to the profession also increases organizational commitment (Gaither, 1998a; Gaither & Mason, 1992; Gaither et al., 2008). Support from management and administrators are positively related to organizational commitment for pharmacists working for pharmaceutical manufacturers (Kong et al., 1992). Organizations that allow professionals to be managed by other professionals (i.e., pharmacists managing pharmacists) support them in maintaining control over their work (Hall & Tolbert, 2009). Employers who emphasize interpersonal relationships and those pharmacists and pharmacy technicians who experienced increased supervisor support felt increased commitment to both the profession and the employer (Desselle & Holmes, 2007; Gaither et al., 2008; Kong, 1995). Pharmacists who believe that the call for pharmacy care would have a positive effect on pharmacy were more committed to their employer and to pharmacy as a career.

With more professionals being employed by health care organizations, and the increased use of interprofessional teams, more conflict is likely to occur. Members of various professions are likely to take different views and approaches to the same issue (Hall & Tolbert, 2009). Attention must be given to these different perspectives. A study on creating high-performing work environments in hospitals found more variation within units than between units (Weinberg et al., 2013). Different types of support may be needed for different types of professionals. As mentioned earlier, team effectiveness can be improved by considering the characteristics of successful teams, and understanding how others see us, knowing each person's unique contribution, and taking ownership for team outcomes (Gordon, 2002). It can be concluded that pharmacists' responses to organizational demands can have important implications for their professional values and ability to find meaningful work. This behooves students and pharmacists alike to work for and with organizations that facilitate fulfillment of their expectations. If the values of the organization are not in line with the values of the health profession, negative personal and organizational behaviors will occur.

■ PHARMACISTS' ORGANIZATIONAL BEHAVIORS

Examining pharmacists' work-related attitudes and behaviors is important if an organization wants to improve the positive and decrease or minimize the negative actions of employees. Increased absenteeism, tardiness, and counterproductive behaviors such as not completing work in a timely manner or theft will decrease organizational productivity and performance significantly. This has the economic consequence of decreasing the profitability of the organization (Barnett & Kimberlin, 1984). An unhappy coworker can also make the work environment unpleasant for other workers. The entire day seems longer and more stressful. Negative organizational attitudes can also compromise patient care. An unhappy or dissatisfied pharmacist may be less motivated to keep skills and knowledge levels current. Management practices play a big role in pharmacists' organization behaviors. Job dissatisfaction and inadequate feedback have been found to be associated with an increased risk of medication errors (Bond & Raehl, 2001; Patterson & Pace, 2016). The physical and mental health of the pharmacist can also suffer, owing to the stress of working in an unappealing pharmacy environment with a heavy workload (Gaither et al., 2008b, 2015; Gidman et al., 2007; Kreling et al., 2006). Studies of pharmacists' organizational behaviors have focused on a variety of work-related attitudes and behaviors. The most common are job satisfaction, organizational commitment, job stress, and job turnover.

Job Satisfaction

Job satisfaction can be defined either as an emotional response (the pleasurable or positive emotional state resulting from the appraisal of one's job or job experiences) (Locke, 1976) or as a comparison between expectations and the perceived reality of the job as a whole (Bacharach et al., 1991). Each individual brings a set of expectations to a job. Research in pharmacy suggests that how closely the job meets expectations, performing more clinical or nondistributive work activities, higher levels of autonomy, recognition, ability utilization, good environmental conditions (e.g., better work schedules, less workload, control over work, good workplace teamwork and communication, adequate staffing, and less stress), professional commitment, being an active preceptor, working in an independent or nonpatient care environment, access to continuing professional development and organizational climate are strong predictors of job satisfaction (Chua et al., 2014; Desselle et al., 2018; Gaither et al., 2008, 2015, Gustafsson et al., 2018; Kuiper et al., 2011; Latessa et al., 2013; Liu & White, 2011; McCarthy et al., 2015; Mott et al., 2004; Munger et al., 2013; Payakachat et al., 2011; Reuppell et al., 2003). Being younger, male, nonwhite, in a staff position, working full-time, high role stress (e.g., role ambiguity, role strain, or role overload), and negative interpersonal interactions with either coworkers, management, or patients (Carvajal et al., 2018; Cavaco & Krookas, 2014; Ferguson et al., 2010; Gaither et al., 2008; Gidman, 2011; Lea et al., 2012; Mott et al., 2004; Prince et al., 2003; Seston et al., 2009) are factors associated with less satisfaction. Increased job satisfaction also predicted pharmacists' confidence that patients understood how to use their medications after receiving counseling from them and the feeling that patient profile reviews were more complete (Chui et al., 2014). In a study of physicians, an organizational emphasis on quality of care enhanced job satisfaction (Williams et al., 2002). The same should be true for pharmacists. Positive interactions with key stakeholders outside the pharmacy department were the largest drivers of job satisfaction for a group of health-system pharmacists (Lane et al., 2010). Enhanced job satisfaction leads to more positive feelings toward the employing organization (organizational commitment) (Rojanasarot et al., 2017).

Organizational Commitment

Organizational commitment has been defined both as an emotional attachment (affective organizational commitment) (Meyer & Maltin, 2010) and as accepting the organization's goals and values, putting forth effort, and wanting to maintain membership (Mowday et al., 1979). Organizational commitment is important because it is related to reduced job turnover intention for pharmacists (Chua et al., 2014; Gaither et al., 2008; Kahaleh & Gaither, 2005; Rojanasarot et al., 2017; Urbonas et al., 2015). Organizational commitment is enhanced when health care professionals receive appropriate compensation and benefits (Gaither & Mason, 1992; Gaither et al., 2008) and have access to important organizational information, resources to perform the job, opportunities for advancement within the organization, and perceived organizational support (structural empowerment) (Kahaleh & Gaither, 2005; Urbonas et al., 2015). This enhancement holds true regardless of practice setting (Kahaleh & Gaither, 2007). Psychological empowerment (e.g., finding meaning, feeling competent, and having independence and influence in a job) positively influences commitment for independent community pharmacists (Kahaleh & Gaither, 2007). High job demands (stress) and unpleasant interpersonal interactions decrease affective organizational commitment for hospital pharmacists (Gaither & Nadkarni, 2012).

Job Stress

Role stress in the form of role conflict, role ambiguity, role overload, and work–home conflict increases job stress (Gaither, 1998b; Gaither et al., 2008). Job dissatisfaction is also associated with increased job stress (Lea et al., 2012; Munger et al., 2013). Role expansion in the form of increased expectations to provide medication use reviews and other nondispensing services without the supporting infrastructure or support of other health care professionals has led to increased job stress, decreased job satisfaction, and increased intentions to leave the profession (Eden et al., 2009; McCann et al., 2009; Rothmann & Malan, 2007). Lack of control over the work environment and decision-making policies are particularly stressful for organizational-employed professionals (Oren, 2012; Gaither et al., 2015; Rojanasarot et al., 2017). High stress levels are related to poor working conditions, which makes it more difficult to have an organizational culture focused on patient safety and organizational improvements (Boyle et al., 2016). Higher environmental stress is also related to perceived ease in finding an alternative job (Rojanasarot et al., 2017). Stress that continues to be ignored can lead to a phenomenon known as burnout. Burnout is found to be associated with staffing inadequacy, high workload, and high levels of mental concentration and effort over time (Chui et al., 2014). It is thought to develop through a series of stages that starts with chronic fatigue and loss of energy; progresses to negativity, cynicism, emotional distress, and loss of social contacts (Weber & Jaekel-Reinhard, 2000). It includes physical manifestations such as insomnia and gastrointestinal problems, along with increased use of drugs and alcohol. It can end with suicidal thoughts and action. If caught at any time, it can be reversed.

Traditionally, burnout has been conceptualized as a problem confined to the individual (i.e., flaws in a person's character, behavior, or productivity). However, growing evidence suggests that burnout is tied to the social environment of the workplace (Maslach et al., 2001). The structure and functioning of the workplace shape how people interact and carry out tasks. Failure to recognize the human side of work increases the risk of burnout. Engagement with work requires a person's full participation in the social environment. Support, recognition, and collaboration help people focus their energy more effectively, justify their involvement and extend their achievements. Consequently, this leads to a more robust organization and lessens burnout (Maslach et al., 2001).

A recent initiative by the National Academy of Medicine is addressing clinician burnout and its effect on patient care (Brigham et al., 2018). More information on how to manage job stress and burnout is found in Chapter 12.

Job Turnover

Job turnover is one of the most pressing concerns of organizations. The decreased productivity from voluntary turnover is very costly to an organization because less experienced workers must be used to replace the more experienced workers who leave. Advertising, recruiting, and training a replacement employee for someone who has left can be costly not only in monetary terms but also in terms of lost productivity owing to the time spent bringing the new employee up to speed. In a time of shortage of available employees, it is important to retain existing employees. Actual job turnover rates of pharmacists have been estimated to be between 14% and 25% per year (Gaither, 1998a; Knapp et al., 2011). In an interview of chain pharmacists who recently left their employers, the main reasons pharmacists gave for leaving were related to working conditions: inflexible and long working hours and inadequate support personnel (Schulz & Baldwin, 1990). Other reasons for leaving an organization relate to job dissatisfaction, role stress, and culture and climate factors (Desselle et al., 2018; Gaither, 1998a; Gaither et al., 2007, 2008; Mott, 2000). Personal variables such as number of children (more), race (whites less), age (older more or less), education (e.g., having an advanced degree), and having a major life event (e.g., getting married, getting divorced, or death in family) can also result in job turnover intention (Gaither et al., 2007). Market conditions such as the number of jobs available are important because this may make it easier to leave one job for another.

As with burnout, job turnover is viewed as a process in which an individual will first think about leaving, search for job alternatives, form an intention to leave, and then actually leave. Therefore, it can be influenced at various stages. Managers may not be able to control all the factors related to job turnover (e.g., major life events or market conditions), but they can be very influential as mentioned earlier and should be on the lookout for ways in which the organization can foster commitment, improve job satisfaction, and decrease role stress. Employers can actively promote job embeddedness by encouraging employees to form social ties with one another and with the nonwork community (Leupold et al., 2013). A study of 145 community pharmacists found that higher job embeddedness along with job satisfaction was related to lower intentions to leave the employer within 1 or 3 years. Another place to start would be with the structure of the organization. Examining the amount of decision-making ability given to pharmacists, the tasks/workload assigned, the reward structure, and communication between management and staff is a good way to determine areas that need improvement. Another factor that may be particularly important for professional employees such as pharmacists is organizational identification.

Organizational identification is defined as the perception of oneness with or belongingness to a group/organization (Ashforth & Mael, 1989). To identify with an organization implies that one sees oneself as a personal representative of the organization and feels that the organization's successes and failures are one's own. Fostering organizational identification may be a very important way to shape health professionals' organizational behavior because outside influences (e.g., professional associations, colleagues, or patients) are important in the formation and maintenance of professional behavior (Dukerich et al., 2002).

The more strongly employees identify with an organization, the more likely they are to engage in organizational citizenship or extra-role behaviors specifically related to the organization (e.g., courtesy, conscientiousness, sportsmanship, civic virtue, and altruism) (Hekman et al., 2009; Konovsky & Pugh, 1994; Trybou et al., 2013). These behaviors are actions that are typically not captured in the normal reward structure of the organization. Employees who have a stronger commitment to remain at their employer, higher job satisfaction, and a positive view of their climate were more likely to participate in organizational citizenship behaviors (Desselle et al., 2018). A study of community pharmacists found that participation in pharmaceutical care activities was associated with greater organizational identification (O'Neill & Gaither, 2007). Higher levels of organizational identification were related to lower job turnover intention. In addition, the way in which an employee believes the organization is viewed by outsiders has a direct impact on both organizational identification and job turnover intention; the more positive the image, the greater is identification. Joe Smart may want to ask some of the patients and even the doctors and nurses who come into the ambulatory care pharmacy how they view the pharmacy and the services it provides. If these "outsiders" have a negative view of the pharmacy, it may be contributing to the tense atmosphere in the pharmacy. In line with the focus on identification and organizational citizenship behaviors, more recent research focuses on the positive organizational behavior of well-being.

Well-being

One of the major factors contributing to the rise in studies examining well-being is the changes which are occurring in organizations and the way in which people work. Technology continues to be a major influence in how people work. Automation can take over work that used to be performed by pharmacists or technicians leading to employment insecurity and competition for jobs. "Precarious work" (labor insecurity) is becoming a more prominent model in the relationship between employers and employees (Traulsen & Druedahl, 2018), with new pharmacists being given contracts that are less than full-time or positions as "floaters" where one does not work in a designated location but moves from location to location based on the need. Technology intensifies work since employees are always connected to their jobs via telephone, text or email. The expectation to maintain constant connection takes a toll on employees' physical and mental well-being (McDonald & Hite, 2018).

The National Academies of Medicine is addressing the issue of clinician well-being given the body of evidence that burnout is endemic in health care providers and negatively affects patient outcomes (Brigham et al., 2018). To address this issue, many are calling for an increased focus by employers on developing resilience (the ability to bounce back from adversity or personal setbacks) in their workers (Luthans et al., 2006). Individuals who are resilient are more emotionally stable when faced with adversity and are more flexible to changing demands and are open to new experiences (Bonanno et al., 2001; Tugade & Fredrickson, 2004). Supportive workplaces are keys in helping employee develop resilience (Mishra & McDonald, 2017). Providing formal programs that further develop employees' skills and competencies and flexible work schedules, in addition to informal networks which include mentoring and support from family and friends, can help build resilience. Employers are also looking at engagement as another way to combat burnout.

Engagement is defined by a positive, fulfilling, work-related state of mind that is characterized by vigor, dedication and absorption and reflects a persistent positive state that is not focused on any particular object, event or individual (Schaufeli et al., 2002). Engagement can be described as a behavior (organizational citizenship) or a trait (conscientiousness) (Macey & Schneider, 2008). It is related to the maintenance of pharmacist professional competence (Austin & Gregory, 2019). This brings us to another important area in pharmacists' organizational behaviors: emotions.

Emotions

Emotions are intense feelings that are directed at someone or something (Greenberg & Baron, 2008). Emotions are sometimes confused with moods, which are pervasive emotions not directed at any particular person or object (Fiske & Taylor, 1991). Moods have been shown to be related to withdrawal behaviors such as absenteeism and turnover (Pelled et al., 1999). Health care organizations put more emotional demands on employees and patients than many other organizations, yet very little is known about what these demands are and the strategies people use to deal with their emotions (Ovretveit, 2001). One study in pharmacy found that the emotional expression of anger, defensiveness, or disgust is related to job dissatisfaction and depression, whereas the expression of resentfulness and disappointment is related to emotional exhaustion, a major component of job burnout (Abunassar & Gaither, 2000).

Health care demands both the suppression and expression of emotion and skills to know and manage feelings appropriately (Ovretveit, 2001). Emotional regulation in the workplace has been termed *emotional labor* and is particularly important to health care professionals. Emotional labor is defined as expressing organizationally desired emotions during service transactions (Hochschild, 1983). The difference between the emotions that an individual expresses and those he or she actually feels can be the basis of emotional exhaustion and burnout.

Individuals who have the ability to take another's perspective or to know what another is feeling (empathic concern) or who generally express or feel positive emotions (positive affect) will have less of a need to expend emotional labor (Zammuner & Galli, 2005). It is also suggested that persons who are more emotionally mature (or possess greater emotional intelligence) will experience greater job satisfaction than those who do not.

Emotional intelligence is the ability or capacity to perceive, assess, and manage the emotions of oneself and of others (Ledlow & Coppola, 2014). The pharmacists in the scenario's ambulatory care pharmacy may be expending high levels of emotional labor. The pharmacy director may want to explore training for pharmacists to enhance their empathic behaviors, which may also decrease their emotional labor and possibly enhance emotional intelligence. The concept of emotional intelligence has also been linked to another important influence on the organizational behavior of employees: the leadership abilities of those in management or administrative positions. The emotional intelligence model of leadership focuses on the relational aspects of a leader (self-awareness, self-management, social awareness, and social skills). This aspect of leadership will be revisited at the end of the next section (Ledlow & Coppola, 2014).

Management versus Leadership

Leadership can be thought of as getting a group of people to move toward a particular vision or ideal (see Chapters 3 and 4). Leadership is concerned with making organizational change and with motivating employees to move toward a shared vision. *Management,* on the other hand, is concerned with handling the complexities involved in running an organization (i.e., planning, control, evaluation, and financial analysis) (Kotter, 1990). Given this distinction, a manager or an administrator may not necessarily be a leader. She may be more concerned with the day-to-day functioning of the organization. The manager may give little thought to the overall goals of the organization and how her department/pharmacy fits into the overall scheme. In addition, managers may not give much thought to the future and to developing a shared vision with employees as to where the organization should be moving. A good manager should also be a leader because one needs to be concerned with the present situation but have an eye on the future. The future should include not only the tasks and activities in which the organization engages but also the development of motivation and future leadership in the staff. This motivation and energy are essential to facilitate the transformation of pharmacy from drug procurement and dispensing into the provision of pharmaceutical care.

◼ LEADERSHIP BEHAVIOR

In an era of increasing corporatization of health care, securing the welfare of patients requires that health professionals participate in the creation of optimal frameworks to deliver care (Stoeckle & Stanley, 1992). No longer should the individual pharmacist say, "I am not the manager or administrator, so I have no role in determining how the pharmacy is structured or organized." Without highly competent and aggressive leadership, the provision of pharmaceutical care and other new roles advocated by the pharmacy profession could be usurped by other health professionals, corporate entities, or technologies (Knoer, 2014). This will require the development of leadership abilities in all pharmacists.

■ THEORIES OF LEADERSHIP

Trait Theories

Much of the early research on leadership focused on identifying personality traits that could distinguish leaders from nonleaders. Intelligence, self-confidence, a high energy level, and technical knowledge about the task at hand are positively correlated with leadership abilities (Robbins & Judge, 2018). The problem with the search for traits of leaders is that it implies that leaders are born and not made. Individuals without these traits could never be leaders. It also ignores the influence and needs of the employees one is trying to lead. Trait theories focus more on leaders and less on followers. Research findings in this area have been inconsistent. Some studies found that one trait was related to leadership ability, whereas another study found that it was not related (Stodgill, 1948; Yukl, 1989). An explanation for this inconsistency is that the trait itself is not important; however, its interaction with the environment is what makes the difference (DeHoogh et al., 2005). Different environments need different types of leadership styles to be successful.

Other research suggests that traits do make a difference when categorized into five basic personality characteristics (Judge et al., 2002): *extroversion*—one's comfort level with relationships; *agreeableness*—an individual's propensity to defer to others; *conscientiousness*—how reliable a person is; *emotional stability*—a person's ability to withstand stress; and *openness to experience*—an individual's range of interests and fascination with novelty (Robbins & Judge, 2018). High energy and self-confidence can be categorized under extroversion and emotional stability. The other main drawback with the trait approach is that it does a better job of predicting who may emerge as a leader than determining what constitutes effective leadership. This has led contemporary researchers to take a behavioral approach to leadership and to focus on the preferred behavioral styles that good leaders demonstrate.

Behavioral Theories

Researchers have observed three very basic leadership styles: autocratic, democratic, and laissez-faire. *Autocratic leaders* make all the decisions and allow for no or very little input from the employees. *Democratic leaders* consult with their subordinates and allow them some input in the decision-making process. *Laissez-faire leaders* allow employees complete autonomy. In such an approach, employees set their own goals and work toward them with no direction from management. Let's say a pharmacy manager would like to implement a disease management program in the pharmacy. An autocratic leader would just inform the employees of the change in approach and then assign the tasks necessary to implement the program. A democratic leader would present the idea to the employees and ask for their input about the appropriateness of the idea and take into consideration their ideas on how to implement the program. Finally, a laissez-faire leader would not mention the idea unless the employees came to him with it. The leader then would allow the employees to develop the entire program and implement the plan. Research suggests that males tend to use a more autocratic style and females use a more democratic style (Eagly & Johnson, 1990). Reasons for this vary, but some suggest that women have better interpersonal skills than males and/or need to use this style of leadership since they may get more resistance from subordinates than males when trying to lead (Eagly at al., 1992). As the number of female pharmacists in management and leadership positions continue to increase (Gaither et al., 2015), it will be interesting to watch if these distinctions hold true. It has been found that all three styles of leadership behavior can be appropriate depending on the situation (La Monica, 1994). These findings led researchers to begin examining the components of leadership behavior and the determination of appropriate behavior for the specific situation.

Situational or Contingency-Based Theories

Hersey's Situational Leadership® model is a leadership theory based on three basic dimensions: task and relationship orientation behavior and follower readiness (Hersey & Blanchard, 1988). *Task orientation behavior* refers to the extent to which a leader engages in one-way communication by defining the roles of individuals and members of the group by explaining (telling or showing or both) what each subordinate is to do, as well as when, where, how much, and by when specific tasks are to be accomplished. This dimension also includes the extent to which the leader defines the structure of the organization (e.g., chain of command, channels of communication) and specifies ways of getting jobs accomplished. *Relationship orientation* behavior refers to the extent to which the leader engages in two-way communication, provides socioemotional support, and uses facilitative versus directive efforts of bringing about group change. This component considers the establishment of effective interpersonal relationships between the leader and the group based on trust. The third component consists of *follower readiness or maturity*. In this case, maturity readiness is related to the group's or individual's willingness or ability to accept responsibility for a task and whether they are currently performing the task at a sustained and acceptable level. Certainly, the possession of the necessary training or experience to perform the task impacts on their ability to perform but what matters most in assessing readiness is whether they are doing the task now rather than what they are potentially capable of doing. As in the example given earlier, a group of pharmacists may be quite willing to develop a disease management program but may be inexperienced at implementing such a program. Each of these dimensions can be located on a continuum that is divided into four quadrants (Waller, Smith, & Warnock, 1989).

1. *High task/low relationship.* The leader determines the roles and goals of the group and closely supervises the task. Communication is one way and usually flows from the leader to the followers. This style, also known as *telling* (S1), is most appropriate when followers are unable/unwilling or insecure (R1).
2. *High task/high relationship.* The leader still closely supervises the task but will also explain why decisions are made. The leader may alter the plan given the followers' reactions. This style, also known as *selling* (S2), is most appropriate when followers' are unable but more willing or secure (R2).
3. *High relationship/low task.* In this case, the leader is more concerned about process and how the group works together to accomplish the task rather than the task itself. In this style, also called participative or *supportive* (S3), the leader still may define the problem but supports the group's efforts at accomplishing the task. Followers in this case are able but unwilling or insecure (R3).
4. *Low task/low relationship.* The leader turns over all decisions and responsibility for task accomplishment, goal attainment, and implementation to followers. The leader may be available for consultation but usually maintains a low profile. In this case, also called *delegation* (S4), followers are very able, willing, and secure (R4).

It is the leader's job to determine the performance readiness of the group and then apply the appropriate leadership style to the situation.

A final component of this model is *leader effectiveness* (La Monica, 1994). A leader's influence over an individual or group can be either successful or unsuccessful. When a leader's behavior fails to influence an individual or group to achieve a specified goal, then the leader must re-evaluate what occurred and redesign a strategy for goal accomplishment. Even when a goal is accomplished, a leader's influence can still range from very effective to ineffective depending on how followers feel about the leader's behavior. If a leader knows the personal strengths of her followers and assigns goals or tasks with them in mind, this can make goal accomplishment quite rewarding for the followers. On the other hand, if the followers feel coerced to accomplish by a leader who uses positional power, close supervision, and rewards and punishments, the followers may be very unhappy and carry negative feelings toward the leader. Leadership effectiveness is very important because effective leadership will lead to followers who are motivated and goal oriented even when the leader is not present. Ineffective leadership will lead to followers who often will relax the drive to accomplish when the leader is absent.

A study of pharmacists who worked in community settings or for national and state pharmacy associations found that the most common leadership style was selling (high task/high relationship), and the next most common was participation (low task/high relationship) (Ibrahim & Wertherimer, 1998; Ibrahim et al., 1997). About 26% of the pharmacists did not have a dominant style. Not surprisingly, most pharmacists scored in the low- (community pharmacists) to-moderate (association executives) range in their ability to adapt their style to the needs of their subordinates (leadership effectiveness). These results suggest that while pharmacists possess a dominant leadership style, there is room for improvement in terms of learning to respond and modify their style to best fit the needs and motivational levels of their staff.

Leader–Member Exchange Theory

Another theory related to the leader–follower relationship is the leader–member exchange (LMX) theory (Green & Uhl-Bien, 1995). This theory suggests that leaders establish special relationships with a small group of followers early on in the tenure of the leader. These individuals make up the leader's in-group, whereas others are considered part of the out-group. It is unclear how these relationships form, but most likely they result from the followers either having similar personality characteristics to the leader or exceptional abilities to perform the job. The in-group gets special attention from the leader and tends to have higher job satisfaction and lower job turnover intention than members of the out-group (George & Jones, 2012). Another study found that the more positive the LMX between nurses and their supervisors, the higher level of extra-role behavior (Trybou et al., 2013). These findings suggest that leaders need

to pay attention to the nature of their relationships with followers because these relationships can greatly affect employee morale.

Leader-Participation Model

One of the more recent additions to contingency-based leadership theories relates leadership behavior and participation in decision-making (Vroom & Yetton, 1973). This model assumes five behaviors that may be feasible given a particular situation. These behaviors are as follows: (1) you solve the problem yourself using the information you have available at the time; (2) you obtain the necessary information from subordinates and then decide on a solution yourself; (3) you share the problem with relevant subordinates individually, getting their ideas and suggestions without bringing them together as a group, and then you make the decision; (4) you share the problem with your subordinates as a group and collectively obtain their ideas and suggestions, and then you make the decision that may or may not reflect your subordinates' influence; and (5) you share the problem with the group and together you generate and evaluate alternatives and attempt to reach consensus on a solution. The leader-participation model then uses a series of eight yes–no questions to determine how much participation should be used. Questions include the following:

- Do I have enough information to make a high-quality decision?
- If the decision were accepted, would it make a difference which course of action was adopted?
- Do subordinates have sufficient additional information to result in a high-quality decision?
- Do I know exactly what information is needed, who possesses it, and how to collect it?
- Is acceptance of the decision by subordinates critical to effective implementation?
- If I were to make the decision by myself, is it certain that my subordinates would accept it?
- Can subordinates be trusted to base solutions on organizational considerations?
- Is conflict among subordinates likely in the preferred solution?

These questions allow the leader to determine which of the five behaviors is most appropriate. Results from research on this model suggest that leaders should consider the use of participatory methods when the quality of the decision is important, when it is crucial that subordinates accept the decision and it is unlikely that they will if they do not take part in it, and when subordinates can be trusted to pay attention to the goals of the group rather than simply their own preferences (Robbins & Judge, 2018). An update of this model adds several more yes–no questions to consider regarding time constraints that limit subordinate participation, costs of bringing subordinates together, minimizing the time needed to make the decision, and the importance of developing subordinates' decision-making skills (Vroom & Jago, 1988).

This approach may be fruitful in pharmacy because new leadership models of organizing health care have been proposed. Governance models that focus on shared decision-making between management and health care professions offer a way to combine both professional and organizational concerns (Young, 2002). The management style of leaders in an era of change is one that has a high regard for people and production and emphasizes shared responsibility, involvement, commitment, and mutual support (Williams, 1986). The most productive and motivated staff members are those who have strong relationships with others with whom or for whom they work (Abramowitz, 2001). By focusing on followers, leaders can empower followers to reach their potential and in turn nurture future leaders (Barr & Dowding, 2016).

Transactional versus Transformational Leadership

Most of the theories presented in this chapter are considered transactional in nature. In other words, they are largely oriented toward accomplishing the task at hand and maintaining good relations with those working with the leader by exchanging promises of rewards for performance (Dessler, 2003). A newer approach to leadership takes a transformational approach. Transformational leaders make subordinates more conscious of the importance and value of their task outcomes and provide followers with a vision and motivation to go beyond self-interest for the good of the organization (Daft, 2016; Osland et al., 2006). They also create an environment that supports exploration, experimentation, risk-taking, and sharing of ideas (Jung et al., 2003), which focuses sharply on the current moment in time (Davidson, 2010). This focus on task outcomes is a major shift in the health care arena because much of the focus of health care has been on the process of care (Borkowski, 2016). It is suggested that health care organizations need both transactional (for control and efficiency) and transformational (for innovation) leadership. A recent survey of health-system pharmacists indicated that pharmacists did possess both transactional and transformational characteristics, but few were interested in becoming the director of pharmacy (Abraham, 2006; White & Enright, 2013). This suggests that more research is needed as to why this type of leadership is unattractive to pharmacists and what can be done to remedy this situation. More information on leadership theories can be found in Chapter 3.

There is always the question of whether leadership is really necessary. As mentioned earlier, advocating for patients and the fulfillment of new roles for pharmacists will require that all pharmacists demonstrate leadership behaviors. Such factors as ability, intrinsic motivation, the nature of technology, and the structure of the organization can affect the performance and satisfaction of its members. Upon graduation, pharmacists possess the basic task knowledge to practice pharmacy. Pharmacists may also try to maintain good working relationships with patients and management because of professional values. These factors can substitute for effective leadership. Goals will be met regardless of what the leader or manager does or does not do. But managers and leaders need to recognize that by no means will motivated pharmacists continue to be motivated and energized in working environments that are negative and highly stressful. It is important for leaders to develop a shared vision with individual units in their organizations and support and empower employees to move toward that vision. An effective leader conducts self-diagnosis and is aware of his or her blind spots, seeks ways to address them, and also surrounds himself or herself with people having complementary strengths.

This circles back to the concept of organizational culture. There is a growing trend to incorporate culture into leadership theories and models (Ledlow & Coppola, 2014). This suggests that leaders need to determine, develop, and maintain an organizational culture that can meet expectations, thrive, and continue to respond to the ever changing and demanding health care environment. This requires leaders to focus on the relational aspects of the emotional intelligence model.

One final note regarding leadership and the increasing diversity in health care organizations. This is in regards to not only the type of personnel working together (e.g., physicians, nurses, pharmacists, technicians, and assistants) but also the demographic characteristics of these workers (e.g., gender, race/ethnicity, and age). Leaders must be able to effectively manage this diversity to maximize individual and group performance. An approach that links diversity to the actual work performed and values it for what it adds to the organization leads to an environment in which the benefits of diversity can be maximized (Ely & Thomas, 2001).

■ REVISITING THE SCENARIO

Joe Smart knew that something was wrong with the internal environment of the ambulatory care pharmacy. What he probably noticed was a lack of leadership on the part of the pharmacy director and how the pharmacists were very task-oriented in their behavior and seemed not to find their work meaningful. It may be that the employees of the pharmacy do not feel like a part of the health system organizational team and are feeling frustrated by a lack of recognition by others. They may also be uncertain of their roles in the future and if they will still be employed. It seems as though not a lot of time has been spent building relationships within or outside the department. Since Joe is the newest employee of the pharmacy, he is a

bit hesitant to get involved, but he may be the perfect person to inquire about the values and goals of the ambulatory care pharmacy and how the pharmacy is structured to meet these goals. This would be a perfect time to examine the culture and climate in the pharmacy to find out why the employees are dissatisfied. Although Joe does not have a leadership position in the organization, he should think about what he could do to improve the environment of the pharmacy. It is everyone's responsibility to make sure that health care is being delivered in the best manner possible, and unhappy staff members probably are not doing their best. Joe also could work on building relationships with others on the staff. This may help the employees talk about what is going on at the pharmacy. Improved dialogue within the pharmacy and with other stakeholders outside the pharmacy department could enhance the sense of community among the employees and their sense of well-being. With the help of more experienced employees, Joe could bring these matters to the attention of the pharmacy director. By taking a proactive stance, Joe is developing leadership skills that will serve him throughout his career.

■ CONCLUSION

An understanding of organizational behavior is needed by pharmacists to function productively in an increasingly complex organizational environment. Looking for employers who facilitate professional goals is necessary for the continued development of new roles for pharmacists. Employers must constantly monitor the work environment for signs of job dissatisfaction, job stress, and burnout in their employees. It is important that health care professionals do not stay away from participating in organizational governance. It is a part of their professional responsibility to ensure that health care is delivered appropriately to patients. Leadership ability can greatly influence pharmacists' attitudes and behaviors. Without a clear and shared vision between management and staff, innovative practices will be difficult to implement.

■ QUESTIONS FOR FURTHER DISCUSSION

1. Why did the focus of organizational behavior in health care change over time?

2. Given that organizations are trying to empower employees at all levels, are organizational charts still necessary? Why or why not?

3. How important is division of labor, span of control, unity of command, departmentalization, and other structural aspects in pharmacy today? Do you see more or less of these structures in pharmacy organizations? What new organizational forms do you see developing in the future?

4. What are some ways in which professionals respond to organizational demands? Are these appropriate? What are other ways of responding?

5. What role do values play in an organization?

6. How might pharmacists find meaningful work and well-being in their organizations?

7. Why is it important for pharmacists and employing organizations to monitor organizational behaviors?

8. How can organizations assist pharmacists in expanding their role without inadvertently increasing their workload to unmanageable levels?

9. What role does emotion and emotional intelligence have in a health care organization? How might we better understand their importance?

10. What are some key features of leadership? Is it important for pharmacists to develop leadership skills? How will you develop your leadership abilities?

REFERENCES

Abraham D. 2006. Pharmacy leadership crisis: Is it the people or the job? Paper presented at American Society of Health-System Pharmacists Midyear Clinical Meeting, Anaheim, CA.

Abramowitz PW. 2001. Nurturing relationships: An essential ingredient of leadership. *Am J Health Syst Pharm* 58:479.

Abunassar SM, Gaither CA. 2000. The effects of cognitive appraisals and coping strategies on job satisfaction, commitment and burnout levels in hospital pharmacists. Paper presented at the 147th Annual Meeting of the American Pharmaceutical Association, Washington, DC.

Ashforth BE, Mael FA. 1989. Social identity theory and the organization. *Acad Manage Rev* 14:20.

Austin W. 2007. The ethics of everyday practice: Healthcare environments as moral communities. *ANS Adv Nurs Sci* 30:81.

Austin Z, Gregory PAM. 2019. The role of disengagement in the psychology of competence drift. *Res Social Admin Pharm* 15:45.

Bacharach SB, Bamberger P, Conley S. 1991. Work-home conflict among nurses and engineers: Mediating the impact of role stress on burnout and satisfaction at work. *J Org Behav* 12:39.

Barnett CW, Kimberlin CL. 1984. Job and career satisfaction in pharmacy. *J Social Admin Pharm* 2:1.

Barr J, Dowding L. 2016. *Leadership in Health Care*, 3rd ed. Thousand Oaks, CA: Sage.

Bonanno GA, Papa A, O'Neill K. 2001. Loss and human resilience. *Applied and Preventive Psychology* 10:193.

Bond CA, Raehl CL. 2001. Pharmacists' assessment of dispensing errors: Risk factors, practice sites, professional functions and satisfaction. *Pharmacotherapy* 21:614.

Borkowski N. 2016. *Organizational Behavior in Health Care*. Sudbury, MA: Jones and Bartlett.

Boyle TA, Bishop A, Morrision B, et al. 2016. Pharmacist work stress and learning from quality related events. *Res Social Admin Pharm* 12:772–783.

Boyle TA, Mahaffey T, Mackinnon NJ, Diehl H, Hallstrom LK, Morgan H. 2011. Determinants of medication incident reporting, recovery, and learning in community pharmacies: A conceptual model. *Res Social Admin Pharm* 7:93.

Brigham T, Barden C, Dopp AL, et al. 2018. A journey to construct an all-encompassing conceptual model of factors affecting clinician well-being and resilience. *NAM Perspectives* Discussion Paper, National Academy of Medicine. Washington DC.

Bunniss S, Kelly DR. 2008. 'The unknown becomes the known': Collective learning and change in primary care teams. *Med Educ* 42:1185.

Bush J, Langley CA, Wilson KA. 2009. The corporatization of community pharmacy: Implications for service provision, the public health function, and pharmacy's claim to professional status in the United Kingdom. *Res Social Admin Pharm* 5:305.

Carlin JE. 2011. *Lawyers On Their Own: The Solo Practitioner in an Urban Setting*. New Orleans, LA: Quid Pro Books.

Carvajal MJ, Popovici I, Hardigan PC. 2018. Gender differences in the measurement of pharmacists' job satisfaction. *Human Resources for Health* 16:33.

Cavaco AM, Krookas AA. 2014. Community pharmacies automation: Any impact on counseling duration and job satisfaction? *Int J Clin Pharm* 36:325.

Cherniss C. 1995. *Beyond Burnout*. New York, NY: Routledge.

Chisholm-Burns MA, Lee JK, Spivey CA, et al. 2010. US pharmacists' effect as team members on patient care: Systematic review and meta-analysis. *Med Care* 48:923.

Chua GN, Yee LJ, Sim BA, et al., 2014. Job satisfaction, organization commitment and retention in the public workforce: A survey among pharmacists in Malaysia. *Int J Pharm Prac* 22:265.

Chui MA, Look KA, Mott DA. 2014. The association of subjective workload dimensions on quality of care and pharmacist quality of work life. *Res Social Admin Pharm* 10:328.

Clark BE, Mount JM. 2006. Pharmacy service orientation: A measure of organizational culture in pharmacy practice sites. *Res Social Admin Pharm* 2:110.

Cohen SG, Bailey DE. 1997. What makes team work: Group effectiveness research from the shop floor to the executive suite. *J Manage* 23:239.

Daft RL. 2016. *Organizational Theory and Design*, 12th ed. Boston, MA: Cengage Learning.

Davidson SJ. 2010. Complex responsive processes: A new lens for leadership in twenty-first-century health care. *Nursing Forum* 45:108.

DeHoogh A, Den Hartog D, Koopmam P. 2005. Linking the big five factors of personality to charismatic and transactional leadership. *J Organizational Behavior* 26:839.

Dessler G. 2003. *Management: Leading People and Organizations in the 21st Century*, 3rd ed. Upper Saddle River, NJ: Prentice-Hall.

Desselle SP, Andrews B, Lui J, Raja GL. 2018. The scholarly productivity and work environments of academic pharmacists. *Res Social Admin Pharm* 14:727.

Desselle SP, Holmes ER. 2007. A structural model of CPhTs' job satisfaction and career commitment. *J Am Pharm Assoc* 47:58.

Desselle SP, Skomo ML. 2010. Factors related to pharmacists' care of migraineurs. *Res Social Admin Pharm* 6:232.

Dharamsi S. 2006. Building moral communities? First, do no harm. *J Dent Educ* 70:1235.

Dragoni L, Park H, Soltis J, Forte-Trammell S. 2014. Show and tell: How supervisors facillitate leader development among transitioning leaders. *J Applied Psych* 99:66.

Dukerich JM, Golden BR, Shortell SM. 2002. Beauty is in the eye of the beholder: The impact of organizational identification, identity, and image on the cooperative behaviors of physicians. *Admin Sci Q* 47:507.

Dye CF. 2017. *Leadership in Healthcare: Essential Values and Skills*, 3rd ed. Chicago, IL: Health Administration Press.

Dyrbye LN, Shanafelt TD, Sinsky CA, et al. 2017. Burnout among health care professionals: A call to explore and address this underrecognized threat to safe, high-quality care. *NAM Perspectives* Discussion Paper, National Academy of Medicine, Washington, DC.

Eagly AH, Johnson BT. 1990. Gender and leadership style: A meta-analysis. *Psych Bull* 108:233.

Eagly AH, Makhijam MG, Klonsky BG. 1992. Gender and the evaluation of leaders: A meta-analysis. *Psyc Bull* 111:3.

Eden M, Schafheutle EI, Hassell K. 2009. Workload pressure among recently qualified pharmacists: An exploratory study of intentions to leave the profession. *Int J Pharm Pract* 17:181.

Ely RJ, Thomas DA. 2001. Cultural diversity at work: The effects of diversity perspectives on work group processes and outcomes. *Admin Sci Q* 46:229.

Feletto E, Wilson LK, Roberts AS, Benrimoj SI. 2010. Building capacity to implement cognitive pharmaceutical services. *Res Social Admin Pharm* 6:163.

Ferguson J, Ashcroft D, Hassell K. 2010. Qualitative insights into job satisfaction and dissatisfaction with management among community and hospital pharmacists. *Res Social Admin Pharm* 7:306.

Fiske ST, Taylor SE. 1991. *Social Cognition*. New York, NY: McGraw-Hill.

Frankl VE. 1962. *Man's Search for Meaning*. New York, NY: Clarion.

Franz TM. 2012. *Group Dynamics and Team Interventions: Understanding and Improving Team Performance*. West Sussex, UK: Wiley-Blackwell.

Freidson E. 1970. *Profession of Medicine: A Study of the Sociology of Applied Knowledge*. New York, NY: Dodd, Mead, p. 73.

Fried BJ, Topping S, Edmondson AC. 2012. Teams and team effectiveness in health care services organizations. In Burns LR, Bradley EH, Weiner BJ (eds.) *Shortell and Kaluzny's Health Care Management: Organization Design and Behavior*, 6th ed. Clifton Park, NY: Delmar, Cengage Learning.

Fulk J, Desanctis G. 1995. Electronic communication and changing organizational forms. *Org Sci* 6:337.

Gaither CA. 1998a. The predictive validity of work/career-related attitudes and intentions on pharmacists' turnover behavior. *J Pharm Mark Manage* 12:3.

Gaither CA. 1998b. An investigation of pharmacists' role stress and the work/non-work interface. *J Social Admin Pharm* 15:92.

Gaither CA. 1999. Career commitment: A mediator of the effects of job stress on pharmacists' work-related attitudes. *J Am Pharm Assoc.* 1999;39:353-361.

Gaither CA, Kahaleh AA, Doucette WR, et al. 2008. A modified model of pharmacists' job stress: The role of organizational, extra-role and individual factors on work-related outcomes. *Res Social Admin Pharm* 4:231.

Gaither CA, Mason HL. 1992. A model of pharmacists' career commitment, organizational commitment and career and job withdrawal intentions. *J Social Admin Pharm* 9:75.

Gaither CA, Nadkarni A. 2012. Interpersonal interactions and job stress in health care: The relationship of job demands and work-related outcomes of pharmacists. *Int J Pharm Pract* 20:80.

Gaither CA, Nadkarni A, Mott DA, et al. 2007. Should I stay or should I go? The influence of individual and organizational factors on pharmacists' future work plans. *J Am Pharm Assoc* 47:165.

Gaither CA, Schommer JC, Doucette WR, Kreling DH, Mott DA. 2015. Final report of the 2014 national sample survey of the pharmacists' workforce to determine contemporary demographic and practice characteristics. Available at http://www.aacp.org/resources/research/pharmacyworkforcecenter/Documents/FinalReportOfTheNationalPharmacistWorkforceStudy2014.pdf. Accessed October 3, 2015.

George JM, Jones GR. 2012. *Understanding and Managing Organizational Behavior*, 6th ed. Upper Saddle River, NY: Pearson Education, Inc.

Gibb JR. 1978. *Trust: A New View of Personal and Organizational Development*. Los Angeles: Guild of Tutors Press.

Gidman WK. 2011. Increasing community pharmacy workloads in England: Causes and consequences. *Int J Clin Pharm* 33:512.

Gidman WK, Hassell K, Day J, et al. 2007. The impact of increasing workloads and role expansion on female community pharmacists in the United Kingdom. *Res Social Admin Pharm* 3:285.

Gordon J. 2002. A perspective on team building. *J Am Acad Bus* 2:185.

Green GB, Uhl-Bien M. 1995. Relationship-based approach to leadership: Development of leader-member exchange (LMX) theory of leadership over 25 years: Applying a multi-domain perspective. *Leadership Q* 6:219.

Greenberg J, Baron RA. 2008. *Behavior in Organizations*, 9th ed. Upper Saddle River, NJ: Prentice-Hall.

Gregory ST, Menser T. 2015. Burnout among primary care physicians: A test of the areas of worklife model. *J Health Care Management* 60:133.

Gustafsson M, Mattsson S, Wallman A, Gallego G. 2018. Pharmacists' satisfaction with their work: Analysis of an alumni survey. *Res Social Admin Pharm* 14:700.

Hall RH. 1968. Professionalization and bureaucratization. *Am Sociol Rev* 33:92.

Hall RH, Tolbert PS. 2009. *Organizations: Structures, Processes and Outcomes*. Upper Saddle River, NJ: Pearson Education, Inc.

Harrison JR, Carroll GR. 1991. Keeping the faith: A model of cultural transmission in formal organizations. *Admin Sci Q* 36:552.

Hartnell CA, Ou AY, Kinicki A. 2011. Organizational culture and organizational effectiveness: A meta-analytic investigation of the competing values framework's theoretical suppositions. *J Appl Psychol* 96:677.

Hekman DR, Bigley GA, Steensma HK, et al. 2009. Combined effects of organizational and professional identification on the reciprocity dynamic for professional employees. *Acad Manage J* 52:506.

Hersey P, Blanchard KH. 1988. *Management of Organizational Behavior: Utilizing Human Resources*. Englewood Cliffs, NJ: Prentice-Hall.

Hochschild A. 1983. *The Managed Heart: Commercialization of Human Feeling*. Berkeley: University of California Press.

Ibrahim MIM, Wertherimer AI. 1998. Management leadership styles of effectiveness of community pharmacists: A descriptive analysis. *J Social Admin Pharm* 15:57.

Ibrahim MIM, Wertherimer AI, Myers MJ, et al. 1997. Leadership styles and effectiveness: Pharmacists in associations vs. pharmacists in community settings. *J Pharm Mark Manage* 12:23.

Jacobs R, Mannion R, Davies HTO, Harrison S, et al. 2013. The relationship between organizational culture and performance in acute hospitals. *Social Sci Med* 76:115.

Jacobs S, Ashcroft D, Hassell K. 2011. Culture in community pharmacy organisations: What can we glean from the literature? *J Health Org Manage* 25:420.

Jepsen DM, O'Neill MS. 2013. Australian hospital pharmacists reflect on career success. *J Pharm Pract Res* 43:29.

Jones JE. 1981. The organizational universe. In Jones JE, Pfeiffer JW (eds.) *The 1981 Annual Handbook for Group Facilitators*. San Diego: Pfeiffer and Company.

Judge TA, Bono JE, Ilies R, Gerhardt MW. 2002. Personality and leadership: A qualitative and quantitative review. *J Appl Psychol* 87:765.

Jung DI, Chow C, Wu A. 2003. The role of transformational leadership in enhancing organizational innovation: Hypothesis and some preliminary conclusions. *The Leadership Quarterly* 14:525.

Kahaleh AA, Gaither CA. 2005. Effects of empowerment on pharmacists' organizational behaviors. *J Am Pharm Assoc* 45:700.

Kahaleh AA, Gaither CA. 2007. The effects of work setting on pharmacists' empowerment and organizational behaviors. *Res Social Admin Pharm* 3:199.

Katzenbach JR, Smith DK. 1993. *The Wisdom of Teams: Creating the High-Performance Organization*. Boston, MA: Harvard Business School Press.

Katzenbach JR, Smith DK. 2005. The wisdom of teams. *Harvard Bus Rev* 83:163.

Knapp KK, Manolakis M, Webster A, et al. 2011. Projected growth in pharmacy education and research: 2010–2015. *Am J Pharm Educ* 75:108.

Knoer S. 2014. Stewardship of the pharmacy enterprise. *Am J Health-System Pharm*. 71:1204.

Kong SX. 1995. Predictors of organizational and career commitment among Illinois pharmacists. *Am J Health Syst Pharm* 52:2005.

Kong SX, Wertheimer AI, McGhan WF. 1992. Role stress, organizational commitment, and turnover intention among pharmaceutical scientists: A multivariate analysis. *J Social Admin Pharm* 9:59.

Konovsky MA, Pugh SD. 1994. Citizenship behavior and social exchange. *Acad Manage J* 37:656.

Korba LM, Gillespie AM, Schmidt RE, et al. 2012. Do consistent corporate cultures have better business performance: Exploring the interaction effects. *Human Relations* 65:241.

Kotter JP. 1990. What leaders really do? *Harv Bus Rev* 68:103.

Kreling DH, Doucette WR, Mott DA, et al. 2006. Community pharmacists' work environments: Evidence from the 2004 national pharmacist workforce study. *J Am Pharm Assoc* 46:331.

Kuiper RL, Conway DLP, Pacitti R. 2011. Job satisfaction in hospital pharmacists. *Am J Health Syst Pharm* 68:115.

La Monica EL. 1994. *Management in Health Care: A Theoretical and Experiential Approach*. New York, NY: Macmillan.

Lane DC, Gaither CA, Kim SC, et al. 2010. Examining the relationship between organizational culture, work attitudes, job roles and organizational change. Paper presented at the American Association of Colleges of Pharmacy Annual Meeting, Seattle, Washington.

Latessa R, Colvin G, Beaty N, Steiner BD, Pathman DE. 2013. Satisfaction, motivation and future of community preceptors: What are the current trends? *Acad Med* 88:1164.

Lea VM, Corlett SA, Rodgers RM. 2012. Workload and its impact on community pharmacists' job satisfaction and stress: A review of the literature. *Int J Pharm Prac* 20:259.

Ledlow GR, Coppola MN. 2014. *Leadership for Health Professionals: Theory, Skills, and Applications*, 2nd ed. Burlington, MA: Jones and Bartlett Learning.

Leupold CR, Ellis LE, Valle M. 2013. Job embeddedness and retail pharmacists' intention to leave. *Psychologist-Manager J* 16:197.

Levinson W, Ginsburg S, Hafferty FW, Lucey CR. 2014. *Understanding Medical Professionalism*. New York, NY: McGraw-Hill Education.

Liu CS, White L. 2011. Key determinants of hospital pharmacy staff's job satisfaction. *Res Social Admin Pharm* 7:51.

Locke EA. 1976. The nature and causes of job satisfaction. In Dunnette M (ed.) *Handbook of Industrial and Organizational Psychology*. Chicago: Rand McNally.

Luthans F, Vogelgesang GR. Lester PB. 2006. Developing the psychological capital of resiliency. *Human Resource Development Review* 5:25.

Macey WH, Schneider B. 2008. The meaning of employee engagement. *Industrial Organizational Psychology* 1:3.

Mahl S, Lee SK, Baker GR, et al. 2015. The association of organizational culture and quality improvement implementation with neonatal outcomes in the NICU. *J Pediatr Health Care* 29:435.

Maslach C, Schaufefeli, WB, Leiter MP. 2001. Job burnout. *Annu Rev Psychol* 52:397.

McCann L, Adair CG, Hughes C. 2009. An exploration of work-related stress in Northern Ireland community pharmacy: A qualitative study. *Int J Pharm Pract* 17:261.

McCarthy Jr BC, McConeghy K, Austin JH. 2015. Remeasuring job satisfaction among pharmacy. *Am J Health-Syst Pharm* 72:997.

McDonald KS, Hite LM. 2018. Conceptualizing and creating sustainable careers. *Human Resource Development Review* 17:349.

Meyer JP, Maltin ER. 2010. Employee commitment and well-being: A critical review, theoretical framework and research agenda. *J Vocational Behav* 77:323.

Mintzberg H. 1983. *Structures in Fives: Designing Effective Organizations.* Englewood Cliffs, NJ: Prentice-Hall.

Mishra P, McDonald K. 2017. Career resilience: An integrated review of the empirical literature. *Human Resource Development Review* 16:207.

Mott DA. 2000. Pharmacist job turnover, length of service, and reasons for leaving, 1983–1997. *Am J Health Syst Pharm* 57:975.

Mott DA, Doucette WR, Gaither CA, et al. 2004. Pharmacists' attitudes toward worklife: Results from the 2000 national pharmacist workforce survey. *J Am Pharm Assoc* 44:326.

Mowday RT, Steers RM, Porter LW. 1979. The measurement of organizational commitment. *J Vocat Behav* 14:224.

Muhlestein DB, Smith NJ. 2016. Physician consolidation: Rapid movement from small to large group practice. 2013-15. *Health Affairs* 35:1638.

Munger MA, Gordon E, Hartman J, et al. 2013. Community pharmacists' occupational satisfaction and stress: A profession in jeopardy? *J Am Pharm Assoc* 53:282.

O'Neill JL, Gaither CA. 2007. Investigating the relationship between the practice of pharmaceutical care, construed external image, organizational identification and job turnover intention of community pharmacists. *Res Social Admin Pharm* 3:438.

Oren L. 2012. Job stress and coping: Self-employed versus organizationally employed professionals. *Stress Health* 28:163.

Osland J, Kolb D, Rubin I. Turner M. 2006. *Organizational Behavior: An Experiential Approach*, 8th ed. Upper Saddle River, NJ: Prentice-Hall.

Ovretveit J. 2001. Organizational behavior research in health care: An overview. In Ashburner L (ed.) *Organisational Behavior and Organisational Studies in Health Care*. Basingstoke, Hampshire, UK: Palgrave.

Patterson ME, Pace HA. 2016. A cross-sectional analysis investigating organizational factors that influence near-miss error reporting among hospital pharmacists. *J Patient Safety* 12:114.

Payakachat N, Ounpraseuth S, Ragland D, Murawski MM. 2011. Job and career satisfaction among pharmacy preceptors. *Am J Pharm Educ* 75: Article 153.

Pelled LH, Eisenhardt KM, Xin KR. 1999. Exploring the black box: An analysis of work group diversity, conflict and performance. *Admin Sci Q* 44:1.

Podsakoff NP, Podsakoff PM, Mackenzie SB, et al. 2014. Consequences of unit-level organizational citizenship behaviors: A review and recommendations for future research. *J Organizational Behav* 35:S87.

Pottie K, Haydt S, Farrell B, et al. 2009. Pharmacist's identity development within multidisciplinary primary health care teams in Ontario; qualitative results from the IMPACT project. *Res Social Admin Pharm* 5:319.

Prince M, Engle R, Laird K. 2003. A model of job performance, job satisfaction and life satisfaction among sales and sales support employees at a pharmaceutical company. *J Pharm Mark Manage* 16:59.

Quinn RE. 1988. *Beyond Rational Management.* San Francisco: Jossey-Bass.

Quinn RE, Rohrbaugh J. 1983. A spatial model of effectiveness criteria: Toward a competing values approach to organizational analysis. *Manag Sci* 29:363.

Reuppell R, Scheider D, Lawton GC. 2003. Initiative for improving pharmacist satisfaction with work schedules. *Am J Health Syst Pharm* 60:1991.

Robbins SP, Judge TA. 2018. *Essentials of Organizational Behavior*, 14th ed. New York, NY: Pearson Prentice-Hall Education.

Rojanasarot S, Gaither CA, Schommer JC, Doucette WR, Kreling DH, Mott DA. 2017. Exploring pharmacists' perceived job alternatives: Results from the 2014 national pharmacist workforce survey. *J Am Pharm Assoc* 57:47.

Rosenthal M, Tsao N, Tsuyuki RT, Marra CA. 2016. Identifying relationships between the professional culture of pharmacy, pharmacists' personality traits, and the provision of advanced pharmacy services. *Res Social Admin Pharm* 12:56.

Rosenthal MM, Houle SKD, Eberhart G, Tsuyuki RT. 2015. Prescribing by pharmacists in Alberta and its relation to culture and personality traits. *Res Social Admin Pharm* 11:401.

Rothmann S, Malan M. 2007. Occupational stress of hospital pharmacists in South Africa. *Int J Pharm Pract* 15:235.

Sagie A, Elizar D. 1996. Work values: A theoretical overview and a model of their affects. *J Org Behav* 17:505.

Sarros JC, Gray J, Densten IL, Cooper B. 2005. The organizational culture profile revisited and revised: An Australian perspective. *Australian J Management* 30:159.

Sasaki H, Yonemoto N, Mori R, Nishida T. 2017. Assessing archetypes of organizational culture based on the competing values framework: The experimental use of the framework in Japanese neonatal intensive care units. *International J for Quality in Health Care* 29:384.

Schaufeli WB, Salanova M, Gonzalez-Roma V, Bakker AB. 2002. The measurement of engagement and burnout: A two sample confirmatory factor analytic approach. *J Happiness Studies* 3:71.

Schein EH, Schein P. 2017. *Organizational Culture and Leadership*. Hoboken, NJ: Wiley.

Schommer JC, Doucette WR, Gaither CA, Kreling DH, Mott DA. 2009. Final report of the 2009 national sample survey of the pharmacists' workforce to determine contemporary demographic and practice characteristics. Available at http://www.aacp.org/resources/ research/pharmacymanpower/Documents/2009%20 National%20Pharmacist%20Workforce%20 Survey%20-%20FINAL%20REPORT.pdf. Accessed October 3, 2015.

Schulz RM, Baldwin HJ. 1990. Chain pharmacist turnover. *J Social Admin Pharm* 7:26.

Seston E, Hassell K, Ferguson J, Hann M. 2009. Exploring the relationship between pharmacists' job satisfaction, intention to quit the profession, and actual quitting. *Res Social Admin Pharm* 5:121.

Stodgill RM. 1948. Personal factors associated with leadership: A survey of the literature. *J Psychol* 25:35.

Stoeckle JD, Stanley JR. 1992. The corporate organization of hospital work: Balancing professional and administrative responsibilities. *Ann Intern Med* 116:407.

Song Z, Lee TH. 2013. The era of delivery system reform begins. *JAMA* 309:35.

Tan EL, Day RO, Brian JE. 2005. Perceptions on Drug and Therapeutics Committee policy implementation. *Res Social Admin Pharm* 1:526.

Taylor FW. 1911. *Principles of Scientific Management*. New York, NY: Harper.

Tosi HL, Rizzo JR, Carroll SJ. 1994. *Managing Organizational Behavior*. Cambridge, MA: Blackwell.

Traulsen JM, Druedahl LC. 2018. Shifting perspectives—Planning for the future of the pharmacy profession taking current labor market trends into consideration. *Res Social Admin Pharm* 14:1189.

Trybou J, Gemmel P, Pauwels Y, et al. 2013. The impact of organizational support and leader-member exchange on the work-related behavior of nursing professionals: The moderating effect of professional and organizational identification. *J Advanced Nursing* 70:372.

Tubbesing BS, Chen FM. 2015. Insights from exemplar practices on achieving organizational structures in primary care. *J Am Board Fam Med* 28:190.

Tugade MM, Fredrickson BL. 2004. Resilient individuals use positive emotions to bounce back from negative emotional experiences. *J Personality Soc Psychol* 86:320.

Urbonas G, Kubiliene L, Kubilius R, Urboniene A. 2015. Assessing the effects of pharmacists perceived organizational support, organizational commitment and turnover intention on provision of medication information at community pharmacies in Lithuania: Structural equation modelling approach. *BMC Health Service Research* 15:62.

Vroom V, Yetton P. 1973. *Leadership and Decision-Making*. Pittsburgh: University of Pittsburgh Press.

Vroom VH, Jago AG. 1988. *The New Leadership: Managing Participation in Organizations*. Upper Saddle River, NJ: Prentice-Hall.

Waller DJ, Smith SR, Warnock JT. 1989. Situational theory of leadership. *Am J Hosp Pharm* 46:2336.

Weber A, Jaekel-Reinhard A. 2000. Burnout syndrome: A disease of modern societies? *Occup Med* 50:512.

Weinberg DB, Avgar AC, Sugrue NM, Cooney-Miner D. 2013. The importance of a high-performance work environment in hospitals. *Health Serv Res* 48:319.

White SJ, Enright SM. 2013. Is there still a pharmacy leadership crisis? A seven-year follow-up assessment. *Am J Health-Syst Pharm* 70:443.

Williams ES, Konard TR, Linzer M, et al. 2002. Physician, practice, and patient characteristics related to primary care physician physical and mental health: Results from the physician worklife study. *Health Serv Res* 37:121.

Williams RG. 1986. Achieving excellence. *Am J Hosp Pharm* 43:617.

Young D. 2002. Shared governance builds leaders, aids patient care. *Am J Health Syst Pharm* 59:2277.

Yukl G. 1989. Managerial leadership: A review of theory and research. *J Manage* 15:251.

Zammuner VL, Galli C. 2005. The relationship with patients: "Emotional labor" and its correlates in hospital employees. In Hartel CE, Zerbe WJ, Ashkanasy NM (eds.) *Emotions in Organizational Behavior*. Mahwah, NJ: Lawrence Erlbaum Associates, pp. 251–285.

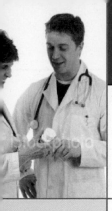

17

HUMAN RESOURCES MANAGEMENT FUNCTIONS

Lauren M. Caldas

About the Author: Dr. Caldas is an Assistant Professor at Virginia Commonwealth University (MCV campus) School of Pharmacy in Richmond. Dr. Caldas received her Doctor of Pharmacy (PharmD) in 2011 from Virginia Commonwealth University. After graduation, she pursued an ASHP/APhA-accredited Community Pharmacy Practice Residency with VCU School of Pharmacy and Kroger Pharmacy. After her residency, she opened the first Marketplace Kroger Pharmacy on the East Coast. She was tasked with hiring and developing the pharmacy team. In 2016, she joined the faculty in Virginia Commonwealth University, where she teaches human resources management and coordinates the Foundations Skills Laboratory, which focuses on community pharmacy practice and non-sterile compounding. She currently practices as an ambulatory care pharmacist at CrossOver Ministries Health, a medical home under a collaborative agreement. Dr. Caldas believes that management, when done well, is extremely difficult, but results in a dedicated staff, a culture of support, and better patient care.

■ LEARNING OBJECTIVES

After completing this chapter, readers should be able to

1. Elaborate on the impact of human resources management in providing high-quality pharmacist services and positive work climate.
2. Define and apply the laws involved in hiring and managing a pharmacy team.
3. Identify critical steps in the recruitment and selection of employees.
4. Compare and contrast job orientation, training, and development.
5. Discuss the strategies for motivating and retaining employees.
6. Explain the strategies of creating a climate of collegial support.
7. Describe the principles and practices of employee performance and feedback, including progressive discipline.

■ SCENARIO

Sakshi Acharya has just accepted a position as pharmacy manager/pharmacist-in-charge (PIC) for a community pharmacy chain. The pharmacy fills approximately 2500 prescriptions per week with two additional pharmacists (one part-time and one full-time), seven technicians (three part-time and four full-time), and one pharmacy intern (a second-year pharmacy student). The pharmacy is open for typical retail hours: 9 am–9 pm weekdays, 9 am–7 pm on Saturday, and 10 am–6 pm on Sunday. The pharmacy manager/PIC's responsibilities in addition to staffing her shift includes: hiring and training her technicians, managing the pharmacy team, meeting corporate policies and programs, and keeping the pharmacy in compliance of state and federal laws governing the practice of pharmacy and employees.

Sakshi has a PharmD degree and 2 years of work experience as a staff pharmacist at another pharmacy in the same chain across town. Her pharmacy district manager has let her know that the pharmacy is in need of a strong leader and will need her to "clean it up and manage the team better." She was also tasked to increase clinical services (10% more immunizations per month and develop medication therapy management services) and increase prescriptions by 5% monthly while maintaining quality patient care and customer satisfaction.

After just 1 month on the job, Sakshi is faced with several personnel problems. The "unofficial" lead technician has left for a hospital job, leaving two full-time technicians attempting to take the role of head technician and leading to numerous conflicts. Both of these technicians have expressed dissatisfaction with their jobs by complaining constantly about the other technician. Two frequent comments made by these two employees are "It's not my job" and "I don't get paid enough for this." The other technicians have expressed discomfort about the conflict between the other two. Some of the discontent has even led to arguments in front of the patients. Two times in the last week patients have complained about the customer service and long wait times since she started

managing. In addition to the technicians' conflict, the pharmacists show little initiative and appear to be only going through the motions of their jobs. The pharmacists will not assist in any of the operations or managing of the technicians, instead insist on leaving any tasks not directed related to dispensing for her days. The part-time pharmacist refuses to vaccinate and either relies on the overlap pharmacist to immunize patients or sends patients away. The technicians are not supervised properly and are allowed to disappear from the department for extended periods. Patients are not prioritized and typically are left unaddressed while the technicians wait to see if another technician will initiate communication. The pharmacy intern has been unavailable to work but will have a school holiday break soon and then be available to help.

The pharmacists and full-time technicians have been with the pharmacy for a range from 5 to 15 years, the part-time technicians have been with the pharmacy for a range of 1 to 6 years and are in varying levels of their training. Prior to Sakshi's arrival, the pharmacy manager, a man who retired recently after 15 years at the same pharmacy, gave minimal feedback or guidance to employees. The former pharmacy manager avoided confrontations, so he typically let personnel problems simmer until they got out of control. Without much guidance from their manager, pharmacy employees developed bad work habits and unprofessional behaviors. Sakshi would like to turn things around in the pharmacy department but is not sure where to begin.

■ CHAPTER QUESTIONS

1. How might poor human resources management in pharmacies cause (a) job stress and burnout, (b) medication dispensing errors, and (c) pharmacist shortages?
2. Describe basic human resources tasks. What are key elements associated with each?
3. Why are job descriptions and performance standards important in human resources management?
4. Why is human resources management a crucial element of a pharmacy's image in the eyes of its patients?

■ HUMAN RESOURCES MANAGEMENT AND PHARMACY PRACTICE

The scenario depicts an all too common situation in health care organizations, in which employees lack direction and guidance in their jobs. As a result, the quality and quantity of work suffers, and the work environment becomes intolerable. Often, the best employees will leave to find work environments that are more tolerable, and the most difficult employees to manage will remain. Without human resources management, even professionals such as pharmacists can lose direction and work below their ability.

The practice of pharmacy management consists of a wide range of complex tasks that involve either managing people or managing nonhuman resources such as property and information. Managing nonhuman resources consists of such activities as inventory control, computer systems design and maintenance, and financial management. This chapter addresses a pharmacy organization's most valued resource: its people. Managing people, known by the formal name of *human resources management* (HRM), is an essential duty for all pharmacists. Almost all pharmacists will manage someone, whether it is other pharmacists, technicians, or student interns. A quality manager will inspire all of those around them to improve themselves and the organization. HRM is important because it can make the difference between a smoothly running pharmacy and a dysfunctional, unsuccessful one. The difference in managers is easily seen with the nature of community pharmacy, where the pharmacists alternate full shifts with the same team of technicians. The same team will perform much differently depending on their manager. A high-performing pharmacy manager will focus on safety and patient care. Their technicians arrive early, work hard, and are enthusiastic about their jobs.

HRM is defined as the process of achieving organizational objectives through the management of people. Tasks associated with HRM include recruiting, hiring, training, developing, and terminating employees. When these tasks are done well, pharmacy employees know their responsibilities and receive sufficient feedback to meet them successfully. When these tasks are done poorly, pharmacy employees are given little or inconsistent direction in their tasks and often are frustrated in their jobs.

HRM is critical to the pharmacy profession because many pharmacists and pharmacy employees probably are capable of much higher performance levels than they are providing currently. The negative consequences of this lost performance can be substantial to both pharmacists and their patients.

Many problems in the pharmacy profession result at least partially from the fact that pharmacists often are poorly managed and led. For example, overwork and stress occur when pharmacy personnel waste time and effort in their jobs owing to unclear directives from management, poor teamwork, insufficient training, inadequate feedback about productivity and quality of work performance, and conflicts between people. If this wasted effort could be channeled into productive activities, then the burden and stress of overwork could be relieved. It can also be argued that many medication errors result from poor personnel management. A manager may contribute to medication errors by emphasizing quantity of work over quality of work or speed over safety. Medication errors may occur when poorly managed pharmacists are permitted to develop poor dispensing habits, provide inadequate supervision of technicians, maintain incomplete medical documentation, or focus on production over patient care. Poorly managed technicians contribute to medical errors when they are improperly trained, take short cuts around software safety measures, or take the "that's not my job" mindset. These types of cultures develop in any organization with detrimental results. After the Columbia Tragedy, the loss of the entire team, National Aeronautics and Space Administration (NASA) had to answer the painful question of "What happened?" This question was addressed by the Columbia Accident Investigation Board (CAIB) in the "A Broken Safety Culture" section. The Board found, "the Shuttle Program's complex structure erected barriers to effective communication and its safety culture no longer asks enough hard questions about risk." (Columbia Accident Investigation Board, 2003). If personnel are supported by better HRM practices, better reporting and fewer errors likely would result, and lives might be saved. This was as true for the NASA's Columbia as it is for pharmacy practice.

This chapter discusses the recruitment, selection, training, coaching, disciplining, and termination of pharmacy employees. It describes the steps involved in HRM and some of the constraints placed on managers and offers recommendations to pharmacists for practice more effective personnel management.

■ LAWS AND REGULATIONS INFLUENCING HRM

The HRM process is influenced by laws and regulations passed by local, state, and federal governments, as well as corporate/company policies. Laws can be separated into the hiring process and management of employees. The following laws are those most commonly addressed in the HRM process; however, it is not an exhaustive list. Pharmacy managers must always also look into to their organization's policies and local/state laws.

Candidate and Employee Protective Laws

Federal Civil Rights Act of 1964: The Federal Civil Rights Act of 1964 is the primary piece of legislation affecting HRM practices (McConnell, 2016). The act and subsequent amendments to the act prohibit discrimination in employment hiring, promotion, compensation, and treatment of protected employee groups. Protected groups are those who might be discriminated against based on their gender, race, age, religion, sexual preference, height, weight, arrest record, national origin, financial status, military record, or disability (Table 17-1).

Laws that amend or supplement the act include (Donnelly et al., 1995; McConnell, 2016):

- *Age Discrimination Act of 1967.* This Act protects employees 40 years of age and older from discrimination. The practical application is that an employer cannot ask a person's age at the interview or cite it as the reason a person cannot be hired. Age cannot be a reason to recommend an employee retire. Even with this protection in place, 64% of workers may have seen or experienced age discrimination in the workplace (Fleck, 2014).
- *The Pregnancy Discrimination Act of 1978.* This Act prohibits discrimination based on pregnancy

Table 17-1.   Federal Civil Rights Act of 1964 Amendments

Year	Amendment	Intended Impact
1967	Age Discrimination Act	Prohibits discrimination based on age. Employers cannot ask an applicant's age at interview or cite it as a reason for not hiring.
1978	Pregnancy Discrimination Act (PDA)	Prohibits the discrimination based on pregnancy or potential for pregnancy. Employers will provide same fringe benefits as others in similar positions.
1990	Americans with Disabilities Act (ADA)	Prohibits discrimination against qualified individuals labeled as disabled. Employers will make reasonable accommodations for these employees to permit access to their jobs.
1991	Title VII of Civil Rights Act	Prohibits discrimination on the basis of race. Employers have the burned of proof that candidate was not discriminated based on race.
1993	Family Medical Leave Act (FMLA)	Protects an employee's job for 12 weeks of unpaid leave for special family duties such as childbirth, adoption of children, illness of family member, or personal illness.

or potential for pregnancy. Individuals shall receive the same fringe benefits, such as health care, as other individuals in the similar positions. The practical application is that an employer cannot ask a candidate if they are or plan to become pregnant (Commission, 1978).

- *Americans with Disabilities Act of 1990 (ADA).* The ADA prohibits employer discrimination against qualified individuals who are labeled as "disabled." This requires employers to make reasonable accommodations for disabled employees to permit access to their jobs.
- *Title VII of the Civil Rights Act of 1991.* This amendment to the original 1964 Act prohibits discrimination on the basis of race and places the burden of proof on the employer. This assigned employers the responsibility to show that the employee or candidate was not discriminated based on race.
- *Family and Medical Leave Act of 1993 (FMLA).* FMLA requires employers of 50 or more employees to guarantee employees 12 weeks of unpaid leave each year for special family duties such as childbirth, adoption of children, illness of family member, or personal illness. This may not apply to smaller independently owned pharmacies who do not meet the minimum 50 employees. The practical application is that the individual's job is protected for at least 12 weeks.

Fair Labor Standards Act (FLSA) of 1938: This law focuses on setting wage and hour protections for employees. Overtime and minimum wage acts, as well as the Equal Pay Act are parts of the FLSA.

- Equal Pay Act: This piece of the FLSA precludes gender-based wage discrepancies among persons in the "same establishment and perform jobs that require equal skill, effort, and responsibility and which are performed under similar conditions." This Act makes exceptions for payment systems based on seniority, merits, quantity or quality of production, or a system that is based on factors other than gender (Commission, 1963). Even with this protection, women often earn less than their peers. Community pharmacy has one of the smallest wage gaps between men and women. In fact, Goldin and Katz (2012) coined it as "the most egalitarian of all professions." However, this does not mean that this to be always the case in pharmacy, and managers should be very diligent about ensuring equal pay across genders.

- Overtime/Minimum Wages: The FLSA requires that employees must make the minimum wage and if working more than 40 hours per week, receive overtime pay. The overtime wages will be at one and one-half times the employee's wage. While pharmacists are exempt from the FLSA's overtime wage, under the professional exemption and salary amount, technicians are generally not (Labor, 2008). This plays a role when devising work schedules for technicians and other support personnel.

Hiring Process Laws

- Immigration Reform and Control Act (IRCA) of 1986: This law's main purpose was to control and deter illegal immigration to the United States. It legalized undocumented aliens who had been continuously unlawfully present since 1982. It also placed sanctions on employees who hire undocumented workers. During the hiring process to comply with this law, most employers will ask for the candidate's social security card or I-9 form at hire date.

Laws on the Horizon or in Transition

- Proposed Overtime Exemptions: The U.S. Department of Labor as part of the FLSA increased the standard salary for full time (i.e., increases the salary for individuals who would not qualify for overtime exemption) from $455 to $913 per week ($23,600 to $47,476 annually). This was observed with recent pharmacy resident salary increases. This rule was taken to Fifth Circuit court and is currently suspended while the Department of Labor refines the standard salary level. However, many organizations have maintained the salary level until a final ruling is decided.
- Pay Equity Laws: As an effort to decrease the gender pay gap, many states have banned salary history

questions during the interview process. The concept is that it continues the gender based pay gap by setting the employee's new salary on their previous salaries, instead of focusing on current position requirements.

- Paid Family Leave: An increase in paid family leave has been seen over the past few years. Certain states currently have paid family leave with at least 19 states proposing similar legislation (Brainerd, 2017). The federal interest has been seen with paid mothers and fathers leave included in the presidential FY2018 proposed budget. The Family and Medical Insurance Leave (FAMILY) Act proposed in both the House and Senate, as well as other methods of compensation proposed in the House and State legislatures.

■ EMPLOYEE PROTECTION ORGANIZATIONS INFLUENCING HRM

Equal Employment Opportunity Commission (EEOC)

The Equal Employment Opportunity Commission (EEOC) was created in 1972 with an amendment to the Civil Rights Act. The EEOC was given the authority to monitor discrimination and file lawsuits to correct discriminatory practices in the workplace. This amendment was also responsible for *affirmative action*, an activist approach to correcting discrimination. Affirmative action encourages employers to actively recruit and give preference to minorities, with the same qualifications, in order to correct previous prejudice in employment. Although highly controversial, affirmative action is practiced commonly in business.

Every process of HRM is influenced in some way by EEOC oversight. Hiring practices require that diversity in the workplace be considered. Interviewing is constrained by limits on questions that may be legally asked of job candidates (defined by the Fair Credit Reporting Act). The Fair Credit Reporting Act (FCRA) is legislation that protects information reported on individuals personal lives, including protection on information collected or used with regard to employment (Cornell Law School). Disciplining employees requires that certain procedures be followed and documentation kept that ensures that discrimination does not occur on the job.

Some managers may chafe at the restrictions, but federal employment laws act primarily to enforce what any good manager should already be doing, for example, developing fair and explicit HRM procedures. Periodically, pharmacy employers have had conflicts with the EEOC. Recent examples are listed below.

- A claim against a pharmaceutical compounding firm in Texas, Pharmacy Solutions, stated that it violated federal law when it fired two female employees because of their pregnancies (EEOC, 2014).
- A CVS pharmacist who claims that he was fired by CVS because of his age was awarded $400,000 in damages by a Federal jury (Gaddy, 2013). A Washington State Community Hospital, Grays Harbor, was forced to pay $125,000 due to the behavior of a supervising pharmacist who sexually harassed pharmacy technicians (Grays Harbor, 2011).

In addition to efforts to address workplace discrimination, employers are increasingly embracing the idea of having a diverse workforce. Workforce diversity can be defined as having an employment environment of acceptance and respect for individuals of all backgrounds and origins. There is an understanding that businesses with a diverse workforce of people will be more competitive and better able to service customers (Dreachslin, 2007). Most pharmacy employers have clear statements embracing workforce diversity on their websites.

Occupational Safety and Health Act of 1970

The Occupational Safety and Health Act of 1970 established the U.S. Occupational Safety and Health Administration (OSHA) to develop and enforce workplace standards designed to prevent work-related injuries, illnesses, and deaths (OSHA, 2007). OSHA is an agency of the Department of Labor (DOL). Of particular relevance to pharmacy are OSHA's ergonomic workplace standards and its rules for preventing exposure to hazardous chemicals and blood-borne pathogens. It covers pharmacy procedures relating to practices like blood glucose testing and administration of immunizations.

A pharmacy manager must be well versed in the laws and organizations involved in HRM to effectively manage their team. At all times from interviewing, coaching, and potentially termination, the HRM hinges on proper compliance with the laws that govern employee protection.

■ RECRUITMENT AND PLACEMENT

Importance of Recruitment and Placement

Recruitment and placement of pharmacy personnel are two of the most important tasks a manager can undertake. If a manager finds and hires competent, self-motivated professionals, issues such as motivation and performance are less of a problem. In practice, the term coaching has replaced the term management in a similar mindset that patient adherence has replaced compliance. The idea of coaching makes the role of the manager to use the employee's strengths to better the organization and the employee together.

The better the hire and placement, the less time the manager will need for motivating and coaching nontechnical duties. Employers need to assess the position they are filling and attempt to hire a person whose strengths match the needs of the position. Gallup has found many times that employees have more loyalty and job satisfaction if they are using their skills effectively. For example, if a pharmacy manager is looking to fill a position for a community pharmacy technician who will be greeting and interacting with patients as the front face of the pharmacy, that manager will need a person who has strengths in communication or even a woo (Gallup's definition: winning others over).

Due to the nature of the profession, pharmacist and pharmacy technicians will have a defined set of skills, so technician training will be minimal after the initial orientation. The area where most pharmacy directors and management spend their time is in managing the nontechnical duties of their employees (i.e., motivation, workplace conflicts, etc.) Gallup has found that hiring the right person for the right position, where they are able to highlight their strengths, will increase job satisfaction and decrease burnout and turnover (Rigoni & Asplund, 2016).

Pharmacy organizations need to exercise great care in recruitment and placement because each employee represents the organization and the profession. All employees who interact with customers help to determine the image they have of your organization. In fact, pharmacy clerks, technicians, and pharmacists are more likely to determine a pharmacy's image than any advertising or promotional events (Holdford, 2003).

Pharmacy employees can be a source of competitive advantage in the marketplace. A good pharmacist can generate significant revenue for a company by maintaining a loyal patient base and drawing others from competitors. In addition, satisfied patients are more likely to recommend a pharmacy to friends and family and purchase greater quantities of merchandise.

Choosing the wrong employee for a position can be quite expensive. If that employee leaves after a short time, the employer must bear the cost of recruiting, selecting, and training a replacement. An average employee costs approximately $1200 in training; however, the skilled labor of pharmacists and pharmacy technicians are likely higher and include the costs of a background check, and all of the hidden costs (such as of loss of productivity while the employee is being trained by others) (Taylor, 2017). Employees are also paid during the orientation and trainings which vary in length. The cost of losing established health care professionals can rise to well over $100,000 (Waldman et al., 2004).

Hiring problem employees accrues even more expenses. Hiring employees who are unproductive or have personal problems can be a nightmare for

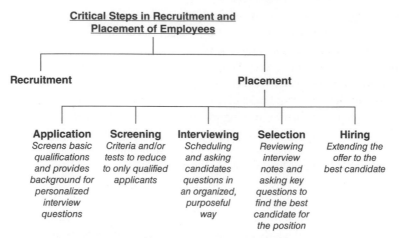

Figure 17-1. Recruiting and Placing Employees.

managers. Many of these employees are able to keep their jobs by riding the line between minimal acceptability and termination. Even problem employees who eventually are terminated can sow conflict within an organization, reduce job enjoyment, increase workplace tension, hinder teamwork, and cause a host of other problems. Problem employees also can take up significant managerial time in counseling, dispute mediation, and oversight. Therefore, it is essential that pharmacy managers do all they can to choose the right employees. The critical steps and selection of employees are illustrated with Figure 17-1.

■ RECRUITMENT

Recruitment consists of all activities associated with attracting qualified candidates to fill job vacancies. The purpose of recruiting is to attract the most qualified candidates to interview for vacant job positions. Recruiting is easier when employers are proactive in their recruitment efforts. Proactive recruitment occurs when employers (1) continually recruit and network, (2) maintain a pleasant work environment where people want to be employed, and (3) establish a positive image in the minds of potential recruits.

Pharmacy employee recruitment should be a continuous activity that takes place regardless of whether a position is open or not. Well-run pharmacies continually develop contacts with potential employees who can be approached once an opening occurs. Contacts can be developed at professional meetings and social gatherings or through work. A pharmacy employer also can cultivate potential employees by hiring pharmacy students for part-time work and mentoring pharmacy students in advanced pharmacy practice experiences (i.e., clerkships or introductory/advanced pharmacy practice experiences.

A desirable work environment also helps in recruiting employees. This includes having an enjoyable work environment and competitive compensation packages. Employers who treat employees well have fewer problems with job turnover because employees do not want to leave. When vacancies occur, they are filled quickly and with less effort because potential employees seek them out. In many cases, jobs are filled quickly through word-of-mouth recommendations from current employees.

Employers who are successful in offering the most desirable jobs often develop a reputation as *employers of choice*. Employers of choice have a positive image in the community and can pick and choose among the best candidates for positions. In addition, employees do not easily leave employers of choice.

Wegmans, a supermarket chain that employs pharmacists, has been one of Fortune Magazine's "Top

100 Employers" for almost two decades (Wegmans, 2014). Among its employee benefits are its flexible scheduling, an employee scholarship program, and the practice of filling leadership positions by promoting from within the company. At Wegmans, there is strong competition for the limited number of job openings that arise, permitting the company to select the most qualified applicants from a ready supply of excellent candidates.

In addition to word-of-mouth recommendations, Internet and traditional advertisements are a common way of recruiting pharmacy employees. The first step in advertising is deciding how wide of a net to cast for potential employees. Will local advertising bring in sufficient numbers of qualified candidates, or should advertising be regional or national? The answer to this question will be influenced by issues of reach and cost; that is, the more people reached by the ads, the greater is the cost. If local advertising is chosen, then advertisements can be placed in hometown newspapers or state professional journals. For regional or national advertisements, employers can use national newspapers (e.g., *New York Times*), national professional associations (e.g., *American Pharmacists Association's Career Center*), or Internet job Websites (e.g., www.monster.com, www.indeed.com). Recent evidence suggests personal recruitment by pharmacists to be very effective in the hiring of quality technicians (Desselle & Holmes, 2017).

Another consideration is targeting an appropriate demographic. For example, if an organization is seeking a pharmacist with considerable years of experience for a management position, it need not advertise in a student pharmacist journal. Instead, it may make more sense to advertise with the local pharmacist organization. On the other hand, if an organization consistently recruits for a large number of positions, it should be conscious about trying to reach populations diverse in age, gender, and race/ethnicity.

After choosing the advertising medium, an advertisement is written. When writing any advertisement, it is important to keep it simple. It should not make false promises and should not use hyperbolic rhetoric or technical jargon. It should only capture the eye of qualified candidates and persuade them to contact the pharmacy. A pharmacy manager will need to review the current organization's policies and procedures to make sure they are compliant with recruiting practices and methods.

■ PLACEMENT

Placement refers to candidate application, screening, interviewing, selection, and hiring processes. In many organizations, pharmacists are assisted in this process by corporate personnel offices. Personnel offices offer valuable assistance in advertising positions, managing applications and paperwork, screening candidates, advising about legal and policy questions, checking references, and extending job offers. They free pharmacy personnel to develop criteria for selecting employees, to interview qualified candidates, and to make the final choice. It is important to emphasize, however, that pharmacists need to monitor and influence the personnel office's performance in the placement process. One reason is that personnel employees do not understand, as well as pharmacists, the requirements of pharmacy practice. They may emphasize different knowledge and capabilities than pharmacists. A second reason is that the personnel office does not have to suffer as much from the consequences of a bad employee choice. Pharmacy personnel will bear the brunt of a bad employee hire. Therefore, it is incumbent on pharmacists to maintain as much control over the process as necessary to ensure a good choice.

Job Description and Analysis

The root, and often underutilized, piece of the entire process is a well-developed job description. The job description should be the result of a job analysis. The job analysis will define the "knowledge, skills, abilities, and behaviors" needed to form the job description (Samuel, 2016). For example, a job analysis for a lead technician would include the listed responsibilities (skills), but also include the preferred traits (or behaviors), knowledge (e.g., certification), abilities, and amount of experience. This allows for a specific and unbiased job description to be created and allows candidates to be evaluated objectively. Additionally, the job description should be the basis of the evaluation process and utilized often. Many managers only reflect on the job description when hiring, but the job description should be the basis in the evaluating employees, as well. After the job description is created, the position should be posted, and the process can begin.

Application

One of the first steps in hiring is for a candidate to fill out a job application. Job applications serve two purposes. The first is to help screen unqualified candidates. Applications can identify whether candidates have the necessary training, degrees, and experience for the job. The second purpose of applications is to provide background about the candidate for the interview.

Screening

Once they have submitted an application, applicants are screened to see if they meet the requirements of the job. Screening is a process that attempts to weed out unqualified applicants from the pool of potential candidates. Common screening criteria include lack of job qualifications (e.g., license, degree, residency, certification, or experience), poorly completed applications (e.g., misspelling, missing information, or sloppy writing), and negative applicant history (e.g., felony conviction, lying on the application, or frequent changes in employment).

Screening tools are also available as standardized tests. It is recommended that these tests undergo validation to demonstrate their appropriateness for selecting the best employees for the position. The EEOC enforces the Uniform Guidelines on Employee Selection Procedure of 1978 when regulating any employee tests (Fleischer, 2005; "Screening by Means of Pre-Employment Testing," 2018).

Interviewing

When qualified candidates are identified, interviews are scheduled. Qualified candidates normally are ranked according to desirability, with the top-ranked candidates receiving initial invitations to interview. If a candidate is not chosen from the first round of applicant interviews, a second round is scheduled, drawing from the remaining pool of applicants.

Preparation for an interview is as important for the interviewer as it is for the candidate. The following is a suggested list of interview preparation steps:

- *Provide information about the position.* It is helpful to provide candidates with specific information about the job description and standards for performance to help them prepare for the interview. The job description will have the knowledge, skills, and abilities needed for the position, as well, as the behaviors necessary for success in the position.
- *Identify interview objectives.* It is important to ask yourself what you want to achieve with the interviews. For example, if you have acute, immediate needs, you may only consider candidates who are available immediately. However, if your interest is long term, you may be willing to wait for an excellent candidate to graduate from pharmacy school or complete a commitment made to another employer. These objectives will help you formulate your interview questions and format.
- *Review the position description and performance standards.* The position description and performance standards will form the basis of your interview questions. Examples of a position description and performance standards are provided in Table 17-2.
- *Develop a list of interview questions.* Pay particular attention to assessing the requirements of the job specified in the performance standards. It is important to have a list questions that will be asked of each applicant. This ensures that each candidate was given the same opportunity to demonstrate their suitability for the job. Questions can be adapted for each candidate (e.g., with additional probes) but should be asked of all candidates.
- *Study the applications and résumés.* Look for accomplishments and credentials on which you want the candidate to expand. Also note frequent job changes, gaps in employment, demotions,

Table 17-2.   Sample Job Description and Performance Standards for a Community Pharmacist

Description

Responsible for preparing medications, dispensing prescriptions, counseling patients, providing patient services such as medication therapy management and immunizations, supervising technicians, and general management of the pharmacy

Qualifications

Advanced Pharmacy degree (PharmD or MS) from an accredited college of pharmacy, licensure, community pharmacy experience preferred

Performance Standards

Dispensing	Dispenses medications in accordance to all state and federal laws
Clinical skills and professional judgment	Integrates clinical, procedural, and distributive judgments using acceptable standards of practice to achieve positive patient outcomes
Productivity	Prioritizes work to ensure that all tasks are completed in a timely manner
Service	Fosters favorable relations between customers and the public
Written documentation and communication	Adheres to all state and federal laws, regulatory agency rules, and pharmacy policies and procedures regarding written documentation
Technician supervision	Provides oversight and feedback to pharmacy technicians that ensures quality care and adherence to departmental policies and procedures
Attendance and punctuality	Meets all pharmacy policies regarding attendance and punctuality

inconsistencies in history, or incomplete information on references about which you want to learn more.

- *Schedule a quiet, uninterrupted interview if possible.* It may be seen as disrespectful to the candidate if you permit interruptions and distractions from giving your full attention to the interview. With the logistics of some work environments, a distraction-free environment may be challenging, so be open and explain at the scheduling and beginning of the interview to the candidate that you will minimize any non-emergency distractions but that you may have a few interruptions.

- *Get pharmacy team or other employee feedback.* Alert coworkers whom you want the candidate to meet so that they can schedule a time to meet. Developing a positive work culture includes having input on candidates from the pharmacy team.

Most interviews follow a relatively predictable number of steps. The first step consists of introductory small talk designed to put the candidate at ease. Rather than jumping immediately into the questioning, a few minutes may be spent developing some rapport with the candidate. After the small talk, interview questions are posed of the candidate. When the questioning phase is finished, the interviewer describes and promotes the job to the candidate. At this point, candidates typically ask questions of the interviewer about the job. At the end of the interview, applicants either meet with other interviewers or are given a tour of the facilities.

Interviews can be conducted in several different ways. The *traditional interview* attempts to engage candidates in a general discussion about themselves. A common question from a traditional interview might be, "Tell me a little about yourself" or "What are your strengths and weaknesses?" *Situation* (or *role-play*) *interviews* direct applicants to describe how they would handle a difficult imaginary situation. For example, "You are the pharmacy manager, and one of your employees has just told you that another worker is stealing merchandise. What would you do?" Situation interviews assess candidates' problem-solving capabilities and communication. *Stress interviews* attempt to replace the polite conversation seen in traditional interviews with a deliberate attempt by the interviewer to unnerve the candidate with blunt questions (e.g., "With your limited experience, why do you think you are qualified for this position?"), interruptions, and persistent pursuit of a subject. It attempts to discern candidate preparation and ability to handle stress. *Behavioral interviews* try to evaluate an applicant's past behavior, experience, and initiative by asking for specifics about past events and the candidate's role in those events. Classic behavioral questions start with "Give me an example when you … " or "Describe your worst … " Behavioral interviewing is based on the assumption that past behavior best predicts future behavior. In many cases, interviewers employ more than one style in an interview (Table 17-3).

Many interviewers have limited experience and are prone to common interview mistakes (Boettge, 2017). A major error for interviewers is lack of planning. Managers who are very busy with immediate problems may be tempted to skimp on interview preparation. However, that savings of time is not a bargain if it leads to a bad hire. Managers need to look at the requirements for the job and the resume's of the applicants to have thoughtful and purposeful questions prepared. Another mistake is the "one-way conversation" which occurs when the interviewer does most of the talking and does not give the candidate an opportunity to speak. The rule of thumb is to have the interviewer only take 20% of the time talking and leave the remaining 80% for the candidate. It is hard to learn much about a candidate when the interviewer is talking. In other situations, interviewers treat the interview as an inquisition designed to squeeze the candidate into revealing his or her flaws and focus on ways to eliminate the candidate from the process. Although this may reveal some insights about the candidate, it is also likely to drive the candidate to another employer. Some interviewers assume that the candidate wants the position, so no attempt is made to sell its benefits. Any of these mistakes can result in either losing a desirable candidate or choosing the wrong one. A final and common mistake is a

Table 17-3. Common Job Interview Question Types

Type of Interview Question	Description/Purpose	Example
Traditional	Asks candidate general information about themselves	Tell me a little about yourself. What are your strengths and weaknesses?
Situational	Asks candidate to describe their response to an imaginary situation	An angry patient demands a refill immediately, how do you handle the situation?
Behavioral	Asks candidate to describe a previous situation assuming past behavior will predict future behavior	Tell me about a time when you had a conflict with a coworker and how it resolved.
Stress	Asks candidate questions intended to unnerve the candidate to assess their stress response	We are looking for a highly qualified individual and you do not have enough experience. Why would you think we would hire you?
Candidate Questions	Asks the candidate which questions they have for the interviewer. This allows the interviewer to assess candidate preparation	Do you have any questions for me?

lack of a structured interview. A structured interview with purpose will help determine the best candidate for the position.

Selecting Candidates

During the interview process, it is important to keep good notes about each candidate. This is essential for keeping details about candidates organized and for documenting the selection process in case any claims of discrimination should occur. It is better to save note taking until immediately after the interview to avoid distracting the candidate during the interview. It is also helpful to develop an interview checklist to structure interview notes. Table 17-4 lists several interview mistakes candidates make frequently that can exclude them immediately from further consideration.

The final choice of the interviewer often comes down to how well a candidate can address the following questions:

- *Can this person perform the basic job?* This addresses the ability of the candidate to contribute to the organization's performance. For instance, a good clinical pharmacist who has little dispensing experience may not be chosen for a position in a community pharmacy setting. Although good clinical skills may be helpful in a community position, basic dispensing capabilities are essential.

Table 17-4.   Interview Mistakes that May Immediately Exclude a Job Candidate from Consideration

- Inappropriate dress or body adornments
- Lack of knowledge about the position and hiring organization
- Tardiness or excessive rescheduling
- Unengaged attitude or flat affect
- Poor response to predictable questions
- Poor body language
- Unclear or irritating speech patterns
- Focusing on self-interest over that of the hiring organization
- Showing under-confidence or over-confidence

- *How well do the candidate's skills and capabilities mesh with the organization's needs?* Sometimes the best employee for a position does not have the greatest credentials or the most talent. In many circumstances, the best employee is the one who can fill skill deficiencies in the organization and complement the talents of other employees. For example, a technician with extensive nonsterile compounding experience may not be the best person to hire for a technician position in a hospital's billing department.
- *Will the candidate make my job easier?* Everyone has some self-interest in the selection of a candidate. Successful applicants often highlight how they will be able to solve problems of individuals and the organization.
- *Would I want to work with this person?* This question deals with the rapport between the applicant and the interviewer. If the rapport is good, the chances of selection are enhanced significantly.

Hiring

In most cases, a candidate cannot be hired until the personnel department completes a reference and background check. If everything is found to be acceptable, a compensation package is put together, and an offer is extended. Once again, it is important that the pharmacy department be involved in the process to ensure that an offer is not mishandled. For example, if an uncompetitive compensation package is put together for the candidate, pharmacy personnel may need to argue for a better one. Once an applicant accepts a position, the hard part of HRM begins.

Hiring is just the first step in the HRM process. Once hired, employees must be given the training and coaching necessary to do their jobs.

■ COACHING (TRAINING AND DEVELOPMENT OF) THE PHARMACY TEAM

A critical job of the manager is to coach the pharmacy team. The idea of coaching is that managers are leveraging the staff members' strengths to improve their ability to succeed in their individual goals and the organization's goals. For the organization, it improves the quality and quantity of work provided by each employee. For the employee, it can make the job more interesting and meaningful and lead to greater morale and sense of accomplishment (Holdford, 2003). Excellent pharmacy service organizations invest in the training and development of their employees.

Coaching consists of both training and developing employees. Training and development serve different purposes. *Training* is meant to improve employee performance with current tasks and jobs, whereas *development* prepares employees for new responsibilities and positions. Therefore, training is essential for meeting current needs, and development is an investment in future needs. The best managers train and develop their staff so that the staff can leave but choose to stay.

Orientation and Job Training

Training comes in two primary forms: orientation and job training. The purpose of *orientation training* is to welcome new employees, present a positive first impression, provide information that will permit them to settle into their new responsibilities, and establish early expectations of performance and behavior (McConnell, 2016). It also involves familiarizing new hires with the company's/department's mission, goals, cultural norms, and expectations. Examples of things covered in orientation training include coworker introductions, a tour of the facilities, discussion of employee benefits, review of departmental policies and procedures, discussion of performance objectives for the job, description of behavioral expectations, demonstration of the computer system, and special organizational training (e.g., HIPAA, sexual harassment, and discrimination). It is a good idea to develop a checklist that covers all orientation topics to ensure that nothing is overlooked. The first days for a new employee are crucial, and early impressions last (McConnell, 2016).

Job training helps current employees learn new information and skills to do their jobs and refresh capabilities that may have diminished over time.

Although pharmacists are highly trained professionals, the changing nature of medical and business practice requires continual training throughout their careers. Job training is a responsibility of both the individual and the organization. For example, a pharmacist might attend a continuing education program offered by a pharmacy school to fill a perceived gap in knowledge about a disease state and its treatment. Alternatively, a pharmacist may be asked by an employer to receive on-the-job training in customer service methods to fulfill a perceived employer need. Job training can be used to develop habits (e.g., time management), knowledge (e.g., new drug treatments), skills (e.g., blood pressure monitoring), procedures (e.g., handling drug insurance claims), and policies (e.g., sexual harassment).

Pharmacy organizations formally or informally may employ a type of training called *job rotation* (also known as *cross-training*). Job rotation is designed to give an individual broad experience through exposure to different areas of the organization. In a hospital pharmacy, for example, newly hired technicians can be trained in filling carts, outpatient dispensing, intravenous admixture preparation, inventory management, billing and crediting, and working in one or more satellite pharmacy units. Such training would diversify technicians' skills, allowing them to work in any number of areas should one be short staffed, and may help improve their self-esteem and sense of contribution to the organization.

Development

Development requires a long-term focus by preparing for future needs of the individual or organization. Professional development typically consists of answering the following questions: (1) What is my present situation? (2) Where do I want to be? (3) What skills, knowledge, and training do I need to get where I want to be?

Development differs from training in that it requires a greater intensity of education and instruction. It calls the pharmacy leader (director or manager) to be invested in their employees and to solicit their goals and assist them in attaining those goals.

Whereas job training might be met sufficiently with continuing education programs, on-the-job instruction, and short courses, professional development may require formal education and structured experiences such as college courses, multiday seminars and certificate programs, residencies, or fellowships.

When coaching employees, it is important to remember the laws that govern HRM and to treat each employee equitably. However, the best managers also find a way to motivate each employee individually. Employee motivation may vary but typically involves: monetary compensation, professional or personal development, work–life balance, the job description itself, and workplace support and environment. Coaching involves a two-way street with the employee and employer. Too often, new managers try to focus on the poorest performers; however, this might not be ideal. While it is true that the bar of acceptance is guided by your poorest performers (e.g., if you allow an employee to consistently be late without consequence, then the new standard acceptable behavior is that employees can be late to the pharmacy), the goal is not to focus on your least motivated and most detached employees.

Urban Meyer, a collegiate football coach with multiple national championships, employed a 10-80-10 rule. This rule can be adapted for pharmacy management. In summary, this rule breaks the employees into three categories: the top 10%, middle 80%, and bottom 10%. These top 10% succeed regardless of their manager or any external motivating factors; these individuals will give their all to the organization and their patients because of an innate internal motivation to be excellent. The bottom 10% is the antithesis of this. As a manager, you will have the biggest return on your time with the 80% whose performance and attitudes are greatly influenced by coaching and feedback. To manage the top 10%, it is best to get out of their way and provide the same encouragement and positive feedback as you do for those you are trying to coach. The bottom 10% is best to begin progressive discipline and encouraged to find employment elsewhere (which will be addressed later in this chapter). The remaining 80% is where you should

set your standard of expectations and coach them to reach their potential and become a top performer.

■ CREATING A CLIMATE OF COLLEGIAL SUPPORT

The climate (more immediate) and culture (more enduring, see Chapter 14) of a workplace can be seen and physically felt by individuals walking into the pharmacy or department. If in doubt, simply notice the difference in one professor's classroom versus another one, and one can feel the different vibes permeating throughout. The same difference can be felt walking into different pharmacies, largely influenced by the climate and culture of the pharmacy.

Is this a pharmacy where the team works well together and supports each other or is it an entirely different pharmacy of frustration and stress. The difference is palpable and set by the pharmacy manager. Managers are an important influence on the productivity and well-being of their employees.

Managers must establish the climate of their pharmacy and lead by example. Disney hired "cast members" for his employees. From the parking attendant to the characters in costume, they were all cast members. The concept was that these individuals when they got to their job would take on the role of the "Happiest place on earth," and morph themselves into this role. The same must happen with the pharmacy manager. A manager is tasked to create the culture of those they manage by encouraging collegial support and giving a clear guidance of the goals of the pharmacy. This guidance is occurring whether purposeful or not, so it is best for the manager to create a climate purposefully. For example, the pharmacy manager, who overrides a wrong NDC code in the pharmacy software system to quickly dispense a patient a medication, has set the pharmacy culture to support speed over safety. Whereas a manager who takes the few minutes to correctly change the NDC in the system, explaining that the correct NDC is very important during recalled medications, has set a very different standard of safety over speed. It is imperative to maintain a strong safety culture, whether managing a 300-bed hospital or sending astronauts to the moon. Managers will influence the climate and culture starting with their actions but also must coach their employees through performance feedback.

■ PERFORMANCE FEEDBACK

Types of Performance Feedback

Performance feedback can be categorized as either informal or formal. Informal feedback comes in a variety of ways, from day-to-day feedback coaching to less manager-controlled feedback such as coworker support system. Formal feedback typically comes in the form of a performance evaluation for a given time period (i.e., annual performance review [see Chapter 20]).

Current research finds that employees learn more from the informal feedback than from waiting for formal feedback (Van, 2013). Immediate feedback regarding a simple change had a much greater impact than a delayed feedback. However, it was found that more strategic processing changes had a larger impact with a delayed feedback than an immediate one (Hattie, 2007). This applies to pharmacy management by making easy coaching recommendations immediately, for example, Sakshi (from the Chapter Scenario) could coach her staff to acknowledge customers within 4 seconds of walking up to the counter. This is a quick fix that could be implemented immediately and gently enforced frequently. However, the larger coaching changes, such as discussing the need to start providing immunization requirements for the staff pharmacist who refused to vaccinate, would be something that should have a more formal feedback focus.

Informal feedback may also take the form of *day-to-day feedback* (also known as immediate feedback). This refers to the verbal and visual messages provided daily to employees through conversations, body language, and behaviors. Daily communication is the most effective performance feedback because it is immediate and often. It also allows employees to make immediate changes and see the impact in real time. The following is a list of suggestions for providing useful daily feedback to employees:

- *Practice management-by-walking-around (MBWA).* This management approach works well for practices where the management may not interact with their entire staff regularly. This consists of getting out the office or from behind the computer/desk and interacting with employees. It is hard to provide feedback to individuals without frequent personal contact. Listen more than talk. Solicit input and advice from others. Employees can add value to the organization leadership by providing ideas for problem-solving issues. Employees may have a better idea of how to solve system problems because they work in the situation on a daily basis. And in turn, employees will become more invested because their input was acknowledged and put into place. For example, a pharmacist might complain that the technicians frequently forget to include the Vaccine Information Sheet (VIS) with each vaccination, causing the pharmacist to have print it, and thus slowing vaccination times. After consulting the technicians, they recommend preprinting the forms on the weekends when the pharmacy is slower and placing them beside the technician vaccine data entry station. Once the manager makes this change, the technicians feel empowered for enacting the change and they hold each other accountable.
- *Focus on the positive.* Encourage people by catching them doing something right, not catching them doing something wrong. Employees get enough corrective feedback. Surprise them with positive comments specific to an action that you want them to continue doing, for example, "I liked how you went out of your way to listen to the concerns of that patient and find exactly the right solution for her needs."
- *Take notes.* When people make suggestions or you make promises, write them down. Provide a deadline for getting back to them about any documented issue. Then keep your promise to get back to them by that deadline.

- *Make individuals see your presence as helpful.* Try not to waste people's time, interrupt their work, nit-pick, complicate things, or do anything that makes their day-to-day job unnecessarily difficult. Each time you add additional responsibilities to employees, consider if you are decreasing their responsibilities anywhere else or whether you are expecting them to do more and more with less time.

Formal feedback comes through the employees' *annual* (or *semiannual*) *performance reviews*. Annual performance reviews act as long-term planning sessions where managers help employees review their previous progress, identify successes and areas that need improvement, and establish goals and objectives for the next year (McConnell, 2016). Annual performance reviews augment and summarize feedback provided by managers on a day-to-day basis. Annual performance reviews are discussed in greater detail in Chapter 20.

The final form of managerial feedback comes from reviews scheduled ad hoc in response to certain particularly good or bad performances. Good *ad hoc performance reviews* are designed to provide recognition for outstanding performance and may be accompanied by some award or gift. Bad ad hoc reviews are designed to address unacceptable employee behavior or performance immediately. These negative ad hoc reviews are part of a process called *progressive discipline*. Coaching, when done well, will be uncomfortable to new managers. The goal is to have the employee's best interest in mind and to strategize upon a way for the employee to succeed, which might include employment elsewhere.

Progressive Discipline

Progressive discipline is defined as a series of acts taken by management in response to unacceptable performance by employees. The role of progressive discipline is to escalate the consequences of poor employee performance incrementally with a goal of improving that behavior. Responses by management to undesirable behavior become progressively severe until the employee either improves, resigns, or is terminated from the position. Although punitive in nature, the purpose of progressive discipline is not to punish. Rather, the aim is to make explicit to an employee the consequences of unsatisfactory behavior in order to encourage improved behavior. Indeed, improved behavior is always the preferred outcome, never the loss of an employee through resignation or termination. However, this method also serves as documentation for termination purposes, to show just cause for termination to comply with the laws the organizations that monitor HRM. Progressive discipline may be initiated in response to employee behaviors such as discourtesy to customers or coworkers, tardiness, absenteeism, unsatisfactory work performance, and violation of departmental policies. Progressive discipline usually consists of the following steps: verbal warning, written warning, suspension, and termination.

Verbal Warning

A verbal warning is a formal oral reprimand about the consequences of failing to perform as expected. A manager might verbally warn a technician that she is performing below expectations in regard to tardiness and that if performance is not improved, further disciplinary action may be warranted. Verbal warnings are relatively common and often the only action needed to correct unacceptable employee performance. Verbal warnings are more constructive and effective in a private setting than in front of coworkers; however, depending on the situation it may be prudent to have another manager or corporate human resources person serves as a witness to the conversation.

Written Warning

If an employee does not respond to a verbal warning, a more formal written warning is issued. A *written warning* is the first formal step in progressive discipline that may result in eventual discharge of the employee. It differs from verbal warnings, which are relatively informal acts that only require the manager to note the time and place of the reprimand and what was discussed. A written warning is a legal document that can end up as evidence in a court case, especially if it is dated and signed by both parties. If an employee is discharged and any disciplinary step is handled inappropriately, the employer can be sued successfully for financial damages by the employee. Therefore, written warnings should be crafted carefully with help from superiors and the human resources department.

The written warning should describe the unacceptable behavior clearly, previous warnings, specific expectations of future behavior to be achieved by a precise deadline, and the consequences of not meeting expectations. For example, "You were verbally warned about tardiness on January 16 of this year. You have continued to be tardy at a rate above that specified in your performance standards. If you are late for work more than twice within the next month, you will be suspended for 1 day without pay." As shown by this example, it is essential for a manager to keep good records of previous warnings because they will be used as the basis for potential written warnings. Employers must hold all of the employees to the same performance standards without exception or be at risk for litigation. For example, if you are giving written warning for one technician who was late because her "alarm didn't go off," you'll need to give a similar written warning for the one whose "car didn't start." The reason for tardiness, if not specified in the FCRA, cannot impact how the policy is applied or it will appear as bias.

Suspension

Suspensions are punitive actions meant to demonstrate the seriousness of a situation. Sometimes written warnings do not result in improved employee performance and need to be backed up by actions. Suspensions are meant to act as a final warning that current behavior is unacceptable. Like written warnings, they must be crafted carefully to include previous warnings, requirements for future actions, and consequences for not improving behavior (e.g., termination).

■ TERMINATION OF EMPLOYEES

Some managers are hesitant to terminate employees because it can be a difficult circumstance for all involved. For the terminated employee, it can have a tremendous impact on self-esteem, reputation, and personal finances. For the manager, it can be an emotionally charged event that results in an unpleasant confrontation and guilt. It also can lead to legal action for the business and individual manager. While it is very difficult to fire someone, it is incorrect when managers claim that laws and rules make doing so impossible. If employees are provided clear performance standards and the procedures for progressive discipline are observed, firing bad employees is quite possible. This means that every step leading up to the termination must be appropriate and documented.

Procedures for terminating employees differ depending on the circumstances. For newly hired employees who are on probation (i.e., a trial period for assessing new employees), the process of progressive discipline ordinarily does not need to be followed. The employee can be terminated at any time during the probationary period if it is clear that the employee will not succeed in the job. The steps of verbal warning, written warning, and suspension are not necessary before termination. The same is true for employees who commit acts that can lead to immediate termination, such as fighting on the job, drug or alcohol use at work, stealing, vandalism, or periods of absence without notice.

For employees who do not fall into the preceding categories, termination should not come as a surprise. Following progressive discipline procedures should give employees explicit expectations of what is going to occur when performance is not improved. Many employees will resign before being terminated. Employees who do not resign are asked to attend a termination meeting.

Prior to the termination meeting, the manager must be certain that all the following statements are true:

- The employee is not being terminated for anything other than poor job performance or breaking major rules (e.g., theft or fighting).
- The reason for termination can be stated in measurable, objective terms to which other employees do meet.

- The employee has been given specific, documented feedback regarding the performance deficiency in measurable, objective terms.
- The organization's policies and procedures regarding discipline have been observed and actions documented.
- The employee has been given ample opportunity to correct the poor performance.
- Employee treatment is consistent with similar situations of employee performance.
- The personnel department has been kept informed throughout the disciplinary process and is currently aware of plans to terminate the employee. If there is no personnel department with whom to confer, a lawyer should be consulted.

Most businesses have a procedure for terminating employees, so the manager simply follows that procedure. Most termination procedures require that a witness be present during the meeting to verify conversations and actions. The employee's codes to the pharmacy software and any company materials are collected and disabled.

The primary goal of the termination meeting is to terminate the employee compassionately and in a manner that maintains the employee's dignity and self-respect. This is better achieved by being direct and to the point by stating something such as, "You have not achieved the performance objectives specified in our last meeting, so we have decided to terminate you from your position."

The employee may respond in multiple ways (e.g., anger, tears), but the manager's response must be neutral. The manager should not argue with or criticize the employee or engage in any negotiations. It is essential to state that the decision is final. Let the employee vent any frustrations, but do not permit abusive or violent behavior. Be ready to discuss a severance package or direct the person to the human resources department, and then end the meeting. It is important to remain calm, objective, and factual. Once the decision for termination has been made, nothing should occur in this meeting to change the outcome of the termination.

Since an employee may be upset and not thinking very clearly after termination, it is useful to offer recommendations on what he or she should do next. For instance, the employer may tell the employee that he does not need to complete his shift and that his belongings will be packed and left for him to pick up the following day at some designated place.

After termination, several final steps need to be concluded. Documentation of final actions should be completed and filed. All people involved should be reminded about the confidentiality of discussions and actions. Finally, the manager should reflect on how the process went and what changes may be necessary to prevent further terminations.

■ REVISITING THE SCENARIO—TACKLING HUMAN RELATIONS

Sakshi Malik's problems in the scenario revolve around HRM. There appear to be three related issues: (1) the need to replace the open technician position and begin to cross-train all pharmacy technicians, (2) employee morale, motivation, and engagement are low, and (3) current employee expectations and behavior are unacceptable. Sakshi has identified several specific employee behaviors that hinder the performance of the pharmacy, including frequent arguments, excessive complaints, pharmacists not supervising technicians, and rude behavior and poor service to patients. The overall expectations the employees have of themselves and their coworkers are the foundations for all of these problems. Sakshi has decided to focus on this first.

Sakshi's first step should be to examine the current job and performance descriptions of the employees to see if they address the problem behaviors described. If they do, then she can use them to illustrate that specific behaviors are documented as unacceptable. For example, if the staff pharmacist's job description is to administer immunizations, Sakshi can address this with her part-time pharmacist. If job descriptions and performance standards do not address problem behaviors, then they need to be updated. With clearly defined duties and performance standards for all employees, Sakshi can start a dialogue with employees about expected behavior using specific examples. For instance, if an employee states that it is not his or her job to address patients at prescription pick-up, Sakshi can review the performance standards that relate to patient care duties and point out that acknowledgment and communication with the patient is just as important if saying "Welcome, we will be right with you" as it is with patient counseling on a drug side effect. It is important for Sakshi to remind and motivate her team of their purpose to serve patients. Sakshi needs to communicate clear expectations of employees and provide feedback in day-to-day discussions, annual reviews, and disciplinary actions.

Sakshi should realize that changing entrenched employees is a long process, so she should be patient and persistent. Some employees may not accept her efforts immediately and may refuse to alter their conduct. She will have to apply pressure through progressive discipline to encourage them to change or find a new employer. If she is consistent and fair, most employees will go along with and even embrace the changes. With successful change, employee morale should also increase and the turnover rate slow down.

■ QUESTIONS FOR FURTHER DISCUSSION

1. What knowledge and skills are employers looking for in pharmacists?
2. What questions might an interviewer ask of a candidate for the job described in Table 17-2?
3. Which interview method do you think is most effective? Least effective? Why?
4. When should the job search process for pharmacist jobs start for pharmacy students? What actions should be taken?
5. How effective would you be at terminating an employee for poor job performance? Why or why not?
6. Think about your last job search and employment. Rate your employer's performance in the areas of
   a. Recruitment and selection
   b. Interviewing
   c. Orientation and training
   d. Performance feedback
7. What type of performance feedback have you received from previous employers? Describe a specific example in which an employer did a particularly good or bad job of providing feedback.

■ CONCLUSION

Good HRM is an important requirement for providing excellent pharmacy services. Pharmacy personnel who are well managed are more likely to be satisfied in their jobs, effective, and productive. Good HRM in health care fields enhances the likelihood that patients will be better served and achieve better health outcomes. Any pharmacist who is serious about serving patients and the profession needs to be committed to good HRM.

REFERENCES

Boettge E. 2017, 06. 10 interviewer mistakes that can cost you time and money: Effective interviewing. *Talent Acquisition Excellence Essentials.* Retrieved from http://proxy.library.vcu.edu/login?url=https://scarch-proquest-com.proxy.library.vcu.edu/docview/1953022914?accountid=14780.

Brainerd J. 2017. *Paid Family Leave in the States* 25(31):1–12. Retrieved from https://fas.org/sgp/crs/misc/R44835.pdf.

Columbia Accident Investigation Board. 2003. Report of Columbia Accident Investigation Board, Volume I, I(August), 1–248. Retrieved from https://doi.org/10.1177/0020852309104177.

Cornell Law School. n.d. Fair Credit Reporting Act. Retrieved January 4, 2019, from https://www.law.cornell.edu/wex/fair_credit_reporting_act_%28fcra%29.

Desselle SP, Holmes ER. 2017. Results of the 2015 National Certified Pharmacy Technician Workforce Survey. *Am J Health Syst Pharm* 74(13):981–991.

Donnelly JH, Gibson JL, Ivancevich JM. 1995. Human resource management. *Fundamentals of Management*, Vol 13. Chicago: Irwin, p. 444.

Dreachslin JL. 2007. Diversity management and cultural competence: Research, practice, and the business case. *J Healthc Manag* 52(2):79–86.

EEOC Sues Pharmacy Solutions for Pregnancy Discrimination. Lanham: Federal Information & News Dispatch, Inc.; 2014 Sep 15.

Fleck C. 2014. Forced Out, Older Workers Are Fighting Back. AARP Bulletin: Work Life Balance. Retrieved from https://www.aarp.org/work/on-the-job/info-2014/workplace-age-discrimination-infographic.html.

Fleischer CH. 2005. *The Complete Hiring and Firing Handbook: Every Manager's Guide to Working with Employees Legally*, 1st ed. Naperville, IL: Sourcebooks, Inc. Retrieved from http://proxy.library.vcu.edu/login?url=http://search.ebscohost.com/login.aspx?direct=true&AuthType=ip,url,cookie,uid&db=nlebk&AN=120011&site=ehost-live&scope=site.

Gaddy D. Local pharmacist receives $400K in age-discrimination suit. McClatchy—Tribune Business News 2013 Nov 9.

Goldin C, Katz LF. 2012. The Most Egalitarian of All Professions: Pharmacy and the Evolution of a Family-Friendly Occupation. *NBER Working Paper*, 705–746. Available at https://doi.org/10.1017/CBO9781107415324.004.

Grays Harbor Community Hospital to Pay $125,000 to Settle Sexual Harassment Lawsuit. Lanham: Federal Information & News Dispatch, Inc.; 2011 Sep 8.

Hattie J, Timperley H. 2007. The Power of Feedback. *Review of Educational Research* 77(1):81–112. Available at https://doi.org/10.3102/003465430298487.

Holdford DA. 2003. *Marketing for Pharmacists*. Washington, DC: American Pharmaceutical Association.

McConnell CR. Umiker's Management Skills for the New Health Care Supervisor, Jones & Bartlett Learning, LLC, 2016. ProQuest Ebook Central, https://ebook-central-proquest-com.proxy.library.vcu.edu/lib/vcu/detail.action?docID=4786081.

Occupational Safety & Health Administration (OSHA), U.S. Department of Labor. 2007. Available at www.osha.gov/; 2019 Jan 7.

Rigoni B, Asplund J. 2016. Global Study: ROI for Strengths-Based Development. Retrieved December 31, 2018, from https://www.gallup.com/workplace/236288/global-study-roi-strengths-based-development.aspx.

Samuel LR. 2016. Harnessing the power of the job description. *Human Resource Management International Digest* 24(6):8–11. doi:http://dx.doi.org.proxy.library.vcu.edu/10.1108/HRMID-09-2015-0143.

Screening by Means of Pre-Employment Testing. 2018. Retrieved December 31, 2018, from https://www.shrm.org/resourcesandtools/tools-and-samples/toolkits/pages/screeningbymeansofpreemploymenttesting.aspx.

Taylor T. 2017. ADP BrandVoice: The Costs Of Training New Employees, Including Hidden Expenses. Retrieved December 28, 2018, from https://www.forbes.com/sites/adp/2017/06/02/the-costs-of-training-new-employees-including-hidden-expenses/#36694122afb2.

U.S. Department of Labor. 2008. U.S. Department of Labor Fact Sheet # 17A: Exemption for Executive, Administrative, Professional, Computer & Outside Sales Employees Under the Fair Labor Standards Act (FLSA). *WHD Wage and Hour Division*, (July).

U.S. Equal Employment Opportunity Commission. Pregnancy Discrimination Act of 1978, University of Hawaii. 1978. Available at https://doi.org/10.1525/sp.2007.54.1.23.

U.S. Equal Employment Opportunity Commission. The Equal Pay Act of 1963 (1963). Retrieved from https://www.eeoc.gov/laws/statutes/epa.cfm.

Van der Rijt J, Van den Bossche P, Segers MSR. 2013. Understanding informal feedback seeking in the workplace. *European Journal of Training and Development* 37(1):72–85. Retrieved from http://proxy.library.vcu.edu/login?url=https://search-proquest-com.proxy.library.vcu.edu/docview/1861433963?accountid=14780.

Waldman JD, Kelly F, Arora S, Smith HL. 2004. The shocking cost of turnover in health care. *Health Care Manage Rev* 29(1):2–7.

Wegmans No. 12 on Fortune's best employer list. Supermarket News 2014.

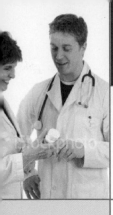

18

THE BASICS OF EMPLOYMENT LAW AND WORKPLACE SAFETY

Leigh Ann Bynum and Erin Holmes

About the Author: Dr. Bynum is an Associate Professor with the Belmont University College of Pharmacy. She received a BA degree in psychology and MS in wellness from the University of Mississippi and a PhD in pharmacy administration from the University of Mississippi. She teaches courses in pharmacy management, human resource management, and the U.S. healthcare system and communications. Dr. Bynum's research focuses on human resource management, the student pharmacist experience, and organization citizenship behaviors.

Dr. Holmes is an Associate Professor with the School of Pharmacy and research associate professor of the Research Institute for Pharmaceutical Sciences, both at the University of Mississippi. Dr. Holmes received her Doctor of Pharmacy (PharmD) degree and MS in pharmacy administration from Duquesne University and PhD in pharmacy administration from the University of Mississippi. She taught pharmacy management for 7 years and currently teaches pharmacy law, personal finance, and health care policy. Her research focuses on organizational behavior, human resource management, and service implementation in community pharmacy practice.

■ LEARNING OBJECTIVES

After completing this chapter, readers should be able to

1. Compare and contrast the role various federal employment laws play in the pharmacy workplace.
2. Describe what is meant by "sexual harassment" and how employers and employees can resolve issues of quid pro quo and hostile work environments.
3. Discuss the concept of drug testing and why it is necessary in the pharmacy workplace.
4. Identify the best ways to resolve pharmacy robbery, burglary, theft, and shoplifting incidents.
5. Describe fundamental issues in occupational safety.

■ SCENARIO

Michael Davis is a brand new pharmacy school graduate, and after receiving his pharmacist license, is immediately promoted to store manager at Bruin Drug and Apothecary, a large chain pharmacy located in the Midwest and Southern United States. Michael is excited about his managerial position. There are two clerks, three pharmacy technicians, and one other pharmacist at Michael's store; all are female except the other pharmacist. After a couple of months, one of the pharmacy technicians approaches Michael and tells him that Mark, the other pharmacist, has been making rather suggestive comments to her and that it makes her feel uncomfortable. Michael regularly plays golf with Mark and really likes him. Michael tells the technician not to worry about it, as he cannot imagine Mark saying anything close to what the technician is telling him.

A couple of weeks later, this same technician tells Michael that she noticed another technician taking some hydrocodone 10-mg tablets and placing them in her purse. After conducting an informal inventory of the hydrocodone in stock and noticing a shortage of 20 tablets, Michael calls both technicians into the break room and confronts the suspected employee. The employee adamantly denies this, but Michael is convinced she committed theft. He tells the suspected employee to wait in the break room while he and the technician making the complaint exit the room. Michael then calls the police. The police arrive 15 minutes later and after questioning the technician, determine that she, in fact, stole the hydrocodone.

■ CHAPTER QUESTIONS

1. What are some of the principal workplace issues that involve federal employment laws?
2. What are some of the skills and abilities managers must possess to ensure a safe and healthy working environment?
3. What are the potential legal issues associated with drug testing in the workplace? Should employers require drug testing of job applicants and employees?
4. What actions should be considered to minimize the risk of robbery, burglary, and theft in the pharmacy?
5. What are the manager's responsibilities related to violence in the workplace and Employee Assistance Programs?

■ FEDERAL EMPLOYMENT LAWS

Health care, in general, is a highly complex environment with numerous laws and regulations that further complicate it. While pharmacists and pharmacy mangers do not necessarily need to be lawyers, they do need to be aware of key legal issues that govern their working environments. This chapter will examine select federal employment laws as well as a number of pertinent issues regarding workplace safety.

Title VII of the Civil Rights Act of 1964 (Title VII) prohibits discrimination against someone on the basis of race, color, religion, national origin, or sex. The law also makes it illegal to retaliate against a person because that person complained about discrimination, filed a charge of discrimination, or participated in an employment discrimination investigation or lawsuit. Additionally, Title VII also requires that employers reasonably accommodate applicants' and employees' sincerely held religious practices, unless doing so would impose an undue hardship on the operation of the employer's business. Discrimination in the workplace can occur in other ways, too, in addition to the five areas listed earlier. For instance, individuals may bring a claim of discrimination based on age, pregnancy, compensation, or disability. As such, other federal employment laws were enacted, such as the Age Discrimination in Employment Act, the Equal Pay Act, and the Americans with Disabilities Act. To protect pregnant individuals, Title VII was amended to include the Pregnancy Discrimination Act. The law forbids discrimination when it comes to any aspect of employment, including hiring, firing, pay, job assignments, promotions, layoff, training, fringe benefits, and any other term or condition of employment. Harassment is a type of discrimination. It is the *unwelcome* conduct that is based on race, color, religion, sex (including pregnancy), national origin, age (40 or older), disability, or genetic information. Petty grievances or isolated events (unless very serious in nature) seldom escalate to illegality. Harassment becomes unlawful when (1) enduring the offensive conduct becomes a condition of continued employment or (2) the conduct is severe or pervasive enough to create a work environment that a reasonable person would consider intimidating, hostile, or abusive. Antidiscrimination laws also prohibit harassment against individuals in retaliation for filing a discrimination charge, testifying, or participating in any way in an investigation, proceeding, or lawsuit under these laws. At first glance, it may appear overwhelming to comply with these federal laws. However, the next few sections will illustrate methods pharmacists can adopt to create, develop, and maintain a workplace free from discrimination. The majority of information for this section comes directly from the United States Equal Employment Opportunity Commission (EEOC) website (http://www.eeoc.gov/). This website is also a valuable resource for pharmacists and student pharmacists who would like more detailed information than can be provided in this chapter.

Title VII of the Civil Rights Act of 1964

Race Discrimination

Discrimination on the basis of an undeniable characteristic associated with race, such as skin color, hair texture, or certain facial features, violates Title VII, even though not all members of the race share the same characteristic. This type of discrimination can also involve treating someone unfavorably because that person is married to (or associated with) a person of a certain race or color or because of a person's connection with a race-based organization or group, or an organization or group that is generally associated with people of a certain race. Title VII also prohibits discrimination on the basis of a condition that predominantly affects one race unless the practice is job-related and consistent with business necessity. For

example, since sickle cell anemia predominantly occurs in African Americans, a policy that excludes individuals with sickle cell anemia is discriminatory unless the policy is job-related and consistent with business necessity. Similarly, a "no-beard" employment policy may discriminate against African-American men who have a predisposition to pseudofolliculitis barbae (severe shaving bumps) unless the policy is job-related and consistent with business necessity.

In a race discrimination lawsuit, the courts will examine whether a particular policy is related to the conditions of employment and consistent with business necessity. This evaluation is conducted on a case-by-case basis but some factors that the courts examine include the following:

- Education
- Employment testing
- Conviction and arrest records

In the profession of pharmacy, pharmacists are required by law to be licensed by their respective licensing board (e.g., state board of pharmacy). So, a nonpharmacist (regardless of race) will not prevail in a race discrimination lawsuit against an employer advertising specifically for a pharmacist position, assuming that the job qualifications require a licensed pharmacist.

Color Discrimination

Title VII prohibits employment discrimination because of "color" as a basis separately listed in the statute. The statute does not define "color." The courts and the EEOC read "color" to have its commonly understood meaning—pigmentation, complexion, or skin shade or tone. Thus, color discrimination occurs when a person is discriminated against based on the lightness, darkness, or other color characteristics of the person. Even though race and color overlap, they are not synonymous. Thus, color discrimination can occur between persons of different races or ethnicities, or between persons of the same race or ethnicity. Although it is a commonly held belief that you must be of a different race or color to discriminate against another, this is not the case. Discrimination can occur when the victim and the person who inflicted the discrimination are of the same race or color.

It is prohibited to harass a person because of that person's race or color. Examples of harassment may include racial slurs, offensive remarks about a person's race, or color or the display of racially offensive symbols. Although the law does not prohibit simple teasing or one-time comments, it is a slippery slope. What may be considered a funny email joke by one person may be considered offensive by another. It is prudent for pharmacists and managers within organizations to be sensitive to everyone within the organization. Remember, the harasser can be the victim's supervisor, a supervisor in another area, a coworker, or someone who is not an employee of the employer, such as a patient or customer.

National Origin Discrimination

Regardless of an employee or job applicant's ancestry, he or she is entitled to the same employment opportunities as anyone else. EEOC enforces the federal prohibition against national origin discrimination (in addition to race, color, sex, and religion) in employment under Title VII. It is unlawful to discriminate against any employee or applicant because of the individual's national origin. No one can be denied equal employment opportunity because of birthplace, ancestry, culture, and linguistic characteristics common to a specific ethnic group, or accent. As with race and color, equal employment opportunity cannot be denied because of marriage or association with persons of a national origin group; membership or association with specific ethnic promotion groups; attendance or participation in schools, churches, temples, or mosques generally associated with a national origin group; or a surname associated with a national origin group. Title VII prohibits offensive conduct, such as ethnic slurs, that creates a hostile work environment based on national origin.

Additionally, the following items are important for employers to keep in mind:

- *Accent discrimination.* An employer may not base a decision on an employee's foreign accent unless the accent materially interferes with job performance.

- *English fluency.* A fluency requirement is only permissible if required for the effective performance of the position for which it is imposed.
- *English-only rules.* English-only rules must be adopted for nondiscriminatory reasons. An English-only rule may be used if it is needed to promote the safe or efficient operation of the employer's business.
- *Coverage of foreign nationals.* Title VII and the other antidiscrimination laws prohibit discrimination against individuals employed in the United States, regardless of citizenship. However, relief may be limited if an individual does not have work authorization. The Immigration Reform and Control Act of 1986 (IRCA) requires employers to prove that all employees hired after November 6, 1986, are legally authorized to work in the United States. IRCA also prohibits discrimination based on national origin or citizenship.

Religious Discrimination

Title VII prohibits employers from discriminating against individuals because of their religion in hiring, firing, and other terms and conditions of employment. The law protects not only people who belong to traditional, organized religions, such as Buddhism, Christianity, Hinduism, Islam, and Judaism but also others who have sincerely held religious, ethical, or moral beliefs. The law also requires employers to reasonably accommodate the religious practices of an employee or prospective employee, unless doing so would create an undue hardship upon the employer. As with race, color, and national origin, harassment is a form of discrimination and may include, for example, offensive remarks about a person's religious beliefs or practices that are so pervasive that it creates a hostile workplace or results in an adverse employment decision. A reasonable religious accommodation is any adjustment to the work environment that will allow the employee to practice his religion. Flexible scheduling, voluntary substitutions or swaps, job reassignments, and lateral transfers are examples of accommodating an employee's religious beliefs.

An employer can claim undue hardship when asked to accommodate an applicant's or employee's religious practices if allowing such practices requires more than ordinary administrative costs, diminishes efficiency in other jobs, infringes on other employees' job rights or benefits, impairs workplace safety, causes coworkers to carry the accommodated employee's share of potentially hazardous or burdensome work, or if the proposed accommodation conflicts with another law or regulation. Undue hardship also may be shown if the request for an accommodation violates the terms of a collective bargaining agreement or job rights established through a seniority system.

It should be noted that what appears as an undue hardship for one pharmacy may not appear as an undue hardship for another pharmacy. As such, there is no definitive standard that determines undue hardship. The courts have held that reasonableness and undue hardship are separate and distinct issues to be considered (Wymer, 2014). Once an accommodation has been determined to be reasonable, then a determination of undue hardship can be made. The EEOC has defined undue hardship as something that "requires more than ordinary administrative costs, diminishes efficiency in other jobs, infringes on other employees' job rights or impairs workplace safety" (SHRM, 2017). Factors relevant to undue hardship may include the type of workplace, the nature of the employee's duties, the identifiable cost of the accommodation in relation to the size and operating costs of the employer, and the number of employees who will need a particular accommodation.

Costs to be considered include not only direct monetary costs but also the burden on the conduct of the employer's business. To prove undue hardship, the employer will need to demonstrate how much cost or disruption a proposed accommodation would involve. An employer cannot rely on potential or hypothetical hardship when faced with a religious obligation that conflicts with scheduled work, but rather should rely on objective information. A mere assumption that many more people with the same religious practices as the individual being accommodated may also seek accommodation is not evidence of undue hardship.

For example, many pharmacies are open on Sunday, a day traditionally reserved for attending church services. This often presents a dilemma for pharmacy managers trying to schedule Sundays. However, what does a pharmacy employer do if all its employees do not want to work on Sunday? The typical answer is "it depends." In general, employers must give time off for the Sabbath or holy days except in an emergency, unless the employee works in key health and safety occupations or the employee's presence is critical to the company on any given day. Since pharmacists and their technicians work in health and safety occupations and often that employee is critical to the company, time off may not always be granted.

One possible way to resolve this potential issue is to address it prior to hiring an employee. Although an employer is prohibited from asking an applicant questions regarding his/her religious beliefs, the employer is allowed to ask the following question: "Are you able to perform all the essential qualifications for the position, qualifications that include working on Sunday?" If the applicant responds "yes," the employer is then allowed to require the employee to work on Sunday. It should be noted, though, that it could appear discriminatory if the same employee (or select employees) are always required to work on Sunday, while other employees (assuming same seniority or less) are not required to work on Sunday. There is some responsibility for the employee here as well. Employees should be advised of the pharmacy policy regarding requests for time off and notify their manager as far in advance as possible for the request time away from work.

Pregnancy Discrimination

In 1978, Title VII was amended to prohibit pregnancy discrimination. This type of discrimination involves treating a woman (an applicant or employee) unfavorably because of pregnancy, childbirth, or a medical condition related to pregnancy or childbirth. An employer may not single out pregnancy-related conditions for special procedures to determine an employee's ability to work. However, if an employer requires its employees to submit a doctor's statement concerning their inability to work before granting leave or paying sick benefits for all employees with all conditions, they may also require employees affected by pregnancy-related conditions to submit such statements.

If an employee is temporarily unable to perform her job because of her pregnancy, the employer must treat her same as any other temporarily disabled employee. For example, if the employer allows temporarily disabled employees to modify tasks, perform alternative assignments, or take disability leave or leave without pay, the employer must also allow an employee who is temporarily disabled because of pregnancy to do the same. Additionally, temporarily disabled pregnant employees must be treated as other temporarily disabled employees as it relates to accrual and crediting of seniority, vacation calculation, pay increases, and temporary disability benefits. Pregnant employees must be allowed to work as long as they are able to perform their jobs. A recent court case (Young v UPS, 2015) has made it more likely that pregnant women who are denied accommodations will be successful in their discrimination claims under the Pregnancy Discrimination Act. At the heart of this case is a young female driver for UPS named Peggy Young. Her doctor restricted her ability to lift (20 lb for the first 20 weeks and 10 lb thereafter) during her pregnancy, yet UPS placed her on unpaid leave rather than provide accommodations stating that her position required her to lift 70 lb. UPS had previously accommodated drivers who were injured on the job or who were considered to have a disability under the ADA, thus leading the court to find in Young's favor (Morris, 2015). Based on this ruling EEOC made slight modifications to their recommendations to ensure employers avoid disparate impact specifically as it relates to light duty. As always, pharmacy managers should seek the most up-to-date information on the law from the EEOC.

On a related note, the Family and Medical Leave Act (FMLA) of 1993 provides up to 12 weeks of unpaid leave to care for the new child (including foster and adoptive parents). To be eligible, the employee must have worked for the employer for 12 months prior to taking the leave and that employer must have 50 or more employees. If during that 12-month period the employee has accrued paid time off per the employer's policy, then they may be paid for that leave.

Sex Discrimination

Sex discrimination involves treating someone (an applicant or employee) unfavorably because of that person's gender. This type of discrimination can also involve treating someone less favorably because of his or her connection with an organization or group that is generally associated with people of a certain sex. Discrimination against an individual because that person is transgender is discrimination because of sex in violation of Title VII. This is also known as gender identity discrimination. Additionally, lesbian, gay, and bisexual individuals may bring sex discrimination claims. These may include, for example, allegations of sexual harassment or other kinds of sex discrimination, such as adverse actions taken because of the person's nonconformance with sex stereotypes.

Sexual harassment is a form of sex discrimination under Title VII. Harassment can include unwelcome sexual advances, requests for sexual favors, and other verbal or physical harassment of a sexual nature. It is important to keep in mind that harassment does not have to be of a sexual nature, however, and can include offensive remarks about a person's sex. For example, it is illegal to harass a woman by making offensive comments about women in general. Although it is common to think of sexual harassment as a male harassing a female, this is not always the case. Both victim and the harasser can be either a woman or a man, and the victim and harasser can be the same sex. In fact, according to the EEOC website, over 17% of the charges filed in 2014 were filed by males (EEOC, 2018). Sexual harassment can occur in a variety of other circumstances as well. For example, the harasser can be the victim's supervisor, an agent of the employer, a supervisor in another area, a coworker, or a nonemployee (pharmacy patient). It is important to note that the victim does not have to be the person harassed but could be anyone affected by the offensive conduct.

Broadly speaking, there are two types of sexual harassment: quid pro quo and hostile work environment. The Latin term "quid pro quo" translates to "something for something." This type of harassment occurs in the workplace when the pharmacist or other authority figure states or implies that the employee will receive something (e.g., a promotion or a raise) in return for some sexual encounter. Conversely, it could also be considered quid pro quo if the authority figure says the person will not be terminated or punished in some way in exchange for a sexual favor. A hostile workplace, on the other hand, may be less overt. The unwanted sexual behavior or communications are a pattern or are pervasive enough to disrupt the employees work. This is more than just a one-time off-color remark which in and of itself may be annoying but is not a pattern and has not disrupted the employees' work.

Prevention is the best tool to eliminate sexual harassment in the workplace. Employers are encouraged to take steps necessary to prevent sexual harassment from occurring. They should clearly communicate to employees that sexual harassment will not be tolerated. They can do so by providing sexual harassment training to their employees and by establishing an effective complaint or grievance process and taking immediate and appropriate action when an employee complains.

Age Discrimination in Employment Act

Age discrimination involves treating someone (an applicant or employee) less favorably because of his or her age. The Age Discrimination in Employment Act (ADEA) forbids age discrimination against people who are aged 40 years or older. It does not protect workers under the age of 40, although some states do have laws that protect younger workers from age discrimination. It is not illegal for an employer or other covered entity to favor an older worker over a younger one, even if both workers are aged 40 years or older. Discrimination can occur when the victim and the person who inflicted the discrimination are both older than 40 years. It is also important to note that an employment policy or practice that applies to everyone, regardless of age, can be illegal if it has a negative impact on applicants or employees aged 40 years or older and is not based on a reasonable factor other than age.

Based on this information, must a pharmacy manager promote a pharmacist over the age of 40 rather than promote a pharmacist who is 30 years of age? The answer is no, provided age was not a factor in the decision. The ADEA is not automatically violated if a pharmacy employee over the age of 40 is not promoted. There are several factors the employer may use in its decision-making process so as to protect the pharmacy (and the pharmacy management/owner) from an ADEA claim. These factors include the following:

- Output
- Productivity
- Education
- Experience (Robinson et al., 2002)

Regarding the previous example, the pharmacy employer must demonstrate that in promoting the 30-year-old pharmacist over the 40-year-old pharmacist, the younger pharmacist performed his job more efficiently, possessed greater education, had more experience as a pharmacist, and/or had a greater number of years with the organization. The presence of these factors is no guarantee that the employer will win a possible ADEA lawsuit, but they do provide a stronger defense. It should be noted that the employer must have documentation to support its claim, chiefly performance evaluations (see Chapter 20).

Equal Pay Act

The Equal Pay Act (EPA) requires that men and women in the same workplace be given equal pay for equal work. The jobs need not be identical, but they must be substantially equal. Job content (not job titles) determines whether jobs are substantially equal. Factors that may be considered when determining if the jobs in question are substantially equal are skill, effort, and responsibility, and working conditions within the same establishment.

- *Skill.* This can be measured by factors such as the experience, ability, education, and training required to perform the job. The issue is what skills are required for the job, not what skills the individual employees may have. For example, two technician jobs could be considered equal under the EPA even if one of the job holders has a master's degree in physics, since that degree would not be required for the job.

- *Effort.* The amount of physical or mental exertion needed to perform the job.
- *Responsibility.* The degree of accountability required in performing the job. For example, a salesperson who is delegated the duty of determining whether to accept customers' personal checks has more responsibility than other salespeople. On the other hand, a minor difference in responsibility, such as turning out the lights at the end of the day, would not justify a pay differential.
- *Working conditions.* This encompasses two factors: (1) physical surroundings like temperature, fumes, and ventilation and (2) hazards.
- *Establishment.* An establishment is a distinct physical place of business rather than an entire business or enterprise consisting of several places of business. In some circumstances, physically separate places of business may be treated as one establishment. For example, if a central administrative unit hires employees, sets their compensation, and assigns them to separate work locations, the separate work sites can be considered part of one establishment.

All forms of pay are covered by this law, including salary, overtime pay, bonuses, stock options, profit sharing and bonus plans, life insurance, vacation and holiday pay, cleaning or gasoline allowances, hotel accommodations, reimbursement for travel expenses, and benefits. If there is an inequality in wages between men and women, employers may not reduce the wages of either sex to equalize their pay.

Title VII also makes it illegal to discriminate based on sex in pay and benefits. Therefore, someone who has an Equal Pay Act claim may also have a claim under Title VII. Title VII, the ADEA, and the Americans with Disabilities Act (covered in next section) prohibit compensation discrimination on the basis of race, color, religion, sex, national origin, age, or disability. Unlike the EPA, there is no requirement under Title VII, the ADEA, or the ADA that the jobs must be substantially equal. At first glance, it may appear that all pharmacy technicians and all pharmacists must be respectively compensated the same amount for working the same hours at the same pharmacy. This, however, is not the case. If the employer can demonstrate that the pharmacists at Pharmacy XYZ, for example, differed in job performance, seniority, or an incentive system (e.g., generic utilization percentage), then pay differentials are allowed. As mentioned earlier, it is imperative that these factors have empirical data to support these claims.

The Americans with Disabilities Act

Title I of the Americans with Disabilities Act (ADA) of 1990 prohibits private employers, state and local governments, employment agencies, and labor unions from discriminating against qualified individuals with disabilities in job application procedures, hiring, firing, advancement, compensation, job training, and other terms, conditions, and privileges of employment. A qualified employee or applicant with a disability is an individual who, with or without reasonable accommodation, can perform the essential functions of the job in question.

An individual with a disability is a person who

- has a physical or mental impairment that substantially limits one or more major life activities;
- has a record of such an impairment; or
- is regarded as having such an impairment.

This definition of disability is rather broad so let us examine each part more closely. First, a "major life activity" can include walking, caring for oneself, seeing, hearing, eating, sleeping, standing, lifting, etc. A "major life activity" can also include the operation of a bodily function, such as the immune system, digestive system, brain, respiratory system, etc. Second, a "record of such an impairment" is defined simply as having a medical record of having a physical or mental impairment. If a medical record exists, then that person is considered to have a disability under the ADA.

Lastly, an individual satisfies the definition of "regarded as having such an impairment" by establishing that he/she has been discriminated against because of an actual or perceived physical or mental impairment. If an employer perceives the person as having a physical or mental impairment and acts in a discriminatory fashion against that individual because of that perception, then it is likely to be determined that there is a disability under the ADA. Also, if the actual physical or mental impairment is obvious/noticeable and the employer discriminates against that person because of it, then you likely have a disability under the ADA.

As obesity rates have soared, the ADA and the United States courts have wrestled with whether to classify obesity as a disability. Prior to 2008, the EEOC guidelines provided that except in "rare circumstances," obesity was not to be considered a disability, and most courts held accordingly. However, the 2008 amendment to the ADA mandated that it be interpreted more broadly. Since that time, the EEOC has taken the position that obesity sufficiently affects major life activities to warrant classification as a disability and several courts have agreed. With the ever increasing rates of obesity in the United States, it is prudent for employers to consider severe or morbid obesity as a disability and provide reasonable accommodations.

Reasonable accommodation may include, but is not limited to, the following:

- making existing facilities used by employees readily accessible to and usable by persons with disabilities.
- job restructuring, modifying work schedules, and reassignment to a vacant position.
- acquiring or modifying equipment or devices, adjusting or modifying examinations, training materials, or policies, and providing qualified readers or interpreters.

An employer is required to make a reasonable accommodation to the known disability of a qualified applicant or employee if it would not impose an "undue hardship" on the operation of the employer's business. Reasonable accommodations are adjustments or modifications provided by an employer to enable people with disabilities to enjoy equal employment opportunities. Accommodations vary depending upon the needs of the individual applicant or employee. Not all people with disabilities (or even all people with the same disability) will require the same accommodation.

As previously stated, an employer does not have to provide a reasonable accommodation if it imposes an "undue hardship." Undue hardship is defined as an action requiring significant difficulty or expense when considered in light of factors such as an employer's size, financial resources, and the nature and structure of its operation. An employer is not required to lower quality or production standards to make an accommodation, nor is an employer obligated to provide personal use items such as glasses or hearing aids.

An employer generally does not have to provide a reasonable accommodation unless an individual with a disability has asked for one. If an employer believes that a medical condition is causing a performance or conduct problem, he/she may ask the employee how to solve the problem and if the employee needs a reasonable accommodation. Once a reasonable accommodation is requested, the employer and the individual should discuss the individual's needs and identify the appropriate reasonable accommodation. Where more than one accommodation would work, the employer may choose the one that is less costly or that is easier to provide.

Many employers are aware of different types of accommodations for people with physical disabilities, but they may be less familiar with accommodations for employees with disabilities that are not visible, such as psychiatric disabilities. Not all employees with mental illness or psychiatric disabilities need accommodations to perform their jobs. For those who do, it is important to remember that the process of developing and implementing accommodations is individualized and should begin with input from the employee. Accommodations vary, just as people's strengths, work environments, and job duties vary. Common reasonable accommodations include altered break and work schedules (e.g., scheduling work around medical appointments), time off for treatment, changes in supervisory methods (e.g., providing written instructions, or breaking tasks into smaller parts), eliminating a nonessential (or marginal) job function that someone cannot perform because of a disability, and telework. These are just examples; employees are free to request, and employers are free to suggest, other modifications or changes.

DRUG TESTING IN THE WORKPLACE

There are a number of Constitutional concerns associated with drug testing in the workplace. The Fourth Amendment to the United States Constitution protects citizens against unreasonable searches and seizures. Many individuals claim that providing a blood or urine sample for drug testing purposes is an intrusive search and seizure. Furthermore, plaintiffs bringing a lawsuit alleging that their Fourth Amendment rights have been violated often assert their right of privacy. It is important to note that pharmacists, as health care professionals and members of a highly regulated industry, have a lessened expectation of (and therefore less right to) privacy. Here, the reasoning is that these workers have voluntarily subjected themselves to licensing and regulation, and this could include drug testing. As such, pharmacists can expect drug testing in the workplace, provided certain conditions exist.

Employers are allowed to conduct drug testing in the workplace. Failure to do so could place the employer at risk for subsequent litigation, especially if the employer was aware that one of its employees had a drug/alcohol problem and did nothing to try and resolve the issue, possibly endangering patients. The Drug-Free Workplace Act provides significant protection for employers by requiring holders of government contracts as well as federal grant recipients in excess of $100,000 to implement programs reasonably expected to reduce and eliminate employee drug use (Robinson et al., 2002). However, private sector employers may also initiate drug-testing programs provided the testing is applied uniformly to all job applicants and employees. This being said, employers are still not allowed to carte blanche discretion when it comes to drug testing its current and future employees. Employers who "select" individuals for drug testing solely on the basis of race, color, sex, religion, national origin, and/or on the basis of a disability run a significant risk of losing a discrimination lawsuit. Random screening is allowed, provided all employees are eligible for the screenings and that the screenings do not result in only certain protected classes (groups protected in Title VII and ADA) undergoing drug testing. Drug testing may also be implemented in circumstances where the employer has a reasonable basis for suspecting that an employee is under the influence of drugs during work hours and when an employer has a legitimate business interest in having the work performed by employees who are not impaired by drugs or alcohol use (Kraslawsky v Upper Deck Co, 1997).

Employee drug testing also has a direct impact on pharmacy students. There is a widespread awareness of the use and abuse of alcohol and drugs on college campuses. Students in the various health professions programs, including pharmacy, are also susceptible to using and misusing these substances (Cates & Hogue, 2012). In fact, Kenna and Wood (2004) found that lifetime prescription opioid and anxiolytic misuse was higher in the student pharmacist population than in the general college student population. Pharmacy students who enter the workforce with a predisposition to abuse either prescription drugs, illicit drugs, or alcohol can jeopardize more than just their careers but also the health of the public (Lord et al., 2009). Given the potential for tragic outcomes resulting from pharmacy students using or abusing drugs or alcohol in patient care areas, it has become common for community pharmacies, hospitals, and other providers to require students to receive drug testing as a condition of their practice experience. With this in mind, more Colleges and Schools of Pharmacy across the United States are considering some type of student drug testing. These programs vary between allowing the experiential sites to conduct testing in accordance with the site policies to limited drug testing for all students at certain points within the curriculum. Some schools have even implemented mandatory random drug screening throughout all years of the professional curriculum (Cates & Hogue, 2012). Given the prevalence of drug and alcohol use, a drug testing policy is worthy of consideration not only by pharmacy managers but also those involved in experiential education.

Robbery, Burglary, and Theft

Since the Centers for Disease Control labeled prescription drug abuse an epidemic in 2010, a number of actions have been taken to limit the supply of prescription drugs to those who seek to abuse them. Drug tracking and monitoring programs as well as education impacting how narcotics are prescribed have all had an influence on the supply side of the drug abuse problem. Unfortunately, the demand side of the prescription drug abuse issue is still problematic. According to the 2016 NSDUH, 62.3% of the population aged 12 or older who reported misuse of pain relievers, cited relief of physical pain as the most common reason for that misuse (SAMHSA, 2016). Drug Enforcement Administration's (DEA) Drug and Theft Assessment (2017) reports that over 50% of those who completed the survey stated that "given by, bought from, or took from a friend or relative." (p7). Regardless of how or why the original diversion occurs, those individuals seeking to illegally use prescription narcotics continue to turn to pharmacies for their supply once their original supply is gone. Unfortunately, this supply is often obtained by breaking into the pharmacy while it is closed or worse, threatening the physical well-being of employees and customers while the store is open.

Pharmacists may experience a number of different losses in association with a robbery or burglary beyond the direct costs associated with replacing the broken or stolen items. They may incur increases in insurance costs and the installation of additional security measures. If there is damage to the facility itself, there may need to be several days where the pharmacy is unable to conduct business as usual. The emotional toll that a robbery or burglary takes on the pharmacist and the rest of the employees and customers can have a negative impact on the business as well. To address the psychological toll, many pharmacies turn to an Employee Assistance Program (EAP) for guidance. EAPs often include short-term counseling and referral services for employees. These programs are discussed more completely in a later section.

Because pharmacies make an attractive target for robberies, burglaries, and thefts, it is imperative that pharmacists do everything they can to try and make the pharmacy a less appealing and more difficult target. While there is not "one size fits all" approach to preventing and handling these crimes once they occur, pharmacy employees and employers who possess an awareness of the issues surrounding these crimes will be better equipped to resolve any difficulties that might arise. Therefore, the aim of this section is to describe pharmacy robbery, burglary, and theft and to suggest tactics and practical tips that may be used to manage the problem as well as to provide resources for the pharmacy manager to consider.

Robbery

Robbery is "the illegal taking of property from the person of another, or in the person's presence, by violence or intimidation" (*Black's Law Dictionary*, 1996). Armed robbery involves the use of a gun or other weapon that can do bodily harm, such as a knife or club. Based on the most recent DEA information, as reported by Pharmacists Mutual (2015), the incidents of pharmacy robberies in the United States are on the rise with 689 being reported in 2011 and 839 in 2014. The current projections indicate that this upward trend will continue. One key point, which cannot be overstated, is that the health and safety of employees and patients is of utmost importance. According to law enforcement professionals, the most important thing to do in order to prepare for a potential robbery is to have a plan in place and to communicate that plan to all staff (Blank, 2018). Considering the fact that many robberies involve individuals who are impaired and/or "drug seeking," the first goal should focus on having the individual spend as little time as possible inside the pharmacy. As such, it is critical for managers and employees to comply with the individual's demands. Controlled substances, money, and merchandise can be replaced; individual lives cannot. To that end, Pharmacists Mutual (2015) suggests the following tips for things you can do prior to a robbery event to keep you safe during that event:

- A pharmacy should plan for a robbery event. Discuss roles and behaviors when and after a robbery occurs.
- Train the staff on what to do when a robbery occurs.
- Consider installing panic buttons which provide an opportunity to notify police without having to make the call. However, make sure you know how the police will respond (e.g., loud sirens and lights or a quiet approach).

- Opening doors with a buzzer and letting people in individually may help but is not totally effective.
- Deploy tracking devices. These devices are disguised to look and feel like narcotic bottles but provide alerts to police notifying them of the location of the device. These devices do not prevent the robbery but may help to catch the thief after the fact. These tracking devices boast a 70% apprehension rate.
- Time safety delays on safes make the robbery event take a little longer. Many would-be thieves do not want to wait so they may move on to another target.

Preventing a robbery from occurring is the first step but once a robbery occurs, it is important to stay calm and comply with the individual's requests. Refer to Table 18-1 for tips on what to do during a robbery.

Table 18-1. What to Do during a Robbery

Remember, the objective is to get the robber out of the store as quickly as possible.
- Try to stay calm. Say to yourself "stay calm."
- *Do exactly as you are told.* No more, no less.
- *Use caution, being careful is not cowardice.*
- Alert the robber to any event or action you know is going to happen that may startle or upset the robber (e.g., someone is due to arrive soon).
- Be observant, make a conscious effort to get a description of the robber, *but* avoid making direct eye contact (the perception is that eye contact promotes recognition).
- Do not make any sudden or quick movements.
- When it is necessary to move or reach to comply with demands, tell the robber what you are going to do and why.
- Listen carefully. Not only in order to obey commands but perhaps to hear a name used or something else said that could be used in the investigation.
- *Do not resist!* Take a step back. Place your hands in front of you with palms held outward.
- Passively try to keep any note or written instructions the robber may have given you. If you can, turn this over to the police later.
- Activate "panic button" or "toe kick" alarms only when you do it secretly. Take no chances!
- Give the robber adequate time to leave. Avoid the urge to give chase! Note the direction of travel when he/she leaves.
- Try to get a description of any vehicle used in the getaway *if* you can do so without compromising your personal safety. Make, model, color, license number, distinguishing features (decals, dents, bumper stickers, hubcaps, etc.).

Data from Pharmacists Mutual Insurance Companies. 2011. Sample policies and procedures (Burglary, Robbery, Shoplifting and Employee Dishonesty Policy & Procedures).

Burglary

Burglary is "the offense of breaking and entering into a structure for the intent of committing a felony" (*Black's Law Dictionary,* 1996). No great force is needed (pushing open a door or slipping through an open window is sufficient), if the entry is unauthorized. In the context of burglary of a pharmacy, force is almost always involved. Unlike robbery, burglary does not involve the threat or use of force against an individual. The most common example of a pharmacy burglary would be a pharmacy that is broken into during the middle of the night, resulting in the loss of medications, money, and/or merchandise. Rates of pharmacy burglary vary across the United States. Although these events tend to cluster around major metropolitan areas, some of the largest claims experienced by Pharmacists Mutual (2015) have happened in rural areas. By far, the most common method of illegal entry (72%) is through a door or window (over half the time entry is made through the front door), although entry through a wall (8%) or roof (4%) is not uncommon (Pharmacists Mutual, 2015). This suggests that pharmacy mangers should consider investing in protective glass, good lighting, and strong doors and windows with burglary resistant locks. If wall and roof burglaries are common in your area, motion or vibration detectors are also good options to consider.

In general, the more barriers criminals face the more likely it is that they will choose another target, or at least be slowed down enough to be caught. Many criminals visit the pharmacy during working hours before deciding to break into the pharmacy after hours, so make your protective features clearly visible. Video surveillance may deter criminals and may help the authorities catch the criminal after the fact. However, the most critical protective feature a pharmacy can provide to limit the extent of a burglary is an effective alarm system (Pharmacists Mutual, 2015). Alarms should be professionally installed and the system must be tested monthly. Investment in the correct technology and placement of that technology can make a tremendous difference in its reliability and in the amount of damage and theft that actually

occurs. It should go without saying that the investment in alarm technology will not pay off if the alarm is not working properly. But, surprisingly, in some reported burglaries, the pharmacist forgot to set the alarm when leaving or the alarm failed due to a lack of maintenance (Pharmacists Mutual, 2015). Despite the manager's best efforts burglaries may still occur. It is important to know what to do when you discover a burglary. Please refer to Table 18-2 for more information.

Theft

Theft (larceny) is "the unlawful taking and carrying away of someone else's personal property with the intent to deprive the owner of it permanently" (*Black's Law Dictionary*, 1996). Although robbery and burglary are types of theft, each is categorized as a different criminal act. The two types of theft that are more commonly seen in the workplace will be addressed in these sections: shoplifting and employee theft (see Chapter 11 on Risk Management).

Shoplifting

Prevention is the key to preventing this type of theft. In fact, training pharmacy employees to detect shoplifters is very important. The following tips are important in trying to prevent shoplifting from occurring:

- Watch for suspicious behavior(s) from customers:
  - Is (are) the customer(s) wearing heavy bulky clothing even though the weather is good?
  - Is the customer constantly looking behind, left or right, or above as if to see if anyone, or anything, is watching?
  - Is a group of customers acting in a boisterous manner as if to call attention to themselves?
  - Is a customer spending an inordinate amount of time looking at the same relatively high-priced merchandise?
  - Is a customer seemingly resentful or uneasy when a sales associate asks if they can assist?

Make mental and/or written notes, including descriptions, of any of the conditions noted earlier. Report any of the preceding conditions to store

Table 18-2.	What to Do upon Discovering a Burglary

Call the police—even if the alarm has been triggered.

Lock the doors. Prevent anyone from entering! Preserve the crime scene for the law enforcement investigators. Don't touch anything the burglar may have touched and block off any areas the burglar(s) was to protect evidence they may have left behind.

Post signs at entries that the store opening will be delayed! If there has been damage to the property, call a contractor to **make repairs as soon as possible.**

Protect property still on the premises from further damages or loss.

When law enforcement arrives, greet them and assist in assessing whether or not the premises are secure. At this point, turn the matter over to the law enforcement officials. **Cooperate fully!**

Refer any inquiries from outsiders (media, etc.) to the responding law enforcement agency.

Do not discuss items or amounts taken with anyone other than law enforcement.

Management—**call the alarm company** vendor to reset or repair the alarm system!

Management—**call a third-party/independent source to assess** the effectiveness of your alarm system. What can and should be done to enhance the system?

Management—call insurance provider to **open a claim file** and get instructions on the claims process. Management—fill out internal burglary report.

Note: If controlled substances are discovered missing, it is imperative to also notify the DEA, the State Board of Pharmacy (depending on the state) and fill out a DEA Form 106.
Data from Pharmacists Mutual Insurance Companies. 2011. Sample policies and procedures (Burglary, Robbery, Shoplifting and Employee Dishonesty Policy & Procedures).

management. Although identification and subsequent prosecution are key methods to deter larceny, it is important to be very diligent before accusing a suspect. There are six widely accepted steps managers and employees should follow when suspecting that shoplifting is taking place. See Table 18-3 for more information.

Employee Theft

Employee theft can range from an employee simply eating a candy bar without paying for it to stealing hydrocodone tablets. As mentioned previously, it is important to prosecute all types of theft in a timely and legally sound manner. Furthermore, it is critical for employers to convey to all employees the expectations of employment, expectations that include zero tolerance for theft. It may appear harsh, at first glance, to tell your employees this information. However, what may appear as "common sense" information to an employer (or even an employee) may not be

viewed the same way by a fellow employee. Thus, in order to protect itself, employers should have a clear company policy for employee theft. Often times, this information is contained in an employee handbook or manual.

The following are some examples of employee theft:

- Taking merchandise without paying for it.
- *Forgery.* Signing company checks or endorsing a customer's check for personal use.
- Pilfering office supplies and converting them to personal use outside the store.
- *Embezzlement.* Conversion of company funds for personal use. Can range from using petty cash for personal use to complicated purchasing/billing/payables.
- Short-changing customers or the register and pocketing the cash.
- Abusing the company's sick leave policies to obtain personal time off while not ill or injured.

Table 18-3.   What to Do if Shoplifting Is Taking Place

To prevent false arrest claims and establish probable cause for detaining a suspected shoplifter, there are **six universally accepted steps** a manager or employee should follow:

1. You must see the shoplifter approach your merchandise or enter your store without any merchandise in their hand(s). This prevents the scenario of falsely detaining a customer who carried an item to be returned or exchanged into your store.

2. You must see the customer select your merchandise. If you can say without doubt that you saw the customer pick up your merchandise before putting it into a pocket or otherwise concealing it, you again protect yourself from that false arrest claim as in #1.

3. You must see the shoplifter conceal, carry away, or convert the merchandise in question. Concealment can be in pockets, in shopping bags, in a child's stroller. It can even be accomplished in full view as in when tags are removed from articles of clothing. A good example of conversion is a shoplifter eating food before paying for it. In some, *but not all,* states, this step is enough to constitute shoplifting.

4. In most states, at this point, you must maintain continuous surveillance of the suspect. You must comply with this step in the strictest sense.

5. You must see the shoplifter fail to pay for the stolen merchandise. Sometimes the thief will walk directly out of the store, but sometimes they will pay for some items but not the concealed one. It is important to see that the concealed item is not retrieved and paid for. There are all sorts of pitfalls for the merchant in this step. Examples include the person concealing or converting a candy bar pays for it along with other items at checkout, the person pays for batteries or a newspaper at the cashier and then picks up the item between the cashier stand and the door on his/her way out. As a double check, ask the cashier if the specific item(s) has/have been paid for.

6. You must see the shoplifter leave the store. Your approach to the thief should be outside the store. This eliminates all arguments that the shoplifter intended to pay for the item(s).

Note: These steps may vary from state to state so please make sure the pharmacy adheres to the particular laws of its state.
Data from Pharmacists Mutual Insurance Companies. 2011. Sample policies and procedures (Burglary, Robbery, Shoplifting and Employee Dishonesty Policy & Procedures).

- Abusing the company's time clock policies by having someone clock in or out for you.
- Overbilling expense accounts.
- Charging personal expenses on company credit cards.

Violence in the Workplace

According to the Bureau of Labor and Statistics (2016), over 16,000 workers experienced trauma from nonfatal workplace violence in 2016. Of those experiencing workplace violence, 70% worked in health care (Bureau of Labor Statistics, 2016). In 2017, Dan Hartley, Ed.D authored a National Institute for Occupational Safety and Health (NIOSH) science blog where he announced "NIOSH is partnering with the Statistical Analysis Center (SAC) to collect information from police departments to provide NIOSH with the data necessary for a study of homicides, robberies, and assaults (simple, aggravated, and sexual) of health care workers, especially pharmacists" (NIOSH, 2017). Through their previous research targeting all workplace violence, they discovered that violence against health care workers and specifically pharmacists had unique characteristics when compared to employees in other workplaces. Not surprisingly, much of the violence against pharmacists involves robbery, burglary, or theft events; however, it is not unusual for a pharmacist to be confronted with angry and potentially violent patients or coworkers. Violence may be defined as incidents of verbal abuse, threats and physical assaults, or an assault with a weapon (FitzGerald & Reid, 2012). Aside from the physical consequences related to violence at work, there are also emotional and psychological concerns. While there is currently very little data on violence against pharmacists available in the literature, anecdotal stories of such incidents abound and research confirms that violence against health care workers in general is on the rise (Kuehn, 2010). As such, it is a worthy endeavor for managers to take steps to prevent violence in the pharmacy.

A zero tolerance policy is an important first step in prevention. It is also worth noting that the attitude of the leadership team has an impact on the potential for violence in the workplace. Managers and other leaders set the tone for the pharmacy culture and have a great deal of influence on those with whom they work. In addition to creating and enforcing policy, mangers must model appropriate ways to deal with difficult situations and patients thus ensuring that anger and violence among staff or from patients is not seen as acceptable behavior. The manager should also evaluate the pharmacy to identify potential risks, thoroughly screen all job applicants for criminal history as well as professional competency, and provide training for staff on how they can identify potential problems early and the steps they should take in the event that there is an angry and potentially violent patient or coworker.

Other Workplace Safety Concerns

More workers are injured in the health care industry sector than any other (Occupational Safety and Health Administration [OSHA], 2019). Health care workers may face a number of safety and health hazards including potential chemical and drug exposures, respiratory hazards, ergonomic hazards from lifting and repetitive tasks, and workplace violence to name a few. Because all employees have a right to a safe workplace, the Occupational Safety and Health Act created the OSHA and established the federal government's role in promulgating and enforcing safety and health standards for places of employment. As such, OSHA has established a number of regulations specific for health care workers. A thorough discussion of the entirety of these regulations is beyond the scope of this chapter. However, one of the more common hazards that pharmacy managers may need to address is that of exposure to bloodborne pathogens and other biological hazards. This is especially important to those pharmacies providing vaccinations or any other service using needles. OSHA has established guidelines to assist employers in reducing or eliminating the hazards of occupational exposure to bloodborne pathogens. An employer must implement an exposure control plan for the pharmacy with details on employee protection measures. The plan must also describe how an employer will use a combination of engineering and work practice controls, ensure the use of personal protective clothing and equipment, provide training, medical surveillance, hepatitis B vaccinations, and signs and labels, among other provisions. The pharmacy's bloodborne pathogens policy must be evaluated annually and employees must receive training at the time of their initial hire and each year thereafter.

Another important law pharmacy managers need to consider is the Clinical Laboratory Improvement Amendments (CLIA). This is a federal law governing the laboratories that test human specimens in health care facilities. When originally adopted, CLIA aimed to regulate laboratories where patient specimens were processed and where the risk to the laboratory worker was significant. With the proliferation of easy-to-use medical tests, more patients are seeking their health care at convenient locations other than the typical clinical lab. This led to what is commonly known as the CLIA waiver program. Under this program, a medical test that has been approved by the United States Food and Drug Administration (FDA) could apply for an exemption to CLIA, permitting the test to be performed in a nonlaboratory setting. The CLIA waiver has opened the door for pharmacists to provide a number of testing programs that have the potential to enhance medical therapy management programs and help to identify patients in need of care earlier in the continuum of care. It is important to note that the pharmacist does not receive the CLIA waiver; instead it is the pharmacy that must receive that waiver. Obtaining a CLIA waiver is a two-part process. The pharmacy must first obtain a CLIA certificate and then must apply for laboratory status at the state level. Because every state manages this process differently, it is important to refer to the state's rules and regulations to determine how to apply (Klepser et al., 2014).

Employee Assistance

Even in well-managed organizations, individual employees will face any number of professional or personal problems that can impact them, others in the workplace, and the organization, as a whole. One resource many organizations have for such issues is confidential EAPs that refer employees for counseling and that train managers in early identification and referral (Smith, 1992). EAPs can be established by contract with independent behavioral health providers. Through a confidential intake, professionals and supervisors can identify employees with problems, and costs can be stabilized by early identification and referral. In addition, employees who are valuable to a company can often benefit from brief interventions and return to work more productive and committed to the organization.

Referral to a company-sponsored EAP program is normally voluntary; however, managers can suggest a referral based on a history of poor work performance or other work-related problems. In extreme cases, such as workplace violence threats or suicidal thoughts, employers may consider a mandatory referral to an EAP. Managers considering a mandatory referral to an EAP should proceed with caution and seek advice from human resource professionals within their organization since requiring EAP services may have implications under the ADA. You will recall that the ADA protects individuals who either have or are perceived to have a disability, including a mental disability. It is possible that requiring the employee to receive an EAP referral could be interpreted in a way that suggests the manager perceives an employee to have a disability even if he or she does not. This is important to recognize should the manager decide to take an action, such as termination, against an employee who refuses the EAP referral or does not comply with treatment may result in claims of disability discrimination based on a perceived disability (SHRM, 2014).

Drug and alcohol problems are personal problems that can significantly affect work performance. Many states have mandatory reporting requirements for pharmacists who have substance abuse problems so that interventions and referrals for treatment and follow-up may be made. Pharmacists and managers have special responsibilities and obligations not to "enable" another's substance abuse through lack of intervention because of the potential harm posed to the public health from an impaired pharmacist. Pharmacists can be at special risk for substance abuse problems because they have universal access to drugs and may have a false sense of invulnerability because of their extensive education regarding the mechanisms and effects of drugs. In addition, the tendency to self-medicate among some pharmacists can cause serious difficulty when applied to addictive medications.

The general procedures for managing impaired pharmacists are summarized as follows:

1. Adhere to mandatory state board reporting requirements for pharmacists who have substance abuse problems but are not receiving treatment
2. Intervention by an organization usually working with the state board
3. Professional assessment
4. Treatment recommendations
5. After-care counseling and monitoring usually involving Alcoholics Anonymous or Narcotics Anonymous, as well as random drug testing for a defined period
6. Reinstatement to practice contingent on successful completion of treatment

For the program to be effective, all employees should be educated about the issue of substance abuse, with special attention paid to early identification, intervention, and responsibilities of management in ensuring intervention and referral for treatment.

In addition to the steps outlined above, the Society for Human Resource Management (2018), suggests that naloxone be made available in the workplace as a part of the overall workplace safety program. Unsurprisingly, much of the attention given to naloxone has been related to the pharmacists' ability to write prescriptions and administer naloxone to their patients; however, as an employer, it is possible to imagine a time in which an employee may also present in an overdose crisis. Laws vary from state to state regarding the inclusion of naloxone as a part of an employee safety program so each pharmacist should become familiar with these laws and adopt clear policies and procedures regarding the training and administration of the drug.

■ REVISITING THE SCENARIO

Michael Davis has a variety of issues facing him as the new pharmacy manager. They include (1) a claim by an employee of sexual harassment and (2) possible theft by one of his pharmacy technicians. As evidenced from the scenario at the beginning of this chapter, Michael did not handle the first issue well, possibly leading to costly litigation against him and the pharmacy. He did, however, handle the second issue appropriately. This section will examine both of these issues separately, suggesting other more appropriate courses of action.

The first issue of concern was the way Michael handled his pharmacy technician's claim of sexual harassment. Any manager should treat a claim of sexual harassment very seriously, immediately investigating the claim to determine its validity. Here, Michael simply dismissed the claim because Mark was his friend and that Michael could not believe Mark would say such things. Properly resolving a claim of sexual harassment is not whether or not a manager could imagine such an event (or events) taking place, but rather,

the results of an unbiased and thorough investigation. In this example, the technician's claim could be false but Michael must investigate before making that determination.

The second issue, a very serious and unfortunately very common issue, is employee theft of hydrocodone tablets. In this case, Michael handled the situation appropriately by attempting to resolve the issue quickly. It is a good idea to have a witness (not the other technician, though) present for interviewing a suspected employee. As an aside, pharmacists who find themselves in Michael's position may be tempted to physically detain a suspect while awaiting law enforcement (e.g., by locking in a room). This

■ QUESTIONS FOR FURTHER DISCUSSION

1. Must a pharmacy manager hire an individual from a "protected class" if there are other individuals from nonprotected classes that apply for a pharmacist position?
2. What are the similarities and differences between the two main types of sexual harassment? How should an employer handle each type?
3. What are some examples of "reasonable accommodations" for a small chain pharmacy? For a large hospital pharmacy? Are they the same? Why or why not?
4. Would you recommend pharmacy employers conduct a drug screen test on its job applicants? Its employees? Its pharmacy students? Give reasons why you would or would not recommend this.
5. What is the best way to "detain" a suspected shoplifter? Suspected theft by an employee?
6. Should a pharmacist chase down a shoplifter? An armed robber? Why or why not?

action is potentially risky both legally and physically. Please alert the police and allow the law enforcement agents to do what is necessary.

■ CONCLUSION

It is important to develop a workplace free from discrimination, where employees are allowed to contribute to the organization's mission and vision and where diverse opinions are valued. Furthermore, it is important to encourage discussion while resolving conflict in a timely and appropriate manner. Employers who are able to address and resolve potential issues before they occur will maintain a tremendous advantage in avoiding legal pitfalls. Although no workplace is guaranteed to be "litigation free," applying these principles will go a long way in helping protect the pharmacist and pharmacy from damaging lawsuits while striving to make patients' needs their top priority.

REFERENCES

Black's Law Dictionary. 1996. St Paul, MN: West Publishing Company.

Blank C. 2018. How to Deal with Pharmacy Robbery: Have a plan in place for what to do—and what not to do. Drug Topics. 162.6 p17.

Bureau of Labor Statistics. 2016. Number of nonfatal occupational injuries and illnesses involving days away from work by industry and selected events or exposures leading to injury or illness, private industry. Available at https://www.bls.gov/iif/soii-chart-data-2016.htm. Accessed January 8, 2019.

Cates ME, Hogue MD. 2012. Experience with a drug screening program at a school of pharmacy. J Am College Health 60(6):476.

FitzGerald D, Reid A. 2012. Frequency and consequences of violence in community pharmacies in Ireland. Occup Med 62:632.

Kenna G, Wood M. 2004. Prevalence of substance abuse by pharmacists and other health professionals. J Am Pharm Assoc 44:684–693.

Klepser ME, Dering-Anderson AM, Klepser SA, Klepser DG. The pharmacist will screen you now. Medscape 2014.

Kraslawsky v Upper Deck Co., 65 Cal.Rptr.2d 297 (Cal. App. 1997).

Kuehn BM. 2010. Violence in health care settings on rise. JAMA 304(5):511.

Lord S, Downs G, Furtaw P, et al. 2009. Nonmedical use of prescription opioids and stimulants among student pharmacists. J Am Pharm Assoc 49:519–528.

Morris L, Calvert CT, Williams JC. 2015. What Young vs. UPS means for pregnant workers and their bosses. Harvard Business Review. March 26, 2015, pp. 2-5.

Occupational Safety and Health Administration (OSHA). Available at www.osha.gov; Accessed January 3, 2019.

Occupational Safety and Health Administration (OSHA). Available at https://www.osha.gov/SLTC/healthcarefacilities. Accessed January 8, 2019.

Pharmacists Mutual Insurance Companies. 2011. Sample policies and procedures (Burglary, Robbery, Shoplifting and Employee Dishonesty Policy & Procedures). Available at http://www.phmic.com/RM/Pages/tools.aspx. Accessed October 17, 2015.

Pharmacists Mutual Insurance Companies. 2015. Pharmacy Crime; A look at pharmacy burglary and robbery in the United States and the strategies and tactics needed to manage the problem. Available at https://www.phmic.com/wp-content/uploads/2016/07/PMC_CrimeReport.pdf. Accessed January 10, 2019.

Robinson RK, Franklin GM, Wayland R. 2002. The Regulatory Environment of Human Resource Management. Fort Worth, TX: Harcourt College Publishers.

Smith J. 1992. EAPs evolve into health plan gatekeeper. Employee Benefit Plan Rev 46:18.

Society of Human Resource Management. 2014. Employee Assistance Program (EAP): Can an employer require an employee to use the services of an employee assistance program? Available at https://www.shrm.org/resourcesandtools/tools-and-samples/hr-qa/pages/cananemployerrequireanemployeetousetheservicesofaneap.aspx. Accessed January 8, 2019.

Society of Human Resource Management. 2017. Religion at Work: The 5 commandments. HR Specialist 15(6): 2-2.

Substance Abuse and Mental Health Services Administration Center for Behavioral Health Statistics and Quality (SAMHSA), National Survey on Drug Use and Health, 2015 and 2016. Available at https://www.samhsa.gov/data/sites/default/files/NSDUH-DetTabs-2016/NSDUH-DetTabs-2016.pdf. Accessed January 17, 2019.

The National Institute of Occupational Safety and Health (NIOSH). 2017. Available at www.cdc.gov/niosh; Accessed January 3, 2019.

The United States Department of Justice and Drug Enforcement Administration (2017). National Drug Threat Assessment. Available at https://www.dea.gov/sites/default/files/2018-11/DIR-032-18%202018%20NDTA%20final%20low%20resolution.pdf. Accessed January 17, 2019.

The United States Equal Employment Opportunity Commission. Available at www.eeoc.gov; Accessed January 3, 2019.

Wymer, JF, Stillwagon, BA. 2014. How much leave is enough? Reasonable Accommodation, Undue Hardship, and the Intersection of the FMLA and ADA. *Employee Relations Law Journal* 40(1):22–30.

Young v United Parcel Service, Inc. Certiorari to the United States Court of Appeals for the Fourth Circuit No. 12–1226. Argued December 3, 2014—Decided March 25, 2015.

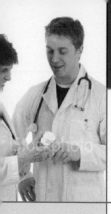

19

PHARMACY TECHNICIANS

Shane P. Desselle, Kenneth C. Hohmeier, and Jan M. Keresztes

About the Authors: Dr. Desselle is professor of Social, Behavioral, and Administrative Pharmacy at Touro University California College of Pharmacy. His research program focuses on optimizing roles for pharmacy technicians, development of mentorship programs, and in promoting strong organizational cultures and positive citizenship behaviors in professional settings. He is a Fulbright Specialist Scholar having completed a project to develop a Center of Assessment for the University of Pristina in Kosovo. Dr. Desselle is Founding Editor-in-Chief of the international peer-reviewed journal, Research in Social and Administrative Pharmacy with graduate students and collaborations worldwide on various projects such as medication safety and medication adherence issues with informal caregivers. Dr. Desselle also is a primary author for the Pharmacy Management Tips of the Week on AccessPharmacy that accompany this textbook.

Dr. Hohmeier is associate professor of Clinical Pharmacy and Translational Science at the University of Tennessee Health Science Center College of Pharmacy (UTHSC) in Nashville, TN. His research primarily focuses on studying the implementation and sustainability of clinical patient-care services in the community pharmacy practice setting as a means to improve patient access to quality, cost-effective health care. Dr. Hohmeier also serves as the Director of Community Affairs for UTHSC College of Pharmacy and is the UTHSC PGY-1 Community-based Residency Program Director, overseeing sites in both chain and independent pharmacy practice across Tennessee. He maintains an active practice site with Kroger Pharmacy in the Nashville area.

Dr. Keresztes has dedicated her career to pharmacy technician issues. For over three decades, she was the coordinator of an ASHP/ACPE Pharmacy Technician Program at South Suburban College in Illinois offering courses to both adults and high school students. Dr. Keresztes has been an active member of the Pharmacy Technician Accreditation Commission (PTAC) with responsibilities to both ASHP and ACPE. Her recognitions include serving as an originator of the Pharmacy Technician Certification Board's (PTCB's) national exam, a founder of the Pharmacy Technician Educators Council (PTEC), and consultant editor for the *Journal of Pharmacy Technology*. Currently, Dr. Keresztes is involved with Talent First PBC, whose primary overall goal is to attract gifted young people from underserved backgrounds to the profession of pharmacy and to examine ways in which the education and effectiveness of pharmacy technicians can be advanced.

■ LEARNING OBJECTIVES

After completing this chapter, readers should be able to

1. Provide a brief historical context behind the employment of technicians and other support personnel in pharmacy.
2. Describe the education, training, and requisite knowledge of technicians, including recent changes at state and federal levels.
3. Describe recent evolutions in the roles of pharmacy technicians.
4. Discuss personnel management issues related to pharmacy technicians specifically and best practices for motivating them and keeping them committed to the profession and to their current employer.
5. Discuss how technicians and other support personnel can be leveraged to improve efficiency in pharmacy operations through workflow redesign and other considerations.
6. Discuss how technicians can be utilized more effectively in implementing new programs while promoting patient safety.
7. Evaluate mechanisms to gather patient feedback through technicians that will help inform the design and successful implementation of new pharmacy services.
8. Identify avenues through which pharmacists can advocate for technicians in the workplace and collectively through boards of pharmacy, professional organizations, and administrators of large employers.

■ SCENARIO

Sadie Metzgar is a district manager for Pharmily, a rapidly growing national chain of drug stores. Pharmily began as a small, regional chain, building a reputation on having the look and feel of independent pharmacies, with its mission and goals centering on customer service and patient wellness. Today, Pharmily is in 29 states and looking to expand into all 50. While Pharmily has thus far leveraged their reputation for high levels of service into its newer markets, they are experiencing challenges in maintaining that same level of service as they expand across the country. Top administrators at Pharmily are sensitive to this and wonder if recent comparisons in both lay press and in consumer ratings (e.g., Yelp and others) between Pharmily and "all the other chains" will hurt their expansion plans. A recent symposium for Pharmily's corporate office executives, regional managers, and district managers unveiled plans for the company to initiate a "Customer-First"

program to better maintain their reputation for service, even as the chain continues its expansion. General guidelines for the program will come from the corporate office, but district managers will have the autonomy to tailor the program in a way that best meets the needs of the region.

Sadie recalled from the symposium various strategies discussed, such as improved efficiency through systems engineering, hiring and maintaining service-oriented personnel, taking initiative on public health endeavors (e.g., immunizations), and new medication adherence programs, all with enhanced customer service in mind. Pharmily's corporate office will even provide funding on a competitive basis to district managers who develop and implement such programs, as well as provide pilot funding for new medication therapy management-related services.

Only 5 years ago, Sadie was a new graduate who took a staff pharmacist position with Pharmily after finishing pharmacy school. She developed a great rapport with pharmacy technicians as she quickly advanced from staff pharmacist, pharmacy manager, and now a district manager. The technicians that she worked with "showed her the ropes" with regards to how the pharmacy operated and how customers received the high levels of service for which Pharmily was known. At the same time, Sadie recalls conversations with technicians who suggested that they did not receive much training after they were hired, and as a result were not performing functions that they've heard that technicians perform at other pharmacies. Sadie recalls her experience at a hospital when she was in pharmacy school where there was a "career ladder" for pharmacy technicians. The hospital provided training for technicians to obtain the skills needed to advance up the ladder (Tech I, II, III, IV, and V). Technicians who obtained the needed skills were eligible for promotion to the next level, which came with increased responsibilities, as well as increased levels of compensation.

Sadie has kept up with current events in pharmacy. Her state board of pharmacy recently expanded the scope of practice for technicians, allowing them to assist pharmacists and interface with patients and other health professionals in new ways. She has read articles in the pharmacy practice literature that demonstrate the effectiveness of deploying technicians more systematically in new programs that promote patient safety. Sadie believes that she can learn from her experiences and the literature to develop several "customer-first" initiatives in her district that Pharmily will approve. The key, she thought, is making the most of the pharmacy's personnel, allowing them to proffer service ideas, and to rely upon her strengths in operations management to implement programs that create a win-win for these employees and the customers of Pharmily.

■ CHAPTER QUESTIONS

1. In what manner has the role of the pharmacy technician evolved over the past 40 years, resulting the technicians now being "front and center" in the implementation of new patient-centered services in pharmacy?
2. What is the current snapshot of the U.S. pharmacy technician workforce? What are their education levels, demographic characteristics, and rate of pay?
3. What does the evidence suggest about which new roles can be delegated at least in part to pharmacy technicians from an operations standpoint?
4. What have regulatory bodies, professional organizations, and employers had to say about redesigning work in pharmacies in a manner that seeks to optimize the use of technicians and all other pharmacy personnel?
5. What can pharmacists do to elicit trust, commitment, motivation, and engagement by pharmacy technicians?

■ BRIEF HISTORY OF PHARMACY SUPPORT PERSONNEL

Pharmacists have long been supported by various personnel. In Europe, hospitals as early as the 1700s employed apothecary assistants and referred to them as the *elaboratorian*, *elaboratory-man*, or *drug-man*, all of which were changed to "dispenser" at a later time (Whittet, 1968). During this time, when British apothecaries began to devote more time to the practice of medicine, they were forced to employ assistant pharmacists, or dispensers, to prepare medicines. To provide adequate controls, the British government enacted the Apothecaries Act of 1815, which gave the Society of Apothecaries the authority to test the fitness and qualification of those who wished to act as "assistants to apothecaries in compounding and dispensing medicines."

In colonial America, pharmacists began as supportive personnel or assistants to physicians. The beginning apprentice performed unskilled duties, but as the apprentice acquired knowledge, they provided more assistance and learned the art and "physic" of pharmacy (Douglas et al., 1986). As is the case with other health professions, pharmacists separated from medical practice, going beyond the role of physician extender into their own unique set of responsibilities in medication preparation and dispensing. Pharmacists went from being trained as apprentices to requirement of baccalaureate degrees, with the first college of pharmacy and the American Pharmacists Association (APhA) founded in the mid-nineteenth century. Those who did not complete their baccalaureate training often became pharmacist helpers (i.e., technicians). Once pharmacy education became the province of universities, pharmacists still needed assistants, and this became even more the case upon creation of the "legend" drug, prefabricated products, and massive increases in the volumes of prescriptions dispensed during the mid-20th century. Pharmacy education was becoming more scientific and clinically oriented, with less emphasis on training in operations and dispensing processes (Hepler & Strand, 1990).

In a similar vein, pharmacy technicians can be viewed as extenders of pharmacists. The U.S. Civil Service Commission had a job description of "pharmacy helper" as early as 1947, and whose qualifications included: skills in the use of the more ordinary pharmaceutical apparatus; good knowledge of the simple pharmacy methods; knowledge of simple mathematics; cleanliness and neatness; ability to follow instructions; and reliability in carrying out assignments (Archambault, 1958). It was recognized that if no one else is there to do the nonprofessional tasks in a pharmacy, then a pharmacist will do it, which is wasteful and results in less time practicing professional pharmacy (Frazier, 1954). A later study found that there was considerable room for improvement in the delegation of responsibilities in pharmacy (Turnbull & Bowles, 1965). Following a recommendation from what was then known as the Department of Health Education and Welfare to incorporate pharmacy services into Medicare, a task force made recommendations to develop curriculum materials for various allied health occupations, including pharmacy, which could be used for an Associate of Arts degree in junior colleges (APhA, 1969). Unfortunately, however, the task force had no actual power

to regulate the training of technicians, and progress toward the standardization of education and training would occur slowly over the next 50 years.

In the 1970s, the Millis Commission report not only stressed the need for pharmacists to become more involved in patient education, it forecasted the utilization of technicians to increase, given more formalized services organized around institutional care (Pharmacists for the Future, 1975). Professional organizations such as the American Society of Hospital Pharmacists (now, American Society of Health-Systems Pharmacists, ASHP) responded with reference to supportive personnel in "Minimum Standards" as being available so as to minimize the use of pharmacists in nonjudgmental tasks (ASHP, 1977). Their House of Delegates also passed a resolution indicating that the Society establish a mechanism to accredit pharmacy technician training programs in U.S. hospitals (ASHP, 1972), although an additional 12 years passed before the regulations and accreditation standards were actually established (ASHP, 1982).

The Association of Pharmacy Technicians (APT) was created in 1979 out of the need for technicians to further advance their own professional causes beyond the associate membership typically offered by other organizations (Whitney, Jr., 1981). In 1988, ASHP organized an invitational task force to address technical personnel in pharmacy. At the conclusion of the conference, the task force made 16 recommendations for pharmacy's future. The concluding statement was "Pharmacy's service to the public is stifled because of the lack of well-defined corps of technical personnel. The profession must take concerted steps toward correcting this deficiency. Further, it should pursue the development of a well-defined corps of technical personnel expeditiously and with a note of urgency" (ASHP, 1989).

■ ADVANCEMENTS, EVEN AMID UNCERTAINTY

In spite of these position statements, literature on the role that technicians would come to play in the evolution of pharmacy practice during the ensuing decades was scant. Researchers in the 1980s and 1990s focused their attention toward pharmacists, studying their leadership capabilities, job satisfaction, commitment to the profession, and attitudes toward patient-centric practice (Cox & Fitzpatrick, 1999; Gaither, 1998; Ibrahim et al., 1997). Pharmacy technicians continued to professionalize, with more professional organizations being formed and with greater involvement in political advocacy to become formally recognized. However, there was little empiric study on how to properly leverage technicians and other support personnel to achieve better organizational outcomes.

During this time, organizations arose that offered certification for pharmacy technicians to create a minimum standard for knowledge to practice. The PTCB, while formally established in 1995, can trace its origins to 1980 when the Michigan Pharmacists Association (MPA) began offering a 1½ day exam with a hands-on lab component. A few years later, the Illinois Council of Health Systems Pharmacy (ICHP) established its own psychometrically valid examination. The APhA and ASHP, along with the National Association of the Boards of Pharmacy (NABP) then endeavored to create one national exam. These organizations, along with MPA and Illinois Council of Health Systems Pharmacists (ICHP) then formed the PTCB.

The certification process is one where technicians engage in self-study in preparation for an examination that addresses some components of pharmacy law, pharmaceutical calculations, basic pharmacology, medication order entry, sterile and nonsterile compounding, quality assurance, inventory management, and medication safety (PTCB, 2018). Several years later, the National Healthcareer Association (NHA) entered the technician certification market with its ExCPT examination procedure similar to PTCB's.

Despite the advent of certification and gains made in pharmacy practice and in technician professionalization, pharmacy technician qualifications, knowledge, and responsibilities remained markedly diverse. Thus, pharmacy technician educators began to meet in 1989 to establish a core curriculum and share tools that would be useful in educating potential pharmacy technician students. In 1990, the national educators became the PTEC and still share ideas both online and at its annual meeting to further promote the professionalization of pharmacy technicians. At the same time PTEC was being formed, a *White Paper on Pharmacy Technicians* by the Council of Credentialing Pharmacy pointed out a pharmacist work force shortage, the momentum to shift practice to pharmaceutical care, societal unmet need, and the desire for safe medication use to have created an increased demand for competent pharmacy technicians (ASHP, 2003). That same White Paper also pointed toward a lack of standardization in education, by which only some individuals had completed an accredited vocational program and/or certification, as well as wide variations in regulation, with some state boards of pharmacy requiring some sort of licensing procedure and others not even maintaining a registry of technicians.

■ A RENEWED FOCUS— STUDIES COMMISSIONED BY CERTIFICATION ORGANIZATIONS

The aforementioned White Paper and several conferences and summits of professional leaders in pharmacy helped to focus pharmacy technician practice. Additionally, PTCB commissioned several studies in hopes of painting an accurate picture of the workplace for technicians, particularly in community pharmacy. Among these was a task analysis undertaken by pharmacists, certified technicians, and technician educators (Muenzen et al., 1999). Around this time in the late 1990s, 90% of community pharmacy technicians were involved in outpatient prescription dispensing, while a majority of hospital pharmacy technicians were involved with inpatient medication dispensing and preparing intravenous (IV) admixtures. Still, there were a number of responsibilities and skill sets, such as communication, organization, and time management that were shared across both settings. Certification was seen as being valuable for imparting broad (rather than task-specific) knowledge. The published task analysis was among the first documents to acknowledge technicians' greater involvement in calculations and particularly in quality assurance activities.

In a follow-up study asking pharmacy technicians across all practice settings to describe their activities, the researchers found a more diverse array of practice activities among respondents (Muenzen et al., 2006). These activities included involvement with inventory control, billing, prepackaging and repackaging medication products, as well as coordinating communication and verifying the work of other technicians, supervisory responsibility, and medication error prevention. This was believed to be indicative that pharmacists were delegating more responsibility to pharmacy technicians and including them to perpetuate a stronger safety culture.

In the early 2000s, PTCB commissioned another study of the certified technician workforce as among the first to examine quality of worklife for pharmacy support personnel (Desselle, 2005a). Certified technicians were earning a median wage of just over $12.00/hour in 2005. They reported moderate levels of job satisfaction and career commitment. They perceived a considerable amount of support from their peers and from supervisors and pharmacists, but less so from their employers (Desselle, 2005b). A follow-up study corroborated these results and found technicians developing close bonds with one another but with concerns that employers viewed technicians as highly replaceable (Desselle, 2016). The prior study found work attitudes related to practice setting, rate of pay and age/experience, but not with gender.

While some pharmacy technicians reported moderate levels of job satisfaction and career commitment, others often complained of low pay, and turnover among technicians was thought to be problematic. A recent study commissioned by PTCB found the median hourly wage for technicians was $15/hour in 2018, an increase of only $3/hour since 2005 (Wheeler et al., 2019). While more state boards of pharmacy are requiring technicians to certification and register, the education and training of technicians still have not been standardized. A study of turnover intentions commissioned by PTCB saw that

relationships with coworkers, good benefits, and flexible work schedule were associated with reasons to stay with the employer, while poor advancement opportunity and insufficient staffing were primary drivers for leaving (Desselle, 2005b). That study found that increments in pay of as little as $0.75/hour were associated with technicians either looking to leave for another job, ambivalence about their pay for their current job, or actually planning to stick around with that job because of the wage/pay (Desselle, 2005a). A subsequent study using the same dataset created a model of pharmacy technician job satisfaction (Desselle & Holmes, 2007). The model suggested that technicians are concerned with future uncertainty about their job and career, and they reported relatively high levels of stress for a job with relatively low pay. However, that same study found that the stress and uncertainty can be buffered or counteracted by having a supportive pharmacist as a supervisor. This says much about the importance of having pharmacists properly delegate, demonstrate empathy for, and promulgate fairness in administering policies when supervising technicians.

At the same time, reports of pharmacy technicians' emerging roles began to appear more widely, albeit primarily as single-institution reports at health-systems pharmacy conferences. These roles were quite diverse. They included some level of managerial tasks, such as managing automation, machinery, supplies, and inventory, but did not include those that demanded clinical judgment (Jackson et al., 1998). Some pharmacy technicians were involved with managerial tasks and assisting pharmacists in drug therapy monitoring clinics (Chevalier & MacDonald, 2003). One institution initiated implementation of the "clinical technician" role, reserved for more senior technicians who would check the work of other technicians, collect patient histories, and assist with some retrospective drug utilization review (DUR) activities (Gasseling et al., 2000). However, these reports were often from singular institutions, and there existed few conceptual models that could be adopted by large and small organizations, particularly in community pharmacy. One paper from a task force organized by the California Society of Health-Systems Pharmacy proposed a career laddering mechanism moving beyond the aforementioned clinical technician role and suggesting a more systematic means of advancing technicians through stages (e.g., Technician I, II, and III) to promote self-development and longer career trajectories within an organization and in the entire profession (Desselle et al., 2015). Referring back to the chapter scenario, Sadie's plans to leverage Pharmily's support personnel could make use of a career laddering mechanism. Such a mechanism would give technicians career goals to aim for, facilitate their own desire for skills development, improve their retention in the company, and position the more senior technicians to take ownership in various customer-first initiatives.

■ EVOLUTION OF TECHNICIAN EDUCATION AND TRAINING

As of 2018, 26 states in the United States regulated technician practice and included at least some sort of language recommending or mandating certification through PTCB or NHA (Pharmacy Technician Certification Board, 2018b). The effects or implications of certification have been studied; and while promoting skills competency, the value of certification is seen more as promoting maturity, diligence, self-confidence, and professionalism among those willing and able to go through a rigorous self-study process (Desselle & Holmes, 2017).

The standardization of technician education, training, and practice have remained elusive. In 2007, the American College of Clinical Pharmacy (ACCP) released a position statement on pharmacy technician education, training, and certification that clarified certain aspects of their practice activities, along with some nomenclature used in describing their practice (American College of Clinical Pharmacy, 2007). A few years later, ASHP began to collaborate with ACPE on accreditation of technician training programs. A pharmacy technician program wanting to be recognized as "accredited" must meet the approval of both the boards of ASHP and ACPE. To assist with this accreditation review process, ASHP and ACPE formed the PTAC in 2014. ASHP's revised standards

document for program accreditation (American Society of Health Systems Pharmacists, 2018b) makes note of several changes from previous educational standards. Most notably are the following:

- Entry-level and advanced-level standards replaced previous referral to only one level of education and training.
- Minimum hour requirements have been added to differentiate entry-level versus advanced-level education.
- There is more emphasis on collaborative behaviors and workflow with the pharmacist.

The standards reflect an evolution of current and future practice expectations. They involve demonstration and/or application of problem-solving, critical-thinking, self-management, time management, interpersonal, active listening, conflict resolution, and even supervisory and innovation skills, along with the application of ethical conduct.

Meanwhile, the certification process has continued to evolve. By the end of 2017, PTCB had certified nearly 650,000 individuals since its inception and projected that there were over 280,000 technicians certified through them that were in active practice. (PTCB, 2018) The most recent version of NHA's exam features components in ethics, assisting pharmacists with Medication Therapy Management (MTM), selecting OTC products based upon a pharmacists' recommendation, performing quality assurance checks, and assisting the pharmacist with identifying potential medication adherence problems (National Healthcareer Association, 2018).

■ PROFESSIONAL ORGANIZATION STATEMENTS ON ADVANCING PRACTICE

ASHP in 2016 published a position statement on the roles of pharmacy technicians (Schultz et al., 2016). The statement recognizes the importance of pharmacy technicians in a safe and effective medication use process. It encourages states to help assure the proper education, training, and assessment of skills through the adoption of uniform laws and licensure. The statement oriented its foundation around ASHP's Pharmacy Practice Model Initiative (PPMI, now rebranded as PAI, the Practice Advancement Initiative) whose goal is to advance the health and well-being of patients by developing and disseminating a practice model that supports pharmacists as direct providers. It delineates roles of an advanced technician to perform such duties as or related to:

- "Tech-check-tech"—technicians checking the work of other technicians in final product verification before it (the medication order or prescription) is given to or reaches the patient.
- Medication history assistance—acquiring during an interview in the context of prospective DUR, the medications that a patient is current taking and has recently taken, including over-the-counter (OTC) and dietary supplements, so that the pharmacist can identify potential interactions or contraindications and determine the appropriateness of the patient's prescribed therapy.
- Quality assurance—known as QA (see Chapter 10), embodies an entire culture and thus a series of activities aimed to reduce errors and improve quality in the medication distribution process. QA encompasses a wide scope of activities including improving speed and efficiency in filling orders/prescriptions, ensuring that inventory is ordered at just the right time and quantity, and seeing that patients are consistently receiving adequate written counseling information.
- Community outreach—encompasses activities aimed to improve medication use and outcomes in entire populations. These are often performed externally to the pharmacy and include educational activities, screenings, and assisting patients with selecting the best pharmacy benefit plan at health fairs and other events.
- Immunization assistance—helping the pharmacist in maintaining adequate stock of vaccines and supplies, coordinating times and managing logistics for patient immunizations, marketing the immunization service, and where allowed, assistance with administration of the immunization directly to the patient.
- MTM assistance—providing help as needed for the pharmacist including patient triage, scheduling office visits for patients with the pharmacist, administering appropriate paperwork to be completed by the patient, and interviewing the patient to determine how they are faring on their drug therapy.
- Drug utilization evaluation and/or adverse drug event monitoring—alerting the pharmacist when entering a prescription/medication order or even being alerted from patient information during an interview that an adverse drug event could be occurring; additionally, assistance with completing FDA MedWatch reports for suspected adverse events.
- Informatics—advising the pharmacist on selection of vendors based upon what systems work well and interface with current programs, evaluating new informatics technology, and maintaining informatics equipment and software (see Chapter 9).

Over a decade after publishing its initial statement on pharmacy education and training, ACCP published an updated White Paper on best practices to incorporate pharmacy technicians into the clinical pharmacist's process of care (Borchert et al., 2018). It produced the following set of recommendations:

1. *Identify the appropriate support personnel to assist with clinical pharmacy tasks on the basis of skills.* Job responsibilities that are not role-specific (e.g., answering telephone calls) should be allocated to existing support personnel (not advanced technicians). Technicians should be included in more advanced roles, such as collaborations with other health care personnel.

2. *Ensure that support personnel are adequately trained and certified.* Beyond certification, training for specific tasks should be provided, largely undertaken by employers.

3. *Incorporate support personnel into appropriate components of the process of care to expand the reach and*

depth of clinical pharmacy services. When supervised by the pharmacist, support personnel can assist in components of collaborative care, including patient assessment, evaluation of medication therapy, development and implementation of a patient care plan, and follow-up evaluation and medication monitoring. These components can be used as a framework to determine how to incorporate support from other personnel to maximize clinical pharmacists' abilities to function at the top of their license.

4. *Incorporate support personnel into ancillary processes that support clinical pharmacy services.* These include such services as practice management, OTC drug counseling, and quality improvement programs. Support personnel can perform a variety of functions such as running monthly reports on drug use patterns and compiling and administering satisfaction surveys to obtain feedback on clinical services. Technicians embedded in practice systems can track safety metrics, and these personnel should be included in a culture of continuous quality improvement (CQI) and safety.

5. *Conduct and disseminate research on the utility and outcomes achieved using support personnel in the clinical pharmacist's process of care.* Current evidence is positive, albeit limited. Future studies should clearly describe the expertise, background, and training of individuals supporting the pharmacist, and the reasons for success or failure should be explored and described.

■ PUTTING STATEMENTS INTO ACTION: EMERGING ROLES OF PHARMACY TECHNICIANS

The above recommendations specify to some degree what had already been taking place, at least for some pharmacy technicians. Their goals are to suggest more specifically how to leverage the use of technicians and other support personnel to assist pharmacists with patient-centric services.

Medication Reconciliation in Transitions of Care

One of the more salient topics of discussion in pharmaceutical and medical care delivery in recent times revolves around transitions of care. In what has always been regarded as a fragmented health care system, practice leaders, payers, and policymakers recognize the need for smooth transitions, for example, when a patient is discharged from the hospital (often more quickly than in years past) into a long-term care facility, home health, rehabilitative unit, hospice care, or other places where they may receive care. The appropriateness of the setting/place where the patient is discharged depends on many factors, including the complexity of their therapeutic regimen and the level of support they receive from informal caregivers. When transitions of care are not sufficiently coordinated or optimized, the patient can easily end up on the wrong medications, wrong dosages, improper dosage forms for the setting in which they are newly residing, or a poorly designed care plan. Medication reconciliation is critical during transitions of care planning, as such activity considers what medications should be discontinued, renewed from previous care, added to the regimen, dosage form changes, and proper supply of, access to, and storage of these medications. One study found technicians useful in medication reconciliation in the emergency room, wherein they were able to acquire patient medication histories and provide initial advice to other emergency room practitioners about medication dosage forms upon patient discharge/admission or triage certain questions/uncertainties appropriately to the pharmacist (Patanwala, 2014). A systematic review on medication reconciliation among pharmacy personnel found that medication discrepancies with higher clinical impact were more likely to be identified by pharmacy personnel (including technicians) than usual care, with no difference between technicians and pharmacists (Mckonnen et al., 2016). An additional study deployed pharmacy technicians as "community health workers" involved in telephone follow-up and home care visits regarding patients' medication postdischarge (Bailey et al., 2016). This also included deployment of a pharmacy technician for medication reconciliation in very specific settings of care, such as a mental health assessment unit (Brownlie et al., 2014).

Patient Medication Adherence Programs

Improving medication adherence might be among the most important roles played by pharmacists and support personnel (Justis et al., 2016). Pharmacies have begun leveraging technicians' frequent interaction with patients to help strengthen medication adherence initiatives (Kadia et al., 2015). This provides the "human touch" and could be more effective than robotic telephone reminders to patients about picking up prescriptions, particularly when the technician can reinforce patients' positive behaviors and reiterate the positive outcomes resulting from adherence. This was demonstrated in a study of technicians assisting the pharmacist to identify patients at high risk for nonadherence (Fera et al., 2018). Findings from these types of studies can be very helpful for Sadie. Sadie recognizes that promoting medication adherence is a largely unmet societal need that can and should be embraced by community pharmacy. The fact that pharmacy technicians are able to not only help to reinforce pharmacists' messages but even help identify those patients at risk for nonadherence to apprise the pharmacist has her thinking about the possibility of a cost-effective program. In such a program, technicians can be further educated/trained to identify these patients, have the pharmacist approach them in a clinically relevant medication adherence program with a personal touch that could both improve the patient's medication-taking behavior and their loyalty to Pharmily stores.

Patient Safety and Medication Access

Medication adherence can be considered under the large umbrellas of public health and patient safety. Pharmacy technicians are taking a more prominent role in these areas. Some of these tasks might appear to be more rudimentary, such as the case with a prior-authorization service, but more often than not, such services involve communication, reinforcement, support, and empathy for the patient (Leinss et al., 2015). Some organizations are now appointing technicians with medication safety tasks such as planning/organizing meetings, researching safety events, and assisting with safety projects (Brown et al., 2016). Part of medication safety is assuring patients' access to needed medications. Technicians have been successfully deployed to assist patients' enrollment in manufacturer-sponsored prescription drug assistance programs (PDAPs) that can help avert substantial out-of-pocket costs for patients who require treatment with a biologic, large-molecule, or other expensive specialty drugs (Gilbert and Gerzenshtien, 2016). Pharmacy technician roles have been activated for involvement in helping to ensure adequate drug supply, such as in the growing problem of drug shortages (See Chapter 27), where they can help coordinate communication between providers, patients, and suppliers of medicines (Mangan et al., 2011). Patient safety efforts also extend to specialized care settings, where technicians have been utilized effectively in assisting pharmacists with postfracture care (Irwin et al., 2014) and in anticoagulation clinics, where they can help monitor adherence, and determine patients' needs for scheduling visits to that clinic (Kuhn et al., 2016).

Public Health Initiatives

Community pharmacies have tremendous potential to make a positive impact in public health. Community pharmacies and pharmacists often host health fairs which address a variety of public health needs such as nutrition, weight management, blood glucose and blood pressure monitoring, cholesterol screenings, and smoking cessation. Pharmacy technicians play important roles in ensuring the success of these programs. One study found technicians to be helpful in a comprehensive program aimed at referring patients to a tobacco quit line (Zillich et al., 2013). The authors stated that novel tobacco intervention approaches are needed to capitalize on the community pharmacy's frequent interface with tobacco users, and that widespread implementation of such feasible efforts could have a substantial impact on the prevalence of tobacco use. Another area in public health gaining considerable traction is that of immunizations. Immunization provision has become a significant part of pharmacy's public health outreach, wherein highly accessible community pharmacies provide immunizations with ease and with very little wait time for the patient. Technicians can perform administrative tasks to assist in the efficiency of immunization programs. At least one state (Idaho) has gone as far as to allow pharmacy technicians to administer immunizations. A pilot project saw thousands of patients immunized by pharmacy technicians without incident (McKiernan et al., 2018).

A recent study provided a framework of care for opioid medication misuse among community pharmacy patients (Cochran et al., 2016). It was suggested that community pharmacy workflows may adapted to address opioid medication misuse by employing the Screening, Brief Intervention, and Referral to Treatment (SBIRT) protocol. The SBIRT protocol integrates screening patients for substance use with one or two 30-minute sessions to explore the patient's motivation for change and possible referral to more intensive care. The authors remarked on the need to include pharmacy support personnel on training for potential recognition of opioid misuse and their integration into the SBIRT model. Likewise, a Deputy Director for the National Institute on Drug Abuse (NIDA) also commented on the need for systematic culture buy-in and education and training for all pharmacy staff, including pharmacy technicians, in meeting the challenge of curbing the opioid crisis (Compton et al., 2018).

Point-of-Care Testing

Another important public health initiative is the availability and applicability of point-of-care testing, which is diagnostic testing at the point of care, thus making the test convenient and immediately available to the patient and providing them with even greater opportunities for effective self-management of diseases. These are often conducted using devices that are portable, transportable, and often hand-held. What began with blood glucose monitors for diabetes has now is comprised of tests for blood gases, urine albumin, coagulation, and others. Pharmacy technicians have been identified as persons who can help streamline pharmacy workflow and assist patients with point-of-care testing in such a manner that improves the outcomes of patients and engenders their loyalty to the pharmacy business (Keller et al., 2015).

■ OTHER TECHNICIAN RESPONSIBILITIES AIMED TO FREE UP PHARMACISTS' TIME

The aforementioned roles, when devised with appropriate job descriptions (see Chapter 17) and workflow designs (see Chapter 8) all can be of importance to help free up the pharmacist's time so that they might evolve their practice into one that is more patient-centric. Additional technician roles have been developed almost as express means of doing so.

Tech-Check-Tech

The most direct application of technicians as "pharmacist extenders" in this way is "tech-check-tech," wherein a technician verifies the work (e.g., the accuracy of filling a medication order) of another technician. This practice varies from state-to-state (board of pharmacy regulations) and from one employer to the next in regard to company policies. There is considerable evidence in favor of implementing tech-check-tech programs. A review of studies in 2011 employing tech-check-tech models suggested accuracy of 99.6%, statistically equal to pharmacists in the final verification of unit dose orders in institutional settings (Adams et al., 2011). Since that time, tech-check-tech programs have become more common in community settings, sometimes under the same name, sometimes under a different one, such as "technician product verification," which is intended to infer a more holistic paradigm of practice involving workflow redesign to enhance the scope of duties of both technicians and pharmacists (Iowa Pharmacists Association, 2018).

A study performed in seven community pharmacies in Iowa confirmed the benefits of implementing tech-check-tech systems (Andreski et al., 2018). They found no changes in medication errors, administrative errors, or overall errors before and after tech-check-tech implementation. The pharmacist's percentage of time spent in dispensing activities significantly decreased from 67.3% to 49.1%, while time spent in direct patient care increased from 20.0% to 34.7%. The total number of patient-oriented services offered from various service categories (e.g., MTM services, follow-up, prescription counseling, patient screening, injection administration) increased from 2.88 to 5.16/hour. Likewise, a study conducted in New Zealand employing a "checking technician" in 12 community and hospital sites used a work sampling approach before and after the checking technician had been in place (Napier et al., 2018). Introduction of the checking technician saw a mean increase of 19% in the pharmacist's time spent in patient-focused activities and a mean 20% decrease in time spent in dispensing activities.

Taking Medication Histories

More recent studies on the accuracy of pharmacy technicians in these types of roles saw a favorable comparison to nurses in taking patient medication histories in an emergency department (Markovic et al., 2017). A 2018 study found similar results in medication history-taking during hospital admission between pharmacy technicians, pharmacists, and nurses (Jobin et al., 2018).

Accepting Verbal Prescription Orders

Phone calls for verbal prescription orders and requests for transfers are routine but time-consuming tasks for pharmacists. Having some familiarity with medications such as common doses and indications, technicians can be delegated the job of accepting verbal prescription orders. Frost and Adams (2017) described doing so to technicians with demonstrated competence in basic medication knowledge and with effective communication skills. As of 2019, there were 17

states that allow technicians to accept verbal orders, transfer prescriptions, or both. In general, it is up to the supervising pharmacist to determine the limitations of the technician's ability to accept orders. States that allow this practice generally require certification or have the ability to hold technicians accountable for mistakes. The need to receive verbal orders is declining with the use of electronic systems, but technicians may be in a position to relieve pharmacists of this task while technology remains in transition.

Referring back the chapter scenario, Pharmily has not had technicians highly involved in accepting verbal prescription orders or requests for prescription transfers. Sadie is aware that there is an absence of clear corporate policies on this matter. Pharmily's expansion into new states would suggest that their stores will be operating under different sets of state regulations. Sadie understand that Pharmily cannot adopt a company-wide policy allowing for technicians' involvement in accepting verbal prescription orders. But she also realizes that the company might need a clearer set of policies and procedures on this matter and that it being precluded in some states does not prevent pilot programs in other states where these practices may be permitted. If the pilot projects work out, then they could be rolled out quickly, giving Pharmily a competitive advantage in those states where accepting verbal prescription orders by technicians becomes permitted.

Assistance With Medication Therapy Management

If pharmacists are to successfully expand their roles to provide MTM and related services, they will need to leverage even more support from pharmacy technicians to free up time to enable them to do so. Two reviews describing technicians roles in MTM were published in 2018. One examined the use of technicians in various elements of MTM services delivery (Gernant et al., 2018). The review included 44 published articles that described the proportion of instances where technicians were involved with medication reconciliation (70%), documentation (41%), and medication therapy review (30%). Roles less frequently described included medication record development (5%), physical assessment (5%), and patient follow-up (2%). The authors noted the need to tailor technician educational (e.g., vocational, certification) programs around medication reconciliation and also noted that there was still considerable room for improvement in their use in MTM programs. A second review found that while studies support technicians performing advanced roles, the benefits to technicians were primarily indirect, such as increased job satisfaction or more desirable work schedule. They suggested that more tangible benefits for technicians (e.g., formal titles, career ladders, enhanced wages) would help optimize their deployment in support of MTM (Mattingly & Mattingly, 2018).

The effective use of technicians in such a manner likely will involve more thoughtful, holistic, and systematic approaches to workflow design even beyond tech-check-tech. Chui et al. (2012) provided an assessment of evaluating and re-organizing work system approaches modeling the systems engineering initiative for patient safety (SEIPS). This model incorporates revised job descriptions and considers organizational culture (see Chapter 16) when designing workflow and job responsibilities.

Sadie Metzger is aware of Pharmily's customer-first organizational culture and it being among the leaders in the chain pharmacy industry in developing MTM services. Unlike the case of accepting verbal prescription orders, many of the roles technicians can play in assisting MTM services are permitted throughout the nation. She understands that the various prescription department layouts, square footage areas, and volumes of prescriptions filled between different Pharmily stores makes it a challenge to devise a rigid workflow design. But she realizes that workflow design concept should incorporate certain principles (such as pharmacist autonomy and optimal use of pharmacy support staff) that are grounded in Pharmily's mission and culture yet allow for flexibility. The important thing is to ensure that pharmacists are comfortable with delegating responsibilities to technicians and that the right technicians are hired and that

they are adequately prepared to assist with Pharmily's Customer-first programs incorporating MTM.

■ THE CURRENT LANDSCAPE OF PHARMACY TECHNICIAN EDUCATION AND PRACTICE

Pharmacy technicians have been successfully incorporated into many care delivery models in pharmacy practice. There is still work to be done to optimize the roles of technicians as payment models, professional inertia, and other factors impede further implementation. Much has been done to hasten the effective utilization of technicians in recent years, as well as the description and evaluation of these models in the peer-reviewed literature. One study provided specific insight into how to restructure technician supervision and reconfigure skill mix in community pharmacy. It organized activities into those that are safe, unsafe, and borderline for support personnel to perform as deemed by both pharmacists and technicians themselves (Bradley et al., 2016). The conclusions suggest that even with legal authority to do so, delegation should be cautioned or even precluded regarding those tasks deemed unsafe until such time wherein more education and training become available. This study also recommends that institutions provide more training and provide an environment to promote self-efficacy, more rapidly alter workflow design and job responsibilities, then bundle them together in configuring work units for support personnel. Additional research suggested that company/employer appraisals are insufficient for revalidation or assessment of fitness to continue practice for pharmacists and technicians alike, but that more attention should be focused upon revalidation efforts for technicians (Schafheutle et al., 2013). It has also been posited that to truly facilitate practice change, greater clarity in technicians' roles, responsibilities, and expected outcomes is needed (Schafeutle et al., 2018).

Sadie Metzger, while contemplating various Customer-first programs, particularly those involving advanced MTM services, should be prioritized by the pharmacists' and staffs' preparedness to take on new responsibilities and that the design of these programs results in improved patient safety. Hiring decisions and training programs for all Pharmily personnel are vital in successfully implementing these programs.

To that end, pharmacists and support staff have to perform relatively stressful jobs (Boyle et al., 2016; Desselle & Holmes, 2017). As previously mentioned, effective management by pharmacists can ameliorate stress and ambiguity among technicians, as well as improve their self-efficacy. Self-efficacy is often a leading factor in determining job performance. An examination into technician self-efficacies identified strategies that could assist employers with further expanding technician practice activities and vocational institutions with modifying educational content (Desselle et al., 2017). This study incorporated an up-to-date task analysis for community and hospital pharmacy technicians, providing their current level of involvement, attitude toward involvement with these responsibilities, and their self-efficacy for continued or further involvement (see Tables 19-1 and 19-2). Pharmacy managers must be adept at facilitating technician self-efficacy and helping them to achieve their own self-actualization (Adams et al., 2018).

Additionally, the profession must continue to address issues regarding education and training, along with agreement on roles and preferably a more ubiquitous or widely recognized career laddering mechanism. One study showed that among certified technicians who had completed a vocational program, more than 1 in 5 did not even know whether that program was ASHP-accredited (Desselle & Holmes, 2017). That same study reported for the first time technicians' reason for entry into the profession, with large proportions of them being recruited directly by a pharmacist and/or referred by a friend or colleague. As such, pharmacists' words of encouragement and inspiration can go a long way toward recruiting (and maintaining) persons into technician practice. That same study also demonstrated that if a technician

Table 19-1. Hospital Pharmacy Technician Involvement In, Attitude Toward, and Self-Efficacy for Performing Various Tasks[a]

Task/Activity	Involvement[b]	Attitude[b]	Self-efficacy[c]
Enter prescription orders in computer	1.38±0.85	2.30±0.84	6.17±3.89
Replenish dose carts and floor stock	3.26±1.14	2.86±0.44	9.17±2.32
Maintain automated dispensing technology	3.07±1.20	2.73±0.58	8.60±2.74
Help to maintain pharmacy equipment	2.98±1.14	2.87±0.35	8.30±2.51
Compound sterile products	2.79±1.28	2.80±0.55	8.07±3.06
Compound non-sterile products	2.63±1.16	2.67±0.66	8.07±2.84
Perform packaging/repackaging activities	2.88±1.14	2.52±0.74	8.10±3.03
Purchasing and inventory management	2.40±1.21	2.77±0.57	6.90±3.55
Communicate with wholesale suppliers and vendors	1.74±1.04	2.40±0.77	5.27±2.77
Oversee activities related to medication assistance programs	1.36±0.73	2.10±0.76	3.67±3.18
Controlled substances system management	2.56±1.22	2.77±0.50	7.50±3.16
Billing and other accounting functions	2.00±1.29	2.48±0.79	5.10±3.39
Engage in continuous professional development	2.84±1.07	2.57±0.63	7.38±2.84
Check the work of other technicians (check-tech-check)	1.98±1.26	2.53±0.73	7.60±3.24

(Continued)

Table 19-1.	Hospital Pharmacy Technician Involvement In, Attitude Toward, and Self-Efficacy for Performing Various Tasks[a] (Continued)		
Task/Activity	Involvement[b]	Attitude[b]	Self-efficacy[c]
Supervise other technicians	1.79±1.03	2.41±0.83	7.10±3.59
Encourage professional development of other technicians	2.14±1.08	2.52±0.74	7.27±3.11
Assist with hiring other technicians	1.62±0.91	2.37±0.81	6.87±3.36
Determine future staffing needs	1.67±1.02	2.28±0.92	6.13±3.62
Reconcile errors or other issues with medication administration records	1.95±1.13	2.43±0.77	5.53±3.71
Update medication administration record or patient's profile	1.69±1.05	2.20±0.93	4.47±3.40
Preparation of clinical monitoring information for pharmacist review	1.31±0.72	1.97±0.93	3.67±3.37
Assist with or facilitate patient transitions of care	1.55±1.00	2.20±0.85	4.73±3.78
Run medication utilization reports	2.05±0.92	2.33±0.84	5.83±3.86
Assist with distribution of medications throughout facility	3.05±1.20	2.70±0.65	7.80±3.41
Follow-up on medication distribution issues or problems	2.63±1.27	2.63±0.72	7.40±3.56
Communicate with nurses and other professionals regarding patient therapy	2.07±1.17	2.37±0.81	5.50±3.70
Ensure proper storage of medications	3.30±0.96	2.77±0.57	8.87±2.27
Participate in protocol or guideline adherence monitoring activities	2.27±1.25	2.23±0.86	5.47±3.56
Communication medication storage issues with nurses	2.81±1.22	2.57±0.68	8.00±2.78
Assume responsibility for quality assurance activities	2.28±1.28	2.23±0.86	6.24±3.44
Participate in disaster preparedness activities	2.16±1.19	2.33±0.80	6.37±3.31
Provide information to patients on drug interactions, side effects, and medication storage	1.48±0.92	2.38±0.86	4.90±3.63
Collaborate with other health professionals to plan, monitor, review, and evaluate the effectiveness of medication therapy	1.64±0.98	2.24±0.87	4.79±3.44
Maintain files of narcotics and habit-forming drugs in accordance with legal requirements	2.02±1.28	2.48±0.83	6.21±3.45
Evaluate labels, packaging, and advertising of drug products	2.24±1.25	2.25±0.84	6.52±3.58
Administer immunizations	1.10±0.37	1.87±0.90	3.41±3.08

[a]Possible respondents (N) = 77. Actual number of respondents ranged from 68 to 75 on various questions.
[b]4-point scale anchored from less (1) to more (4) involved or more positive
[c]10-point scale
Source: Adapted with permission from Desselle SP, Holmes ER. 2017. Results of the 2015 National Certified Pharmacy Technician Workforce Survey. Am J Health-Syst Pharm 74:981–991.

Table 19-2. **Community Pharmacy Technician Involvement In, Attitude Toward, and Self-Efficacy for Performing Various Tasks[a]**

Task/Activity	Involvement[b]	Attitude[b]	Self-efficacy[c]
Collect or communicate patient information	3.57±0.83	2.91±0.29	8.95±1.81
Assess prescription for completeness, accuracy, authenticity, and legality	3.63±0.72	2.95±0.26	8.95±1.58
Input prescriptions into computer	3.44±0.98	2.84±0.46	8.73±2.20
Provide prescription to patient	3.41±1.02	2.72±0.60	8.93±2.35
Triage patient needs for referral to Pharmacist	3.10±1.14	2.68±0.63	8.20±2.77
Identify any problems with prescription (e.g., dosage, patient instructions, missing information, medication name, other)	3.33±0.88	2.89±0.36	8.71±1.72
Discuss over-the-counter medication options with patients	2.21±1.13	2.38±0.72	6.55±3.11
Repackage or reconstitute non-sterile products	2.62±1.30	2.56±0.72	7.61±3.35
Compound prescriptions	1.76±1.03	2.30±0.82	5.76±3.74
Inventory management	3.04±1.09	2.73±0.54	8.31±2.45
Manage medications currently in stock, including organization, storage, and stock rotation	3.38±0.97	2.78±0.52	8.87±2.17
Maintain automated dispensing technology and other equipment	2.37±1.26	2.38±0.82	6.52±3.52
Communicate with insurance companies regarding patient eligibility and other issues	3.09±1.15	2.71±0.55	7.86±2.97
Explain use of medical equipment, appliances, or other devices to the patient	1.91±1.00	2.34±0.74	5.84±3.19
Communicate lifestyle changes to patients	1.70±1.06	2.23±0.84	5.04±3.61
Engage in your own continuous professional development	3.07±0.98	2.70±0.58	8.18±2.48
Supervise other technicians	2.24±1.27	2.34±0.83	6.91±3.33
Discuss effectiveness of treatment plan for returning patients	1.72±1.12	2.23±0.88	4.96±3.77
Accounting and record-keeping	2.55±1.22	2.50±0.73	7.14±3.20
Disposal of expired or adulterated medications	2.90±1.12	2.71±0.60	8.16±2.56
Assist with prescription assistance programs	2.23±1.28	2.33±0.79	6.28±3.67
Assume responsibility for quality assurance activities	2.44±1.26	2.50±0.73	6.70±3.27
Assume responsibility for disaster preparedness	1.79±1.13	2.20±0.83	5.57±3.54
Receive prescriptions from medical doctors or other prescribers	2.29±1.35	2.48±0.78	6.79±3.55
Check patients' medication histories	3.07±1.05	2.67±0.59	8.05±2.68
Ensure proper dosage and drug compatibility before dispensing	2.71±1.24	2.63±0.69	7.07±3.33
Label liquid medicines, ointments, powders, and other medicines before dispensing	3.48±0.96	2.81±0.51	8.80±2.21

(Continued)

Table 19-2. Community Pharmacy Technician Involvement In, Attitude Toward, and Self-Efficacy for Performing Various Tasks[a] (Continued)

Task/Activity	Involvement[b]	Attitude[b]	Self-efficacy[c]
Provide information to providers and patients on drug interactions, side effects, and medication storage	2.08±1.22	2.47±0.79	6.07±3.50
Collaborate with other health professionals to plan, monitor, review, and evaluate the effectiveness of medication therapy	1.61±1.03	2.23±0.87	4.91±3.71
Maintain prescription files of narcotics and habit-forming drugs in accordance with legal requirements	2.76±1.22	2.66±0.65	7.79±2.90
Evaluate labels, packaging, and advertising of drug products	2.28±1.24	2.24±0.79	6.23±3.53
Administer immunizations	1.17±0.65	2.03±0.95	3.91±3.69
Accept verbal prescription orders from a physician or other prescriber	1.45±0.92	2.23±0.90	5.32±3.83
Transfer a prescription from on pharmacy to another	1.63±1.09	2.23±0.90	5.66±3.86
Check the work of other technicians (check-tech-check)	2.51±1.23	2.50±0.73	7.51±3.17
Enter prescription data remotely from home	1.23±0.70	1.91±0.93	5.10±4.06

[a]Possible respondents (N) = 312. Actual number of respondents ranged from 290 to 302 on various questions.
[b]4-point scale anchored from less (1) to more (4) involved or more positive
[c]10-point scale
Source: Adapted with permission from Desselle SP, Holmes ER. 2017. Results of the 2015 National Certified Pharmacy Technician Workforce Survey. *Am J Health-Syst Pharm* 74:981–991.

viewed their training as valuable, no matter the type of training (e.g., on-the-job, certification, and/or vocational education) that the technician reported higher levels of commitment to the profession.

Another component of technician education and training being frequently discussed for inclusion into training programs is in ethics and ethical reasoning. One concern that has arisen regarding technicians having greater roles in practice is their access to and potential responsibility for narcotics and other abusive drugs. While effective arguments have been made for including technicians in patient opioid misuse programs, there is also evidence to suggest that technicians have been far more likely than pharmacists to be involved in medication diversion (Draime et al., 2018). This should be addressed in ethics training but also should raise awareness

among pharmacy managers and employers the need for adequate training, selection, and hiring processes to minimize such occurrences (see Chapter 17). A recent study affirmed the need for ethical reasoning skills in technician education and highlighted the effectiveness of easily implemented interventions to do so (Hogan & Dunne, 2018).

International Perspectives

Technician practice continues to evolve around the world. Pharmacist and technician leaders in the United States can learn much from what is going on elsewhere. A worldwide overview of pharmacy technicians revealed that (Koehler & Brown, 2017b):

- Pharmacists have been able to extend their clinical role with greater use of support personnel.

- Where successful partnerships around education, registration, and regulation have emerged there has been detailed attention to change management and stakeholder engagement, with improved patient care as the focus.
- In more recent years, pharmacy support workforce roles have expanded in some countries, moving from administration and supply to checking the work of other technicians, on toward deeper levels of involvement with patient adherence programs.
- The most recent literature explores the need to further develop the leadership skills of the support workforce.

In various parts of the world, pharmacy technicians carry significant responsibilities including drug distribution and supply chain management in underdeveloped countries that have a shortage of primary health care professionals (Koehler & Brown, 2017a). Technicians have been especially crucial in the supply chain management of drugs from the World Health Organization (WHO) Essential Medicines List. Some countries have put pharmacy technicians at the forefront of various public health initiatives such as that seen in the United Kingdom (Zachariah et al., 2016). In their Health Living Champions program, pharmacists serve as a key primary care provider and are entrusted with responsibilities to promote proper diet (weight management), smoking cessation, and appropriate use of alcohol products. Pharmacy technicians help to market these services, identify potential patients in triage, and coordinate activities and logistics necessary for the program to be successful. In Denmark, pharmacy technicians are referred to as pharmaconomists. These individuals acquire a 3-year educational degree with a residency component all in the one educational institution provider in that country. Pharmaconomists have wider scopes of practice, nearly resembling those of pharmacists, except for the ability to own a pharmacy and certain other select responsibilities (Desselle et al., 2018b). The United States and other countries can learn from various international models, while considering differences

in the population, health systems, and other factors before deciding if and how to implement these models.

While there has been an emphasis on leadership education and training among pharmacists, pharmacy technicians will in all likelihood increase their level of involvement in change management and in supervisory roles. To that end, a thorough and sophisticated competency framework has been suggested which could greatly assist leaders and educators in the United States as they consider additional education and training requirements (Koehler et al., 2018). The pharmacy manager can support the development of technicians and other support staff by encouraging their participation in continuing education (CE), sponsoring their attendance at CE events, having them self-assess their ethical decision-making and leadership skills (see Chapters 3 and 4), and providing incentives (e.g., movie tickets, books, sponsorship of re-certification) for technicians who demonstrate innovation. Sadie Metzger might consider providing a small pool of funds that pharmacy managers could use to offer rewards for technicians who demonstrate initiative and/or high degrees of proficiency in Pharmaily's Customer-first programs.

■ PUTTING IT ALL TOGETHER FOR EFFECTIVE SUPERVISION OF TECHNICIANS

As emphasized throughout this chapter, pharmacy technicians are essential to both daily operations of a pharmacy and advancing the pharmacist's role in providing direct patient care, especially when pharmacists are able to effectively delegate. Through formal, on-the-job training and credentialing, technicians are increasingly important members of the pharmacy team who ultimately allow pharmacists to effectively practice at the top of their license. This means that beyond developing an expertise in pharmacotherapy, a successful pharmacist must be skilled at leading and engaging their technician team to provide optimal patient care. Fortunately, years of experience have uncovered insights, and these insights can be combined with evidence-based management research to provide pharmacists with an approach to successfully lead practice transformations utilizing technicians (Martin et al., 2016).

Regardless of whether a pharmacist is a part-time staff employee or a corporate pharmacy leader, they will have some supervisory responsibility over pharmacy technicians. Supervising other people is challenging and complex, and when done well can result in favorable organizational outcomes (e.g., employee satisfaction, reduced job turnover, higher productivity, and higher employee engagement [see Chapters 3 and 5]). Current evidence suggests that less than desirable work-related outcomes in pharmacy may be largely mitigated through a supportive pharmacist supervisor. The idea that the relationship between leader (pharmacist) and team member (pharmacy technician)

being highly predictive of success is described in the theory of Leader Member Exchange (LMX) (Scandura et al., 1986). This theory describes the nature of delegation of duties and authority to those team members (e.g., technicians) who are empowered by the leader (e.g., pharmacist) because of how the leader's performance is enhanced when the team under their supervision performs well (Figure 19-1).

Core to the idea of LMX is the relationship between leader (pharmacist) AND member (pharmacy technician) (Gotfredson et al., 2016). This is in contrast to other theories that deal with traits specific to the leader OR the follower. Given that the relationship between these two parties is the focus, then it is the relationship which should be the pharmacist's target for enhancing results of the team. These relationships are categorized into two broad categories based on the pharmacist's perception of member performance: in-group (high LMX) and out-group

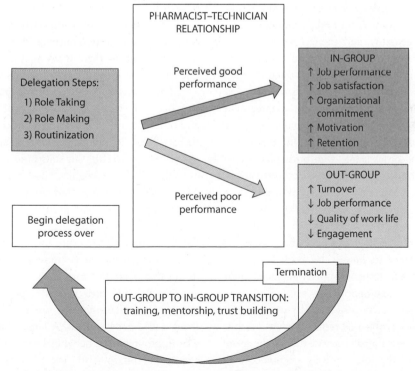

Figure 19-1. Leading technicians using the leader member exchange (LMX) theory.

(low LMX). As one might imagine, those technicians who are in the in-group for a particular pharmacist go above-and-beyond and often take on extra work, whereas members of the out-group do not. Out-group members perform to their job description, but they do not contribute beyond this because of the lower-level relationship, and consequently lower trust between their leader and themselves (for more on trust between leader and member, see Chapter 3). Unlike out-group members, in-group technicians enjoy a fruitful and reciprocal relationship with their pharmacist. For example, a technician who takes on pharmacist-delegated inventory responsibilities because of extra workload placed on the pharmacist may be assigned a work schedule with fewer nights and weekends, further improving the technician's perception of quality of worklife while simultaneously ameliorating the pharmacist's workload.

So, how do these groups arise? Leaders go through a three-step process, often unknowingly, in assigning in versus out groups (Graen et al., 1987). Step 1 is the process of role-taking whereby the pharmacist may identify a new task to delegate to the technician (e.g., inventory management), and the technician accepts this delegated role. This delegation process tests the technician's commitment and leads to Step 2, role-making. In the role-making phase, the newly delegated role is established through mutual agreement between both parties, and clear role parameters are developed. Finally, during routinization, the newly delegated task becomes stable with both pharmacist and technician knowing what to expect, and further growing a high LMX relationship. For example, a pharmacist may no longer review weekly inventory controls because the technician to whom this was delegated has accepted the extra work and performed it well. The pharmacist knows the work is of high quality and comes to respect this technician for their work, and when a new opportunity arises for a new medication reconciliation program, the pharmacist's first thought is to involve this technician. As a result, the technician receives a pay increase due to the more complex nature of the role, annually attends conferences to learn the latest research, and best practices in medication reconciliation, further leading to feelings of appreciation for the work they do. When a new job offer comes to the technician, they only consider it momentarily and eventually decline because they are fulfilled in their current position.

If team success relies on in-group member performance, would it not make sense to aim for all team members to be within the in-group? Absolutely. When applying LMX to improve pharmacy performance, the pharmacist's goal must be to grow the in-group. When one looks more broadly at the entirety of the team's success, a more successful pharmacy team is one where the pharmacist has the largest number of technicians in the "in-group." This takes mentorship, trust, and training when progressing through the three-step role-making process. Pharmacists should challenge technicians often with new roles that support the mission of the organization and remove workload from the pharmacist. When these delegated roles are not performed adequately, rather than assigning the technician to an "out-group," a pharmacist should instead work to build trust through mentorship and training with the goal of ultimately moving through the remaining two steps of role making and routinization. Importantly, there is no magic bullet here—no one way to move technicians into an "in-group."

The means to achieving this larger in-group will vary by technician, pharmacist, organization, culture, and other factors. However, as mentioned previously, there are certain practices that will always translate well with your technician staff (and for pharmacists, as well), which is recognize good performance (with private/personal and a judicious amount of public praise), incent good performance with rewards, encourage self-development, sponsor attendance at CE programming, advocate for "bigger" things such as higher wages and career laddering mechanisms even if you have relatively little direct control over those, and provide the "little things" type of benefits over which you do have control, such as occasional food treats and other surprises. A large pharmacy technician in-group will be beneficial to the pharmacy manager, other pharmacists, the pharmacy's customers, other health professionals, and your patients.

■ REVISITING THE SCENARIO

Sadie Metzger visited the Pharmily store where she was a staff pharmacist. Two of the three technicians and one of the two pharmacists who were there just over a year ago were still employed at the same store. She exchanged pleasantries with them and got up to speed on one another's personal and professional lives. Sadie wanted to originate a brief "listening tour" to solicit ideas and to float her own initial ideas past some of the technicians and pharmacists she knew about some 'Customer-First' initiatives she had in mind. Her initiatives would involve some workflow changes and role clarification for technicians to assume more administrative responsibility over quality assurance programs and immunizations, while experimenting with alternative communication formats to engage customers, while pharmacists spent more time with implementing several new clinical services being rolled out by Pharmily. Sadie figured that the technicians with whom she would speak could give her plenty good advice on how various strategies might work with their patients and that listening to these technicians would help them realize just how valuable their contributions are to the future success of Pharmily.

■ QUESTIONS FOR FURTHER DISCUSSION

1. What sort of experiences have you had working alongside pharmacy technicians with expanding roles? Has it gone smoothly? Why or why not?

2. How do you think that further advancing technician roles will impact job availability and job scope of practice by pharmacists?

3. Where do you think the United States is compared to other countries in regard to technician regulation and scope of practice? Will other worldwide trends make their way to the U.S.? Why or why not?

REFERENCES

Adams AJ, Martin SJ, Stolpe SF. 2011. "Teach-check-tech": A review of the evidence on its safety and benefits. *Am J Health System Pharm* 68:1824–1833.

Adams AJ. 2018. Pharmacist delegation: An approach to pharmacy technician regulation. *Res Social Adm Pharm* 14:505.

American College of Clinical Pharmacy (ACCP). 2007. Position statement. Pharmacy technician education, training, and certification. Available at www.accp.com/docs/positions/positionStatements/Technician_Position_Statement.pdf; Accessed on September 22, 2018.

American Pharmacists Association (APhA). 1969. Report of the Task Force: Practitioner's and subprofessional's role in pharmacy. *J Am Pharm Assoc* NS9:416.

American Society of Health Systems Pharmacists (ASHP). 2018. Accreditation Standards for pharmacy technician education and training programs. Available at https://www.ashp.org/-/media/assets/professional-development/technician-program-accreditation/docs/ashp-acpe-pharmacy-technician-accreditation-standard-2018.ashx?la=en&hash=36EAA6511105A6C6BFEA4F30E193892F19E2C385. Accessed October 3, 2018.

American Society of Health Systems Pharmacists (ASHP). 2003. White Paper on pharmacy technicians 2002: Needed changes can no longer wait. *Am J Health-Syst Pharm* 60:37–51.

American Society of Health Systems Pharmacists (ASHP). 1989. Final Report of the ASHP Task Force on Technical Personnel in Pharmacy. *Am J Health-Syst Pharm* 46:1420–1429.

American Society of Hospital Pharmacists (ASHP). 1982. ASHP Outcomes Competencies for Institutional Pharmacy Technician Training Programs. *Am J Hosp Pharm* 39:317–320.

American Society of Hospital Pharmacy (ASHP). 1977. Minimum Standard for Pharmacies in Institutions. *Am J Hosp Pharm* 34:1356–1358.

American Society of Hospital Pharmacists (ASHP). 1972. Report of the Council on Education and Manpower. *Am J Hosp Pharm* 29:617.

Andreski M, Myers M, Gainer K, Pudlo A. 2018. The Iowa new practice model Advancing technician roles in increase pharmacists' time to provide patient care services. *J Am Pharm Assoc* 58:268–274.

Archambault G. 1958. Qualifications and responsibilities of la help in hospital pharmacy. *Am J Hosp Pharm* 6:210–215.

Bailey JE, Surbhi S, Bell PC, et al. 2016. SafeMed: using pharmacy technicians in a novel role as community health workers to improve transitions of care. *J Am Pharm Assoc* 56:73–81.

Borchert JS, Phillips J, Thompson ML, Livingood A, Andersen R, et al. 2018. Best practices: Incorporating pharmacy technicians and other support personnel into the clinical pharmacist's process of care. *J Am Coll Clinical Pharm.* 2, 74-81.

Boyle TA, Bishop A, Morrison B, et al. 2016. Pharmacist work stress and learning from quality related events. *Res Social Adm Pharm* 12:772–783.

Bradley F, Willis SC, Noyce PR, et al. 2016. Restructuring supervision and reconfiguration of skill mix in community pharmacy: Classification of perceived safety and risk. *Res Social Adm Pharm* 12:733–746.

Braverman J. 1969. Subprofessionals in pharmacy: An international perspective. *J Am Pharm Assoc* NS9:273–277,280.

Brown KN, Bergsbaken J, Reichard JS. 2016. Medication safety pharmacy technician in large, tertiary care, community hospital. *Am J Health Syst Pharm* 73:188–191.

Brownlie K, Schneider C, Culliford R, et al. 2014. Mediation reconciliation by a pharmacy technician in a mental health assessment unit. *Int J Clin Pharm* 36:303–309.

Chevalier BA, MacDonald SA. 2003. Expanding the pharmacy technicians" role in medication teaching. *Am J Health System Phar* 60:709–710.

Cochran G, Gordon AJ, Field C, et al. 2016. Developing a framework of care for opioid medication misuse in community pharmacy. *Res Social Adm Pharm* 12:293–301.

Compton WM, Jones CM, Stein JB, et al. 2018. Promising roles for pharmacists in addressing the U.S. opioid crisis. *Res Social Adm Pharm* [Epub ahead of print] Available at https:doi:org/10.1016.j.sapharm.2017.12.009. Accessed April 7, 2019.

Cox ER, Fitzpatrick V. 1999. Pharmacists' job satisfaction and perceived utilization of skills. *Am J Health Syst Pharm* 56:1733.

Desselle SP. 2005a. Survey of certified pharmacy technicians in the United States: A quality-of-worklife study. *J Am Pharm Assoc* 45:458–465.

Desselle SP. 2005b. Job turnover intentions among certified pharmacy technicians. *J Am Pharm Assoc* 45:676–683.

Desselle SP. 2016. An in-depth examination into technician worklife through an organizational behavior framework. *Res Social Adm Pharm* 12:722–732.

Desselle SP, Benton D, Hacker J, et al. 2015. Proposal for pharmacy technician education, training, practice, and career laddering: A proposal to advance pharmacy and promote patient safety. *Calif J Health-Syst Pharm* 26:29–40.

Desselle SP, Hoh R, Holmes ER, et al. 2018. The caring behaviours of Danish pharmaconomists: Insight for pharmacy technician practice around the world. *Intl J Pharm Pract* Available at https://doi.org/10.1111/ijpp.12478.

Desselle SP, Holmes ER. 2007. Structural model of certified pharmacy technicians' job satisfaction. *J Am Pharm Assoc* 47:58–72.

Desselle SP, Holmes ER. 2017. Results of the 2015 National Certified Pharmacy Technician Workforce Survey. *Am J Health-Syst Pharm* 74:981–991.

Douglas AS, Kramer EL, Bruner WR. 1986. Utilization of technicians. *J Pharm Technol* 2:28.

Draime JA, Anderson DC, Anderson TS. 2018. Description and comparison of medication diversion in pharmacies by pharmacists, interns, and pharmacy technicians. *J Am Pharm Assoc* 58:275–280.

Fera T, Kanel KT, Bollinger ML, et al. 2018. Clinical support role for a pharmacy technician with a primary care resource center. *Am J Health Syst Pharm* 75:139–144.

Frazier W. Utilization of nonprofessional personnel the hospital pharmacy. 1954. *Bull Am Soc Hosp Pharm* 11:257–261.

Frost TP, Adams AJ. 2017. Expanded pharmacy technician roles: Accepting verbal prescriptions and communicating prescription transfers. *Res Social Adm Pharm* 13:1191–1195.

Gaither CA. 1998. The predictive validity of work/career-related attitudes and intentions on pharmacists' turnover behavior. *J Pharm Mark Manage* 12:3.

Gasseling LR, Hughles T, McGuire EA, et al. 2000. Clinical technician, a partner in pharmaceutical care. Paper presented at: American Society for Health-System Pharmacists Midyear Clinical Meeting; December 5, 2000; Las Vegas, NV.

Gernant SA, Nguyen MO, Siddiqui S, et al. 2018. Use of pharmacy technicians in elements of medication therapy management delivery: A systematic review. *Res Social Adm Pharm* 14:883–890.

Gilbert EM, Gerzenshtein L. 2015. Integration of outpatient infectious diseases clinical pharmacy services and specialty pharmacy services for patients with HIV infection. *Am J Health Syst Pharm* 73:757–763.

Graen GB, Scandura TA. 1987. Toward a psychology of dyadic organizing. *Research Org Behav* 9:175–208.

Hepler CD, Strand LM. 1990. Opportunities and responsibilities in pharmaceutical care. *Am J Hosp Pharm* 47:533–543.

Hogan S, Dunne J. 2018. Evaluating the effectiveness of a focused debate on the development of ethical reasoning skills in pharmacy technician students. *Am J Pharm Educ* 82:Article 6280.

Ibrahim MIM, Wertherimer AI, Myers MJ, et al. 1997. Leadership styles and effectiveness: Pharmacists in associations vs. pharmacists in community settings. *J Pharm Mark Manage* 12:23.

Irwin AN, Heilman RM Gerrity TM, et al. 2014. Use of a pharmacy technician to facilitate post-fracture care provided by clinical pharmacy specialists. *Am J Health Syst Pharm* 71:2054–2059.

Iowa Pharmacists Association. Technician Product Verification. 2018. Available at https://www.iarx.org/files/2018_LegDay/2018_TPV_1-page.pdf. Accessed September 28, 2018.

Jackson ML, Bickham P, Clark T. 1998. Technician management of automation and inventory. Paper presented at: American Society of Health-System Pharmacists Midyear Clinical Meeting; December 8, 1998; Las Vegas, NV.

Jobin J, Irwin AN, Pimetel J, et al. 2018. Accuracy of medication histories collected by pharmacy technicians during hospital admission. *Res Social Adm Pharm* 14:695–699.

Justis L, Crain J, Marchetti ML, et al. 2016. The effect of community pharmacy technicians on industry standard adherence performance measures after cognitive pharmaceutical services training. *J Pharm Technol* 32:230–233.

Kadia NK, Schroeder MN. 2015. Community pharmacy-based adherence programs and the role of pharmacy technicians: A review. 31,51-57.

Keller ME, Kelling SE, Bright DR. 2015. Pharmacy technicians and point of care testing. *J Pharm Technol* 31:143–148.

Koehler T, Brown. 2017a. Documenting the evolution of the relationship between the pharmacy support workforce and pharmacists to support patient care. *Res Social Adm Pharm* 13:280–285.

Koehler T, Brown A. 2017b. A global picture of pharmacy technicians and other pharmacy support workforce cadres. *Res Social Adm Pharm* 13:271–279.

Koehler TC, Bok H, Westerman M, et al. 2018. Developing a competency framework for pharmacy technicians: Perspectives from the field. *Res Social Adm Pharm* [Epub ahead of print] 14:https://doi.org/10.1016/j.sapharm.018.06.017.

Kuhn H, Park A, Kim B, et al. 2016. Proportion of work appropriate for pharmacy technicians in anticoagulation clinics. *Am J Health Syst Pharm* 73:322–327.

Leinss R, Karpinski T, Patel B. 2015. Implementation of a comprehensive medication prior-authorization service. *Am J Health Syst Pharm* 72:159–163.

Mangan MN, Powers MF. 2011. Drug shortages and the role of the pharmacy technicians: A review. *J Pharm Technol* 27:247–250.

Markovic M, Mathis AS, Ghin HL, et al. 2017. A comparison of medication histories obtained by a pharmacy technician versus nurses in the emergency department. *P&T* 42:41–46.

Martin R, Guillaume Y, Thomas G, et al. 2016. Leader–member exchange (LMX) and performance: A meta-analytic review. *Personnel Psychol* 69:67–121.

Mattingly AN, Mattingly TJ. 2018. Advancing the role of the pharmacy technician: A systematic review. *J Am Pharm Assoc* 58:9–108.

McKiernan KC, Frazier KR, Nguyen M, et al. 2018. Training pharmacy technicians to administer immunizations. *J Am Pharm Assoc* 58:174–178.

McKonnen AB, McLachlan AJ, Brien JA. 2016. Pharmacy-led medication reconciliation programmes at hospital transitions: A systematic review and meta-analysis. *J Clin Pharm Ther* 41:128–144.

Muenzen PM, Greenberg S, Murer MM. 1999. PTCB Task Analysis identifies role of certified pharmacy technicians in pharmaceutical care. *J Am Pharm Assoc* 39:857–864.

Muenzen PM, Corrigan MM, Mobley-Smith MA, et al. 2006. Updating the pharmacy technician certification examination: A practice analysis study. *J Am Pharm Assoc* 46:e1–36.

Napier P, Norris P, Braund R. 2018. Introducing a checking technician allows pharmacists to spend more time on patient-focused activities. *Res Social Adm Pharm* 14:382–386.

National Healthcare Association (NHA). Pharmacy technician certification. 2018. Available at https://www.nhanow.com/certifications/pharmacy-technician. Accessed August 28, 2018.

Patanwala AE. Emergency pharmacy practice and medication reconciliation. 2014. *Am J Health Syst Pharm* 71:2167–2168.

Pharmacists for the Future: Report of the Study Commission on Pharmacy. 1975. Ann Arbor, MI: Health Administration Press.

Pharmacy Technician Certification Board (PTCB). 2018. Pharmacy Technician Certification Exam Blueprint. Available at https://www.ptcb.org/docs/get-certified/new_ptce_blueprint.pdf?sfvrsn=6. Accessed September 9, 2018.

Pharmacy Technician Certification Board (PTCB). 2018b. CPhT Map and Regulatory Snapshot. Available at https://ptcb.org/who-we-serve/pharmacy-technicians/cphts-state-regulatory-map#.W9tPW7ivCAM. Accessed November 2, 2018.

Scandura TA, Graen GB, Novak MA. 1986. When managers decide not to decide autocratically: An investigation of leader–member exchange and decision influence. *J Appl Psychol* 71:579–584.

Schafheutle EI, Hassell K, Noyce PR. 2013. Ensuring continuing fitness to practice in the pharmacy workforce: Understanding the challenges of revalidation. *Res Social Adm Pharm* 9:199–214.

Schultz JM, Jeter CK, Keresztes JM, Martin NM, Mundy TK, Reichard JS, Van Cura JD. (2016). ASHP Statement on the Roles of Technicians. *Am J Health Syst Pharm.* 73,928-930.

Turnbull RT, Bowles GC. 1965. Current trends in the utilization of hospital pharmacy personnel. Am J *Hosp Pharm* 22:597–605.

Wheeler JS, Renfro CP, Wang J, et al. 2019. Assessing pharmacy technician certification: A national survey comparing certified and noncertified pharmacy technicians. *J Am Pharm Assoc* [Epub ahead of print] DOI: https://doi.org/10.1016/j.japh.2018.12.021.

Whittet TD. 1968. The place of technicians in pharmacy: The position in Great Britain. *Drug Intell* 2:266–269.

Whitney, Jr. HAK. 1981. Pharmacy technicians establish an independent national organization. *Drug Intell Clinical Pharm* 15:281.

Zachariah N, Portlock J, Rutter P, et al. 2016. Healthy living champions network: An opportunity for community pharmacy's sustained participation in tackling local health inequalities. *Res Social Pharm Adm* 12:1010–1015.

Zillich AJ, Corelli RL, Zibikowski SM, et al. 2013. A random trial evaluating 2 approaches for promoting pharmacy-based approaches to the tobacco quit line: Methods and baseline findings. *Res Social Adm Pharm* 9:27–36.

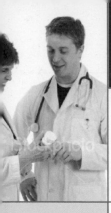

20

PERFORMANCE APPRAISAL SYSTEMS

Shane P. Desselle and Leticia R. Moczygemba

About the Authors: Dr. Desselle is professor of Social, Behavioral, and Administrative Pharmacy at Touro University California College of Pharmacy. His research program focuses on optimizing roles for pharmacy technicians, development of mentorship programs and in promoting health organizational cultures and citizenship behaviors in professional settings. He is a Fulbright Specialist Scholar having completed a project to develop a Center of Assessment for the University of Pristina in Kosovo. Dr. Desselle is Founding Editor-in-Chief of the international peer-reviewed journal, *Research in Social and Administrative Pharmacy* with graduate students and collaborations worldwide on various projects such as medication safety and medication adherence issues with informal caregivers. Dr. Desselle also is a primary author for the Pharmacy Management Tips of the Week on AccessPharmacy that accompany this textbook.

Dr. Moczygemba is an associate professor and associate director of the Texas Center for Health Outcomes Research and Education at The University of Texas College of Pharmacy. Her research program focuses on working with communities and health systems to mitigate health disparities by developing patient-centered interventions to optimize medication-related health outcomes. She has worked to advance the health care of homeless individuals, older adults, and those living in rural areas through the development, implementation, and evaluation of care models that integrate pharmacists with health care teams. She teaches in the health care systems course in the Doctor of Pharmacy (PharmD) program and is engaged in interprofessional education initiatives with a focus on quality improvement (QI) and patient safety.

■ LEARNING OBJECTIVES

After completing this chapter, readers will be able to

1. Discuss the rationale behind the implementation of a systematic performance appraisal system.
2. Discuss the implementation of a performance appraisal system within a pharmacy organization.

3. Identify various types of performance appraisal processes and evaluate the strengths and weaknesses of each type.
4. Discuss contemporary performance feedback and appraisal processes such as 360-degree feedback.
5. Discuss issues of reliability and validity within the context of evaluating a performance appraisal system.
6. Describe how to conduct a performance appraisal interview and how to handle disagreements that may arise during or subsequent to the interview.
7. Discuss the linkage of performance appraisal results with the proper allocation of organizational rewards.
8. Discuss the importance of formal and informal feedback and describe best practices for providing informal feedback and praise to employees to maximize their work satisfaction, commitment, and productivity.

■ SCENARIO

"What?" asked Marcus Green, emphatically. "You've got to be kidding! That's just not fair. I've been here for $3^1/_2$ years, and I've received only one raise—and that may as well have been nothing. Why did she get another raise? She's probably making more money than I am, and she's only been here for a little more than 1 year." With a look of consternation, Marcus lowers his voice and asks his colleagues at the lunch table, "Where did you hear this from, anyway? Ah, never mind. I don't want to discuss it any further," Marcus chimed as he finished scarfing up the remainder of his lunch and left the table in a huff.

Marcus's fellow pharmacy technicians at Community Hospital were equally upset that Susan Bostik allegedly had received another raise, but they were not sure that they had done the right thing by telling Marcus about it. Marcus, having worked at Community Hospital for nearly 4 years, generally was regarded as the "best tech" in the pharmacy. He filled orders twice as fast as anyone else, always showed up on time, and came to work on short notice when others called in sick, even though he was perhaps a bit more prone to making a dispensing error and was well known for being a "hothead." Susan Bostik, on the other hand, seemed to be the "boss's pet." Indeed, she was regarded as a very pleasant person who got along

with everyone, especially the Pharmacy Director, Cynthia Broedl, with whom she shared an appreciation for poetry and theater.

Marcus continued to stew over his plight throughout the afternoon. He didn't really *feel* like looking for another job, making phone calls, filling out forms, and going on interviews. But he also did not understand why other technicians seemed to be rewarded at Community Hospital pharmacy more frequently with raises than he did. He wondered just what about his performance was not up to par. He did not recall being formally evaluated in over 2 years, when he and Ms. Broedl had a few words on his suggestion that he often had to "pick up the slack" for pharmacists "not doing their jobs." Meanwhile, Terrence Whitfield, the Assistant Pharmacy Director, appeared in Cynthia's office to discuss his relief that the apparent exodus of staff occurring during the previous few months appeared to be over.

■ CHAPTER QUESTIONS

1. What is a performance appraisal system? What does formal appraisal have to do with employee motivation, productivity, and turnover?
2. What is the difference between absolute, relative, and goal-oriented systems for appraising employee performance?

3. What kinds of appraisals typically are performed in pharmacy environments? How might these appraisal systems be improved?

4. How are formal performance appraisal mechanisms implemented? What are some strategies to maximize the effectiveness of the appraisal interview?

5. How should performance appraisals be linked to the allocation of organizational rewards? What are some innovative reward strategies that can be used to optimize employee satisfaction and productivity?

6. What is the difference between formal and informal performance feedback? Why is frequent and regular informal feedback so important? What are some methods to provide informal feedback?

■ WHAT ARE PERFORMANCE APPRAISALS?

Virtually every practitioner and many students reading this text have either participated in or know of a discussion similar to the one taking place at the beginning of the scenario. Pharmacists and pharmacy support staff are typically hardworking, honest people who want the best for their patients and their organizations. However, they are made of the same fabric as everyone else and desire equitable treatment and fair compensation for their work.

The scenario begs the question of precisely what qualities signify a "good" pharmacist or pharmacy technician. Are promptness, dedication, and hard work the attributes most revered by administrators, or are collegiality and amicability? What is more important—the quantity or the quality of the work performed? The scenario raises some additional concerns. Do some employees get preferential treatment because they have things in common with those in administrative positions? How do other employees in the pharmacy feel about the way they are being treated and compensated by their employer? Why have so many employees left the pharmacy department at Community Hospital of late? Do the Pharmacy Director and Assistant Pharmacy Director

know how Marcus feels and that he is contemplating quitting as well? What do the pharmacists at Community Hospital think about the situation?

As humans, we are concerned primarily for the interests of ourselves, our families, and our closest loved ones. Each person's concern for self, manifesting within the cornucopia of personalities that exist among us, practically ensures occasional discontent among employees. And discontent, coupled with the consistency of life changes (e.g., employees will bring on new family members, get sick or perhaps die, find new opportunities, or retire and leave the workforce) guarantees some level of turnover within all organizations that is beyond the control of management. The lack of a well-planned, well-executed, and equitable performance appraisal system can be a major source of discontent among employees of any pharmacy operation. However, putting such a system in place is well within management's control.

Strictly defined, a *performance appraisal* is a formal assessment of how well employees are performing their jobs. But a performance assessment is also much more than that. It is a way of formally communicating the organization's mission and goals, a foundation on which to establish informal channels of communication, a method on which to base organizational rewards, and a tool to improve the performance of each and every employee within the organization. Unfortunately, performance appraisal is a frequently neglected function. Managers have cited performance appraisals (also known as *performance reviews*) as their least favorite activity (Cappelli & Conyon, 2018). Constructing, implementing, and monitoring a performance appraisal system presents many formidable challenges.

■ THE RATIONALE FOR A FORMAL PERFORMANCE APPRAISAL SYSTEM

As Chapters 16, 17, and 18 pointed out, human resources are among a pharmacy's most valuable assets. Employee wages are the greatest operating expense for almost every pharmacy (see Chapter 21). Employees, however, should not be viewed simply as an expense, but as an essential asset for organizational success. The ramifications of executing a good performance appraisal system extend to most human resources decisions. In fact, evidence suggests that poor performance appraisal systems result in employees' lower job satisfaction, lower organizational commitment, and higher quit intentions (Brown et al., 2010). The scenario depicting Marcus Greene's plight is not at all uncommon. Employees need to feel that their contributions to the organization are valued and appreciated, and if they feel otherwise, lower job satisfaction is only the beginning of a possible cascade of negative consequences. Table 20-1 summarizes some important points about the need for performance appraisals.

Legal

Performance appraisals are necessary to document employees' progress toward achieving goals and heeding the advice of administrators on how to improve performance. Documentation is necessary to demonstrate fairness in promotion and termination (discharge) practices. Title VII of the Civil Service Reform Act ushered in heightened concern regarding appraisal issues (Martin & Bartol, 1991). Title VII is a federal statute that applies to and sets forth constitutionally protected classes as they pertain to employment, including religion, national origin, race or color, and gender (Blackwell et al., 1996). An employee can initiate a Title VII claim based on disparate treatment, disparate impact, or retaliation (see Chapter 18). As will be described later in this chapter, certain types of performance appraisal systems facilitate documentation of critical incidents such as those pertaining to harassment and hostile work environment (disparate treatment), which has been shown to be problematic for women in pharmacy (Broedel-Zaugg et al., 1999) and for other health care workers whose primary language is not English (Akomolafe, 2013).

In such situations, the claimant would have to demonstrate that a hiring, promotion, or discharge had a significant adverse impact on a member of a protected class. Should a pharmacy be accused of any

---

Table 20-1.   Rationale for Implementing Effective Performance Appraisals

Legal
- Title VII of the Civil Service Reform Act
- Age Discrimination in Employment Act

Communicative
- Ensures understanding of performance expectations by managers and staff
- Provides a formal means for employees to voice concerns and make suggestions for system improvement
- Indicates management's commitment to open dialogue and fairness

Productivity of Labor
- Provides direction to employees on how to improve
- Establishes an environment conducive to self-motivation
- Assists employees with career planning
- Promotes satisfaction and elicits commitment of employees
- Mitigates turnover

Equity in Rewards
- Provides a means for accurate and equitable distribution of organizational rewards
- Provides recognition for past service
- Helps to establish support for terminating "problem" or underachieving employees

Other Managerial Functions
- Supplies evidence to review organizational and systems problems
- Provides data on recruitment and selection procedures
- Identifies deficiencies in orientation and training programs

Financial Position
- Assists in reducing operating costs
- Avoids costly litigation
- Reduces replacement costs

one of these, there are a limited number of defenses, most notably the bona fide occupational qualification (BFOQ). With the BFOQ, the pharmacy must demonstrate that the employee claimant could not perform essential job duties safely and effectively. Having implemented a formal performance appraisal system, the pharmacy possesses critical documentation that an employee's performance was lacking and that the employee was provided adequate warning that failure to improve would result in certain consequences (termination/discharge, failure to obtain a promotion or pay increase, etc.) (Mitchell & Koen, 2016).

Communicative

An employee typically will come to know what is expected of him during the performance appraisal process. These expectations may or may not have been communicated adequately during the hiring, training, or informal feedback processes. The performance appraisal process affords managers the opportunity to inform employees of the importance of their roles and responsibilities to the organization and how their performance will be measured, thus mitigating the possibility of *role stress* among employees (Hills, 2014). Role stress is typically viewed as having two components: role ambiguity and role conflict. *Role ambiguity* exists when an employee is unsure about his responsibilities. *Role conflict* is the simultaneous occurrence of two or more role expectations (Bowling et al., 2017). The prevalence of role conflict and role ambiguity have been studied in pharmacy (Desselle & Tipton, 2001). It is not difficult to envision their occurrence. In hospital pharmacies, technicians often experience stress over who maintains responsibility for cleaning the laminar flow hood, delivering medications to the floors, and filling stat orders. In community pharmacies, conflicting roles for pharmacists may involve demands from administrators to increase prescription volume while also expecting an increase in the time spent performing clinical functions like patient education and medication therapy management.

If it becomes apparent to an administrator that productivity among their staff is suffering, information can be gathered during the performance appraisal process that can lead to constructive changes in non-personnel aspects of the business (e.g., workflow design). In any event, the dialogue emanating from the appraisal process provides data *for* administrators, as well as data to employees *from* administrators.

Performance appraisals have been increasingly used to communicate and inculcate an organization's values to employees. An appraisal system can be designed to reflect a company's mission by incorporating performance criteria deemed important to the organization (Park & Huber, 2007). These criteria may be written as specific competencies among employees needed to transform an organization's entire approach to its business (Kalb et al., 2006). Many pharmacy organizations stress a need to improve the quality of the medication use process and increase medication safety as part of their culture. As such, they are incorporating these values into their performance appraisal systems (Heinitz et al., 2018). Community Hospital had not formally reviewed Marcus' performance with him in over 2 years, so if the organization had decided to put more weight on activities related to medication safety in employees' evaluations, this had not yet been communicated, at least not to Marcus Greene.

Productivity of Labor

A principal reason for conducting appraisals is to enhance performance. During the appraisal process, employees should be provided feedback on their strengths and areas of performance that require improvement. Suggestions for improvement may be in reference to general areas of competence or to very specific roles or functions. This feedback, coupled with other components of the appraisal (equitable distribution in rewards and career planning), provides specific goals that an employee may strive to attain in the future. It is said that managers cannot motivate employees, but rather can establish an environment conducive to self-motivation (McConnell, 2010). Thus, a supervisor cannot force or trick employees into being good performers. A well-planned performance appraisal can make employees aware of what they have to do to be judged as good performers and leaves it up to them to strive and achieve these goals.

The feedback and open dialogue present in performance appraisals are valuable to the career planning process. Career planning helps employees formulate personal goals and evaluate strategies for integrating their goals with the goals of the organization. This is important because very few people work in the same jobs their entire career, often changing jobs within one organization and/or changing organizations. When these changes are poorly conceived, both the individual and the organization suffer (Heavner et al., 2016). Career planning informs employees that they are valued enough by their organizations to be considered in their long-range plans. Career planning increasingly has been suggested for use among pharmacy technicians (Desselle & Holmes, 2007) and pharmacists (Gaither et al., 2007). Chapter 17 provides additional detail on career planning.

Employees are more likely to be satisfied with their jobs if they have directed feedback and specific goals for which to aim. It has been shown that satisfaction with the performance appraisal process itself is closely linked to overall job satisfaction (Blau, 1999), which precedes commitment to the employer (Weer & Greenhaus, 2017) and averts costly turnover (Mone & London, 2018). A high level of turnover often leaves an organization temporarily short staffed, which creates even more stress for current employees. It also results in administrators having to invest extra time in recruiting, selecting, and training new employees rather than engaging in activities more productive to the organization. If Community Hospital were to lose Marcus Greene, the operations and productivity of the pharmacy may be impacted in ways that might not be easily remedied. Marcus may have his drawbacks and limitations, as all employees do. However, the performance appraisal process can assist employees in working through those limitations, even leveraging them into strengths with the proper feedback and job structuring. This could create a "win-win" for Community Hospital and for Marcus.

Equity in Rewards

One of the key factors in providing an environment conducive to self-motivation is to distribute rewards equitably. The allocation of rewards (e.g., promotions and salary increases) cannot be arbitrary or even be perceived as arbitrary by staff, as might be the case with Marcus Green in the scenario. Evidence suggests that employees in service organizations, such as pharmacies, who have equitable performance appraisal and reward systems treat customers more fairly (Smith, 2017).

Many performance appraisal systems allow the manager to either rate employees on a given set of attributes or provide them feedback on how they might compare to benchmarks or work standards created by the department or organization. The quantification of performance into a score or ranking creates a foundation from which to base rewards. The culmination of a series of performance appraisals taken over several years can be used as support for recognizing top performers with extraordinary rewards (such as a gift, plaque, or reimbursement for travel to a conference) that exceed annual merit increases.

■ OTHER HUMAN RESOURCE MANAGEMENT (HRM) FUNCTIONS

The performance appraisal process inherently generates data for administrators. Poor performance of a group or an entire unit of personnel may be indicative of poor direction from an immediate supervisor or a lack of adequate resources for employees to perform their jobs. If not stemming from an organizational or systems problem, deficiencies among a significant number of employees could indicate that management has been ineffective in recruiting and selecting employees or perhaps in orientation and training, particularly if the underachieving employees are new hires (see Chapter 17).

Financial Position

Enhanced productivity translates into efficiency and the reduction of labor costs. For example, Community Pharmacy A may be able to dispense 200 prescriptions per day on average with 10 fewer employee hours worked per week than Community Pharmacy

B without any excess stress or burden. The 10 fewer hours is less costly to Pharmacy A and thus enhances profitability. In addition, having well-constructed performance appraisals can save an organization a significant amount of money by avoiding damage awards from litigation brought on by employees in the types of wrongful termination suits described previously. Finally, if the performance appraisal system is effective in holding turnover to a minimum, this saves the organization money that would have been dedicated to recruiting and training new employees.

■ TYPES OF PERFORMANCE APPRAISALS

A variety of performance appraisal systems are in use. These systems are summarized in Table 20-2. Performance appraisal methods are typically categorized into three broad types: absolute, relative, and outcome oriented (Shahzileh & Aghajan, 2015).

Absolute Systems

Absolute systems require the rater to indicate whether or not the employee is meeting a set of predetermined criteria for performance. This usually involves the use of a scale or index. Absolute systems are the most commonly employed of the three types of performance appraisal methods (Rue et al., 2015). The main advantage that absolute systems have over other types of appraisal methods is the feedback that is derived inherently from the process. Allowing employees to see how they are evaluated among criteria deemed important by their organization enables them to learn about their strengths and areas that may require improvement.

There are two types of absolute systems that do *not* employ any sort of scaling procedure. One is the *essay method,* in which the rater responds to a series of brief open-ended questions concerning the employee's performance, such as, "What are the employee's strengths?" and "How does this employee get along with coworkers?" By allowing the rater to include what they think is most valuable; the data can

be richer than those obtained from the use of scales. However, it is more difficult to translate these data into numeric quantities for the purpose of allocating rewards and communicating organizational goals. In addition, differences among raters in their detail and writing abilities can subject the process to charges of bias. A second method, the *critical-incident appraisal,* may mitigate some concerns over subjectivity because it requires that the rater keep a written record of significant incidents (both positive and negative) as they occur. These incidents provide a basis for the evaluation. As mentioned previously, while documentation of certain critical incidents is important, anyway, using this system can serve as the basis for employee discipline and/or protection from litigation. The data are still subject to interpretation, however, and maintaining such detailed records can be cumbersome. Employees who do a "steady" job may complain that this type of evaluation fails to capture their strongest suit.

The *checklist* is one of three types of summated rating scale methods. In a summated rating scale, a rater indicates the employee's level of performance along a list of criteria. The ratings assigned to each criterion are then summed to provide a total score for the employee. With the checklist, the rater simply answers a set of yes/no questions concerning whether or not the employee exhibited certain characteristics. The employee receives a point when the rater assigns an affirmative response to a desirable characteristic or a negative response to an undesirable characteristic. While indicative of specific behaviors and easy for the rater to complete, the checklist ignores levels of performance along each performance criterion. Thus, it is less precise and does not generate as much feedback as other summated scale methods.

The *graphic rating* appraisal, on the other hand, has the rater assess the employee's level of performance on a scale, usually from one to five or one to seven. Some graphic rating scales may include written descriptions along with the numerical ranges. An example of such is given in Table 20-3.

Although it has the advantage of lending greater precision and feedback, the graphic rating appraisal,

Table 20-2.   Performance Appraisals and their Advantages and Disadvantages

System	Brief Description	Advantages	Disadvantages
Absolute			
Essay	Rater prepares a written statement describing the employee's strengths and weaknesses	May provide rich data	Differences across raters, lack of objectivity
Critical incident	Rater maintains a record of incidents indicative of both positive and negative behaviors of the employee	Derived from documented data	Burdensome and subject to interpretation
Checklist	Rater answers with a yes or a no to a series of questions about the employee's behavior	Easy to complete, indicative of specific behaviors	Less precision
Graphic rating	Rater indicates various employee traits and behaviors on a scale	Often based on trait measures	Leniency, central tendency, use of traits
Behaviorally anchored rating scales	Rater employs highly descriptive scales to indicate employee's tendency to demonstrate desirable behaviors	Quantitative, conducive to supplying feedback	Central tendency, burdensome
360-degree feedback	Employees rate themselves, and comparisons are made with ratings by various stakeholders	Multiple points of view, facilitates reflection	Very time consuming, subject to role conflict
Forced choice	Rater ranks a set of statements describing the employee's performance	Mitigates bias	Irksome to raters, feedback is challenging
Relative			
Alternation ranking	Rater selects most and least valued employee from remaining pools of employees	Eliminates leniency and central tendency	Limited feedback, perceptions of bias
Paired comparisons	Each employee is compared with every other employee one at a time on each criterion	May appear to be less subjective than alternation ranking	Limited feedback
Forced distribution	Rater categorizes employees into one of three groups according to how well they meet expectations tendency	Eliminated leniency and central tendency	Limited feedback, skewing
Outcome Oriented			
Management by objectives	Rater establishes goals for the employee to achieve during the next period, and employee is evaluated on his/her success	Highly participatory and incentive driven	Employees evaluated by different standards
Work standards approach	Rater sets a standard or an expected level of output and compares each employee's performance to the standard	Evaluation is more standardized	Standards may be viewed as unfair

Table 20-3.   Sample Items on a Graphic Rating Scale Evaluation Form

Quantity of work—the amount of work an employee does in a workday

Does not meet minimum requirements	Does just enough to get by	Volume of work is satisfactory	Very industrious, does more than is required	Has a superior work production record

Dependability—the ability to do required jobs well with a minimum of supervision

Requires close supervision; is unreliable	Sometimes requires prompting	Usually completes necessary tasks with reasonable promptness	Requires little supervision; is reliable	Requires absolute minimum of supervision

Job knowledge—information an employee should have on work duties for satisfactory job performance

Is poorly informed about work duties	Lacks knowledge of some phases of job	Is moderately informed; can answer most questions about the job	Understands all phases of job	Has complete mastery of all phases of job

Attendance—faithfulness in coming to work daily and conforming to work hours

Is often absent without good excuse or frequently reports for work late, or both	Is lax in attendance, or reporting for work on time, or both	Is usually present and on time	Is very prompt, regular in attendance	Is always regular and prompt; volunteers for overtime when needed

Accuracy—the correctness of work duties performed

Makes frequent errors	Careless, often makes errors	Usually accurate, makes only average number of mistakes	Requires little supervision; is exact and precise most of the time	Requires absolute minimum of supervision

Adapted with permission from Byars LL, Rue L: *Human Resource Management*, 6th ed. New York: McGraw-Hill; 2000.

like many absolute systems, is prone to rater biases. One is *central tendency*, which occurs when the rater appraises everyone at or near the median of the scale or rates everyone similarly for fear of causing angst or feelings of injustice among employees. With *leniency*, the rater not only judges each employee similarly but also rates each on the high end of the performance scale. Leniency is common in many appraisal systems. Raters might inflate their ratings more for low performers than for others because they believe this will help achieve harmony and boost morale. The primary reasons identified were under the auspices of achieving harmony and boosting motivation. However, this can backfire. If better performers believe that they are not being recognized accordingly for their efforts, then the result can be more disharmony. This might be a component of what is going on with the case of Marcus Greene.

Some graphic rating appraisals may consist mostly of traits as criteria rather than particular performance indicants. While traits may manifest into certain behaviors, they are innately part of every person's character. To this end, managers should avoid evaluating an employee on characteristics such as appearance, knowledge, or friendliness without specifying how this translates into actual performance. The *halo effect* occurs when a rater allows a single prominent characteristic of an employee to influence her judgment on each separate item in the appraisal. For example, a pharmacy technician who is very friendly may be rated more highly on performance than someone not as outwardly amicable, despite the latter outperforming the technician on other aspects of the job. While the halo effect can be problematic for any type of appraisal system, it can be especially problematic when traits are used in a graphic rating scale. In the scenario, Susan Bostik might not be favored overtly; however, she could be the beneficiary of some halo effect originating from her pleasant demeanor.

There is growing research on rater biases in employee performance appraisal. Back in 2000, Scullen et al. conducted a thorough evaluation of job performance ratings. They found leniency to be prevalent but even more so the halo effect. Specifically, when peers are asked to rate one another (as part of a 360-degree or some other procedure discussed later in the chapter) and when peers are asked to rate their bosses, the halo effect was even more prominent than leniency. That is, the rater takes a particular characteristic they really like or dislike about the ratee, which clouds all other judgments, or aspects of their performance. It was observed that while biases exist at all levels, gaining input from various sources in evaluating someone was deemed more accurate than with one rater doing so. Even while the halo and other effects when very problematic can almost obviate a good evaluation system, research has indicated that professionals should turn to standards administered by professional organizations to assist in developing appropriate criteria that minimize bias (Weenink et al., 2017). An example of this is the Oath of a Pharmacist, which encompasses topics such as maintaining relevant knowledge and skills, protecting personal and health information, and adhering to high moral, ethical, and legal standards (American Association of Colleges of Pharmacy,

2008). Another study demonstrated cultural biases at play with the halo effect, and how these can be mitigated to some degree with multisource ratings and flatter versus more hierarchical organizational structures (Ng et al., 2011).

The *behavior-anchored rating scale* (BARS) method of performance appraisal is designed more specifically to assess behaviors necessary for successful performance. Most BARS methods use the term *job dimension* to mean those broad categories of duties and responsibilities that make up a job, requiring development of unique scales for each dimension. Managers often develop BARS in collaboration with employees well versed in the responsibilities that comprise the dimensions of job performance. An example of how a BARS may look for a community pharmacy clerk in dealing with patients is illustrated in Table 20-4. The BARS system lends itself to providing quality feedback, particularly if supplemented with qualitative comments on how to improve. A drawback is the time and effort required to develop an effective BARS appraisal; however, evidence suggests BARS to be effective in rating both clinical behaviors (Smith et al., 2011) and quite especially for "non-technical" or soft skills such as caring and customer service (Watkins et al., 2014).

More common to larger organizations than community or institutional pharmacies, *360-degree feedback,* also known as *multi-rater assessment,* involves the use of a summated rating scale or brief closed-ended questions requiring the employee to rate himself and compare these ratings with those afforded to him by supervisors, peers, customers, patients, suppliers, and/ or colleagues on a similar instrument. This mitigates an employee's concern that one particular rater may be biased against him, and engenders a degree of reflection by any employee who receives feedback from so many points of view. Moreover, supervisors are relieved from being the only party to evaluate performance, as they learn from other evaluators in the process, particularly about contributions that may not be evident during their interactions with the employee. Employees may also be more accepting of negative feedback when it is consistent among multiple raters

Table 20-4.   Example of a Behaviorally Anchored Rating Scale for "Providing Customer Service" in a Community Pharmacy

Scale	Values	Anchors
1	Poor	Does not interact well with customers, who frequently complain about the employee; employee instigates conflict with customers.
2	Below average	Courtesy is inconsistent; is not responsive to customer needs.
3	Average	Is polite and friendly with customers but lacks creativity in meeting customer needs.
4	Above average	Is polite, friendly, and professional in dealing with customers; is adept at meeting customer needs and strives to improve in this area.
5	Excellent	Has managed to develop a bond with customers, who anticipate coming to the pharmacy and interacting with this employee; is innovative in creating ways to satisfy customers.

(Campion et al., 2015). Aside from the time it takes to gather and collate all of the data used in 360-degree feedback, another disadvantage from the employee's point of view is the role conflict that may arise owing to differing demands placed by various stakeholders in the process. This problem is further exacerbated when there is a lack of inter-rater reliability among evaluators, as is often the case in many organizations (Cormack et al., 2018). Increasing the number of raters can increase the reliability of 360-degree feedback (Campion et al., 2015). It also assists with maintaining anonymity of the raters, which has been found to be helpful and appreciated (Castanelli & Kitto, 2006). In health care specifically, the use of 360-degree feedback systems have been associated with leadership development due to their promotion of self-awareness and emotional intelligence (Gregory et al., 2018) and for enhancing the performance of interprofessional teams (Kamangar et al., 2015).

Another type of absolute method that seeks to mitigate bias or perceptions of bias is *forced-choice rating*. Forced-choice rating is used more often in larger organizations with formal human resources departments. With this method, the rater is presented with a set of statements that describe potentially how the employee might be performing on the job and ranks each statement on how well it describes that employee's behavior. The weights

and scoring, known and performed by the human resources department, are unknown to the rater. An example is given in Table 20-5.

Relative Systems

Rather than requiring the rater to evaluate employees on a predetermined set of characteristics or standards,

Table 20-5.   Sample Set of Statements in a Forced-Choice Rating Scale

Instructions: Rank the following statements according to how they describe the manner in which this employee carries out duties and responsibilities. Rank 1 should be given to the most descriptive and rank 5 to the least descriptive. No ties are allowed.

Rank	Description
_____	Is easy to get acquainted with
_____	Places great emphasis on people
_____	Refuses to accept criticism
_____	Thinks generally in terms of money
_____	Makes decisions quickly

Adapted with permission from Byars LL, Rue L: *Human Resource Management*, 6th ed. New York: McGraw-Hill; 2000.

relative systems require the manager to make comparisons among employees. Relative systems have an advantage over absolute systems in that central tendency and leniency effects are minimized. The likelihood of the halo effect occurring is also reduced. The fact that employees are pitted against one another, so to speak, makes it easier to base organizational rewards on merit. Moreover, social comparison theory implies that it may be more efficacious for raters to compare an employee to other employees rather than use absolute rating standards, and some research suggests that certain types of relative systems showed greater validity and precision over absolute systems (Goffin et al., 2009). It has been shown that relative measures induce raters to consider social comparison information and behavioral information when making their responses more than absolute measures, which might be problematic, but yet shows higher correlations of accuracy with relevant criteria (Olson et al., 2007).

Relative systems have a significant drawback in that they do not generate substantive feedback to employees. If, for example, an employee is rated below two-thirds of her colleagues on overall performance, what does this mean to the employee? What behaviors are being demonstrated that resulted in this ranking? What behaviors could be demonstrated that would result in improved performance and a higher ranking during the next evaluation? This adds to the manager's challenge of establishing an environment for employee self-motivation. An employee may be performing well but still ranked below a majority of colleagues, and vice versa. These are among the reasons that these types of performance evaluations are undergoing scrutiny and various mutations. While relative systems inform employees where they stand in comparison to the whole of their colleagues in a department or in an organization, it should be kept in mind that generally the rankings of each employee are not made public. Rather, each employee is made aware of their performance in comparison to a selected group, as a whole, on certain indicators or benchmarks.

Three types of relative performance appraisal systems are used. One is called *alternation ranking,* a method in which the rater chooses the most and least valuable persons from a list of employees with similar jobs. Both names are crossed off, and then the procedure is repeated until every employee on the list has been ranked. With its ability to eliminate central tendency and leniency and with its ease of implementation, alternation ranking may appear appealing. However, aside from its failure to generate feedback, the halo effect could come into play. Moreover, employees may be concerned with the potential for bias and inaccuracy by the evaluator, especially when criteria for performance have not been delineated clearly.

The method of *paired comparisons* has the rater comparing each employee against every other employee, one by one, on either specific aspects of performance or on overall performance. During each comparison, the rater places a checkmark by the name of the employee who was considered to have performed better. The employee with the most checkmarks is considered to be the best performer. While more precise and perhaps seemingly less ambiguous to employees, paired comparisons still may fail to generate substantive feedback and is more burdensome to implement than other relative systems.

The *forced distribution* method requires the rater to compare the performance of employees and place a certain percentage of them into various groupings. It assumes that the performance level in a group of employees will be distributed according to a bell-shaped or normal distribution curve. While lending itself well to the allocation of organizational rewards, levels of actual performance may be skewed by forcing their distribution into a bell-shaped curve, ignoring the possibility that perhaps most or all employees are performing well or performing poorly. Forced distribution, as well as other relative systems, may fail to demonstrate system deficiencies that can be improved by management.

As previously mentioned, absolute systems have strengths, but also limitations. The lack of feedback was discussed, but there are additional drawbacks. While the exact rankings of employees are not (at least should not be) publicly aired, the inherent "competition" could spur uncollegial behaviors (e.g., taking credit for someone else's work) and an overly competitive culture, which can be bad for morale.

Outcome-Oriented Systems

Where absolute and relative systems focus on behaviors, outcome-oriented systems are concerned with evaluating end results. These systems involve setting quantifiable goals for the succeeding period, to be followed with a performance review at its conclusion. Outcome-oriented systems can be used to generate feedback, but equity issues arise because rewards are allocated according to how well goals are met, and employees with similar jobs may receive substantially different sets of goals and expectations for performance. Because these systems are used more frequently for persons in autonomous positions (e.g., attorneys, college professors, pharmacists), flexibility has to be built in to allow for contingencies that resulted in an employee changing his goals or not being able to meet them. On the other hand, an employee can always come up with excuses as to why certain goals were not met.

The most commonly employed type of outcome-oriented system is *management by objectives* (MBO), also known as *results management, performance management,* and *work planning and review.* The MBO process typically consists of six steps (Rue et al., 2015):

1. Establishing clear and precisely defined statements of objectives for the work to be done by an employee.
2. Developing an action plan indicating how these objectives will be accomplished.
3. Allowing the employee to implement the action plan.
4. Measuring objective achievement.
5. Taking corrective action when necessary.
6. Establishing new objectives for the future.

The establishment of objectives is critical to the success of MBO. The objectives must be challenging but attainable. They should be expressed in terms that are objective and measurable and should be written in clear, concise, unambiguous language. Table 20-6 presents examples of how some poorly stated objectives for pharmacists might be better stated. It is important

Table 20-6.	Examples of How to Improve Work Objectives in Pharmacy
Poor:	To maximize the number of prescriptions dispensed
Better:	To increase the average daily prescription volume by 10% at the end of the year
Poor:	To make as few dispensing errors as possible
Better:	To commit no dispensing errors that result in an untoward event during the next 6 months
Poor:	To get all medications up to the floors more quickly
Better:	To get unit-dose medications to the floors within 30 minutes after the order arrives to the pharmacy
Poor:	To make sure that nurses are happy with the clinical services you provide
Better:	To achieve a mean score of at least 80 out of 100 on a survey measuring nurses' satisfaction with the clinical services provided

that the objectives be derived through collaboration and consent of the employee. In this respect, the objectives and action plan can serve as a basis for regular discussions between the manager and the employee.

A concern of MBO is the potential incongruence among the goals and objectives of employees with similar jobs, especially when it comes to allocating organizational rewards. One study confirmed that when using such an approach, persons with higher accountability come under more intense scrutiny during performance evaluations (Roch & McNall, 2007). Other research shows the importance of feedback, and attribution of the feedback to factors within the employee's control to improve self-efficacy, which in turn can assist her with creating more accurate, yet cautiously ambitious goals (Tolli & Schmidt, 2008).

While shortcomings of an MBO system can be overcome to some degree by basing the rewards on the outcomes themselves, use of another method, the *work standards approach,* can further mitigate the problem. The work standards approach is a form of goal setting in which each employee is compared with some sort of standard or an expected level of output. In other words, the objectives are the same or similar for each employee in the group. Without as much input from each employee, however, the standards established may be viewed as unfair, and employees may not have as much incentive to strive to attain them.

■ SPECIAL CONSIDERATIONS FOR APPRAISAL SYSTEMS IN PHARMACY

A community pharmacy is typically a for-profit organization that must be concerned with its financial position to remain solvent over the long term. Community pharmacies also must conduct their business in an ethical manner. Moreover, it can hardly be argued that pharmacists and support personnel must practice altruism, putting patients ahead of personal motives (Roth & Zlatic, 2009). Like any organization, a pharmacy will be more likely to achieve its goals when its employees derive gratification from performing their jobs. The pharmacy profession has experienced numerous environmental changes that affect the work experiences of pharmacy personnel. These include higher prescription volumes, greater complexity in payment reform, increasing professional emphasis on patient-centered care, and implementation of automated dispensing technologies (Gaither et al., 2015). These trends behoove pharmacy managers to take special care in developing effective performance appraisal systems. One first has to determine whether a similar performance appraisal should exist among technicians and pharmacists working within the same organization. Certain similarities in the jobs of pharmacists and support personnel exist. In addition, there are certain values (e.g., dependability, dedication, altruism) that the organization may want to assess in all its employees regardless of their position or status. There are, however, certain aspects of

pharmacists' jobs and those of support personnel that may call for alternative systems or at least different components of a similar system. Most notable of these is the level of autonomy and responsibility they share.

Considerations for Support Personnel

A pharmacy organization's effectiveness is often linked to the productivity of its technicians and other support personnel. Pharmacy technicians, for example, are now beginning to take responsibility for more nonclinical functions, including drug preparation, order entry, and managing pharmacy informatics (Desselle & Holmes, 2017; Gernant, 2018). Some states have adopted tech-check-tech programs whereby the filling accuracy is checked by a technician rather than a pharmacist (Adams et al., 2011), and there have also been reports about expanded technician roles in the delivery of medication reconciliation (Sen et al., 2014). The profession has recognized the need for thorough job descriptions, training manuals, equitable pay, and productivity-monitoring systems among pharmacy support personnel (Mattingly & Mattingly, 2018). More on performance appraisal and other aspects of technician supervision can be found in Chapter 19.

Considerations for Pharmacists

Evaluating pharmacist performance may be more challenging than evaluating technician performance because of pharmacists' greater levels of autonomy and responsibility. This may be further compounded by the presence of disparate roles various pharmacists may play within an organization and an emphasis on more direct patient care activities such as comprehensive medication management and disease state management. It may be fruitful to gather information from customers, including patients and other health care professionals, when evaluating pharmacists for the services they provide. This may be accomplished through informal feedback, surveys, or even through critical incidents appraisal previously described. While it is beyond the scope of this chapter to describe them in detail, a few types of performance appraisal systems have been suggested for pharmacists, particularly those whose responsibilities are more clinical in nature (Schumock et al., 1990; Young, et al., 2018). These systems are usually the result of a job analysis for pharmacists in a particular organization and that which go even further than desired behaviors in general (e.g., providing high quality patient service, providing proper oversight to medication distribution processes), but enumerate specific responsibilities that pharmacists are involved. For example, in one organization a pharmacist might have responsibility over several tasks related to an opioid misuse reduction program or an immunization service. In these cases, some employers have begun including these areas more specific to the pharmacist's job in the performance appraisal process.

Other Types of Bias to Consider

In addition to various biases discussed earlier in this chapter, there are evaluator discrepancies that could arise due to race/ethnicity and gender and intergenerational dynamics also come into play. While each individual is unique, certain values emanating from major events occurring during development years permeate each generation, and thus can become a source of conflict, or rater bias. The rater must be culturally competent and trained in various facets of conducting performance evaluations. The chapter scenario does not provide the ages of those employed; however, there could very well be intergenerational or other dynamics at play when considering the different values placed by employees on different aspects, or components of performance. Unless the organization communicates what it values most, there will be misconceptions and battle lines drawn between employees with competing values.

■ THE FUTURE OF PERFORMANCE APPRAISAL SYSTEMS

While the debate between the advantages and disadvantages of various systems will likely continue for some time, there are some trends worth noting. More organizations are seeking a wider array of input to make more accurate assessments of employee performance and provide more ample feedback to improve patient outcomes, such as 360-degree mechanisms to improve patient satisfaction (Hageman et al., 2015). Employees have expressed favorability toward systems with high differentiation of rewards, frequent feedback, and large comparison groups (Blume et al., 2009). Using an absolute system, anonymity is all but lost as the comparison groups grow smaller. When rater teams are used, and they are required to reach a consensus, greater accuracy is manifest in part from rater motivations being negated (Roch, 2007).

Another issue widely agreed upon is the need for specific and additional training for raters, or those evaluating and motivating the performance of others. One study demonstrated that even in the presence of less behaviorally oriented or more vague job dimensions performance measures, raters can overcome bias and subjectivity with the proper training (Roch et al., 2009). There is additional evidence to suggest that at least some personality-related cues and traits can be evaluated more precisely with the proper training (Powell & Goffin, 2009). Also important in this process is training rates, as organizations continue to identify means of enhancing both rater and ratee reactions to the appraisal system (MacDonald & Sulsky, 2009). Organizations are continually seeking ways to improve the process, and one method currently being evaluated and implemented in some organizations is a reflection component by the employee shortly after the formal review process (Anseel et al., 2009). A more direct form of training for raters is frame-of-reference training, which separates what is considered good organizational citizenship behaviors by employees from more specific behaviors to be evaluated. Frame-of-reference training also provides effectiveness levels of alternative behaviors in comparison to those most desired and thus increases accuracy in evaluations (Uggerslev & Sulsky, 2008).

It should be noted that the trends in performance appraisal systems are finally catching up with other aspects of management. For example, many are advocating a QI model of performance appraisal system rather than a quality assurance (QA) system (Edwards, 2009). In the traditional QA model, performance was judged to be effective or ineffective, and either reme-diation or punishment is offered to poor performers. In the QI model, the performance appraisal system is viewed as one tool to shift the curve of performance for an entire department or organization upward. This concept is commensurate with the aforemen-tioned goals in frame-of-reference training and with the ideals of continuous QI in operations manage-ment described in Chapter 10.

THE PERFORMANCE APPRAISAL INTERVIEW

Regardless of the type of system selected, the written appraisal should be accompanied by a formal inter-view of the employee. It is during the interview that the results of the written appraisal are discussed. The success of the performance appraisal hinges signifi-cantly on the interview. Some of the same biases that manifest in evaluations of performance can also arise in the interview itself. Research has shown that posi-tive feedback can adversely affect those with poor self-image and vice-versa (Budnick et al., 2015). It cannot be expected of the interviewer to be entirely adept at social psychology, but it would be wise of them to understand in general how different employ-ees could react under stressful circumstances and be prepared with situational leadership as needed (see Chapter 3). If the supervisor is mindful of taking a few precautionary steps and follows some helpful guidelines, most appraisal interviews will come off without a hitch.

Preparing the Employee for the Interview

An appointment should be made with the employee well in advance, at least 3 to 4 weeks. The employee should be provided with a copy of the position description and corresponding performance stand-ards, a copy of the evaluation form used in the appraisal process, a copy of the report of the previous formal review, departmental/organizational objectives for the current and subsequent year, and instructions on how to prepare for the meeting. The employee may be instructed to prepare comments on how well objectives set during the last review were met and to prepare a list of new objectives. The employee may also be asked to discuss what she considers her most valuable contribution to the organization to be since the last review, barriers to her achieving current goals, and what the organization or supervisor can do to facilitate her progress (McConnell, 2010). In some organizations, employees are asked to complete a self-evaluation on an instrument similar to the one used by the employer. This may help identify gaps in per-ceptions of effectiveness in certain areas and reinforce strengths and limitations in others.

Planning for the Interview

The supervisor should enter the interview well informed of prior appraisals and be intimately famil-iar with the responsibilities of the employee's job. The supervisor should also have appropriate documenta-tion and evidence to support claims of the employee's performance, particularly in areas of deficiency but also in areas of strength. To prepare for the interview, the supervisor should have answered the following questions (Rue et al., 2015):

1. What results should the interview achieve?
2. What good contributions is the employee making?
3. Is the employee working up to his potential?
4. Is the employee clear about the organization's per-formance expectations?
5. What strengths does the employee have that can be built on or improved?
6. Is there any additional training available that can help the employee improve?

Conducting the Interview

The interview should be conducted in the following sequence: (1) review and update the position descrip-tion and performance standards, (2) discuss the per-formance ratings assigned to the employee using the prescribed appraisal form, (3) highlight strengths and accomplishments since the previous appraisal,

(4) discuss objectives that were not reached since the previous review, and (5) discuss future performance and assist with career planning.

Supervisors should establish a comfortable, professional atmosphere and maintain a positive tone when conducting the interview. They should be careful not to stereotype or prejudge employees. There may be occasions in which the rater simply does not like the person whom she is evaluating but must be careful to remain focused on the relevant behaviors and performance. Nonetheless, circumstances will arise in which the supervisor has to address performance deficiencies with an employee. Some suggestions for addressing these situations are as follows (McConnell, 2010, p. 233):

- Limit criticism to one or two major problems. Do not search for significant problem areas when none exist.
- Reserve critical remarks until after some of the positives have been accentuated.
- Maintain open dialogue with the employee. Offer the employee opportunities for self-criticism and to accentuate positive contributions and citizenship behaviors to the organization and to peers. Allow the employee to offer how performance can be improved, including perceived need for support and/or other types of resources from the organization along with a time frame for how performance (even entire departmental performance) can be improved.
- Avoid the use of terms that potentially could be misconstrued, such as *attitude, work ethic, professionalism,* and *weakness.*

Remain firm but supportive. Use assertiveness skills by reinforcing points of agreement, handling disagreements diplomatically, and avoiding defensiveness.

The interview should be concluded with an expression of confidence that the employee will be able to meet the new objectives. The supervisor also should thank the employee for her time spent in the interview and for her contributions to the organization.

■ ENSURING VALID RESULTS FROM THE PERFORMANCE APPRAISAL SYSTEM

A pharmacy manager must carefully consider the advantages and drawbacks of each type of appraisal system. Aside from those specifically designed for pharmacy organizations described in this chapter, the prevailing consensus among employers is that summated rating scales, particularly derivations of BARS methods, are the best systems to employ. Regardless of the type of system selected, managers must be mindful of ensuring that the system is reliable and valid and is helping the organization to achieve its objectives. *Reliability* is another word for consistency, inferring that the system produces similar results in multiple iterations. For example, given a certain employee's level of performance, any rater should view the performance similarly. If a system is unreliable, then it cannot be valid. *Validity* implies that the system is measuring what it purports to measure.

Implementing the System

A primary consideration when implementing a system is how frequently to conduct the formal appraisal. Rating periods usually are annual, either on the employee's anniversary of hire date or during a rating period in which all employees are evaluated, the latter of which is easier to implement. Evidence suggests, however, that better results are obtained from more frequent evaluations, such as semiannually or quarterly (Martin & Bartol, 1998). Everyone in the organization should be well informed about the role each person plays in the appraisal process and how the appraisal results are used.

Monitoring the System

The effectiveness of the appraisal system itself should be monitored (Somon et al., 2017). Certain indicators can be helpful, including the quality of performance standards, effective use of appraisal results, tracking of the raters, and elimination of adverse impact. *Quality of performance standards* refers to the standards being specific, challenging, realistic, dynamic, understandable, and consistent with organizational goals. *Use of performance appraisal results* refers to how well these results are tied with rewards and recognition and to what extent the appraisal process has contributed to improved performance among all employees. Tracking the raters consists of reviewing the ratings awarded by individual raters and giving them feedback concerning the quality of their ratings, which may be overly stringent, lenient, or biased in some way in comparison with other raters. *Adverse impact* refers to a performance appraisal system whose use results in significantly lower ratings for members of any protected group described previously.

■ PERFORMANCE AND ORGANIZATIONAL REWARDS

Organizational rewards consist of both intrinsic rewards (those internal to the individual and derived from involvement in the job, such as achievement, feelings of accomplishment, informal recognition, satisfaction, and status) and extrinsic rewards (those controlled and distributed by the organization, such as formal recognition, incentive pay, fringe benefits, and promotions). Proper allocation of both is critical for varied reasons. Evidence rejects a popular view that satisfaction leads to performance (Rue et al., 2015). It does suggest, however, that (1) rewards based on current performance enhance subsequent performance and (2) job dissatisfaction leads to turnover, absenteeism, tardiness, accidents, grievances, and strikes. Research also supports the notion that while extrinsic rewards do not in themselves cause satisfaction, perceived deficiencies or inequities can result in dissatisfaction among employees (Tunji-Olayeni et al., 2018). A national survey of chain and independent pharmacists found that pharmacists had low levels of satisfaction with recognition from supervisors, including getting a promotion or pay raise based on performance. This was important because their satisfaction

was correlated with their intention to look for a new position (Munger et al., 2013).

In addressing employees' base and merit pay, managers must consider internal, external, and individual equity. Internal equity concerns what an employee is being paid for doing a job compared with what other employees in the same organization are being paid to do their jobs. External equity concerns what employees in an organization are being paid compared with employees in other organizations performing similar jobs. Individual equity addresses the rewarding of individual contributions and is related closely to linking pay with performance. Internal and external equity are factors considered more in determining base wage and fringe benefits, or those rewards are based merely on employment and seniority with an organization. Pharmacy managers must ensure that pharmacist and support staff salaries and benefits (e.g., vacation, paid holidays, health insurance, child care, and pension plans) are competitive with those offered in similar pharmacy settings and even other types of pharmacy settings in the region.

Managers also must address individual equity and allocate certain rewards (pay increases, promotions, and formal recognition) in a manner that corresponds with the right types of behaviors. Such behaviors include but are not limited to working extra hours when required, volunteering for unenviable tasks or assignments, substituting for others willingly, and pleasing customers. More specifically, rewarding behaviors listed and evaluated in the performance appraisal system eliminates ambiguity about what constitutes good performance. Other suggestions for allocating rewards are as follows (Rue et al., 2015):

- *Consider the presence of performance constraints.* The employee's performance should not be hampered by things beyond his control.
- *Provide a clear distinction between cost-of-living, seniority, and merit pay increases.*
- *Enlist trust among employees.* Similarly, employees should not be misled into thinking that their rewards were based on merit, only to find out later

that the increases were across the board. This could result in distrust and dissatisfaction.

- *Make merit pay substantial.* While operating within the organization's budget, merit pay has to be worthwhile. Employees will not appreciate being evaluated very highly and praised only to see very small pay increases as a result.
- *Be flexible in scheduling rewards.* It is easier to establish a credible pay-for-performance plan if all employees do not receive pay adjustments on the same date.
- *Effectively communicate merit and total pay policy to employees.* In addition, do not prohibit employees from discussing pay because this may be a violation of the National Labor Relations Act.

There are detractors to using performance appraisals as a means to allocate rewards. It has been suggested that appraisals used in this way create "winners" and "losers," ultimately, a zero-sum game for an organization, which should not use systems to make miniscule distinctions in pay adjustments (Kennedy & Dresser, 2001). Monetary rewards are said to work best when completely unanticipated by the employee, rather than based upon the appraisal feedback. Moreover, while managers' ability to reward with pay is limited, there are no such constraints on other forms of recognition.

■ MOTIVATION AND OTHER REWARDS NOT TIED TO BASE PAY

Chapters 3, 16, and 17 discuss motivation of employees through leadership and support. Support by the supervisor goes a long way toward keeping employees satisfied. In fact, supervisor and organizational support has proved to be an effective deterrent to pharmacists' uncertainty about their future in an organization and a buffer against the stress that accompanies work (Desselle & Tipton, 2001). Pharmacy managers should also keep this in mind when dealing with support personnel. Managers may believe that support personnel do not value intrinsic rewards, but this is certainly not true. Managers should be cognizant of the desire for autonomy and personal growth by all employees.

Informal Feedback: Providing Consistent, Constructive Criticism and Giving Praise

Support from supervisors need not be confined to the formal appraisal period. Informal feedback should be rendered on a consistent basis. Not only is feedback helpful in improving performance, employees have several motives for seeking feedback, including reduction of uncertainty, goal achievement, protection of ego, self-esteem, and desire to be responsive (Anseel et al., 2007). Employees should be instructed immediately when they demonstrate behaviors detrimental to the organization or if they are not performing to standards, as long as it is done in a professional manner. For example, the supervisor should never criticize an employee in the presence of others. Offering praise to an employee for a job well done should be done in public, however, as long as the employee truly deserves such praise, the praise is not overdone, and it is not overly repetitive (Swift & Peterson, 2018). Supervisors also should consider following up praise with an official memo and boasting of the employee to colleagues so that it may get back to her indirectly. Other suggestions include complimenting the employee as soon as possible after the behavior, addressing the person by name when giving praise, complimenting a specific action, and explaining why the action being praised was important to you and the organization (Byers, 2010).

Supervisors should avail themselves of opportunities to provide performance feedback whenever possible. Seldom should either laudatory or critical comments during the formal appraisal process come as much of a surprise to employees. Supervisors can seek training on how to provide consistent and continuous feedback without giving employees the impression that they are losing autonomy. When the supervisor handles these situations deftly and develops a positive relationship with the employee, the latter will have a positive reaction toward any type of feedback and are more likely to believe that the organization is promoting fairness among its employees (Feys et al., 2008).

Other Benefits

Pharmacy managers may consider the use of other strategies to recognize and reward good performers:

- Offer to pay for attendance at local continuing education programs.
- Provide funding for attendance at national conferences.
- Offer to offset the cost of professional recognition and certification processes for pharmacists and technicians.
- Fund membership in a professional association.
- Buy lunch.
- Allow someone to represent you at an important meeting.
- Assign tasks with greater levels of responsibility if the employee is ready to handle them.

■ REVISITING THE SCENARIO

Administrators may consider the fact that Marcus has made more errors than other technicians to be of greater consequence than his promptness and vigorous effort. Marcus may contend that a greater frequency of errors is bound to occur as a result of him filling a greater number of medication orders. The technicians may not be clear on who is responsible for certain tasks. Pharmacy staff may be concerned that management plays favorites among the employees. Overall, it would appear as though Community Hospital does not have a formal system of evaluation in place, or at least is not abiding by it. This is problematic for all the reasons discussed throughout the chapter.

Marcus is confused and frustrated for having seldom been evaluated formally. Has management avoided subsequent appraisals because the last one did not run so smoothly? Has this been the case with other employees as well? None of these questions is necessarily an indictment of management at Community Hospital pharmacy because there is much

information not known in the scenario. However, best human resources practices tell us that all employees at the pharmacy should be evaluated formally at least once a year, informed of behaviors that are viewed as desirable, instructed on how they may improve performance, and shown how various aspects of performance translate into the allocation of organizational rewards.

■ CONCLUSION

Supervisors often view performance appraisals as an undesirable task, but careful planning and implementation should make them less onerous. Performance appraisals are closely linked to employee motivation, performance, commitment, and turnover. Numerous

■ QUESTIONS FOR FURTHER DISCUSSION

1. What types of skills do you think are necessary for selecting and implementing a performance appraisal system? What about for conducting an appraisal interview?
2. How would you feel about having responsibility for determining whether or not an employee will receive merit pay?
3. Has your performance ever been assessed formally at a job? How was that experience? What do you think the supervisor could have done better when assessing your performance?
4. How would you react if you were told that your performance was not measuring up to the expectations of an organization?
5. Does everyone with similar jobs in a pharmacy deserve the same level of pay raises, or should they be based more on performance?
6. Do you know anyone who has left a job because, in part, of the kinds of issues raised in the chapter scenario?

systems are available, each of which has its strengths and drawbacks. The formal appraisal must be accompanied by frequent and substantive informal feedback. The appraisal interview is the key to the success of the appraisal system. The allocation of organizational rewards must be linked closely to the results of the appraisal process.

REFERENCES

Adams AJ, Martin SJ, Stolpe SF. 2011. "Tech-check-tech": A review of its safety and benefits. *Am J Health Syst Pharm* 68:1824.

Akomolafe S. 2013. The invisible minority: Revisiting the debate of foreighn-accented speakers upward mobility in the workpace. *J Cultural Diversity* 20:7.

American Association of Colleges of Pharmacy. *Oath of a Pharmacist*. 2008. Available at https://www.aacp.org/sites/default/files/oathofapharmacist2008-09.pdf. Accessed December 31, 2018.

Anseel F, Lieens F, Levy PE. 2007. A self-motives perspective on feedback-seeking behavior: Linking organizational behavior and social psychology research. *Intl J Manage Reviews* 9:211.

Anseel F, Lievens F, Schollaert E. 2009. Reflection as a strategy to enhance task performance after feedback. *Org Behav Hum Decision Processes* 110:35.

Blackwell S, Szeinbach S, Garner D, Smith M. 1996. Legal issues in personnel management. *Drug Top* 140:74.

Blau G. 1999. Testing the longitudinal impact of work variables and performance appraisal satisfaction on subsequent overall job satisfaction. *Hum Relat* 52:1099.

Blume BD, Baldwin TT, Rubin RS. 2009. Reactions to different types of forced distribution performance evaluation systems. *J Bus Psychol* 24:91.

Broedel-Zaugg K, Shaffer V, Mawer M, Sullivan D. 1999. Frequency and severity of sexual harassment in pharmacy practice in Ohio. *J Am Pharm Assoc* 39:677.

Bowling NA, Khazon S, Alarcon GM, et al. 2017. Building better measures of role ambiguity and role conflict: The validation of new stressor scales. *Work Stress* 31:1.

Brown M, Hyatt D, Benson J. 2010. Consequences of the performance appraisal system. *Pers Rev* 39:396.

Budnick CJ, Kowal M, Santuzzi AM. 2015. Social anxiety and the ironic effects of positive interviewer feedback. *Anxiety Stress Coping* 28:71.

Byers M. 2010. Nicely done! The power of genuine compliments. *J Mich Dental Assoc* 92:26.

Campion MC, Campion ED, Campion MA. 2015. Improvements in performance management through the use of 360 degree feedback. *Ind Org Psychol* 8:85.

Cappelli P, Conyon MJ. 2018. What do performance appraisals do? *Industr Labor Relations Rev* 71:88.

Castanelli D, Kitto S. 2006. Perceptions, attitudes, and beliefs of staff anaesthetists related to multi-source feedback used for their performance appraisal. *Nurs Manag* 14:356.

Cormack CL, Jensen E, Durham CO, Smith G, Dumas B. 2018. The 360-degree evaluation model: A method for assessing competency in graduate nursing students: A pilot study. *Nurse Educ Today* 64:132.

Desselle SP, Holmes ER. 2007. A structural model of CPhTs' job satisfaction and career commitment. *J Am Pharm Assoc* 47:58.

Desselle SP, Holmes ER. 2017. Results of the 2015 National Certified Pharmacy Technician Workforce Survey. *Am J Health Syst Pharm* 74:981.

Desselle SP, Tipton DJ. 2001. Factors contributing to the satisfaction and performance ability of community pharmacists: A path model analysis. *J Soc Admin Pharm* 18:15.

Edwards MT. 2009. Measuring clinical performance. *Physician Exec* 35:40.

Feys M, Libbrecht N, Anseel F, Lievens F. 2008. A closer look at the relationship between justice perceptions and feedback reactions: The role of the quality of the relationship with the supervisor. *Psychol Belg* 48:156.

Gaither CA, Nadkarni A, Mott DA, et al. 2007. Should I stay or should I go? The influence of individual and organizational factors on pharmacists' future work plans. *J Am Pharm Assoc* 47:165.

Gaither CA, Schommer JC, Doucette WR, et al. 2015. Final Report of the 2014 National Sample Survey of the Pharmacist Workforce to Determine Contemporary Demographic Practice Characteristics and Quality of Work-Life. Alexandria, VA: Pharmacy Workforce Center, Inc.

Gernant SA, Nguyen MO, Siddiqqui S, Schneller M. 2018. Use of pharmacy technicians in elements of medication therapy management: A systematic review. *Res Social Adm Pharm* 14:883.

Goffin RD, Jelley RB, Powell DM, Johnston NG. 2009. Taking advantage of social comparisons in performance appraisal: The relative percentile method. *Hum Resour Manage* 48:268.

Gregory J, Ring D, Rubash H, Harmon L. 2018. Use of 360-degree feedback to develop physician leaders in orthopaedic surgery. *J Surg Orthop Adv* 27:85.

Hageman MG, Ring DC, Gregory PJ, Ruhash HE, Harmon L. 2015. Do 360-degree feedback survey results relate to patient satisfaction measures? *Clin Orthop Rel Res* 473:1590.

Heavner MS, Tichy EM, Yazdi M. 2016. Implementation of a pharmacist career ladder program. *Am J Health Syst Pharm* 73:1524.

Heinitz K, Lorenz T, Schulze D, Schorlemmer J. 2018. Positive organizational behaviour. Longitudinal effects on subjective well-being. *PLoS One* 13(5):e019858.

Hills LD. 2014. How to boost a low-morale medical team. Twenty-five strategies. *J Med Pract Manage* 30:37.

Kalb KB, Cherry NM, Kauzloric J, et al. 2006. A competency-based approach to public health nursing performance appraisal. *Public Health Nurs* 23:115.

Kamangar F, Davari P, Parsi KK, et al. 2015. 360-degree evaluations on physician performance as an effective tool for interprofessional teams: A critical analysis of physician self-assessment as compared to nursing staff and patient evaluations of providers. *Clin Orthop Relat Res* 473:1590.

Kennedy PW, Dresser SG. 2001. Appraising and paying for performance: Another look at an age-old problem. *Empl Benefits J* 26:8.

MacDonald HA, Sulsky LM. 2009. Rating formats and rater training redux: A context-specific approach for enhancing the effectiveness of performance management. *Can J Behav Sci Revue* 41:240.

Martin DC, Bartol KM. 1991. The legal ramifications of performance appraisal: An update. *Employee Relat Law J* 17:257.

Martin DC, Bartol KM. 1998. Performance appraisal: Maintaining system effectiveness. *Public Person Manag* 27:223.

Mattingly AN, Mattingly TJ. 2018. Regulatory burden and salary for pharmacy technicians in the United States. *Res Social Adm Pharm* Available at https://doi.org/10.1016/j.sapharm.2018.07.009. Accessed July 22, 2019.

McConnell CR. 2010. *Umiker's Management Skills for the New Health Care Supervisor*. Sudbury, MA: Jones and Bartlett.

McNall LA, Roch SG. 2009. A social exchange model of employee reactions to electronic performance monitoring. *Hum Perform* 22(3):204–224.

Mitchell MS, Koen CM. 2016. Making "termination" mean it's REALLY over. Part 2—proper documentation. *Health Care Manager* 35:113.

Mone EM, London M. 2018. *Employee Engagement through Effective Performance Management: A Practical Guide for Managers*. New York: Taylor-Francis.

Munger MA, Gordon E, Hartman J, Vincent K, Feehan M. 2013. Community pharmacists' occupational satisfaction and stress: A profession in jeopardy? *J Am Pharm Assoc* 53:282.

Ng, KY, Koh C, Ang S, Kennedy JC, Chan KY. 2011. Rating leniency and halo in multisource feedback ratings: Testing cultural assumptions of power distance and individualism-collectivism. *J Appl Psychol* 96:1033.

Olson JM, Goffin RD, Haynes GA. 2007. Relative versus absolute measures of explicit attitudes: Implications for predicting diverse attitude-relevant criteria. *J Personal Soc Psychol* 93:926.

Park EJ, Huber DL. 2007. Balanced scorecards for performance management. *J Nurs Adm* 37:14.

Powell DM, Goffin RD. 2009. Assessing personality in the employment interview: The impact of training on rater accuracy. *Hum Perform* 22:465.

Roch SG. 2007. Why convene rater teams: An investigation of the benefits of anticipated discussion, consensus, and rater motivation. *Org Behav Hum Decision Processes* 104:29.

Roch SG, McNall LA. 2007. An investigation of factors influencing accountability and performance ratings. *J Psychol* 141:523.

Roch SG, Paquin AR, Littlejohn TW. 2009. Do raters agree more on observable items? *Hum Perform* 22:409.

Roth MT, Zlatic TD. 2009. Development of student professionalism. *Pharmacotherapy* 29:749.

Rue LW, Ibrahim NA, Byars, LL. 2015. *Human Resource Management*, 11th ed. New York, NY: McGraw-Hill.

Schumock GT, Leister KA, Edwards D, et al. 1990. Method for evaluating performance of clinical pharmacists. *Am J Hosp Pharm* 47:127.

Scullen SE, Mont MK, Goff M. 2000. Understanding the latent structure of job performance ratings. *J Appl Psychol* 85:956.

Sen S, Siemianowski L, Murphy M, McAllister SC. 2014. Implementation of a pharmacy technician-centered medication reconciliation program at an urban teaching medical center. *Am J Health Syst Pharm* 71:51.

Shahzileh ZH, Aghajan AM. 2015. Performance appraisal: Review and case study. *Intl J Bus Excellence* 8 Available at https://doi.org/10.1504/IJBEX.2015.071279. Accessed July 22, 2019.

Smith JE, Gianni LM, Garner BR, Malek KL, Godley SH. 2011. A behaviourally-anchored rating system to monitor treatment integrity for community clinicians using the adolescent community reinforcement approach. *Psychol Assess* 23:44.

Smith LL. 2017. The performance appraisal process: Best approaches to support organizational justice for employees. College Park, MD. Doctoral dissertation.

Somon B, Campagne A, Delorme A, Berberian B. 2017. Performance monitoring applied to system supervision. *Front Hum Neurosci* 11:360.

Swift P, Peterson JB. 2018. Improving the effectiveness of performance feedback by considering personality traits and task demands. *PLoS One* Doi: 10.1371/journal.pone.0197810.

Tolli AP, Schmidt AM. 2008. The role of feedback, causal attributions, and self-efficacy in goal revision. *J Appl Psychol* 93:692.

Tunji-Olayeni PF, Olawabi JD, Amusan LM, Nduka D. 2018. Job satisfaction of female construction professionals in male dominated fields. *Int J Mech Engineer Technol* 9:72.

Uggerslev KL, Sulsky LM. 2008. Using frame-of-reference training to understand the implications of rater idiosyncrasy for rating accuracy. *J Appl Psychol* 93:719.

Watkins SC, Roberts DA, Boulet JR, McEvoy MD, Weinger MB. 2014. Evaluation of a simpler tool to assess nontechnical skills during simulated critical events. *J Child Adolesc Subst Abuse* 23:185.

Weenink JW, Kool RB, Hesselink G, Bartels RH, Westert GP. 2017. Prevention of and dealing with poor performance: An interview study about how professional associations aim to support healthcare professionals. *Int J Qual Health Care* 29:838.

Weer CH, Greenhaus JH. 2017. Managers' assessments of organizational career growth opportunities. *J Career Develop* Available at https://doi.org/10.1177/0894845317714892. Accessed July 22, 2019.

Wick JY. 2008. Using pharmacy technicians to enhance clinical and operational capabilities. *Consult Pharm.* 23(6):447–458.

Young MC, Rosenthal MM, Manson KR, Houle SKD. 2018. Do community pharmacist performance evaluations capture the modern pharmacist's role? Mapping competencies assessed in Canadian community pharmacy performance evaluation templates against the General Level Framework. *J Am Pharm Assoc* Available at https://doi.org/10.1016/j.japh.2018.08.006. Accessed July 22, 2019.

SECTION IV

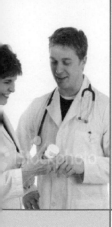

MANAGING MONEY

SECTION IV

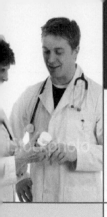

21

FINANCIAL REPORTS

Rashid Mosavin

About the Author: Dr. Mosavin is Dean and Professor of the College of Pharmacy and Health Sciences at Texas Southern University. He received a B.S. in Pharmacy from the University of Kansas, a Ph.D. in Pharmaceutical Sciences from the University of Wisconsin—Madison, and an MBA from the University of Chicago. He is an experienced pharmacy educator and administrator who has also worked in the pharmaceutical industry, hospital pharmacy, and ambulatory care pharmacy settings. His research interests encompass economic evaluation of health care delivery systems and the role of pharmacists in these systems (especially as it relates to management of chronic diseases by pharmacists). Another key area of his research is analysis of economic gains achieved by health information technology implementation in ambulatory care pharmacy practice. Dr. Mosavin teaches business plan writing and independent pharmacy finance while advising students and pharmacists in the National Community Pharmacists Association (NCPA).

■ LEARNING OBJECTIVES

After completing this chapter, readers should be able to

1. Describe the importance of accounting principles in pharmacy practice.
2. Compare and contrast the fundamental objectives of a balance sheet and an income statement.
3. Demonstrate the relationship between a balance sheet and an income statement for a given fiscal year.
4. Describe the utility of financial ratios and interpret basic financial ratios used in community pharmacy practice.
5. Describe and integrate the financial information depicted in a balance sheet and an income statement in community pharmacy practice.
6. Define the flow of funds involved in community pharmacy practice, including expenses, prescription adjudication, receipt of payment, and revenue generation.
7. Describe the basic financial and productivity reports used in hospital pharmacy practice.

■ SCENARIO

It was a beautiful summer day when Marco and Diana met at a coffee shop near where they had gone to pharmacy school. It had been just a couple of years since they had graduated, but they had a lot to catch up on. Marco had always wanted to own a community pharmacy but was currently working in a chain community pharmacy to gain experience and save money. Diana had recently finished a cardiology fellowship and had accepted a clinical faculty position at a large teaching hospital. Diana was interested in hospital pharmacy management and was hoping eventually to be given some administrative and leadership responsibilities in the pharmacy department.

Over the past 2 years, Marco and Diana had begun to gain an appreciation for the need to track the use of money. On a personal level, Marco was beginning to pay off his student loans. Not only was he successfully paying off his loans, he was actually beginning to save some money for his future. While Diana was able to defer payment on her loans during her residency and fellowship, she had to learn to manage her own money wisely, given that she earned substantially less during the past 2 years than many of her friends who took pharmacist positions immediately on graduation. Both were beginning to understand that to become a successful hospital pharmacy administrator or independent pharmacy owner, one needs to also understand how money moves through an organization. Just as Marco and Diana have had to carefully track their own finances to meet their personal financial goals, tracking the uses and flow of money is an essential element in operating any type of pharmacy. They hoped that if they could understand the flow of money in personal finance, they would be able to learn the financial management principles necessary to succeed as pharmacy administrators.

Marco and Diana decided to meet once a month for the next 3 months. Over the course of these meetings, they planned to learn more about accounting, financial reports, and their uses in pharmacy practice.

■ CHAPTER QUESTIONS

1. Why is it essential for pharmacy students to understand the fundamentals of financial accounting?
2. Even though they may not be responsible for the organization's financial performance, why is it important for pharmacists to have a basic understanding of the financial reports in their workplace?
3. How do financial reports in hospital pharmacy practice differ in the type and scope of information they contain from the financial reports of a community pharmacy?
4. How would mastering financial reports make a pharmacist a more effective manager?

■ INTRODUCTION

As mathematics is the language of the physical sciences, accounting is the language of business. The American Institute of Certified Public Accountants defines *accounting* as "the language of business because it deals with interpreting and communicating information about a company's operations and finances. It allows executives to make informed business decisions—decisions that help those companies become more successful (AICPA, 2019)." Although society may perceive accounting as a mundane task involving the endless juggling of numbers, the truth is that accounting provides the framework for critical decision-making processes essential for the success of any organization. Accounting is the dynamic process by which corporations, small businesses, and even individuals determine and report how they finance their activities and use their money. A major use of accounting is to track the flow of money (cash or credit) between financing and investing activities. Familiarity with financial reports is essential to understanding the flow of money. Financial reports are prepared on the basis of generally accepted accounting principles (GAAP). Determining profitability, future growth, and tax liability are examples of the vital functions accounting plays in the day-to-day operations of any type of organization or even at the personal level.

Here is a simple example that defines a few terms fundamental to understanding of an organization's financial health. If one's goal is to drive for a service like Uber or Lyft, one needs to obtain a car. The car is an *asset*. By definition, assets are things that a business owns that can be used to generate income (e.g., driving paying passengers to their destinations). Obtaining the money needed to acquire an asset requires *financing*. Financing for the car may come from a combination of personal savings, gifts, a bank loan, or even money borrowed from friends and relatives. These sources of financing can be further classified as *liabilities* (money owed to others) and *owner's equity* (the owner's own funds). Whatever the total amount invested in an asset, it always must equal the amount financed for its acquisition. If one paid $25,000 for the car, the value of the asset is recorded as $25,000. Now let us say that one financed this asset by putting up $10,000 of their own money and getting a $15,000 loan from a bank. In accounting language, this *investment* in the *asset* ($25,000 for the car) is financed by *owner's equity* ($10,000 of the owner's own money) and a *liability* (the $15,000 loan owed to a bank).

This brings us to the most important rule in accounting, often referred to as the *accounting equation:*

$$\text{Assets} = \text{owner's equity} + \text{liabilities}$$

This rule always holds, whether you own a small community pharmacy or a major multinational corporation. Mastering this relatively simple equation will help one understand even the most complex financial concepts!

■ REVIEW OF ACCOUNTING PRINCIPLES

Accounting principles are essential tools that can be applied in all areas of pharmacy practice (Finkler et al., 2019). This is because any pharmacy, just as

any other type of organization, engages in three fundamental activities:

1. Obtaining financing
2. Making investments
3. Conducting a profitable operation

Obtaining Financing

To start a business, one needs to acquire assets. Financing activities to acquire assets involve obtaining funds from owners as well as creditors (i.e., banks). When owners fund the activities of a corporation, they become shareholders of the corporation. Shareholders have a claim on the company's assets, and their investments in the company are rewarded by either regular distributions from the company to the owners (also known as *dividends*) or by an increase in the value of the company's total assets owing to profitable operations.

Creditors, on the other hand, provide funds to the company but do not receive dividends. They require the company to repay the funds with interest over a specified period of time. This period of time can range from days from vendors that supply companies with inventory or raw materials to years from banks that grant long-term loans. There are many other types of financing, the discussion of which is beyond the scope of this chapter. Interested readers can learn more by reading *Investments* (11th edition) by Bodie et al. (2017) and *Principles of Corporate Finance* (12th edition) by Brealy, Myers, and Allen (2017).

Making Investments

The types of investments a company makes depend largely on the type of business it is conducting. In pharmacy settings, funds are invested in acquisition of inventory, equipment and supplies, information systems, dispensing systems, buildings, and land. Acquiring the resources necessary to employ the appropriate number of pharmacists, pharmacy technicians, and other staff also can be viewed as an investment activity.

Conducting a Profitable Operation

After an individual or organization obtains financing, and then invests those funds to acquire needed assets, the final step is to engage in operations. In general, the operating activities of pharmacies include purchasing, distribution (i.e., prescription-filling activities), clinical activities, and administration. In many pharmacies, marketing is also a significant operation activity, in that it is required so that others can learn of the goods and services that the pharmacy offers (see Chapters 24 and 25).

■ THREE ESSENTIAL FINANCIAL STATEMENTS

Most organizations use a number of different financial statements. However, there are three types of financial statements that are essential to the operations of any organization. Before learning about these essential financial statements, though, it is important to define the term *fiscal year*. A fiscal year is a unit of time—a year as the term implies—that businesses use to record their financial interactions. A fiscal year can start on January 1 and end on December 31, or it can start on any other date and end 1 year later. Businesses (such as retail department stores) that experience heavy sales during the month of December usually begin their fiscal years in March or April. Businesses have to pay their taxes to the Internal Revenue Service (IRS) based on dates set by IRS rules regardless of the calendar dates of their fiscal year. IRS rules on corporate taxes are beyond the scope of this discussion, but readers can learn more by visiting the IRS Web site at www.irs.gov (Internal Revenue Service, 2019). Search the site for Publication 538, Accounting Periods, and Methods.

The three financial reports that are essential to the operation of any organization are the *balance sheet*, the *income statement*, and the *statement of cash flows* (Table 21-1). Please note that several other types of financial reports are also generated by organizations that are not discussed in this chapter. A publicly traded organization, that is an organization whose shares are traded on a stock market, is required to file a number of other financial reports with the Securities and Exchange Commission (SEC).

Table 21-1.	Three Main Types of Financial Statements
Type	**Use**
Balance sheet	Snapshot of the firm's investments (assets) and how they are financed (liabilities and owner's equity)
Income statement	Connects the beginning and ending balance sheets in any given period by providing the details of operating activities (such as sales and expenses)
Statement of cash flow	Connects the beginning and ending balance sheets by indicating the impact of the company's investments, financing, and operations on cash flows

One of these reports is Form 10-Q, which describes the organization's quarterly financial performance. The methodology used to prepare these and other financial reports is established by the Financial Accounting Standards Board (FASB) (2019), a nongovernmental agency dedicated to establishing standards in accounting practice.

For investor protection, Congress passed the Securities Act of 1933 and the Securities Exchange Act of 1934. These acts provided government oversight on US capital markets to prevent the kind of fraud that had resulted in the 1929 stock market crash. In 1934, Congress established the SEC to enforce the new laws and to provide stability for US capital markets (United States Securities and Exchange Commission, 2019).

The Balance Sheet

Table 21-2 shows the balance sheet for Whole Health Partners Pharmacies (WHP). The *balance sheet* provides a snapshot of an organization's assets, liabilities, and shareholder equity at any particular point in time. While organizations generally prepare a balance

Table 21-2. Whole Health Partners Balance Sheet

November 1	Year 0 ($)	Year 1 ($)
Assets		
Current assets		
Cash	50,000	100,000
Accounts receivable	0	200,000
Inventories	200,000	300,000
Noncurrent assets		
Building	300,000	300,000
Equipment	50,000	50,000
Total assets	**600,000**	**950,000**
Liabilities		
Current liabilities		
Accounts payable to wholesalers	200,000	170,000
Salaries payable to employees	0	30,000
Noncurrent liabilities		
Bonds payable	100,000	250,000
Total liabilities	**300,000**	**450,000**
Shareholders' equity		
Common stock	300,000	300,000
Retained earnings	0	200,000
Total shareholders' equity	**300,000**	**500,000**
Total liabilities and shareholders' equity	**600,000**	**950,000**

sheet at the end of a fiscal year, they may prepare this statement at any point in time (e.g., at the end of a month or a quarter). In holding with the accounting equation described earlier, the balance sheet's total assets must equal the total liabilities plus shareholders' equity at all times.

As of November 1, Year 0, WHP had not yet started operations. However, WHP had acquired all the assets it needed to begin operations. When we examine WHP's balance sheet after 1 year of operations (Year 1), we notice changes in assets, liabilities, and shareholders' equity. WHP's goal, like that of most businesses, is to increase its assets through profitable operations throughout the fiscal year. Assuming that WHP is able to keep its liabilities unchanged, an increase in assets would result in an increase in shareholders' equity, and that will make for one happy pharmacist owner! Remember that owner's equity

represent the funds that an owner puts up to start the business. WHP's balance sheet indicates that the owners started with $300,000 of their own money. At the end of Year 1, the owners have increased this amount by $200,000 to $500,000 owing to profitable operations during Year 1. The owners could leave this extra $200,000 of profit to be used in the business (known as *retained earnings*), or they could take some or all of the money to pay themselves (known as *dividends*).

The Income Statement

The balance sheet in Table 21-2 shows the values of assets, liabilities, and shareholders' equity, but because it is only a snapshot, it does not reveal much about what caused these values to change over the course of the year. The balance sheet also does not tell us how income was generated and what types of expenses were incurred during the accounting period.

Table 21-3.	Whole Health Partners Income Statement for Year 1 ($)
Revenue	
Sales—prescription	2,000,000
Sales—nonprescription	500,000
Total revenue	**2,500,000***
Expenses	
Cost of goods sold	1,800,000
Administrative expenses	350,000
Income tax expense	50,000
Total expenses	**2,200,000**
Net income	**300,000**

*Includes $1,200,000 in total credit sales.

Table 21-4.	Whole Health Partners Statement of Retained Earnings for Year 1 ($)
Retained earnings Year 0	0
Net income Year 1	300,000
Dividends distributed to shareholders	100,000
Retained earnings Year 1	200,000

The *income statement* is a dynamic document that provides information about money coming into an organization (*income*) and money necessary to obtain that income (*expenses*). The difference between income and expenses is commonly referred to as *net income*, *net profit*, or *earnings*. The income statement tells the reader what happens to an organization over a period of time. While organizations generally create income statements that span their fiscal year, they often create income statements that describe revenues, expenses, and net income over shorter periods of time, such as quarters, months, weeks, or even over a single day.

Table 21-3 shows WHP's income statement for Year 1. The income statement shows all the operating activities that resulted in either revenues or expenses. It also shows the net income for Year 1. It is important to understand that the terms *net income* and *earnings* are used interchangeably in financial reports. You will note that the net income for Year 1 is $300,000. The balance sheet (Table 21-2) shows retained earnings of $200,000. This is the portion of the net income that the owners have reinvested in the business. Where did the rest ($100,000) of the net income go? It was redistributed among owners as dividends (as depicted in Table 21-4). The connection between the net income value from the income statement and retained earnings from the balance sheet is an example of how these

two reports are linked. In this particular example, the details of this linkage can be examined by the statement of retained earnings (Table 21-4).

The Statement of Cash Flows

Throughout the fiscal year, the inflows and outflows of cash are recorded in the *statement of cash flows*. These recorded values generally fall into three categories: operating, investing, and financing. Table 21-5 shows WHP's statement of cash flows. It is customary in accounting to represent negative values (i.e., cash outflows) in parentheses. By the end of Year 1, WHP has increased its cash by $50,000. The last line in the

Table 21-5.	Whole Health Partners Statement of Cash Flows for Year 1 ($)
Operating	
Revenues providing cash	2,300,000
Expenses using cash	2,150,000
Cash flow from operating	150,000
Investing	
Acquisition of noncurrent assets	0
Sales of noncurrent assets	0
Cash from investing	0
Financing	
Issue of bond	0
Dividends	(100,000)
Net change in cash	(100,000)
Net change in cash	50,000
Cash—end of Year 0	50,000
Cash—end of Year 1	100,000

statement of cash flows, indicating the amount of cash available at the end of a fiscal year, is always the same as the amount of cash recorded on the balance sheet for the beginning of the following fiscal year. Once again, you should note the fluid nature of these reports and the degree to which they are linked.

■ FINANCIAL RATIOS

Organizations, investors, creditors, and even individuals use financial ratios to examine an organization's financial performance. Some financial ratios, such as net income/average total assets, provide useful information on the profitability of the organization. Other ratios can be calculated that provide insight into the liquidity of the organization (how much cash is available to pay the bills) or how well the organization is converting its accounts receivable to cash. Data are taken from the balance sheet and income statement for calculating most ratios. Although financial ratios can be used to quantify many aspects of an organization, they should not be used in isolation from other financial reports. In general, financial ratios allow users of financial information to make comparisons between:

- A single organization and the entire industry average
- Differences within an organization over time (e.g., months, quarters, years)
- Two or more units within a single organization (e.g., pharmacies within the same chain)
- Two or more organizations with each other (e.g., comparisons between chain pharmacy corporations)

Financial ratios should be compared to a reference point (such as historical values of the same company). Financial ratio analysis is only as valid as the financial information on which it is based. If the information provided in the financial statements has not been independently verified (audited), the results of a financial ratio analysis are not likely to give the reader an accurate assessment of the financial performance of that organization. While financial ratio analysis can provide valuable insight to the performance of any organization, it is important that the users of financial ratios are also mindful of their limitations.

When calculating financial ratios for terms shorter than 1 year (i.e., day, week, month, quarter), keep in mind that seasonal factors may distort many ratios. For example, over-the-counter (OTC) cold and cough sales may be higher during the winter months than any other time of the year and therefore result in more favorable ratios for the quarter spanning the winter months.

Firms may also use different, yet still commonly accepted, accounting methods to prepare their balance sheet and income statement. Therefore, it is imperative to understand how the values used in calculating the ratios were obtained. Remember that standards set by FASB are based on acceptable accounting methods and these methods may vary in how they measure revenues collected (cash vs. credit) or expenses paid (cash vs. accounts payable).

Financial ratios are classified according to the information they provide. Table 21-6 provides a list

Table 21-6.	Financial Ratios
Name	**Formula**
Profitability ratios	
Gross profit margin	(Sales−cost of goods sold)/total sales
Net profit margin	Net income (after tax)/ total sales
Return on assets	Net income/average total assets
Return on equity	Net income/average owner's equity
Liquidity ratios	
Current	Current assets/current liabilities
Quick	Quick assets/current liabilities
Turnover ratios	
Inventory turnover	Cost of goods sold/ average inventory
Receivables turnover	Credit sales/average account receivable

of selected financial ratios used in various pharmacy settings. Different ratios give different pictures of the company's performance and serve different analytical needs. Profitability ratios, liquidity ratios, and turnover ratios are described below. For further discussion of other financial report ratios, please refer to Finkler et al. (2019).

Profitability Ratios

Since an inherent goal of any business (both for-profit and not-for-profit organizations) is to be profitable (i.e., to generate revenues in excess of their expenses), we can view profitability ratios as measures of overall success in the daily operations of a business. More specifically, profitability ratios provide a method to measure the overall financial success of a company. Examining profitability ratios allows managers to assess the company's level of success in generating profits. The most commonly used profitability ratios in pharmacies are the *gross profit margin* and the *net profit margin.*

Gross profit margin = [sales – cost of goods sold

(COGS)] ÷ total sales

By considering the cost of goods sold (COGS), this ratio provides information on the company's ability to generate gross profits. Higher gross profit margin ratios are desirable because they indicate the availability of funds for the company's other expenses. The typical range for this ratio in community pharmacy practice is 20% to 25% as reported by NCPA (2018). Two main factors that influence profitability ratios, and in particular the gross profit margin ratio, are drug prices and reimbursement formulas in third-party contracts (see Chapter 23). Pharmacy managers have to monitor reimbursement and drug price changes regularly to ensure a viable gross profit margin ratio.

Net profit margin = net income (after taxes)

÷ total sales

Net profit margin indicates the fraction of net profit that is generated for every dollar of sales. As mentioned earlier, as a profitability ratio, it could be used to determine how well the organization manages its operating expenses. It could also be used to compare the performance of two or more pharmacies within a chain or to assess the performance of a pharmacy against industry performance. Community pharmacies tend to have net profit margins between 2% and 5%, with higher percentages always being desirable. An analysis performed by the National Community Pharmacy Association (NCPA) found that independent community pharmacies averaged a net profit of 3% between 2007 and 2016 (NCPA, 2018).

Return on assets (ROA) = net income

÷ average total assets

This ratio provides information on the company's ability to generate profits using the company's assets. As stated in the introduction, profits can only be generated from the company's assets. Therefore, effective use of assets results in a high ROA ratio. The industry norm for community pharmacies is about 5% as reported by CSIMarket (2019). The ROA varies significantly across different industries.

Return on equity (ROE) = net income

÷ average owner's equity

Return on equity, also known as *return on investment* (ROI), is a measure of how well the company can make profits from funds provided by owners or investors. High ROE levels are desirable because investors—similar to companies—are interested in maximizing their profits. ROA and ROE sometimes are used to gauge the manager's performance. All else equal, managers who make better financial decisions are better able to produce higher ROA and ROE ratios for their organizations. Remember that investors have the option to invest in other industries or simply the stock market if they feel that they will receive a higher ROI on their investment. Thus the return rates generated by an owner's investment in a pharmacy should always be gauged against the returns the owner could have generated if they had invested their funds in other vehicles with similar levels of risk.

Liquidity Ratios

Liquidity ratios provide information on the business's ability to meet its short-term financial obligations. The most popular liquidity ratios are the *current ratio* and the *quick ratio*.

The *current ratio* is the ratio of current assets to current liabilities.

Current ratio = current assets ÷ current liabilities

An organization with a high current ratio is taking fewer risks in meeting its financial obligations. For example, having a lot of cash in the bank and few debts (*liabilities*) to pay results in a high value for current assets, a low value for liabilities, and therefore a high current ratio. While high current ratio values generally are considered desirable, values greater than 5.0 are considered by some to be too high. This might be a sign of a company that is too conservative, leaving too much of its money in the bank rather than investing it in ways that could help the organization grow (e.g., building new pharmacies or expanding existing services). A low current ratio (<2.0) indicates that the organization has low current assets (especially cash) relative to its current liabilities (often bills that are due in 30–60 days). This is not a desirable position for any organization because the inability to pay current liabilities may result in bankruptcy.

An alternative to the current ratio is the *quick ratio* (also known as the *acid test*). For this ratio, *quick assets* are defined as assets that are easily converted to cash. Therefore, inventories and prepaid expenses (such as prepaid rent and insurance policies) are not included in calculating assets. Because the quick ratio considers only assets that are easily converted to cash (and therefore can be used to pay bills, etc.), it provides a better picture of a company's liquidity and its ability to meet its financial obligations.

Quick ratio = (current assets – inventories
– prepaid expenses)
÷ current liabilities

The standard quick ratio that any organization strives to obtain is at least 1.0. Simply put, having a quick ratio of greater than 1.0 means that the organization has more quick assets than it has current liabilities. On the other hand, having a quick ratio of less than 1.0 means the cash that organization has on hand would not be sufficient to pay all its current liabilities, particularly its short-term bills and other obligations.

Now that we have the definition of current ratio and quick ratio, let us calculate these ratios for WHP (see Table 21-2, Year 1). The current ratio at the end of Year 1 is $450,000 ÷ $200,000 = 2.25, which appears to be acceptable. However, the amount of quick assets on hand at the end of Year 1 is only $150,000 (current assets – inventories). The resulting quick ratio is $150,000 ÷ $200,000 = 0.75. One concludes from the calculation of these two ratios that WHP has a large inventory ($300,000) and may have difficulty satisfying its short-term debts. A quick ratio of less than 1 is very alarming. This example also illustrates the point that financial ratios should not be considered in isolation because a single ratio rarely will provide a comprehensive picture of the organization's financial health.

Turnover Ratios

Turnover ratios measure the efficiency with which an organization uses its assets. They are also referred to as *efficiency ratios* or *asset utilization ratios*. The two most commonly used turnover ratios are *inventory turnover* and *receivables turnover*.

Inventory turnover ratio = COGS ÷ average
inventory (at cost)

The inventory turnover ratio measures how quickly, on average, an organization's inventories are sold. The data for this ratio come from two different financial statements. COGS is found on the income statement, and the average inventory comes from the balance sheet. Let us assume that a community pharmacy reported COGS of $1,200,000 for a given year and an average inventory of $100,000 over the course of that year. This results in an inventory turnover ratio of 12.0. In other words, the pharmacy is able to sell (and therefore replace) its entire inventory, on average, once a month. If you divide 365 by the inventory turnover ratio, you will have a ratio known as the *days inventory on hand.* This ratio indicates the number of days worth of inventory that is on hand. In the example above, 365/12 = 30.42 days. Clearly, lower values for this ratio would mean more effective inventory management.

Low inventory turnover ratios (6.0 or below) indicate that the organization's inventory is too large for its operations and that cash that could be better spent elsewhere is tied up in inventory. High inventory turnover ratios are generally desirable because this means that the organization was able to sell and replace its inventory with high efficiency and therefore generate higher revenues and profits. Although a high inventory turnover ratio generally is desirable, it can also result in the loss of sales and profits if the average inventory is kept too low. Remember that one can achieve a high inventory ratio by keeping a very small inventory. As the denominator value decreases, the ratio will increase, assuming that all else is unchanged. However, the pharmacy will face chronic shortages during its daily operations that may result in patient dissatisfaction. Patients may choose other pharmacies for better service (Nelson, 2017).

Receivables turnover ratio = credit sales
÷ average accounts receivable

This ratio measures how quickly receivables (money owed to the organization by others) are turned into cash. Credit sales are reported on the balance sheet under accounts receivable. In addition, they are reported as notes to income statement. These figures can be provided daily by the credit card processing companies that the pharmacy uses to perform credit card transactions. A high receivable turnover ratio shows that the organization can collect its receivables efficiently while keeping the total amount it is owed by others at any given time relatively low. You notice from the balance sheet that WHP has $200,000 in accounts receivable in year 1. From the income statement you note that $1,200,000 of total revenue was in credit sales. This results in a receivable turnover ratio of 6 indicating that the pharmacy is able to collect its receivable on average every 2 months. If you

divide 365 by the receivable turnover ratio, you will have a ratio known as the *average collection period.* The average collection period indicates the number of days (on average) that credit sales remain in accounts receivable before they are collected.

The receivable turnover ratio and the average collection period are particularly important in community pharmacy practice. In the 1950s and 1960s, the majority of expenditures on prescription drugs were paid by patients with cash out of their own pockets. Today, third-party payers (e.g., private insurance, Medicaid, and Medicare Prescription Drug Plans [PDPs]) are responsible for paying the vast majority of these expenditures (see Chapter 23). Unlike patients, who pay their copayments at the pharmacy when they pick up their prescriptions, third-party payers often take up to 90 to 120 days before they reimburse the pharmacy for prescriptions dispensed. This lag period increases the accounts receivable and depletes the cash reserves of the pharmacy. This becomes a significant problem for independent pharmacies that do not have large cash reserves to cover their expenses (current liabilities) during this period.

Although community pharmacies pay close attention to third-party payer contracts to ensure that they understand the reimbursement timetables, in many instances they are not able to influence the third-party practices. For example, being a pharmacy provider for Medicaid patients is a profitable business for many pharmacies across the nation. However, the contracted pharmacies have very little influence on reimbursement schedules set by the Centers for Medicaid and Medicare Services (CMS). See Chapter 23 to learn more about the financial implications of pharmacy reimbursement contracts with third-party payers.

■ FINANCIAL REPORTS IN COMMUNITY PHARMACY PRACTICE

Financial reports used in independent pharmacy practice are very similar to those used in chain community pharmacies. Managers in chain community pharmacies pay attention to the same financial ratios and key indicators on balance sheets and income statements. It was with this knowledge that Marco and Diana decided to spend some time with WHP's owner to gain more insight into the preparation and review of financial reports in community pharmacy practice.

Almost all prescriptions filled in a community pharmacy are paid for through a third-party payer, and nearly all of them are adjudicated online. Table 21-7 shows a section of WHP's Daily Plan Payment report. As depicted in this report, the manager is able to monitor the daily number of prescriptions filled for each plan, the total amount paid by each third-party payer, the total copayments made by patients, and total cost of drug products used to dispense these prescriptions. From this information, the gross margin for each payer can be calculated (as shown in the last column). Daily inspection of this report identifies plans with low reimbursement rates. In addition, when a low gross margin is detected, the manager examines the cost of prescription products dispensed to ensure that the pharmacy has received the best prices from the wholesaler. This is especially true for multisource medications (e.g., generics).

The revenues and expenses from the Daily Plan Payment report are compiled each month and entered into the income statement report (typically by the organization's accountant or bookkeeper, not by the pharmacists themselves). WHP begins its fiscal year on November 1. In addition to the yearly income statement and balance sheet, WHP's accountant

prepares a monthly income statement and balance sheet to provide managers with a more precise picture of the financial status of the pharmacy. Before we examine these reports, we have to consider an important point about the preparation of the monthly income statement.

The revenues on the monthly income statement have to be revised once reimbursements have been received from third-party payers. The reason for making adjustments is that most payers make adjustments to each claim and charge the pharmacy administrative fees. These fees are typically processing fees that Pharmacy Benefit Manager (PBM) companies charge pharmacies for processing each prescription. Please see Chapter 23 for more detailed description of these administrative fees. Therefore, the actual amount paid to the pharmacy for prescriptions dispensed is almost always lower than the amount indicated on the Daily Plan Payment report. If the manager fails to revise the revenues, the income statement will show artificially inflated revenue. This can have a number of adverse consequences for a pharmacy, including inaccurate financial reports and higher income taxes. In other words, if the revenues are recorded from online adjudications, the pharmacy will pay taxes for revenues it never earned. The pharmacy generally receives the reimbursement check with an Explanation of Benefits (EOB) or Pharmacy Reconciliation Report (PRR) form. This form will show the details of the reimbursement (i.e., beneficiaries' names, prescription numbers, amounts paid for each prescription, and all adjustments and administrative fees deducted).

Table 21-7.   Whole Health Partners Plan Payment Report for Thursday, July 30, 2019[a]

Plan ID	Plan Name	Rx's	Rf's	Total Plan Pay ($)	Copay ($)	Cost ($)	Gross Margin (%)
AETNA	AETNA	10	32	851.03	335.30	1,010.18	15
ANTHEM	ANTHEM	7	2	1,096.65	15.00	1,014.49	9
BLCS-D	Blue Cross-D	93	119	14,155.35	432.16	15,316.89	(5)
CIGNA	CIGNA	31	10	1,290.78	562.12	1,426.73	23

[a]Only an excerpt of the entire plan is shown.

WHP's manager points out that for every $1,000 in third-party reimbursement, the pharmacy may lose $30 to $40 in administrative and other fees. This is a 3% to 4% reduction in revenue that should be reconciled on the income statement.

Table 21-8 shows the balance sheet for the last 2 months of WHP's last fiscal year (September and October 2019) and the first month of the next fiscal year (November 2019). After careful examination of the information in Table 21-8, notice that the retained earnings of $825,000 in October is reduced to $798,000 in November. What has caused the retained earnings to drop by $27,000? Did the owners redistribute the funds to themselves as dividends? Table 21-9 depicts the income statement for the last 2 months and the entire 2019 fiscal year. In looking over the yearly income statement (fourth column in Table 21-9), note that WHP recorded a loss of $27,000. In November 2019, the previous year's loss was taken out of the retained earnings. Therefore, the new fiscal year began with $27,000 less in shareholders' equity. Consequently, a reduction in retained earnings on the balance sheet does not provide the reader with concrete evidence of the status of the pharmacy's financial health. Once a change in retained earnings is observed on the balance sheet, one has to further examine the income statement to get a "true" sense of the pharmacy's financial status.

Examining the income statement in Table 21-9, we observe that WHP recorded a significant loss for October 2019. In looking closely at the income and expenses for that month, note that the COGS and total expenses for the month of October are significantly higher than for the previous month. What has caused such a dramatic change in just 1 month? While there can be many potential reasons for such a change, remember that October is the last month of WHP's fiscal year. Pharmacies often make extra drug purchases and pay more of their expenses before ending their fiscal year. Many managers believe that spending more money at the end of a fiscal year allows them to have more cash throughout the rest of the year to use for financing and investing activities. However, keep in mind that all necessary inventory purchases and other expenses have to take place and be recorded so that the net income for the year is not artificially inflated. This is another reason why it is important to evaluate more than a single income statement or balance sheet when evaluating the financial performance of any organization.

■ FINANCIAL REPORTS IN HOSPITAL PHARMACY PRACTICE

Financial reports used to manage the department of pharmacy in hospitals are often quite different from those used in community pharmacy practice. The budget for a hospital pharmacy department is primarily composed of drug costs and labor (pharmacists, technicians, and administrators) and is a part of the global budget of the entire hospital. Drug costs are generally the larger of the two components, although this varies with the size of the hospital, the size of the pharmacy department, and the types of clinical and distributive services the hospital provides. Interested readers should review the book *Financial Management for Health-System Pharmacists* by Andrew Wilson (2009) for more information about financial statements used in hospitals and hospital pharmacies.

The four management principles discussed in Chapter 2 (plan, organize, lead, and control) are relevant in the financial planning of a hospital's pharmacy department. The financial stability of the department will depend on planning and implementation of financial management programs that span these four principles.

A hospital's chief pharmacy officer or director of pharmacy is responsible for the creation of policies and procedures to manage expenditures. These include, but are not limited to, group purchasing, utilization review protocols, and cost-effective clinical pharmacy services (Schneider et al., 2018). In their efforts to manage expenditures, hospital pharmacy administrators are faced with a set of unique challenges unlike those seen in community pharmacy. While all pharmacies have experienced large increases

Table 21-8.   Whole Health Partners Balance Sheet

Assets	September 2019 ($)	October 2019 ($)	November 2019 ($)
Current assets			
Petty cash	1,500	1,500	1,500
Cash in bank	105,000	133,000	75,000
Accounts receivable	680,000	658,000	776,000
Allow for doubtful accounts	(16,000)	(16,000)	(16,000)
Inventory—prescription	378,000	441,000	440,000
Inventory—other	17,000	20,000	19,000
Prepaid federal income tax	33,000	44,000	44,000
Prepaid state income tax	16,000	15,000	15,000
Total current assets	1,214,500	1,296,500	1,354,500
Noncurrent assets			
Automobiles	50,000	50,000	50,000
Machinery and equipment	130,000	130,000	130,000
Office equipment	140,000	140,000	140,000
Leasehold improvements	97,000	97,000	97,000
Accumulated depreciation	(308,000)	(310,000)	(313,000)
Total noncurrent assets	109,000	107,000	104,000
Total assets	**1,323,500**	**1,403,500**	**1,458,500**
Liabilities			
Current liabilities			
Accounts payable	223,000	393,000	369,500
Line of credit—Wells Fargo	60,000	55,000	55,000
Payroll taxes payable	0	30,000	0
Sales tax payable	500	500	1,000
Federal income tax pay—current	90,000	0	100,000
State income tax pay—current	25,000	0	35,000
Total current liabilities	398,500	478,500	560,500
Noncurrent liabilities			
Note payable	40,000	40,000	40,000
Loan payable	50,000	50,000	50,000
Total noncurrent liabilities	90,000	90,000	90,000
Total liabilities	**488,500**	**568,500**	**650,500**
Shareholders' equity			
Common stock	10,000	10,000	10,000
Retained earnings	825,000	825,000	798,000
Total shareholders' equity	**835,000**	**835,000**	**808,000**
Total liabilities and shareholders' equity	**1,323,500**	**1,403,500**	**1,458,500**

Table 21-9.   Whole Health Partners Income Statement

Income	September 2019 ($)	October 2019 ($)	Fiscal Year 2019 ($)
Sales—current prescriptions	702,000	864,000	9,313,000
Sales—taxables	5,000	8,000	80,000
Total income	**707,000**	**872,000**	**9,393,000**
Cost of sales			
Purchases—prescriptions	623,000	920,000	7,600,000
Purchases—other	400	1,000	18,000
Purchases—supplies	0	600	2,000
Total cost of sales	**623,400**	**921,600**	**7,620,000**
Gross profit on sales	**83,600**	**(49,600)**	**1,773,000**
General and administrative expenses			
Advertising	1,400	1,500	25,000
Automobile	2,900	2,900	25,000
Bank charges	0	600	14,000
Billing services	0	4,000	26,000
Benefits	7,000	7,000	82,000
Depreciation	2,000	2,000	26,000
Dues and subscriptions	150	150	500
Interest expense	4,000	3,800	15,000
Insurance—general	400	8,000	50,000
Legal and accounting	1,000	2,500	29,000
Licenses	500	500	6,000
Maintenance and repairs	0	3,500	7,000
Meals and entertainment	1,000	2,400	22,000
Office expense	1,500	6,500	4,500
Office salaries	52,000	52,000	650,000
Officer salaries	19,000	100,000	422,000
Outside services	9,000	12,000	100,000
Postage	400	400	1,500
Pension plan expense	2,400	50,000	54,000
Promotion	400	400	1,500
Rent	8,000	8,000	95,000
Taxes—payroll	3,800	4,900	70,000
Telephone	1,900	2,600	20,000
Travel	0	0	4,000
Utilities	1,100	1,000	10,000
Total general and administrative expenses	**119,850**	**277,150**	**1,800,000**
Net income	**(36,250)**	**(326,750)**	**(27,000)**

in the costs of drug products since the 1990s (often >10% per year), hospitals, unlike community pharmacies, generally cannot pass on higher drug costs to consumers in the form of higher prices for their goods and services. Medicare and other payers often use *prospective payment systems* in hospitals, in which they are provided with fixed payments based on a patient's diagnosis or the number of lives they agree to provide services for over a given period of time. While community pharmacies generally can improve their profitability by selling more goods and providing more services, hospital pharmacies generally cannot "sell" their goods and services because their payers are paying a set amount regardless of how many drugs the hospital dispenses or clinical services it provides. While community pharmacies generally are considered to be *profit centers,* hospital pharmacy departments are considered to be *cost centers* because they do not generate revenue directly and only help to contribute to their hospitals' overall profitability by using drug therapy and clinical pharmacy services to help lower the overall cost of caring for patients. The hospital pharmacy administrator manages the performance of this cost center by evaluating complex financial reports that compare actual with budgeted values and the variance between budgeted and actual costs.

The hospital pharmacy administrator uses an expense report prepared on a monthly or weekly basis. In this report, all pharmacy department expenses are categorized into at least five major sections. Each expense is also given a unique code so that not only the pharmacy department but also the hospital's central accounting office can access and monitor expenses. The expense report indicates the amount budgeted for each expense, the actual expense incurred, the variance between budgeted and incurred expenses, and the variance percentage. Table 21-10 shows an abbreviated, simplified expense report for the pharmacy department of a large tertiary care hospital.

The pharmacy expense report consolidates the expenses for the month and compares the actual expenses against the budgeted expenses for the month. The value of this report lies with the comparisons of

the total expense for the current year and the variances for the monthly and yearly expenses for the previous year. This allows the manager to identify potential trends or expenses that could be outliers and evaluate how to bring the expenses back to budget. For example, uncertainty on the cost and the release date of newly approved drugs and personnel variances such as staff overtime due to poor managing of the schedule can be effectively analyzed and corrective action taken. Categories with a positive value for variance (and variance percentage) indicate that department has spent more money than it had budgeted for those categories. Positive values for variance (and variance percentage) for year-to-date figures also indicate that department is spending more funds this year as compared with the previous year. Conversely, negative variance values are indicative of lower than budgeted expenditures and certainly desirable from the manager's perspective.

An important element of financial cost analysis in the pharmacy department is the development of productivity assessment reports. Most pharmacy department administrators prepare a productivity report for each pay period in which the number of full-time equivalents (FTEs) and the quantity of outputs (such as clinical services provided by pharmacists) are analyzed. These reports are useful because they enable managers to use historical data to create budgets and monitor trends over time.

Besides the pharmaceuticals, labor is the other major expense of a pharmacy. The FTE and overtime report helps the manager determine if the correct number of employees are working for a given pay period, as well as the total for the year. It is important to look at the total expense for the year, as this will smooth out pay period variations in staffing that can take place due to vacation coverage and holidays. Evaluating the amount of labor that is caused by overtime will help the manager determine if the department has the correct mix of full-time, part-time, and per diem employees, which can be used appropriately to decrease the amount of overtime for the department. Table 21-11 depicts the FTE and overtime productivity report of the pharmacy department.

Table 21-10. Pharmacy Department Expense Report—Actual versus Budgeted

Payroll	August 2019—Monthly				2019—Year to Date (YTD)				Monthly Last Year		YTD Last Year	
	Actual ($)	Budget ($)	Variance ($)	Variance (%)	Actual ($)	Budget ($)	Variance ($)	Variance (%)	Actual ($)	Variance (%)	Actual ($)	Variance (%)
Ancillary												
Manager/Supervisor	37,916	37,520	396	1.1	301,204	300,160	1,044	0.3	36,541	3.6	298,587	0.9
Technicians/Interns	68,521	70,250	−1,729	−2.5	568,240	562,000	6,240	1.1	67,526	1.5	562,458	1.0
Pharmacists	210,354	210,500	−146	−0.1	1,682,504	1,684,000	−1,496	−0.1	210,586	−0.1	1,602,485	4.8
Administrative	3,825	3,805	20	0.5	29,864	30,440	−576	−1.9	3,912	−2.3	28,862	3.4
Subtotal ancillary	320,616	322,075	−1,459	−0.5	2,581,812	2,576,600	5,212	0.2	318,565	0.6	2,492,392	3.5
Employee benefits												
Benefits—medical/dental	21,058	21,500	−442	−2.1	175,481	172,000	3,481	2.0	22,015	−4.5	176,982	−0.9
Vacation/Sick leave	9,572	8,500	1,072	12.6	67,524	68,000	−476	−0.7	9,632	−0.6	66,057	2.2
Payroll taxes	72,545	73,000	−455	−0.6	594,214	584,000	10,214	1.7	71,523	1.4	584,672	1.6
Subtotal employee benefits	103,175	103,000	175	0.2	837,219	824,000	13,219	1.6	103,170	0.0	827,711	1.1
Subtotal payroll	423,791	425,075	−1,284	−0.3	3,419,031	3,400,600	18,431	0.5	421,735	0.5	3,320,103	2.9
Nonpayroll	($)	($)	($)	(%)	($)	($)	($)	(%)	($)	(%)	($)	(%)
IV and irrigations solutions	4,528	7,510	−2,982	−39.7	58,796	60,080	−1,284	−2.1	4,689	−3.6	61,865	−5.2
IV supplies	8,650	6,585	2,065	31.4	51,248	52,680	−1,432	−2.7	8,542	1.2	49,879	2.7

Chemotherapy drugs	72,505	75,000	−2,495	−3.3	632,541	600,000	32,541	5.4	61,535	15.1	602,045	4.8
Noninjectable drugs	165,258	158,652	6,606	4.2	1,284,576	1,269,216	15,360	1.2	151,897	8.1	1,225,483	4.6
Injectable drugs	637,265	625,800	11,465	1.8	5,012,478	5,006,400	6,078	0.1	588,963	7.6	4,701,756	6.2
Office supplies	1,850	1,925	−75	−3.9	13,458	15,400	−1,942	−12.6	1,763	4.7	12,647	6.0
Equipment repair	754	800	−46	−5.8	4,215	6,400	−2,185	−34.1	651	13.7	3,897	7.5
Subtotal direct materials	890,810	876,272	14,538	1.7	7,057,312	7,010,176	47,136	0.7	818,040	8.2	6,657,572	5.7
Other nonpayroll												
Other nonpayroll Business meetings/travel/meals	564	600	−36	−6.0	3,524	4,800	−1,276	−26.6	423	25.0	4,635	−31.5
Reference materials/subscriptions	358	450	−92	−20.4	3,049	3,600	−551	−15.3	348	2.8	3,524	−15.6
Training expenses	495	350	145	41.4	1,786	2,800	−1,014	−36.2	267	46.1	2,227	−24.7
Other miscellaneous expense	865	650	215	33.1	5,432	5,200	232	4.5	792	8.4	5,189	4.5
Subtotal other nonpayroll	2,282	2,050	232	11.3	13,791	16,400	−2,609	−15.9	1,830	19.8	15,575	−12.9
Subtotal nonpayroll	893,092	878,322	14,770	1.7	7,071,103	7,026,576	44,527	0.6	819,870	8.2	6,673,147	5.6
Total expenses	1,316,883	1,303,397	13,486	1.0	10,490,134	10,427,176	62,958	0.6	1,241,605	5.7	9,993,250	4.7

Table 21-11.   Full-Time Equivalents (FTEs) and Overtime Productivity

	Actual	Budget	Variance
Paid FTEs per pay period	39	38	1
YTD paid FTEs	38.5	38	0.5
Overtime analysis			
Overtime dollars per pay period	$3,521	$2,500	$1,021
Percent overtime per pay period	6.5%	5.0%	1.5%
YTD payroll overtime dollars	$98,754	$85,246	$13,508
YTD percent overtime of total payroll	5.9%	4.5%	1.4%

YTD, year to date.

The table shows actual versus budgeted and percent variance of FTEs. In addition, the report provides information on the cost of overtime pay for the pay period and year to date. For an in-depth discussion of productivity monitoring in hospital pharmacy practice, see Rough et al. (2010a, 2010b). There are a number of productivity ratios that can be used in the inpatient pharmacy to determine the productivity of the department. Table 21-12 depicts the names and definitions of seven of the most commonly used productivity ratios in hospital pharmacy practice. Hospital pharmacy directors pay very close attention to these productivity ratios to manage the allocation of their labor and other resources.

Table 21-12.   Productivity Ratios

Patient days	The total number of days patients are in the hospital occupying a bed for a given time period
Case mix index (patient acuity factor)	An indicator of the level of severity of the patients which are classified by disease, diagnostic or therapeutic procedures performed, method of payment, duration of hospitalization, and intensity and type of services provided by the facility for a given time period
Full-time equivalents (FTEs) per occupied bed	A measurement of the number of full-time workers who used to care for each bed occupied by a patient
Drug cost per patient day	The cost of the drugs purchased by the pharmacy divided by the number of patient days of the facility
Labor cost per patient day	The cost of the labor (salary and benefits) divided by the number of patient days of the facility
Hours paid by job code	Evaluation of the hours worked and paid by job classification (technicians, pharmacists, clerical, and management). This ratio indicates the appropriate use of labor force.
Paid-to-work ratio	The total number of paid hours (includes worked, sick, holiday, and vacation hours) compared to the total number of work hours that are paid. Measured per pay period for the entire department, it reveals if vacation approvals are resulting in excessive over-time pay.

■ QUESTIONS FOR FURTHER DISCUSSION

1. Marco has found two other pharmacists willing to invest in purchasing an existing community pharmacy. This pharmacy has been open for only 2 years and is located in the lobby of an ambulatory care clinic affiliated with a 200-bed community hospital. This year, the pharmacy is projected to have sales of $2 million.
   a. To prepare for purchasing negotiations, what financial documents should Marco review? Name specific financial indicators that Marco should pay special attention to as he reviews these documents.
   b. Based on the material in this and other chapters in this book, what strategies should Marco employ to increase prescription volume, increase pharmacy revenues, and ensure the pharmacy's long-term success?
2. A few years after Marco and his associates purchase this pharmacy, the director of the affiliated hospital pharmacy retires. Marco announces this news to Diana and encourages her to apply for the position. Diana begins to update her résumé and prepare a letter of intent.
   a. What type of questions should Diana ask during an interview to gain insight into the pharmacy department's financial status? What key financial indicators should hospital administration share with Diana to convince her of the pharmacy department's financial strengths?
   b. Based on the material in this chapter and other chapters in this book, what strategies should Diana employ to ensure the pharmacy department's long-term success?

Finally, hospital pharmacy administrators pay special attention to external financial reports. Professional associations such as the American Hospital Association and the American Society for Health-System Pharmacists publish reports that show the national trends in pharmaceutical expenditures and labor productivity in hospitals (American Hospital Association, 2019; Hoffman et al., 2012). Pharmacy managers can gauge the efficiency of their operations by comparing their financial and productivity ratios and with national averages.

■ CONCLUSION

Familiarity with basic accounting concepts and preparation of financial reports is essential knowledge for every pharmacist. The financial success of any organization depends on proper management of its funds. Those who understand how organizations finance operations, generate revenue, and allocate financial resources will have an easier task understanding many of the factors that affect their success. Marco and Diana truly enjoyed their meetings learning about financial reports and their importance in pharmacy practice. They also found financial analyses a fun and rewarding exercise.

■ GLOSSARY

Bond A long-term debt type of security generally issued by corporations or governments to generate cash. The *coupon rate* is the interest rate paid to the bondholder. The *maturity date* is when the face value of the bond will be paid to the bondholder.

Cost center A unit of an organization for which costs are recorded and analyzed. In general, cost centers add to the overall cost of the organization but contribute to the profits of the organization indirectly. Some examples of cost centers are customer-service centers and research and development departments.

Dividend Distribution of a portion of a company's net income to its shareholders.

Current ratio A liquidity ratio that reflects a company's ability to satisfy its short-term financial obligations.

Case mix index (CMI) A relative value assigned as an indicator of the severity of the patients' condition by diagnostic groups in hospitals.

Quick ratio A liquidity ratio that reflects a company's ability to satisfy its short-term obligations with its most liquid assets.

Inventory turnover A ratio that reflects the number of times in a fiscal year that a pharmacy's inventory is sold and replaced.

Receivables turnover A ratio that reflects a pharmacy's ability to collect its debt and extend credit to its customers.

Gross profit margin Also known as *gross margin*, this represents the amount of money left in a firm once the cost of goods sold is subtracted from revenues. It reflects the company's ability to pay for its other expenses.

Net profit margin A profitability ratio that indicates the fraction of net profit generated for every dollar of sales. It is calculated by dividing net income after taxes by total sales.

Patient days A unit used in health care accounting of the total number of days patients are in the hospital for a given period of time.

Return on assets A profitability ratio reflecting a company's ability to generate net income as a percentage of its total assets.

Return on equity A profitability ratio reflecting a company's ability to generate net income as a percentage of total investments by shareholders.

■ ACKNOWLEDGMENTS

I would like to thank Dale J. Timothy, RPh, MBA, director of Inpatient Pharmacy at Kaiser Permanente Riverside Medical Center in Riverside, CA, for his contributions to the "Financial Reports in Hospital Pharmacy Practice" Section of this chapter. I would also like to thank Dr. Robert Beeman, owner of Beeman Pharmacies in San Bernardino, CA, for his consultations and contributions to the "Financial Reports in Community Pharmacy Practice" section of this chapter.

REFERENCES

American Hospital Association. 2019. Health Care Statistics and Market Research Data. Available at www.aha .org. Accessed January 7, 2019.

American Institute of Certified Public Accountants (AICPA). 2019. Becoming a CPA. Available at www .aicpa.org. Accessed January 7, 2019.

Bodie Z, Kane A, Marcus A. 2017. *Investments*, 11th ed. New York, NY: McGraw-Hill.

Brealy R, Myers S, Allen F. 2017. *Principles of Corporate Finance*, 12th ed. New York, NY: McGraw-Hill/Irwin.

CSIMarket Inc. 2019. Available at www.CSIMarket.com. Accessed March 18, 2019.

Financial Accounting Standards Board. 2019. "Standards" Available at www.fasb.org. Accessed January 7, 2019.

Finkler S, Calabrese T, Ward D. 2019. *Accounting Fundamentals for Health Care Management*, 3rd ed. Burlington, MA: Jones and Bartlett Learning.

Hoffman J, Li E, Doloresco F, et al. 2012. Projecting future drug expenditures 2012. *Am J Health Syst Pharm* 69:405.

Internal Revenue Service. 2019. "Forms & Pubs" Available at www.irs.gov. Accessed January 7, 2019.

National Community Pharmacists Association (NCPA). 2018. NCPA Digest. Alexandria, VA: National Community Pharmacists Association.

Nelson D. 2017. *Taking Stock: Inventory Management Best Practices for Community Pharmacies*. Chesterbrook, PA: AmerisourceBergen.

Rough S, McDaniel M, Rinehart J. 2010a. Effective use of workload and productivity monitoring tools in health-system pharmacy, part 1. *Am J Health Syst Pharm* 67:300.

Rough S, McDaniel M, Rinehart J. 2010b. Effective use of workload and productivity monitoring tools in health-system pharmacy, part 2. *Am J Health Syst Pharm* 67:380.

Schneider P, Pederson C, Scheckelhoff D. 2018. ASHP national survey of pharmacy practice in hospital settings: Dispensing and administration—2018. *Am J Health Syst Pharm* 75:1203.

United States Securities and Exchange Commission. 2019. Available at www.sec.gov. Accessed January 7, 2019.

Wilson AL. 2009. *Financial Management for Health Systems Pharmacists*. Bethesda, MD: American Society of Health-Systems Pharmacists.

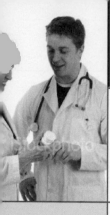

22

BUDGETING

David A. Gettman

About the Author: Dr. Gettman is a professor in the Department of Pharmaceutical, Administrative, and Social Sciences at the D'Youville College School of Pharmacy. He received his BS in pharmacy from the University of Montana, an MBA from the College of William and Mary, and PhD in pharmacy health care administration from the University of Florida. He has practiced pharmacy in numerous settings, including community, hospital, nursing home, hospice, and in the U.S. Navy and Air Force. In addition to pharmacy management, Dr. Gettman has taught pharmacy law, health care ethics, health care delivery, pharmacoepidemiology, pharmacoeconomics, biostatistics, and research design. The author of numerous publications, he has made over 150 presentations to professional health care groups at the state, national, and international levels.

■ LEARNING OBJECTIVES

After completing this chapter, readers should be able to

1. Explain the relationship between financial planning and the master budget.
2. List and explain five purposes of budgeting systems.
3. Describe the similarities and differences in the operational budgets prepared by pharmaceutical manufacturers, health system pharmacies offering value-added services, community pharmacies selling merchandise, and nonprofit pharmacy organizations.
4. Explain the concept of activity-based budgeting (ABB) and the benefits it brings to the budgeting process.
5. Describe each of the budget schedules that make up a master budget.
6. Discuss the role of assumptions and predictions in budgeting.
7. Describe a typical pharmacy organization's process of budget administration.
8. Understand the importance of budgeting product lifecycle costs.
9. Discuss the behavioral implications of budgetary slack and participative budgeting.

■ SCENARIO

Mary Quint, pharmacy student, has just started a 6-week elective advanced pharmacy practice experience (APPE) at Home TPN Care. On this APPE, Mary is working with Anne Smith, PharmD, who manages the production and distribution of total parenteral nutrition (TPN).

Home TPN Care is part of a local university's health system that includes a large teaching hospital, several clinics, and numerous ancillary services. Procurement, receiving, insurance verification, claims processing, and cash application operation activities all take place at the Home TPN Care facility, located 5 miles away from its main hospital. Home TPN Care consistently generates a positive net margin that contributes to the health system's margin targets and support of nonrevenue-generating activities. Clinical, patient care, quality, and process improvement programs are integrated into the health system's strategic plan.

Home TPN Care is a licensed pharmacy and home infusion provider responsible for providing a wide range of products and services to safely and effectively facilitate care to patients in the convenience and comfort of their homes. Since 2001, Home TPN Care has been providing infusion medications, nutritional therapy, specialty drugs, high-tech infusion nursing, and care management services throughout the region. An interdisciplinary team of pharmacists, nurses, and dietitians, along with technical, administrative, and support staff, provides pharmacy manufacturing (i.e., compounding), equipment management, dispensing, delivery, and care management services to ensure that patient home regimens are safe and effective throughout the course of therapy. The staff has direct access to up-to-date and complete medical and patient drug information that facilitates effective and efficient collaboration with physicians and other caregivers within the organization. To ensure a smooth transition to home care, Home TPN Care has a training and education team. This team consists of nurses and dietitians who work with patients and the referring health care team to ensure that home care needs are identified prior to hospital discharge and infusion nurses who provide care for patients in their homes.

Although Home TPN Care resides within the home care service division in the health system's organizational structure, an administrative relationship exists between Home TPN Care and the health system's department of pharmacy services. Thus, many administrative, pharmacy practice, and educational activities are collaborative and integrated. There is Home TPN Care representation on several pharmacy department committees. In addition, most of the Home TPN Care's health care professionals hold academic appointments within the university, reflecting a commitment to teaching, experiential training, and research.

Mary Quint has been advised that during this APPE she will need to assist Dr. Smith to develop a master budget, or profit plan, for Home TPN Care. It quickly became apparent that she would need to review the materials she studied in her pharmacy management course about budgeting before she could tackle this important challenge.

■ CHAPTER QUESTIONS

1. How does a budget facilitate communication and coordination in a pharmacy organization?
2. What is a master budget, and what are the parts of a master budget?
3. What is meant by the term *operational budgets*?
4. How does ABB help explain the logic of budgeting?
5. How does e-budgeting make use of the Internet?
6. What is the purpose of a budget manual?
7. Is padding the budget unethical?
8. What is budgetary slack, and what problem(s) can it cause?
9. What are three issues that create challenges for multinational pharmacies in preparing their budgets?

■ INTRODUCTION

Developing a budget is a critical step in planning any economic activity. This is true for any type of pharmacy operation, for individual pharmacists, and for governmental agencies that regulate both pharmacies and individual pharmacists. As individuals, we all must budget our money to meet day-to-day expenses and plan for major expenditures, such as buying a car or paying for college tuition. Similarly, pharmacies of all types and governmental agencies must make financial plans to carry out routine operations, to plan for major expenditures, and to help in making financial decisions.

As pharmacy organizations grow, they need systems to track financial, clinical, and other types of data. They also need to provide this data when, where, and to whom it is needed, in formats that managers find useful. People in pharmacy organizations also must communicate regarding this data with one another to create performance targets and set expectations about the financial and nonfinancial operations of the organization.

By formalizing the communication and coordination of operating and financial plans, the *master budget* makes sure that everyone's plans are consistent and that the total output of all those plans yields a result that makes sense for the organization. The master budget collects all of the operating plans and translates them into a financial picture of the results of the planned operations, along the way identifying the resources required to accomplish those plans and the costs of those resources.

■ PURPOSES OF BUDGETING SYSTEMS

A *budget* is a detailed plan, expressed in quantitative terms, which specifies how resources will be acquired and used during a specified period of time. The procedures used to develop a budget constitute a *budgeting system*. Budgeting systems have five primary purposes: planning; facilitating communication and coordination; allocating resources; controlling profit and operations; and evaluating performance and providing incentives.

Planning

The most common purpose of a budget is to quantify a plan of action. The budgeting process forces people who make up an organization to anticipate or react to changes in the environment and to plan ahead. For example, in the recent past, a patient with a chronic hepatitis C virus (HCV) infection faced a number of adverse health outcomes, including the possibility of liver transplantation. Managing these outcomes could result in costs for a payer of $500,000 or more over the patient's lifetime. However, newer oral drugs for chronic HCV infection have advantages in response rates and convenient dosage forms. They can greatly improve outcomes and eliminate the need for a liver transplant. However, these medications are expensive. For example, the pharmaceutical company Gilead Sciences had charged $84,000 for a 12-week treatment of Sovaldi™, and it priced another drug, Harvoni™, at $94,500. However, Gilead has released a generic version of Harvoni™ in January 2019, pricing it at $24,000 (Inserro, 2019).

Planning is also very important at the level of the practicing pharmacist. A good example involves the planning for vaccinations at pharmacy-based clinics. Cho and colleagues (2011) describe a mass vaccination clinic budgeting tool that clinic managers may use to estimate clinic costs and to examine how costs vary depending on the availability of volunteers or donated supplies and on the number of patients vaccinated per hour. The tool can also contribute to planning efforts for universal seasonal influenza vaccination. For novel vaccines (e.g., rotavirus, respiratory syncytial virus, human papilloma virus, and herpes zoster), another author describes a more tailored planning approach based on the individual characteristics and use of each product (Cannon, 2007).

Facilitating Communication and Coordination

For any organization to be effective, each manager throughout the organization must be aware of plans made by other managers. The budgeting process must pull together the plans, financial, as well as operational, of each manager in an organization. For example, pharmaceutical companies who market products with "blockbuster" potential are often developed by groups of researchers and project managers around the world. These managers require coordinated financial information at the local, national, and global levels (Cowlrick et al., 2002).

Moving closer to the level of the practicing pharmacist, communication and coordination are also very important. For example, the use of radiofrequency identification tags (RFID) to monitor drug movement is a relatively recent phenomenon (see Chapter 27). With the increases in drug counterfeiting and diversion across the world, pharmaceutical companies are striving to maintain top safety standards to keep their product in safe hands. Progressively, companies are coming to realize the value of containing data in an e-pedigree that can help them improve the reconciliation processes, such as returns and recalls. RFID technology can help with these issues and reduce costs, improve patient safety, and improve supply chain management effectiveness by increasing the ability to track and locate supplies, as well as monitoring theft prevention, distribution management, and patient billing (Coustasse et al., 2013).

Allocating Resources

All resources are limited, including those used by pharmacists and pharmacies. Budgets provide one means of allocating resources among competing uses. Hospitals, for example, must make difficult decisions about allocating their revenue among services (e.g., pharmacy, laboratory, and nursing), maintenance of property and equipment (e.g., beds, laminar flow hoods, and vehicles), and other community services (e.g., child care services and programs to prevent alcohol and drug abuse). In particular, allocating resources to pharmacy initiatives to improve patient safety often competes with initiatives from nursing and other areas where dollars are also needed to improve patient care (Tierney, 2004).

Controlling Profit and Operations

A budget is a plan, and plans are subject to change. Nevertheless, a budget serves as a useful benchmark with which actual results can be compared. For example, a community pharmacy can compare its actual sales of prescriptions for a year against its budgeted sales. Such comparisons can help managers evaluate the pharmacy's effectiveness in selling prescriptions. Pharmacy managers must be prepared and make changes when facing a financial crisis, such as when facing an unanticipated decline in sales or revenues or

an increase in expenses. Managers facing these situations must take the initiative to acquire the necessary data, to translate data into relevant information, to seek benchmarks for comparison, and to take corrective action. Once the crisis has passed, attention must be given to updating and maintaining databases, supporting the staff, and improving morale. Scenario planning can help to identify measures that might be taken should another crisis develop (Demers, 2001).

Evaluating Performance and Providing Incentives

Comparing actual results with budgeted results also helps pharmacy managers evaluate the performance of individuals, departments, or entire corporations. Since budgets are used to evaluate performance, they can also be used to provide incentives for people to perform well. Many third-party payers of patient care services utilize the fee-for-service (FFS) model, with formulas used to determine how much a provider will receive each time they provide a health service or sell a health product. Some movement is being made toward pay-for-performance (P4P) models within health care and particularly for pharmacy. Lenz and Monaghan (2011) concluded after their study that pharmacists should begin to explore ways they can participate in a high-performance health care system by moving to a P4P model of reimbursement rather than FFS or product-based dispensing reimbursement because P4P models of reimbursement could be beneficial to the patient, the payer, and the pharmacist. But, Rosenthal et al. (2017) conducted a study more recently that revealed a hesitation to radically transform payment for pharmacists' patient services toward a P4P model; and that efforts to implement P4P should therefore be gradual and accompanied with a robust evaluation plan.

■ TYPES OF BUDGETS

Different types of budgets serve different purposes. A *master budget*, or *profit plan*, is a comprehensive set of budgets covering all phases of a pharmacy organization's operations for a specified period of time.

Budgeted financial statements, often called *pro forma financial statements*, show how the pharmacy organization's financial statements will appear at a specified time if operations proceed according to plan. Budgeted financial statements include a budgeted income statement, a budgeted balance sheet, and a budgeted statement of cash flows.

A *capital budget* is a plan for the acquisition of capital assets, such as buildings and equipment. A *financial budget* is a plan that shows how the pharmacy business will acquire its financial resources, such as through the issuance of stock or incurrence of debt.

Budgets are developed for specific time periods. *Short-range budgets* cover a year, a quarter, or a month, whereas *long-range budgets* cover periods longer than a year. *Rolling budgets* are continually updated by periodically adding a new incremental time period, such as a quarter, and dropping the period just completed. Rolling budgets are also called *revolving budgets or continuous budgets*.

■ THE MASTER BUDGET: A PLANNING TOOL

When developing a budget, it is helpful to think of the production process for goods or services as a big machine: certain inputs are fed into the machine, various resources are then applied to convert those inputs into something different, and the output from the machine is what people are willing to buy. These are exactly the things that an organization needs to plan for in its budget: the quantity and cost of inputs, the quantity and cost of resources needed for conversion, and the units and revenues of outputs that can be sold. When managers develop budgets, it is important to recognize that the order of this planning process is reversed. The sales planning process and sales budget are created first, because the need for products and services to fill sales orders is what drives the company's production plans and the related production budget. The production budget, in turn, tells the organization how much of each input and conversion resource is needed. Combining this information with

the organization's input and resource cost estimates yields the appropriate budgets.

This logic and the resulting budgets are shown in Figure 22-1. The *master budget*, the principal output of a budgeting system, is a comprehensive profit plan that ties together all phases of a pharmacy's operations. The master budget consists of many separate budgets, or schedules, that are interdependent. It is a complicated process, but if one understands the budgets and relationships described in Figure 22-1, one will be well on his or her way to understanding budgeting.

Sales of Services or Goods

Because the market demand for a good or service drives the production process, the starting point for any master budget is a *sales revenue budget.* The sales revenue budget is based on a *sales forecast* for goods or services. For many pharmacy departments, this budget begins with a sales forecast for prescription drug spending. Community pharmacies base these estimates on past prescription counts and changes in trends that may influence the numbers of prescriptions filled in their pharmacies. Hospital pharmacies monitor bed counts and patient acuity levels when forecasting their production of pharmacy goods and services. Online and mail-order pharmacies forecast the number of patients visiting their sites and the percentage that will make purchases. Manufacturing and merchandising pharmacies forecast sales of their goods. Additionally, pharmacy managers need to keep abreast of how changes in government expenditures (e.g., Medicare prescription drug coverage) might change the distribution of drug spending among payers and affect aggregate spending (Poisal et al., 2007).

Sales Forecasting

The accuracy of the entire budgeting process depends on getting the sales budget right. Sales forecasting is a critical step in the budgeting process, and it is very difficult to do accurately.

Various procedures are used in sales forecasting, and the final forecast usually combines information from many different sources. Many pharmacy

SALES BUDGET   **OPERATIONAL BUDGETS**   **BUDGETED FINANCIAL STATEMENTS**

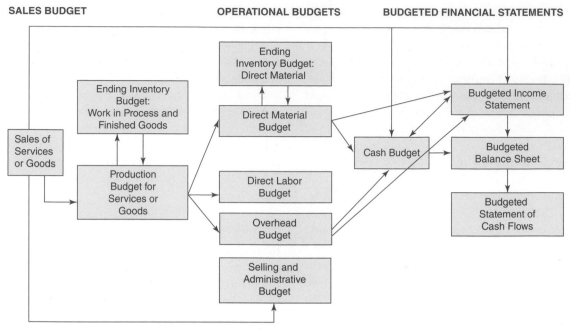

Figure 22-1. Master budget components.

corporations have a market research staff whose job is to coordinate the corporation's sales forecasting efforts. Typically, everyone from key executives to the firm's sales personnel will be asked to contribute sales projections.

Major factors considered when forecasting sales include the following:

1. Past sales levels and trends
   - For the firm developing the forecast (e.g., Walgreen's)
   - For the entire industry (e.g., the chain drug store industry)
2. General economic trends
   - Is the economy growing? How fast?
   - Is a recession or economic slowdown expected?
3. Economic trends in the pharmaceutical industry
   - Changes in the types of goods and services offered by pharmacies
   - Changes in the competitive environment between pharmacies
   - Changes in the demographic characteristics of pharmacy customers

4. Other factors expected to affect sales in the pharmaceutical industry
   - Is an unusually cold winter expected, which would result in increased demand for cold remedies in chain drug stores located in northern climates?
   - An increase or decrease in the incidence or prevalence of a particular condition or illness
5. Political and legal events
   - Impact of new laws on sales of pharmacy goods and services (e.g., Medicare Part D, Affordable Care Act)
   - Prescription to over-the-counter switches
6. The intended pricing policy of the pharmacy
7. Planned advertising and other promotional activities
8. Expected actions of competitors
9. New goods or services contemplated by the pharmacy or other pharmacies
   - Medication therapy management (MTM) services may increase the demand for some medications, while decreasing demand for others
10. Market research studies

The starting point in the sales forecasting process is generally the sales level of the previous year. Then the market research staff considers the information described above along with input from key executives and sales personnel. In many pharmacy organizations, elaborate econometric models are used to incorporate all the available information systematically. Statistical methods, such as regression analysis and probability distributions for sales, may also be used, particularly in large, multi-unit organizations (Shim et al., 2012). A great deal of effort goes into the sales forecast because it is such a critical step in the budgeting process. Developing a sales forecast is like shooting an arrow. If the archer's aim is off by only a fraction of an inch, the arrow will go further and further astray and miss the bull's eye by a wide margin. Similarly, a slightly inaccurate sales forecast, coming at the very beginning of the budgeting process, will likely disrupt all the other schedules comprising the master budget.

Operational Budgets

Based on the sales budget, a pharmacy organization develops a set of operational budgets that specify how its operations will be carried out to meet the demand for its goods or services. The budgets constituting this operational portion of the master budget are illustrated in Figure 22-1. Operational budgets differ because they are adapted to the operations of individual pharmacies in various industries. However, operational budgets are also similar in important ways. In each pharmacy, they encompass a detailed plan for using the basic factors of production—material, labor, and overhead—to produce a product and/or provide a service (Ward, 2015).

Pharmacy Organizations with Manufacturing

A pharmacy organization that conducts manufacturing operations develops a *production budget*, which shows the number of product units to be manufactured. Coupled with the production budget are ending *inventory budgets* for raw material, work in process, and finished goods. For example, home infusion pharmacies plan to have some inventory on hand at all times to meet peak demand while keeping production

at a stable level. From the production budget, this pharmacy develops budgets for the direct materials, direct labor, and overhead that will be required in the production process. A budget for selling and administrative expenses is also prepared.

Pharmacy Organizations with Merchandising

A pharmacy organization with merchandising may not manufacture products. Instead, it purchases products manufactured by others and sells them to end users, adding value through a combination of distribution and retail operations. The operational portion of the master budget of a pharmacy organization with merchandising is similar in a pharmacy organization with manufacturing, but instead of a production budget for goods, a merchandiser develops a budget for merchandise purchases. For example, a chain drug store pharmacy will not have a budget for direct material because it does not engage in production but they will have a costs of goods sold (COGS) budget (Cafferky & Wentworth, 2014). Furthermore, the chain drug pharmacy will develop budgets for labor (or personnel), overhead, and selling and administrative expenses.

Pharmacy Organizations with Patient Care Services

Based on the sales budget for its patient care services, a service-oriented pharmacy organization develops a set of budgets that show how the demand for those services will be met. A service-oriented pharmacy organization prepares a production budget for the production of its services and the related operational budgets, but the precise nature of these budgets depends on the specific patient care services. Pharmacy departments in hospitals are focusing their efforts on improving the efficiency of product-related functions mainly through automation and redeploying staff to value-added clinical functions. Services added under these transformations include intravenous-to-oral conversion, dosage adjustments for patients with renal impairment, MTM services, and participation in rounds in all areas of the hospital. The introduction of clinical pharmacy services as part of hospital-wide reengineering programs has been associated with positive benefit–cost ratios and a substantial net cost savings (Schumock et al., 1999).

Summary of Operational Budgets

Operational budgets differ since they are adapted to the operations of individual pharmacy organizations. However, operational budgets are also similar in important ways. In each organization, they encompass a detailed plan for using the basic factors of production—material, labor, and overhead—to produce a good and/or provide a service.

Financing Budgets

After developing its sales and operational budgets, a pharmacy organization knows where its money will be coming from and where it will go. But several timing issues affect when they can collect the cash. To plan for this, pharmacy organizations develop a set of financing budgets, shown in Figure 22-1, that project their cash flow and identify likely cash shortfalls and surpluses.

Cash Receipts Budget

Every pharmacy organization prepares a series of financing budgets. The cash receipts budget provides information about the cash flows into the pharmacy organization based on sales of its goods or services (as well as from cash contributions and grants, in the case of not-for-profit organizations). These inflows will often not precisely match budgeted sales. Reasons can include the following:

- The timing of sales and collections can differ from patient to patient. Between organizations, it is common to have payment terms specifying that cash will not change hands until 30 days or more after the sales date.
- Different payment methods convert to cash at different speeds. Cash payments can usually be deposited to the bank the same day as the sale. Proceeds from credit cards can take several days to be received, and payments from checks may take even longer.

- Some sales are never collected. Uncollectable accounts receivable due to bounced checks, counterfeit money, credit and debit card fraud, and customers who default on their obligations are all challenges that pharmacy organizations confront.

Cash Disbursements Budget

As shown in Figure 22-1, the cash disbursements budget depends on the spending plans reflected in several operational budgets, making it a quite complex budget. To further complicate matters, the timing of cash flows out of the pharmacy organization does not precisely align with the expenditures reflected in the operational budgets. The pharmacy organization will not pay cash immediately for most of its expenditures. Rather, it will pay its suppliers according to standard commercial arrangements, often delaying payment 30 days or more past the delivery date.

Cash Budget

The cash budget summarizes the various cash inflows and outflows from operations. The cash budget plays a critical role in planning the pharmacy organization's cash needs. Frequently, there is a mismatch in timing between when cash must be paid to produce goods and services and when cash can be collected from the patients and payers who purchase them. By predicting its net cash position at frequent points during the planning period, the pharmacy organization can plan ahead. It can arrange sources of borrowing for times when cash outflows exceed inflows, and it can plan to pay off borrowings and make investments when the cash flow reverses. The ability to foresee and avoid cash emergencies makes the cash budget a very important and powerful tool.

Not-for-profit Organizations

The master budget for a not-for-profit organization includes many of the components shown in Figure 22-1. However, there are some important differences. Many not-for-profit organizations provide services free of charge. Hence, there may be no sales budget as shown in Figure 22-1. However, such organizations do begin their budgeting process with a budget that describes the level of services to be provided. For example, the budget for a free clinic would describe the planned levels of various public services, such as the hours of operation for the outpatient pharmacy. Not-for-profit organizations also prepare budgets showing their anticipated funding. A free clinic budgets for revenue from both public (e.g., support from government agencies) and private sources (e.g., donations).

Budgeted Financial Statements

The final portion of the master budget, depicted in Figure 22-1, includes a budgeted income statement, a budgeted balance sheet, and a budgeted statement of cash flows. These budgeted financial statements show the overall financial results of the pharmacy organization's planned operations for the budget period. Notice that they are not the beginning of the master budgeting process, they are the end result.

■ ACTIVITY-BASED COSTING AND ACTIVITY-BASED BUDGETING

The concepts that underlie activity-based costing (ABC) can be used to better understand the budgeting process. ABC uses a two-stage cost-assignment process. In Stage 1, overhead costs are assigned to cost pools that represent the most significant activities. The activities identified vary across pharmacy organizations, but examples include such activities as purchasing, material handling, prescription processing, scheduling, inspection, quality control, and inventory control.

After assigning costs to the activity cost pools in Stage 1, cost drivers are identified that are appropriate for each cost pool. Then, in Stage 2, the overhead costs are allocated from each activity cost pool to cost objects (e.g., prescriptions, value-added services, and patients) in proportion to the amount of activity consumed. Figure 22-2 portrays the two-stage allocation process used in ABC systems.

ABC systems can be complicated. So, to illustrate the ABC process, Blakely-Gray (2018) offers a simple example. Let's figure out how much you are spending on utilities to create a product. To do this, you estimate that your utility bill is $20,000 for the year. You determine that the cost driver impacting your utility bill is the number of direct labor hours worked. The number of direct labor hours worked totaled 1000 hours for the year. Divide your total utility bill by your cost driver (the number of hours worked) to get your cost driver rate. Your overhead application rate is $20 ($20,000/1000 hours). For this particular

Stage 1 Resource costs are assigned to activities.	Resource costs are assigned to activity Cost pools associated with significant activities (e.g., purchasing or employee scheduling)

Stage 2 Overhead costs are assigned to cost objects.	Costs are assigned from each activity cost pool to each cost object in proportion to its consumption of the activity. Each activity has its own cost driver. (e.g., customers served)

Figure 22-2. Activity-based costing (ABC) system.

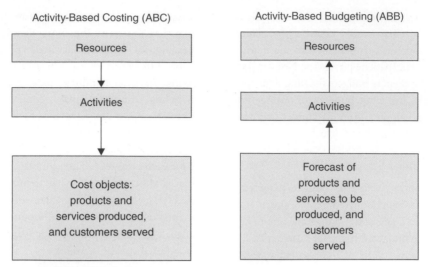

Figure 22-3. Activity-based costing (ABC) versus activity-based budgeting (ABB).

product, you used utilities for 3 hours. Multiply the hours by the cost rate of $20 to get $60.

Applying ABC concepts to the budgeting process helps to explain the logic of budgeting. Sometimes, the process is even referred to as *activity-based budgeting*. Conceptually, ABB takes the ABC model and reverses the flow of the analysis, as depicted in Figure 22-3. The first step is to specify the products and services produced and patients served. Then the activities that are necessary to produce these products and services are determined. Finally, the resources necessary to perform the specified activities are quantified.

ABB is more likely to be utilized by newer companies without historical budgeting information on which to rely. Also, ABB is more useful for companies undergoing material changes, such as those with new subsidiaries, significant customers, business locations, or products. So, to illustrate the ABB process, Kenton (2018) offers a simple example. A company anticipates receiving 50,000 sales orders in the upcoming year. The cost to process a single order is $2. Therefore, the ABB for the expenses relating to processing sales orders for the upcoming year is $100,000 ($50,000 * $2).

■ USING ACTIVITY-BASED BUDGETING TO PREPARE THE MASTER BUDGET

The process of constructing a master budget requires the pharmacy manager to use a variety of schedules that are displayed in Table 22-1. Manufacturing pharmacy organizations have several characteristics that complicate the budgeting process. Foremost among these are inventories, which add several additional steps to adjust for planned changes in inventory levels. Both inventories of finished products and inventories of raw materials and components require additional budgeting steps.

In many cases, manufacturing pharmacy organizations (e.g., community pharmacies that specialize in compounding, hospitals that prepare sterile intravenous admixtures) also have more complex cash flows because of the many transactions involved in their conversion processes and because of the many different ways they sell their products. Frequently, manufacturing pharmacy organizations also have large investments in property and equipment that require periodic reinvestment. The process of constructing a master budget for a manufacturing pharmacy

Table 22-1.   Schedules Used to Construct a Master Budget

Schedule	Description
Sales budget	Displays the projected sales in units for each quarter and then multiplies the unit sales by the sales price to determine sales revenue
Purchases budget	Shows services or goods from outside the organization in order to create its own services or goods
Production budget	Shows the number of units of services or goods that are to be produced during a budget period
Direct material budget	Shows the number of produced units and the cost of material to be purchased and used during a budget period
Direct labor budget	Shows the number of hours and the cost of the direct labor to be used during the budget period
Manufacturing overhead budget	Shows the cost of overhead expected to be incurred in the production process during the budget period
Selling, general, and administrative (SG&A) expense budget	Lists the expenses of administering the firm and selling its units (e.g., prescriptions)
Cash receipts budget	Details the expected cash collections during a budget period
Cash disbursements budget	Details the expected cash payments during a budget period
Cash budget	Details the expected cash receipts and disbursements during a budget period
Budgeted schedule of cost of goods manufactured and sold	Details the direct material, direct labor, and manufacturing overhead costs to be incurred, and shows the cost of the goods to be sold during the budget period
Budgeted income statement	Shows the expected revenue and expenses for the budget period, assuming that planned operations are carried out
Budgeted statement of cash flows	Provides information about the expected sources and uses of cash for operating activities, investing activities, and financing activities during a particular period of time
Budgeted balance sheet	Shows the expected end-of-period balances for the company's assets, liabilities, and owner's equity, assuming that planned operations are carried out

organization requires the pharmacy manager to use a variety of additional schedules.

Assumptions and Predications Underlying the Master Budget

A master budget is based on many assumptions and estimates of unknown parameters. Some estimates tend to be quite accurate, while other predictions are much more difficult to make accurately. A typical pharmacy organization's master budget reflects

predictions involving salaries, wage rates, electric and other utility rates, and insurance and property tax rates. Some of these predictions, e.g., property tax rates, would likely be quite accurate. Other predications would be more difficult. For example, the cost of natural gas for heating purposes is hard to predict because it depends on the weather.

Making predictions and agreeing on assumptions are valuable parts of the budgeting process. Pharmacy managers are forced to identify and agree on the assumptions that will be part of the year's financial plan. And after making the predictions, the risk of being wrong can sometimes be mitigated by pharmacy managers' actions.

Financial Planning Models

Pharmacy managers must make assumptions and predictions in preparing budgets because pharmacies, like any other business or organization, operate in a world of uncertainty. That is why the master budget is just one part of financial planning. Another part of financial planning is the financial planning model. A *financial planning model* is a set of mathematical relationships that expresses the interactions among the various operational, financial, and environmental events that determine the overall results of an organization's activities. A financial planning model is a mathematical expression of all the relationships expressed in the flowchart of Figure 22-1.

In a fully developed financial planning model, all of the key estimates and assumptions are expressed as general mathematical relationships. Then, the model is run on a computer many times to determine the impact of different combinations of these unknown variables. "What if" questions can be answered about such unknown variables as inflation, interest rates, the value of the dollar, demand, competitors' actions, union demands in forthcoming wage negotiations, and a host of other factors. The widespread availability of economical spreadsheet tools and cloud-based financial planning tools has made financial planning models a common management tool.

■ BUDGET ADMINISTRATION

In small organizations, the procedures used to gather information and construct a master budget are usually informal. The pharmacy owner or manager may be the sole person charged with gathering the required information, creating the various budgets, and evaluating their organization's performance against their budget. In contrast, larger organizations use a formal process to collect data and prepare

the master budget. Such organizations usually designate a budget director or chief budget officer. This is often the organization's controller (or comptroller in government organizations). The budget director works with departments of employees to specify the process by which budget data will be gathered, collect the information, and prepare the master budget. To communicate budget procedures and deadlines to employees throughout the organization, the budget director often develops and disseminates a budget manual. The budget manual states who is responsible for providing various types of information, when the information is required, and in what form the information is to take. For example, the budget manual for a community pharmacy chain may specify that each regional director is to send an estimate of the coming year's sales, by product line, to the budget director by September 1. The budget manual also states who should receive each schedule when the master budget is complete.

A budget committee, consisting of key senior executives, is often appointed to advise the budget director during preparation of the budget. The authority to give final approval to the master budget usually belongs to the board of directors or a board of trustees in not-for-profit organizations. Usually the board has a subcommittee whose task is to carefully examine the proposed budget and recommend approval or any changes deemed necessary. By exercising their authority to make changes in the budget and grant final approval, governing boards can wield considerable influence on the overall direction the organization takes.

e-Budgeting

As pharmacy organizations operate across multiple locations both nationally and internationally, the Internet is playing an increasingly important role in the budgeting process. e-Budgeting is an increasingly popular, Internet-based budgeting tool that can help streamline and speed up an organization's budgeting process. The "e" in e-budgeting stands for both electronic and enterprise-wide. Employees throughout an organization and at all levels can submit and retrieve budget information electronically via the Internet (Shim et al., 2012b).

e-Budgeting can occur in two different ways. In the first, a pharmacy organization runs a central financial planning application (software) on the pharmacy organization's computers, and then employees throughout the organization use the Internet to access the centralized application (the enterprise-hosted model). In an increasingly popular alternative approach, a financial planning software provider hosts the application on its website and the pharmacy organization's employees use the Internet to access the application and record data there. Unlike the enterprise-hosted model, this provider-hosted approach, often called a cloud or SaaS (software-as-a-service) solution, has the advantages of frequent, centralized updating of the e-budgeting software by the software vendor combined with the outsourcing of the technology issues associated with hosting and running the software. However, it also has one very important disadvantage: the pharmacy organization's proprietary financial data resides outside the company's walls. This is a serious data security risk, but one that financial planning software providers are increasingly mitigating to the satisfaction of their clients via extensive security procedures (Button, 2015).

Managers in pharmacy organizations using e-budgeting have found that it greatly streamlines the entire budgeting process. In the past, these organizations have compiled their master budgets on hundreds of spreadsheets, which had to be collected and integrated by the corporate controller's office. One result of this cumbersome approach was that a disproportionate amount of time was spent compiling and verifying data from multiple sources. Under e-budgeting, both the submission of budget information and its compilation are accomplished electronically. Thus, e-budgeting is just one more area where the Internet has transformed how the workplace operates in the era of e-business. Examples of this type of software include OutlookSoft, Cognos, and Web-FOCUS.

■ INTERNATIONAL ASPECTS OF BUDGETING

As the economies and cultures of countries throughout the world become intertwined, more companies are becoming multinational in their operations. For example, Walgreen Co. has reached beyond the borders of the United States with an unprecedented international expansion by buying a 45% stake in Alliance Boots, a European retail pharmacy chain, creating a new company known as Walgreens Boots Alliance (WBA) (Cherney, 2014). Firms like WBA with international operations face a variety of additional challenges in preparing their budgets. First, a multinational firm's budget must reflect the translation of foreign currencies into the organization's official corporate currency, which is usually determined by the location of the corporate headquarters or the stock exchange on which the organization has its primary listing. Although multinationals have sophisticated financial ways of hedging against such currency fluctuations, the budgeting task is still more challenging. Second, it is difficult to prepare budgets when inflation is high or unpredictable. Most countries occasionally experience periods of high inflation, and some countries have experienced hyperinflation, sometimes with annual inflation rates well over 100%. Finally, the economies of all countries fluctuate in terms of consumer demand, availability of skilled labor, laws affecting commerce, and other factors. Companies like WBA with offshore operations face the task of anticipating such changing conditions in their budgeting processes (Shumsky, 2018).

■ BUDGETING PRODUCT LIFECYCLE COSTS

A relatively recent focus of the budgeting process is to plan for all the costs that will be incurred throughout a product's lifecycle, before a commitment is made to the product. Product lifecycle costs encompass the following five phases in a product's lifecycle:

1. Product planning and concept design
2. Preliminary design

3. Detailed design and testing
4. Production
5. Distribution and customer service

For example, for a pharmaceutical manufacturer to justify a new drug's introduction, the sales revenues it will generate must be sufficient to cover all these costs. Thus, planning these costs is a crucial step in making a decision about the introduction of a new drug. This is particularly true for firms with products that may have very short lifecycles. When product lifecycles are as short as a year or 2, the firm does not have time to adjust its pricing strategy or production methods to ensure that the product turns a profit. Management must be fairly certain before a commitment is made to the product that its lifecycle costs will be covered. Most of a product's lifecycle costs are committed rather early in the product's life. By the time the planning, design, and testing phases are complete, roughly 85% of the product's lifecycle costs have been committed, while only about 5% actually have been incurred (Silva, 2015). Given the early commitment that must be made to significant downstream costs in a product's lifecycle, it is crucial to budget these costs as early as possible.

■ BEHAVIORAL IMPACT OF BUDGETS

A budget affects virtually everyone in an organization—those who prepare the budget, those who use the budget to facilitate decision-making, and those who are evaluated using the budget. The human reactions to the budgeting process can have considerable influence on an organization's overall effectiveness.

A great deal of study has been devoted to the behavioral effects of budgets (Michelle & Talib, 2017; Sherman, 2017). Two key issues that a pharmacy manager should clearly understand are budgetary slack and participative budgeting.

Budgetary Slack: Padding the Budget

The information on which a budget is based comes largely from people throughout an organization.

For example, the sales forecast for a community pharmacy chain relies not only on research and analysis by market research staff but also incorporates the projections of sales personnel, including pharmacy managers. If a regional sales manager's performance is evaluated on the basis of whether the sales budget for the region is exceeded, what is the incentive for the sales manager in projecting sales? The incentive is to give a conservative estimate, or to *underestimate* the anticipated levels of sales. The sales manager's performance will look better in the eyes of administrators when a conservative estimate is exceeded than when an ambitious estimate is not met.

On the other hand, when an administrator is asked to provide a cost projection for budgetary purposes, there is an incentive to *overestimate* costs. When the actual cost incurred proves to be less than the inflated cost projection, the administrator appears to have managed in a cost-effective way.

These illustrations are examples of padding the budget. *Budget padding* means intentionally underestimating revenue and/or overestimating costs. The difference between the revenue or cost projection that a person provides and a realistic estimate of the revenue or cost is called *budgetary slack*. For example, if a pharmacy manager believes the annual utilities cost will be $18,000 but gives a budgetary projection of $20,000, the manager has built $2,000 of slack into the budget.

Why do managers pad budgets with budgetary slack? There are three primary reasons. First, managers often perceive that their performance will look better in their superiors' eyes if they can "beat the budget." Second, budgetary slack is often used to cope with uncertainty. A pharmacy manager may feel confident in his or her cost projections. However, the pharmacy manager also may feel that some unforeseen event during the budgetary period could result in unanticipated costs. For example, an unexpected laminar flow hood breakdown could occur. One way of planning ahead for unforeseen events such as a laminar flow hood breakdown is to pad the budget. If nothing goes wrong, the pharmacy manager can beat the cost budget. If some negative event does occur, the pharmacy manager can use the budgetary slack to absorb the impact of the event and still meet the cost budget (Huang & Chen, 2009).

The third reason why cost budgets are padded is that budgetary cost projections are often cut by others in the resource-allocation process. Thus, the process of preparing budgets can result in a vicious cycle. Budgetary projections are padded because they will likely be cut, and they are cut because they are likely to have been padded (Leavins et al., 1995).

How does an organization solve the problem of budgetary slack? First, it can avoid relying on the budget as a performance evaluation tool. If a pharmacy manager is beleaguered by a higher level administrator every time a budgetary cost projection is exceeded, the likely behavioral response will be to pad the budget. In contrast, if the pharmacy manager is allowed some discretion to exceed the budget when necessary, there will be fewer tendencies toward budgetary padding. Second, pharmacy managers can be given incentives not only to achieve budgetary projections but also to provide *accurate* projections. This can be accomplished by asking pharmacy managers to justify all or some of their projections and by rewarding pharmacy managers who consistently provide accurate estimates as opposed to rewarding managers who perform under their cost projections and punishing managers who exceed their cost projections (Chen & Jones, 2004). And, finally, across the board budget cuts during the budgeting process should be avoided in favor of more targeted approaches that are based on spending justifications.

Is Padding the Budget Unethical?

A budget (such as a pharmacy department budget) is often used as the basis for evaluating a pharmacy manager's performance. Actual results are compared with budgeted performance levels, and those who outperform the budget are often rewarded with promotions and/or salary increases. In many cases, bonuses are tied explicitly to performance relative to the budget. For example, the top-management personnel of a department may receive a bonus if departmental profit exceeds budgeted profit by a certain percentage.

Serious ethical issues can arise in situations where a budget is the basis for rewarding managers. For example, suppose a pharmacy department's top-management personnel will split a bonus equal to 10% of the amount by which actual departmental profit exceeds the budget. This may create an incentive for the departmental budget officer, or other managers supplying data, to pad the departmental profit budget. Such padding would make the budget easier to achieve, thus increasing the chance of a bonus. Alternatively, there may be an incentive to manipulate the actual departmental results to maximize management's bonus. For example, year-end sales could be shifted between years to increase reported revenue in a particular year. Budget personnel could have such incentives for either of two reasons: (1) they might share in the bonus or (2) they might feel pressure from the managers who would share in the bonus.

Put yourself in the position of the pharmacy department manager. Your bonus, and that of your boss, one of the organization's vice presidents, will be determined in part by the department's income in comparison to the budget. When your department has submitted budgets in the past, upper management has usually cut your budgeted expenses, thereby increasing the department's budgeted profit. Moreover, it makes less likely that you and your departmental colleagues will earn a bonus.

Now your boss is pressuring you to pad the expense budget, because "the budgeted expenses will just be cut anyway at the upper management level." Is padding the budget ethical under these circumstances? What do you think? And, how could you resolve the situation?

Participative Budgeting

Most people will perform better and make greater attempts to achieve a goal if they have been consulted in setting the goal. The idea of participative budgeting is to involve employees throughout an organization in the budgetary process. Such participation can give employees the feeling that "this is our budget" rather than the all-too-common feeling that "this is the budget you imposed on us." After a 5-year growth spurt, participative budgeting has entered its awkward adolescence, full of bold achievements, flashes of potential, and some stumbles (Lerner, 2017).

While participative budgeting can be very effective, it can also have shortcomings. Too much participation and discussion can lead to vacillation and delay. Also, when those involved in the budgeting process disagree in significant and irreconcilable ways, the process of participation can accentuate those differences. Finally, the problem of budget padding can be severe unless incentives for accurate projections are provided.

■ REVISITING THE SCENARIO

Mary Quint, pharmacy student, has been working with Dr. Anne Smith, and now knows that a budget is often used as the basis for evaluating a pharmacy manager's performance. Actual results are compared with budgeted performance levels, and those who outperform the budget are often rewarded with promotions or salary increases. In many cases, bonuses are tied explicitly to performance relative to a budget.

Serious ethical issues can arise in situations where a budget is the basis for rewarding managers. For example, suppose Home TPN Care's top-management personnel will split a bonus equal to 10% of the amount by which the actual business unit profit exceeds the budget. This may create an incentive for the pharmacy manager supplying data to pad the profit budget. Such padding would make the budget easier to achieve, thus increasing the chance of a bonus.

Alternatively, there may be an incentive to manipulate the business unit's actual results to maximize management's bonus. For example, year-end sales could be shifted between years to increase reported revenue in a particular year. Budget personnel could have such incentives for either of two reasons: (1) they might share in the bonus or (2) they might feel pressure from the managers who would share in the bonus.

Mary Quint has put herself in the position of Home TPN Care's controller during this APPE and learned a great deal about what it would be like to be a manager like Dr. Anne Smith. Her bonus, and that of her boss, the health system's Vice President, will be determined in part by Home TPN Care's income in comparison with the budget. She can see from budgets submitted in the past that the organization's management usually has cut the unit's budgeted expenses, thereby increasing the business unit's budgeted profit. This, of course, makes it more difficult for her business unit to achieve the budgeted profit. Moreover, it makes it less likely that she and her business unit colleagues will earn a bonus. Now her boss is pressuring her to pad the expense budget because "the budgeted expenses will just be cut anyway at the organizational level." Is padding the budget ethical under these circumstances?

■ CONCLUSION

The budget is a key tool for planning, controlling, and decision-making in virtually every organization. Budgeting systems are used to force planning, to facilitate communication and coordination, to allocate resources, to control profit and operations, and to evaluate performance and provide incentives. Various types of budgets are used to accomplish these objectives.

Since budgets affect almost everyone in an organization, they can have significant behavioral implications and can raise difficult ethical issues. One common problem in budgeting is the tendency of people to pad budgets. The resulting budgetary slack makes the budget less useful because the padded budget does not present an accurate picture of expected revenue and expenses.

■ QUESTIONS FOR FURTHER DISCUSSION

1. Give an example to explain how a budget could be used to allocate resources in a hospital pharmacy.
2. Give an example of how general economic trends would affect sales forecasting in the pharmaceutical industry.
3. Give three examples of how an independent community pharmacy could use a budget for planning purposes.
4. Discuss the importance of predictions and assumptions in the budgeting process.
5. How can the pharmacy department of a large urban hospital help to reduce the problems caused by budgetary slack?
6. Why is participative budgeting often an effective pharmacy management tool?
7. List the steps you would go through in developing a budget to meet your independent community pharmacy expenses.

REFERENCES

Blakely-Gray. 2018. Activity-based costing for small business. Accounting training, tips, and news. Available at https://www.patriotsoftware.com/accounting/training/blog/activity-based-costing-small-business/. Accessed February 28, 2019.

Button K. 2015. Considering the cloud. *CFO* 31:41–43.

Cafferky ME, Wentworth J. 2014. Breakeven analysis: the definitive guide to cost-volume-profit analysis. New York: Business Expert Press, p. 222.

Cannon HE. 2007. Pharmacy management of vaccines. *J Manag Care Pharm* 13(7):S7–S11.

Chen CC, Jones KT. 2004. Budgetary slack and performance in group participative budgeting: The effects of individual and group performance feedback and task interdependence. *Adv Manage Account* 13:183–221.

Cherney M. 2014. Walgreen deal adds to bonds' banner year. *Wall Street J* 264:110, C4.

Cho BH, Hicks KA, Honeycutt AA, et al. 2011. A tool for the economic analysis of mass prophylaxis operations with an application to H1N1 influenza vaccination clinics. *J Public Health Manag Pract* 17:E22–E28.

Coustasse A, Tomblin S, Slack C. 2013. Impact of radio-frequency identification (RFID) technologies on the hospital supply chain: a literature review. *Perspect Health Inf Manag* 10:1d.

Cowlrick I, Dumon J, Bauleser M. 2002. Managing medical information effectively facilitates the quality and time to delivering the final product. *Drug Info J* 36:825.

Demers RF. 2001. Operational and financial principles of "managing up." *Am J Health Syst Pharm* 58:S7.

Huang CL, Chen ML. 2009. The effect of attitudes towards the budgetary process on attitudes towards budgetary slack and behaviors to create budgetary slack. *SBP* 37(5):661–671.

Inserro A. 2019. 2019 Brings end to Hepatitis C virus treatment rationing in Oregon. Available at https://www.contagionlive.com/news/2019-brings-end-to-hepatitis-c-virus-treatment-rationing-oregon. Accessed February 28, 2019.

Kenton W. 2018. Activity-Based Budgeting (ABB). Investopedia. Available at https://www.investopedia.com/terms/a/abb.asp. Accessed February 29, 2019.

Leavins JR, Omer K, Vilutis A. 1995. A comparative study of alternative indicators of budgetary slack. *Managerial Finance* 21(3):52–67.

Lenz TL, Monaghan MS. 2011. Pay-for-performance model of medication therapy management in pharmacy practice. *JAPhA* 51(3):425–431.

Lerner J. 2017. Conclusion: time for participatory budgeting to grow up. *New Political Science* 39(1):156–160.

Michelle TC, Talib A. 2017. Behavioral aspects of budgeting. *IJDR* 7(10):16318–16322.

Poisal JA, Truffer C, Smith S, et al. 2007. Health spending projections through 2016: Modest changes obscure Part D's impact. *Health Aff* 26(2):w242–w53.

Rosenthal MM, Desai N, Houle SKD. 2017. Pharmacists' perceptions of pay for performance versus fee-for-service remuneration for management of hypertension through pharmacist prescribing. *Int J Pharm Pract* 25(5):388–393.

Schumock GT, Michaud J, Guenette AJ. 1999. Reengineering: An opportunity to advance clinical practice in a community hospital. *Am J Health Syst Pharm* 56(19):1945–1999.

Sherman F. Behavioral Aspects of Budgeting in Managerial Accounting. 2017. Bizfluent. Available at https://bizfluent.com/info-8561309-behavioral-aspects-budgeting-managerial-accounting.html. Accessed March 1, 2019.

Shim JK. Siegel JG. Shim AI. 2012. Regression Analysis: Popular Sales Forecast System. Budgeting Basics and Beyond. 4th Edition. Hoboken, NJ: Wiley, pp. 289–300.

Shumsky T. 2018. Walgreens Boots Alliance: Zero-Based Budgeting Stars in Walgreens' Cost Cutting Push. MarketScreener. Available at https://www.marketscreener.com/WALGREENS-BOOTS-ALLIANCE-19356230/news/Walgreens-Boots-Alliance-Zero-Based-Budgeting-Stars-in-Walgreens-Cost-Cutting-Push-27786456/. Accessed February 28, 2019.

Silva H, Sonstein S, Stonier P, et al. 2015. Alignment of competencies to address inefficiencies in medicines development and clinical research: Need for inter-professional education. *Pharm Med New Zealand* 29(3):131–140.

Tierney M. 2004. Lessons from patient deaths: An Ontario pharmacist responds to Calgary's patient safety review. *Can Pharm J* 137(8):9.

Ward WJ. 2015. Health Care Budgeting and Financial Management. 2nd ed. Santa Barbara, CA: Praeger. pp. 113–138.

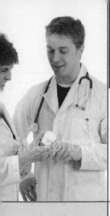

23

THIRD-PARTY PAYER CONSIDERATIONS

Julie M. Urmie and Benjamin Y. Urick

About the Authors: Dr. Urmie is an associate professor in the Health Services Research Division at the University of Iowa College of Pharmacy. She received a BS in pharmacy from the University of Wisconsin and worked as a community pharmacist prior to returning to the University of Wisconsin for graduate school, where she received an MS in pharmacy administration and a PhD in social and administrative sciences in pharmacy. Her teaching interests include insurance and reimbursement in pharmacy, health insurance, the US health care system, health policy, and pharmacy management. Her main areas of research are prescription drug insurance and consumer preferences related to health care use.

Dr. Urick is a research assistant professor at the Center for Medication Optimization at the University of North Carolina Eshelman School of Pharmacy. His academic interests lie at the intersection of pharmacy practice, health care, and health policy. His primary research focuses on the role of community pharmacists in the evolving health care system and the use of secondary data to measure health care quality and spending. His current research includes evaluation of pharmacy services interventions, scientific reliability of provider-level quality measures, and factors which influence medication-related health care quality.

■ LEARNING OBJECTIVES

After completing this chapter, readers should be able to

1. Discuss the history of third-party reimbursement for prescription drugs and its impact on pharmacy management.
2. Understand the basic principles of third-party reimbursement for prescription drugs and define commonly used reimbursement terminology.
3. Evaluate the financial impact of third-party reimbursement on the pharmacy using an average net profit comparison, a differential analysis, and a pro forma analysis.
4. Identify the broad range of factors that a pharmacy manager should consider when evaluating a third-party contract.
5. Discuss issues related to third-party reimbursement for prescription drugs.

■ SCENARIO

Natalie Hawkins, the pharmacy manager at Good Service Pharmacy in Tipton, IA, is concerned because she has been losing Better Health Medicare Part D plan patients to other pharmacies which are part of the Better Health preferred pharmacy network. If patients go to a preferred pharmacy, they can save $15 per prescription per month in copayments so there is a strong incentive for patients to choose preferred pharmacies. She opens her mail and sees that Better Health Medicare Part D has sent a new contract wherein she can now join the preferred network. Under the contract, her pharmacy has an opportunity to join Better Health's preferred pharmacy network but reimbursement rates will be lower. Alternatively, they can keep the current reimbursement rate and remain a non-preferred pharmacy, but risk continuing to lose Better Health patients. The new contract also has direct and indirect remuneration (DIR) fees that are based on the pharmacy's performance. For this contract, performance is defined using a combination of adherence measures and generic drug utilization rate (GDUR). If the pharmacy can score in the top 20% of all pharmacies on enough measures, Better Health will consider them a high-performing pharmacy. Her current contract with Better Health is AWP—15% for brand and—25% for generic with a *maximum allowable cost* (MAC) list, plus a $0.75 dispensing fee (DF) with a 3% DIR fee. To be a Better Health preferred provider, she would have to accept a reimbursement rate of AWP—17% for brand and AWP—27% for generic, plus a $0.50 DF with a 5% to 7% DIR fee based on pharmacy performance.

Better Health currently provides prescription drug coverage for 15% of their patients, and Natalie worries about the financial impact of continuing to lose those customers if she does not join the preferred pharmacy network. Natalie also thinks about Mrs. Anderson, a 78-year-old woman with Better Health Insurance, who has been coming to her pharmacy for over 20 years. Natalie has spent many hours over the years talking with Mrs. Anderson about her medications, and Mrs. Anderson has stated her rent has gone up recently and she needs to pinch every penny she can. Natalie cannot imagine having to tell her that they aren't a preferred pharmacy so she will have to pay more for her prescriptions if she continues to use Good Service Pharmacy. As the pharmacy manager, Natalie knows that it is her responsibility to decide whether to become a preferred pharmacy, but as a new manager, she worries about how to make an informed decision that balances the financial needs of the pharmacy with other considerations. Natalie wonders:

1. Is it better for Good Service Pharmacy to accept a lower reimbursement rate to become a Better Health preferred pharmacy? How much will the net profit on an average Better Health prescription decrease under the contract terms for preferred pharmacies? Will the pharmacy lose money on each Better Health prescription it dispenses?

2. If Good Service Pharmacy becomes a preferred pharmacy, what would be the difference in profit if the plan determines the pharmacy to be a high performer vs. low performer based on adherence scores and GDUR?

3. Overall, would Good Service Pharmacy be better off financially by joining the Better Health preferred pharmacy network?

4. What other factors need to be considered? Could the contract be renegotiated? What effect would signing or declining the contract have on its customers?

5. Good Service Pharmacy will likely lose revenue regardless of whether or not they join the Better Health preferred pharmacy network. Is there any way for Good Service Pharmacy to make up the lost revenue? Or decrease its expenses?

■ OVERVIEW OF THE IMPACT OF THIRD-PARTY REIMBURSEMENT IN PHARMACY

This scenario is a common occurrence in pharmacies of all sizes and types across the country. Although the scenario focuses on an independent pharmacy, all pharmacies that dispense outpatient prescriptions face similar decisions. Pharmacists working at chain pharmacies, clinics, and outpatient hospital pharmacies may not directly make decisions about third-party contracts, but contract-related decisions are being made at a corporate level under the same environmental pressures faced by independent pharmacy owners. All pharmacists feel the effects of these decisions, so it is important for all pharmacists to understand third-party reimbursement. A *third party* is defined as an organization that reimburses a pharmacy or patient for all or part of the patient's prescription drug costs. Since the vast majority of prescriptions dispensed in pharmacies today are paid for by third parties, it is essential that pharmacy managers and pharmacists understand the effect of third parties on pharmacy operations.

Pharmacies have third-party patients and private-pay patients. Private-pay patients, sometimes referred to as *cash patients*, are people who do not have any health insurance coverage or people who have health insurance that does not cover prescription drugs. Some patients with prescription drug insurance may choose to pay cash if the cash price is less than their copayment; this has become more common due to rising patient cost sharing and the prevalence of $4 generic prescriptions or other discount pricing offered by some pharmacies. Other patients may have prescription insurance, but have a deductible or limit in benefits. From the pharmacy's perspective, patients who pay the pharmacy directly for their prescriptions and later are reimbursed by their insurance company often are indistinguishable from private-pay patients. This type of prescription drug insurance, called *indemnity insurance*, used to be common, but it has now been replaced largely by *service benefit plans*. Under a service benefit plan, the patient may pay the pharmacy a predetermined portion of the prescription cost, but the pharmacy is reimbursed directly by the third party for most of the prescription cost.

Third parties may be public or private. Private third parties typically are insurance companies, although other private entities sometimes pay for a patient's prescriptions. For example, some pharmaceutical manufacturers provide free or discounted prescriptions through pharmaceutical manufacturer assistance programs. Public third parties are government entities that pay for prescriptions through a government program, for example, Medicaid, Medicare Part D, or a state prescription drug assistance program. Medicaid is the government program that provides health care for the poor. The program is funded jointly by federal and state governments, with each state determining its own prescription drug reimbursement rates. Medicaid was expanded in many states under the Affordable Care Act of 2010 (ACA). A trend in Medicaid is for states to have private insurance companies manage their Medicaid programs. In 2017, almost 70% of Medicaid beneficiaries were in plans managed by a private insurance company (Medicaid and CHIP Payment and Access Commission, 2017). Medicare, the government program that provides health insurance for the elderly and disabled, implemented a voluntary Medicare Part D outpatient prescription drug benefit in 2006. Medicare Part D has had a significant impact on pharmacies because many former private-pay patients now have Part D coverage. Medicare Part D is a mixed public and private third party because the government regulates the benefit, but private third parties deliver the benefit.

Most third parties hire pharmacy benefit managers (PBMs) to provide prescription claims processing and other services. Examples of third parties that hire PBMs are insurance companies, employers, Medicare Part D plans, and state Medicaid programs. PBMs establish pharmacy networks as part of their claims management services, so many pharmacy third-party contracts are with PBMs. In addition to processing claims for prescriptions filled at pharmacies, other services PBMs provide include rebate negotiation with pharmaceutical manufacturers, drug benefit design, formulary development and management, drug utilization management, and disease-state/case management. Most PBMs also offer mail-order pharmacy services.

The past three decades has been a time of tremendous growth in third-party payment for prescriptions. The percentage of prescription drug expenditures reimbursed by a third party increased from 44% in 1990 to 86% in 2017 (Martin et al., 2019). Initially, most of the growth was in private third-party payment, but more recently the trend has been away from private insurance payment and toward public insurance payment. This trend was accelerated by Medicare Part D and the ACA. The percent of *prescriptions* paid for by third parties is slightly higher than the percent of *prescription drug expenditures* paid by third parties due to patient cost sharing (e.g., copayments, deductibles). In 2017, 89% of prescriptions dispensed at independent pharmacies were paid for by a third party: 53% by government programs and 36% by other third-party payers (NCPA, 2018).

This shift toward predominantly third-party payment for prescription drugs has had a significant impact on pharmacy management. Pharmacies determine what price they want to charge private-pay patients, but as discussed further in the following paragraph, the reimbursement level for third-party prescriptions is determined by a contract between the third party and the pharmacy. Pharmacies usually are not allowed to charge patients more than the contracted reimbursement rate, so in practice, the revenues that a pharmacy receives for the vast majority of prescription medications are not determined by the prices that they charge, but instead by the reimbursement terms set in contracts with various third parties. This decreases the flexibility that pharmacy owners and managers have to price prescription drugs dispensed at their pharmacies.

Owners and managers decide what third-party contracts to accept, but once the contract is accepted, the revenue generated for dispensing a prescription is determined by the contract between the pharmacy and the third party. A significant concern in pharmacy is the level of reimbursement specified in these contracts. The reimbursement varies considerably across contracts, so pharmacy managers must make informed decisions about which contracts to accept. An important piece of information to know for each contract is the average *gross margin*, sometimes called *gross profit*, defined as the difference between the reimbursed price and the ingredient cost of the dispensed product. The average gross margin for independent community pharmacies in 2017 was 21.8%,

a decrease from 24.0% in 2010 (NCPA, 2018). There is considerable apprehension about ongoing decreases in third-party reimbursement for prescription drugs. Another concern associated with third-party prescriptions is that they generally cost more to dispense than private-pay prescriptions because of the extra steps involved in dispensing a third-party prescription. For third-party prescriptions, the pharmacy staff must verify patient eligibility, submit and reconcile claims, wait for payment, and comply with third-party rules and requirements, such as formularies. Knowing how to calculate the average cost of dispensing (COD) prescriptions is an important managerial tool that will be discussed in more detail later in this chapter.

Lower third-party reimbursement combined with higher third-party COD means that average net profit generally is lower for third-party prescriptions than for private-pay prescriptions. This implies that pharmacy owners and managers need to evaluate carefully the financial impact of accepting third-party contracts. Tools for this evaluation are discussed later in this chapter. Pharmacy managers also need to consider many nonfinancial factors when making third-party contract decisions; these factors also will be discussed in this chapter.

■ PHARMACY NETWORKS

Third-party payers have pharmacy networks for which pharmacies must accept the third party's reimbursement rate to participate in the network. Third-party payers either require that patients obtain their prescriptions from a network pharmacy, or they may allow patients to use non-network pharmacies, but then require the patient to pay more out of their own funds for their prescriptions. Third-party payers also may only allow patients to get more than a one-month supply for maintenance medications at a network pharmacy. These incentives for patients to use network pharmacies put considerable pressure on pharmacies to participate in third-party networks. Third-party payers also may have a preferred pharmacy network within their broader pharmacy network. Patients have reduced copayments or other incentives to use the preferred pharmacies. Pharmacies choosing to be preferred pharmacies have the opportunity to obtain additional prescription volume, but usually at the cost of lower prescription drug reimbursement rates.

Third-party payors have considerable leverage when it comes to negotiating with pharmacies on reimbursement rates and other terms of network participation. This stems from the fact that there are usually many pharmacies which serve a given area, but relatively few third-party payers. Individual pharmacies need to participate in a third-party payer's network much more than a third-party payer needs any individual pharmacy to participate in their network in order to provide adequate levels of service to their beneficiaries. This challenge has been magnified by many mergers among PBMs and health insurance companies in the past decade, the most recent being the CVS Health merger with Aetna (Abelson and Singer 2012; Livingston, 2018; Pear, 2015; Wilde et al., 2015). Pharmacy owners and managers often face the same dilemma as Natalie does in this chapter scenario, deciding whether the pharmacy should accept lower preferred pharmacy reimbursement rates in exchange for higher prescription volume. Some third-party payers choose to include a limited number of pharmacies in their preferred networks, so an individual pharmacy may be excluded from a preferred network, even if they are willing to accept their terms.

In recent years, there has been a proliferation of preferred pharmacy networks, particularly in Medicare Part D. The percent of Medicare Part D plans with a preferred pharmacy network increased from 7% in 2011 to 99% in 2018 (Fein, 2017). In Medicare Part D, patients are allowed to use non-preferred pharmacies, but they will face higher cost sharing. Large chain pharmacies, as well as pharmacies that serve large geographic areas, are likely to have more bargaining power than single independent pharmacies or pharmacies that compete with many others in a small area. The pharmacy access standards that Medicare requires for plans participating in Part D may increase bargaining power for pharmacies located

in areas with no other pharmacies. For example, if there is only one pharmacy in a rural or underserved area of a state, and the access standards require at least one network pharmacy in that part of the state, then that pharmacy should be able to negotiate better reimbursement terms.

■ PHARMACY SERVICES ADMINISTRATIVE ORGANIZATIONS

Most independently owned pharmacies outsource their third-party contract negotiation to pharmacy services administrative organizations (PSAOs). PSAOs act as intermediaries between the third-party payers and the smaller pharmacies. They help smaller pharmacies to gain more bargaining power by negotiating on behalf of many pharmacies. The number of pharmacies represented by the major PSAOs ranged from 700 to 5900 in 2017 and the largest PSAOs are owned by drug wholesalers (Fein, 2018a). PSAOs provide valuable and timesaving services, but it is important to assess whether they are making the contracting decisions that best represent the interests of your pharmacy. As discussed later in this chapter, many factors go into evaluating a third-party contract, so having a good understanding of how a contract will affect your pharmacy is essential to make strategic decisions.

■ THIRD-PARTY REIMBURSEMENT FOR PRESCRIPTION DRUGS

The payment for a third-party prescription is based on a reimbursement-rate formula that is specified in the contract between the pharmacy and the third-party payer. The reimbursement-rate formula almost universally consists of two parts: the *product cost portion* and the *DF*. The *product cost portion* is intended to pay the pharmacy for the cost of the drug product, and the *DF* is intended to cover the COD the prescription. The total reimbursement rate (product cost + DF) should be higher than the costs of obtaining and dispensing the drug to provide some profit to the pharmacy. In reality, many third-party contracts currently provide product reimbursements that are higher than the actual pharmacy cost to obtain the drug, but provide DFs that are less than most pharmacy's actual COD a prescription. A more recent trend is a total reimbursement rate (product cost + DF) that is below the pharmacy's cost to purchase the drug product (Murry et al., 2018).

Most third-party contracts state that the reimbursement rate for a prescription is the lower of two prices: (1) the price from the reimbursement-rate formula and (2) the usual and customary (U&C) pharmacy price. The U&C price, also referred to as the *cash price*, is the price that the pharmacy would charge a private-pay patient for the prescription.

Understanding pharmacy reimbursement requires knowledge of an alphabet soup of acronyms. A list of commonly used reimbursement terms, acronyms, and definitions is provided in Table 23-1. *Actual acquisition cost* (AAC) is the price that the pharmacy pays to purchase the drug product. Third parties would like to base their reimbursement on AAC, but AAC varies across pharmacies and may change frequently, making it administratively difficult to base reimbursement on an individual pharmacy's AAC. As a result, the product cost portion of the third-party reimbursement rate is an estimate of AAC and is called the *estimated acquisition cost* (EAC).

Example 1: Reimbursement Formula Using AWP

AWP − 18% + $1.00 dispensing fee

To establish EAC, many third parties use a standardized drug cost estimate that often is based on the *average wholesaler price (AWP)* or the *wholesaler acquisition cost (WAC)*. Theoretically, AWP is the price that the wholesaler charges to pharmacies, but in reality, AWP

Table 23-1. Third-Party Reimbursement Terms

Actual acquisition cost (AAC)	The price that the pharmacy pays the drug wholesaler or manufacturer to obtain the drug product.
Average actual acquisition cost (AvAC) or (AAAC)	An average of the prices paid by different pharmacies for drug products. Must be determined via pharmacy survey.
Average manufacturer price (AMP)	The average price received by a manufacturer from wholesalers for drugs distributed to the retail class of trade.
Average wholesaler price (AWP)	A list price for what drug wholesalers charge pharmacies. This is an overestimate of what the wholesaler actually charges the pharmacy.
Estimated acquisition cost (EAC)	The third-party's estimate of what the pharmacy pays the drug wholesaler or manufacturer.
Generic drug utilization rate (GDUR)	The percent of prescriptions at a pharmacy that are dispensed with a generic drug. Also called generic dispensing rate.
Generic effective rate (GER)	The average third-party reimbursement rate for generic prescription drugs across all generic drug products.
Maximum allowable cost (MAC)	The maximum cost that the third party will pay for a multisource drug. This typically is an average of the generic drug price from several manufacturers.
Wholesaler acquisition cost (WAC)	A list price for what pharmaceutical manufacturers charge drug wholesalers. This is an overestimate of what manufacturers actually charge wholesalers.

is the *list* price rather than the actual price. Just as the sticker price for a car is generally an overestimate of the price someone actually pays for the car, AWP is generally an overestimate of the price pharmacies pay for the drug product. Historically, AWPs have been published for all drug products, so AWP provided a convenient, standardized basis for determining a pharmacy's EAC. Third parties do not know the exact amount of discount that pharmacies receive, but they recognize that pharmacies receive some discount from AWP. As a result, the EAC used by third parties typically has been AWP less some percentage. The percentage off of AWP that third parties have negotiated into their product cost reimbursement formulas has steadily increased over time, resulting in lower reimbursements for drug products to pharmacies. For example, in the mid-1980s, brand name product reimbursement rates were commonly in the AWP less 5% to 10% range, whereas by the mid-1990s, rates often were about AWP less 15% (AMCP, 2007). The discount off of AWP also may vary by the days supply dispensed, with larger discounts for 90 day supplies. A 2018 study reported an average discount of AWP less 20% for 30-day supply brand name drugs and AWP less 22% for 90-day supply brand name drugs (PBMI, 2018).

Example 2: Reimbursement Formula Using WAC

WAC + 1% + $1.00 dispensing fee

An alternative way for third parties to establish EAC is by using the WAC. WAC used to be the actual price that drug wholesalers paid pharmaceutical manufactures to purchase drug products, and thus was proprietary information unavailable to third parties. Over the years, WAC has evolved to become an alternative list price. Wholesalers now purchase drug products at some percent off the WAC, and there are some standardized WAC lists available for use by third parties, although the information may not be as accessible as AWPs. The EAC typically will be the WAC plus a small percentage.

An alternative replacement for AWP-based reimbursement formulas is average actual acquisition cost, here called AvAC or AAAC to distinguish it from the AAC. The AvAC reflects an average cost for which pharmacies obtain drug products. Although AvAC may be a more accurate estimate of a pharmacy's AAC than AWP or WAC, it also is subject to some problems. AvAC typically must be assessed by surveying pharmacies. As a result, it is labor intensive to collect AvAC and difficult to verify the accuracy of AvACs reported by pharmacies. Another issue is that an individual pharmacy's AAC may be quite different from the AvAC, as different pharmacies negotiate different purchasing terms from their wholesalers. However, this problem is also an issue with WAC- and AWP-based reimbursement. The National Association of State Medicaid Directors (NASMD) recommended that Medicaid move toward AvAC reimbursement with a single national benchmark being used for AvAC (NASMD, 2010). Since 2013, the federal government has conducted national pharmacy surveys to create a national AvAC list to use for Medicaid, called the National Average Drug Acquisition Cost (NADAC) list. As of September 2018, 43 state Medicaid programs used NADAC or some other form of AvAC as their reimbursement basis for ingredient cost (CMS, 2018a). This is a considerable increase from 2015 when only 9 states used some form of AvAC as their reimbursement basis (CMS, 2015). In most state Medicaid programs using AvAC as the ingredient cost reimbursement basis, the DF component of the reimbursement formula more closely reflects the average pharmacy's COD and generally ranges from $10 to $12 depending on state and pharmacy prescription volume (CMS, 2018a).

The EAC for generic drugs sometimes is determined differently from the EAC for brand-name drugs. AWP is a particularly inaccurate estimate of AAC for generic drugs because, as mentioned previously, pharmacies generally purchase generic drug products at a large discount from AWP. There can also be wide variations in the price for the same generic drug product across different generic manufacturers. One way third-party payers handle this problem is to have a separate reimbursement-rate formula for generic drugs that specifies a larger discount from AWP than for brand-name drugs. A 2018 study reported average generic reimbursement rates of AWP less 56% for 30 days supply and AWP less 61% for 90 days supply (PBMI, 2018). A commonly used alternative method is to specify an MAC for each generic product. The MAC is an average cost to obtain the generic drug product. The federal government calculates and publishes a list of MACs for selected generic drug products, called the federal upper limit (FUL). The Deficit Reduction Act of 2005 mandated a change to an *average manufacturer price* (AMP)-based reimbursement for the Medicaid program's multisource MAC list. AMP is defined as the average price received by a manufacturer from wholesalers for drugs distributed to the retail class of trade. The *retail class of trade* refers to entities that purchase drugs for sale to the general public. Some third parties use the federal MAC lists, and some establish their own MAC list. The MAC also may be used for all multisource drugs in some third-party plans. *Multisource drugs* are drug products that have at least one generic equivalent available. In this case, the MAC is the reimbursement level for both the brand-name product and the generic equivalent. The result of this type of MAC policy is that the pharmacy may need to collect the difference between the MAC and the brand-name cost from the patient if the patient requests the brand-name product and the plan allows the brand name drug to be dispensed. Because of the use of MAC lists to set generic reimbursement, contract AWP rates are not a reliable indicator of generic drug reimbursement.

Pharmacy owners and managers have many concerns about the processes third-party payers use for MAC reimbursement. Private third-party payers use proprietary methods to determine their MAC rates, so pharmacies often do not know how the MACs are determined and may not have access to the MAC lists. This lack of transparency for MAC lists makes it difficult for pharmacies to make fully informed decisions about which third-party payer contract to accept. There also are concerns that MAC lists often are not updated in a timely manner following drug price changes, and that MAC rates are set too low. One study found that the ingredient cost reimbursement for generic prescription drugs was below the pharmacy's AAC for 15.1% of all generic prescriptions they dispense, with the rate of below cost reimbursement ranging from 4.1% to 25.9% across payers (Murry et al., 2018). These below cost MACs are sometimes referred to as "*underwater MACs.*"

Another term related to generic drug reimbursement is *generic effective rate (GER)*. GER is the average reimbursement rate across all generic drug products and is defined in terms of AWP minus a percentage. For example, a third-party payer reporting a GER of AWP − 85% implies that their average MAC across all generic drug products is an 85% discount off of AWP. Theoretically, knowing a third-party payer's GER should help the pharmacy evaluate the likely profitability of the contract. However, the reported GER is an average discount off of AWP across all generic products, so the specific generic reimbursement will vary depending on the product mix at the pharmacy. Pharmacy owners and managers need to be aware that the MAC rates for more commonly used generic drugs may be lower as a percent of AWP than the MAC rates for less commonly used drugs (Deninger, 2016). For example, if the GER for a plan is AWP − 85%, but the most commonly used generic drugs at a pharmacy are reimbursed at a rate of AWP − 95%, pharmacy profitability will be less than expected.

The uncertainty created by proprietary MAC lists makes reimbursement projections for generic drugs difficult to predict. It is challenging, therefore, to make revenue projections because generic drugs comprise 80–90% of the typical pharmacy's dispensed products. The technical term for the percent of prescriptions dispensed at the pharmacy that are generic is the GDUR. Also known as the generic dispensing rate, the GDUR is often provided either directly from the dispensing system or from third-party applications which use pharmacies' dispensing or claims data to track adherence or help manage patient care. Alternatively, this can be calculated using reports generated by the dispensing system.

DIRECT AND INDIRECT REMUNERATION

DIR fees have become a problematic part of third-party reimbursement, particularly for Medicare Part D plan reimbursement. The Centers for Medicare and Medicaid Services (CMS) defines what types of fees and other price concessions are considered DIR but generally they occur after the point of sale, with point of sale meaning when the prescription is dispensed. DIR fees collected by Medicare Part D plans increased from $13.4 billion in 2013 to $35.1 billion in 2017; pharmacy price concessions were 11.4% of the total DIR amount in 2017 (Fein, 2018b). The majority of DIR fees (84%) are rebates that pharmaceutical manufacturers pay to third-party payers (Fein, 2018b), but pharmacies are outside this rebate system and thus are only concerned with the DIR fees from pharmacy price concessions. Part D plans are required to report DIR fees to CMS. Pharmacy DIR fees are not paid by a pharmacy at the time that a prescription is dispensed, but are remitted to the Part D plan at a later date. These fees can be a percentage of the ingredient cost or a flat fee (see examples given further). DIR fees sometimes are charged for inclusion in a preferred pharmacy network, but plans frequently have DIR fees for participating in both non-preferred and preferred networks; the preferred networks typically have higher DIR fees. Most Part D plans also have a performance component to their DIR fees, where lower DIR fees are charged to pharmacies that meet various performance criteria. The specific performance criteria vary by plan, but examples of different types of performance criteria are discussed in the value-based payment section further in text. DIR fees are challenging for pharmacies, because they make it difficult to evaluate contracts and accurately assess prescription gross margin in a timely manner. There also are tax implications for pharmacies. DIR fees have an impact on patients because patient cost-sharing is calculated based on the point of sale prices, rather than the post-DIR price. In their proposed Part D rule for the 2020 plan year, CMS stated that they are considering including DIR fees in the point of sale price calculation in order to lower beneficiary costs (CMS, 2018b).

Example 1: DIR Fee as a Percent of Ingredient Cost

A Part D plan's reimbursement formula is AWP − 18% + $1 DF and a 6% DIR fee. If a pharmacy dispenses a prescription for that Part D plan with an AWP of $75, they receive $62.5 (AWP − 18% + $1) when the claim is reconciled, but later the pharmacy will have to pay back $3.69 to the plan ($61.5 × 0.06). The net payment to the pharmacy for dispensing the prescription is $58.81.

Example 2: Flat DIR Fee

A Part D plan's reimbursement formula is AWP − 16% + a $0.50 DF and a $5 DIR fee. If a pharmacy dispenses a prescription for that Part D plan with an AWP of $50, they receive $42.50 (AWP − 16% + 0.50) when the claim is reconciled, but later that pharmacy will have to pay back $5 of that amount to the Part D plan. The net payment to the pharmacy for dispensing the prescription is $37.50.

VALUE-BASED PAYMENT OR PAY FOR PERFORMANCE

Value-based payment, sometimes called pay-for-performance, has become widespread in health care and much more common in pharmacy contracts with third-party payers. Payers want to incentivize health care providers to improve their performance. There are many possible models for value-based payment in pharmacy (Pringle et al., 2016; Urick et al., 2018; Urick and Urmie 2019). Early types of value-based payment involved paying "bonus" dispensing fees if pharmacies met GDUR or formulary compliance rate goals, but value-based payment formulas now have become much more sophisticated and are based on a wide variety of cost and quality outcomes. Medicare Part D plans have incentives to improve their star quality ratings and those incentives often are reflected in their pharmacy reimbursement formulas. Medicare Part D plans are rated on patient adherence to diabetes, cholesterol, and hypertension medications. As a result, many plans are now holding pharmacies accountable for improving quality, and, as of 2018, more than 60% or Part D beneficiaries were enrolled in plans that use quality measurement to modify pharmacy payments or fees (Sega, 2018).

The Pharmacy Quality Alliance (PQA) is an organization whose mission is to promote appropriate medication use and develop medication performance measures. More information about different medication-related quality measures which could be used to assess pharmacy performance can be found at the PQA website (https://www.pqaalliance.org). Most community pharmacies now have access to scores on the Electronic Quality Improvement Platform for Plans and Pharmacies (EQuIPP) (see https://www .equipp.org for more information) or another electronic platform that measures their performance on common outcomes used for value-based reimbursement. For more information on pharmacy quality measurement, see Chapter 10.

■ EVALUATING THE FINANCIAL IMPACT OF THIRD-PARTY REIMBURSEMENT

This section describes several ways to examine how third-party reimbursement affects a pharmacy's financial performance. Although other factors are also important and will be discussed later in this chapter, it is essential to understand the impact of different third-party plans on a pharmacy's net profit. One important step in evaluating a third-party contract is to examine the average net profit per prescription. An average net profit comparison may be used to evaluate the effect of a change in reimbursement for a particular third-party plan or to evaluate reimbursement rates across third-party plans and private-pay prescriptions. An important part of this analysis is calculating the average COD a prescription.

Recognizing that there are many fixed costs in pharmacies, another evaluation technique that will be discussed is differential analysis. This analysis accounts for the fact that many pharmacy expenses change little as the prescription volume increases or decreases. Finally, pro forma analysis will be discussed. This analysis factors in the different volumes of prescriptions in different third-party plans and includes elements of both the differential analysis and the average net profit comparison.

Calculating the Cost of Dispensing a Prescription

As mentioned previously, the DF is intended to cover the COD a prescription. In actuality, determination of the DF is rather arbitrary, and the amount of the fee provided in many PBM reimbursement contract is lower than the actual COD. The 2018 NCPA Digest reported an average COD of $10.79 for independent pharmacies (NCPA Digest, 2018). A recent statewide survey for the Iowa Medicaid program found that the median COD was $10.07 (Myers and Stauffer, 2018). Third-party dispensing fees are in the $0.50 to $13 range, with the higher fees usually occurring in state Medicaid programs or other payers who use the average actual acquisition cost (AvAC or AAAC) as the basis for drug ingredient cost reimbursement.

Calculating the average COD is a fundamental pharmacy management tool. The COD includes the *fair share* of all a pharmacy's costs related to dispensing a prescription *over and above* the cost of the drug product. Knowing the COD is necessary to evaluate third-party contracts, and it is also useful in tracking pharmacy expenses. Costs can be separated into two different types of costs: fixed and variable. *Fixed costs* are costs that do not change as prescription volume changes (e.g., computer or other equipment purchases, pharmacy license, and depreciation). *Variable costs* are costs that change directly as prescription volume changes (e.g., prescription vials). When differential analysis is discussed, it will be necessary to identify the average variable costs of dispensing a prescription. A variation is *semi-variable costs*, which only change with large changes in prescription volume. An example of a semi-variable cost would be pharmacist labor costs. Pharmacists will not be hired or fired for small changes in prescription volume, but if there are large changes in prescription volume, it may be necessary to change the number of pharmacists employed by the pharmacy or reduce pharmacist hours (e.g., full time to part time).

Another way to classify costs is direct vs. indirect. *Direct costs* are costs that are completely attributable to the prescription department (e.g., the costs of prescription vials and labels). Pharmacist labor is considered a direct expense unless the pharmacist has managerial responsibilities in nonprescription departments or spends significant time on non-dispensing tasks such as professional services. *Indirect costs* are costs that are shared between the prescription department and the rest of the store. Rent, clerical labor costs, utilities, and promotional expenses for the pharmacy are examples of indirect expenses. Methods for allocating indirect expenses to the prescription department are discussed in Table 23-2.

The overall process to calculate a COD is to identify the direct and indirect costs associated with the prescription department, allocate the fair share of indirect costs to the dispensing process, and then divide the total prescription department expenses by the number of prescriptions dispensed during the same time period. It often is convenient to use a full year as the time frame. Note that the same process also may be used to calculate the cost of a different service, such as medication therapy management (MTM) or vaccinations. To calculate the COD, you will need the most recent income (revenue and expense) statement or a pro forma income statement for the pharmacy and information on the number of prescriptions dispensed during the same time period as the statement. More information on income statements is provided in Chapter 21, and pro forma income statements are discussed later in this chapter. The calculations use the income statement and other relevant information for Good Service Pharmacy that is provided in Table 23-3. This table also contains information about the percentage of expenses allocated to the

prescription department. This information will be used to illustrate part of the process of calculating a COD, but it is not typically contained in an income statement and must be calculated separately. Table 23-2 shows the process for calculating the COD for Good Service Pharmacy. It should be noted that although the COD is calculated for the entire prescription department, the COD often varies as the percentage of prescriptions paid for by private or third-party sources changes.

It is useful to know the COD for third-party prescriptions and even the COD for a specific third-party plan, but often the necessary information for these calculations is unavailable or too time-consuming to obtain. In this example, the overall average COD for Good Service Pharmacy is $8.42 per prescription.

Average Net Profit Comparison

The basic formula for calculating an *average net profit comparison* is included in Table 23-4. The average cost of goods sold (COGS) per prescription is subtracted from the average price (for private-pay prescriptions) or average reimbursement rate to give the average gross margin. Gross margin may also be referred to as *gross profit*. The average COD is subtracted from the gross margin to yield the average net profit per prescription. The average net profit can be calculated for all prescriptions dispensed at the pharmacy, for selected third-party plans, or for a particular third-party plan before and after a change in reimbursement. The same formula is used on an aggregate basis to conduct a pro forma analysis. Table 23-4 shows an average net profit comparison for the current and new Better Health reimbursement rates from the scenario. In this example, assume that the COD will not change and that the average COD for Better Health prescriptions is the same as for all other prescriptions. Also assume that the average COGS will not change. When conducting an average net profit comparison across different third-party plans, the most accurate approach would be to calculate the average COGS separately for each plan because each plan may have a very different prescription drug mix. In reality, it is often assumed that the average COGS is the same

Table 23-2.   Calculating the Average Cost of Dispensing Per Prescription

Step 1: Identify costs associated with the prescription department

Labor expenses

Labor expenses need to be allocated between the prescription department and the rest of the pharmacy. These expenses typically are allocated based on the percent of time spent in the prescription department. Natalie Hawkins, the pharmacy manager at Good Service Pharmacy, estimates that she spends 75% of her time in the prescription department. Assume that the employee pharmacist and the four pharmacy technicians spend 95% of their time in the prescription department, so 95% of their wages are allocated to the cost of dispensing. The other workers (1.5 FTE) spend about 50% of their time in the prescription department. Using these percentages and the wage information contained in the notes under the Income Statement, the total amount of labor costs allocated to the prescription department is $435,702.

Direct expenses

Some expenses are directly related to prescription drug dispensing and should be allocated 100% to the prescription department. For Good Service Pharmacy, the direct expenses that are listed on the Income Statement are prescription supplies (labels, caps, vials, etc.). The annual total of these direct expenses is $11,326. *Note: Other direct expenses that may appear in a pharmacy Income Statement include delivery expenses, professional liability insurance, continuing education expenses, transaction fees, and professional license fees.*

Indirect expenses

The rest of the expenses are indirect expenses that are not as clearly linked to a particular department. Occupancy expenses such as rent, utilities, and other facility costs are often allocated using a square-footage allocation method. Under this method, costs are allocated to the prescription department using the percentage of the store square footage occupied by the prescription department. For Good Service Pharmacy, this percentage is 25.8.

The typical allocation method for other indirect expenses, such as computer systems and advertising, is percent of sales. Since the prescription department generated 81.9% of the total sales, 81.9% of each of the other expenses will be allocated to the prescription department. *Note: The percent of sales allocation method may also be used for occupancy expenses. This method usually results in a higher cost of dispensing than the square-footage allocation method because prescription departments typically generate a large percentage of sales but occupy a small percentage of the store square footage.*

The total of indirect expenses allocated to the prescription department is $83,007 ($21,087 in occupancy expenses and $61,920 in other indirect expenses). All the allocation percentages and amounts are displayed in the far right columns in Table 23-3.

Step 2: Sum all the prescription department costs

Labor expenses	$435,702
Direct expenses	$11,326
Indirect expenses	$83,007
Total expenses	$530,035

Step 3: Divide the prescription expenses by the number of prescriptions dispensed

Average cost of dispensing per prescription: $530,035/62,920 = **$8.42**

Table 23-3.   Income Statement for Good Service Pharmacy, 2019

| | Prescription Department | | | |
	2019 ($)	Sales (%)	Allocation for COD	Allocation for COD (%)
Sales				
Prescription sales[1]	2,679,334	81.9%		
Other sales	592,317	18.1%		
Total sales	3,271,651	100.0%		
Cost of goods sold[2]	2,531,974	77.4%		
Gross margin	739,677	22.6%		
Expenses		0.0%		
Labor	517,335	15.8%	435,702	
Rent	58,059	1.8%	14,979	25.8%
Utilities/other facility costs	23,673	0.7%	6,108	25.8%
Prescription vials/labels	11,326	0.4%	11,326	100
Computer	7,498	0.2%	6,141	81.9%
Advertising	25,781	0.8%	21,115	81.9%
All other expenses	42,325	1.3%	34,664	81.9%
Total expenses	685,997	21.0%		
Net profit (before taxes)	53,680	1.6%		

COD, cost of dispensing; COGS, cost of goods sold.

Notes:
1. Number of prescriptions dispensed in 2019 = 62,920.
2. Prescription COGS = 83.6% of the total COGS.
3. Labor costs (wages plus benefits averaging 25% of total salary): Pharmacy manager = $169,000 (75% in prescription department); employee pharmacist = $133,120 (95% in prescription department, 1 employee pharmacist FTE); pharmacy technicians = $166,400 (95% in prescription department, 4 technician FTEs); and other staff = $48,815 (50% in prescription department, 1.5 support staff FTEs).
4. The pharmacy department occupies 25.80% of the store square footage.

to simplify the analysis. When conducting an average net profit comparison, the need for accurate COGS data must be balanced with practical constraints.

Note: In practice, it may be difficult to determine the average COGS. The information on the COGS that is provided in the computer records often is not an actual reflection of the true COGS. One way to calculate the average COGS is to examine invoices that the pharmacy receives from their wholesaler. However, the invoice price also may be somewhat inaccurate because the pharmacy may receive extra discounts or rebates from the wholesaler at the end of the year or during some other time

period if the pharmacy reaches target purchase levels (see Chapter 27).

The net profit comparison of the current and new Better Health reimbursement rates reveals that Good Service Pharmacy is already losing money under the current rate and it would lose even more ($4.49 on an average Better Health prescription) if it accepted the new contract. Although this result would seem to make the decision about accepting the contract clear, this analysis is only one of several relevant financial analyses, and other factors need to be considered. It may also be useful to conduct an average net profit comparison across other third-party plans

Table 23-4.   Conducting an Average Net Profit Comparison

If total reimbursement is known, that could be used to calculate average reimbursement. If it's not known, then the following steps can be used to estimate reimbursement and make comparisons between different reimbursement formulas.

Step 1: Estimate COGS, AWP, and generic drug utilization rate

There are three key pieces of information needed to estimate total reimbursement based on the formulas presented at the beginning of this chapter: cost of goods sold (COGS), generic drug utilization rate (GDUR), and average wholesaler price (AWP). With these pieces of information, estimates can be made of the total reimbursement received under any AWP-based contract. For reimbursement formulas like Better Health's that apply different reimbursement rates for brand and generic products, it is best to consider COGS and AWP separately for brand and generic products. Good Service Pharmacy estimates their COGS and AWP per prescription dispensed for generics to be $6.86 and $84.37, and for brand name products to be $185.47 and $245.36.

In addition to COGS and AWP, Good Service Pharmacy has to estimate the GDUR for Better Health pharmacy. For this scenario, assume that Good Service Pharmacy looks up their GDUR for Better Health patients using the Electronic Quality Improvement Platform for Plans and Pharmacies (EQuIPP) platform and finds it to be 85%.

Step 2: Calculate the new average reimbursement rate

Now use this data to estimate average reimbursement under the new contract. Average reimbursement for brand and generics will have to be calculated separately, then a weighted average will be created using the GDUR. For the purposes of comparison, we will assume that Good Service Pharmacy does not receive any performance-related direct and indirect remuneration (DIR) bonuses.

The calculation for brand name reimbursement is as follows:

Non-Preferred Pharmacy Formula for Brands: AWP − 15% + $0.75 DF, DIR Fee = 3%

Average Non-Preferred Reimbursement = ($245.36 − 0.15[$245.36]) × (1 − 0.03) + $0.75 = $203.05

Preferred Pharmacy Formula for Brands: AWP − 17% + $0.50 DF, DIR Fee = 7%

Average Preferred Reimbursement = ($245.36 − 0.17[$245.36]) × (1 − 0.07) + $0.50 = $189.89

The calculation for generic drugs is more complicated and requires estimating the generic effective rate (GER) based on historic dispensing data or other available data. When using the GER to estimate reimbursement, replace the AWP discount in the contract (in this case, AWP − 25% to AWP − 27%) with the GER. Assume that the GER for the pharmacy if it remains non-preferred is 85%, and if it joins the network it will be 87%. Using the same formulas as above, but plugging in numbers for generics, Good Service Pharmacy finds average non-preferred reimbursement to be $13.03 and average preferred reimbursement to be $10.70.

The calculation for the weighted average reimbursement is as follows:

Weighted Average = Brand Reimbursement × (1 − GDUR) + Generic Reimbursement × (GDUR)

Non-Preferred Average Reimbursement = $203.05 × (1 − 0.85) + $13.03 × (0.85) = $41.53

Preferred Average Reimbursement = $189.89 × (1 − 0.85) + $10.70 × (0.85) = $37.58

(Continued)

Table 23-4.   Conducting an Average Net Profit Comparison (*Continued*)

If one assumes that the COGS and GDUR will remain constant across the two scenarios, then only one COGS needs to be calculated. The calculation for the weighted average COGS is as follows:

Weighted Average = Brand COGS × (1 − GDUR) + Generic COGS × (GDUR)

Weighted Average COGS = $185.47 × (1 − 0.85) + 6.86 × (0.85) = $33.65

Step 3: Calculate the average net profit

Subtract the average COGS per prescription from the average reimbursement to obtain the average gross margin. Then subtract the average COD that was calculated earlier from the gross margin to obtain the net profit.

Results of an Average Net Profit Comparison

	Formula	Current B.H. Rate ($)	Preferred Network B.H. Rate ($)
	Price/Reimbursement	41.53	37.58
−	COGS	33.65	33.65
=	Gross margin	7.88	3.93
−	Cost of dispensing (COD)	8.42	8.42
=	Net profit	−0.54	−4.49

and private-pay prescriptions at Good Service Pharmacy to see how Better Health compares.

Differential Analysis

Another analysis to consider is a *differential analysis*. The average net profit comparison makes it appear as if accepting the new Better Health contract would be a very bad idea because the pharmacy would lose an average of $4.49 per prescription. However, this analysis does not account for the fact that some pharmacy expenses are fixed and will not change if there is a change in prescription volume. Prescription departments almost always have a large percentage of fixed expenses, and this tendency results in economies of scale[1] because the average fixed cost per prescription decreases as the number of prescriptions increases. One example of this is pharmacist labor costs. In general, having a prescription department requires at least one

full-time pharmacist, and the average COD will be much different if this pharmacist dispenses 100 prescriptions per day or 300 prescriptions per day.

A differential analysis compares the differential (marginal) revenue with the differential (marginal) COD a prescription for a selected third-party plan. The differential revenue minus the differential cost is called the *contribution margin*. The differential revenue is the average gross margin, and the differential cost is the variable cost per prescription. The decision rule is to accept all third-party plans that generate a contribution margin greater than zero. This analysis is particularly useful when deciding whether to accept a contract that would increase the prescription volume. In the scenario, we assumed that Good Service Pharmacy would not have more Better Health patients if it accepts the preferred pharmacy contract; rather, it is assumed that they will lose 10% of their Better Health prescription volume if they do not join the preferred network. However, it is possible that the pharmacy will increase their prescription volume if they join the Better Health preferred pharmacy network, so Table 23-5 shows an example of a differential analysis

---

[1] Economies of scale occur when the average cost per unit decreases as the number of units produced increases.

Table 23-5.   Conducting a Differential Analysis

Step 1: Calculate the differential revenue (average gross margin)

The marginal revenue is the average gross margin per prescription. Recall from Table 23-4 that the average gross margin under the new Better Health contract is $3.93 per prescription.

Step 2: Calculate the differential cost (average variable cost)

The differential cost is the average variable cost. To calculate this cost, it is necessary to divide the average COD into the fixed and variable components. The most obvious variable costs are prescription vials and labels. If the total prescription vial and label cost is divided by the number of prescriptions, the cost for the vial and label is $0.18 for each prescription. It is assumed that the indirect expenses do not vary directly with prescription volume; for example, the rent and advertising costs will not change just because the prescription volume changes.

Determining whether the labor expenses are fixed or variable is somewhat challenging and may be different for different scenarios; that is, a 5% change in prescription volume will have different effects on labor expenses than a 50% change in prescription volume. For this analysis, the effect of 25% increase in Better Health prescription volume will be considered. Recall that 15% of current prescriptions are filled for Better Health patients, therefore a 25% increase in Better Health volume is equal to a 3.75% increase in overall prescription volume. The pharmacy currently has two pharmacist FTEs and pharmacy manager believes that the pharmacy needs all of these pharmacists because of the number of hours the pharmacy is open. As a result, pharmacist labor will be treated as a fixed expense. The pharmacy manager believes that the pharmacy technician hours could be increased if the prescription volume increased, so technician labor is treated as a variable expense. Assume that the pharmacy technician labor expenses will be increased by 3.75% if the prescription volume is increased by 3.75% (a 1:1 ratio), so the average variable technician cost is the total prescription department technician expense divided by the number of prescriptions ($182,488/62,920). This equals $2.90 per prescription. There are no other variable costs other than the prescription vials and the technician labor, so the total variable cost per prescription is $3.08 ($0.18 + $2.90).

Step 3: Calculate the contribution margin

The contribution margin is the differential revenue (DR) minus the differential cost (DC):

$$DR - DC = \$3.93 - \$3.08 = \$0.85$$

The contribution margin is positive, suggesting joining the preferred network would be beneficial if it resulted in increased prescription volume, provided that the existing pharmacists could handle the increase in volume.

for the new Better Health contract if Better Health volume increases by 25%.

A pro forma analysis combines information in the average net profit comparison and the differential analysis to give a more complete picture of the financial implications of joining the Better Health preferred pharmacy network, accounting for both changes in reimbursement and changes in prescription volume.

Pro Forma Analysis

The decision about accepting a third-party contract will be clearly affected by whether 5% or 50% of the pharmacy's prescriptions are dispensed under that third-party plan. The *pro forma analysis* incorporates this important factor. A pro forma analysis is a projection of what the income statement for the pharmacy would look like if the pharmacy joins preferred network vs. the pharmacy stays out of the preferred network. In the case of Good Service Pharmacy, if it doesn't join the newly expanded preferred network, it expects that it will lose about 10% of Better Health prescriptions but have higher per-prescription margins. Alternatively, if Good Service Pharmacy joins the network, it will at least maintain its current prescription volume but it will have a substantial reduction in prescription margins for Better Health patients. Natalie, the pharmacy owner, also knows that improving pharmacy performance can improve profits under the preferred network contract. The pro forma analysis provides a comparison of the total net profit under all three scenarios: Do Not Join, Join (Low Performing), and Join (High Performing).

To conduct a pro forma analysis, it is necessary to construct three income statements using information from the current income statement and knowledge about the pharmacy and the third-party contract being evaluated. Information from the average net profit comparison and the differential analysis also is needed. An example of a pro forma analysis for Good Service Pharmacy is presented in Table 23-6. The results show that although both scenarios result in less net profit than the current situation, joining the preferred network would result in between $22,463 and $30,013 less profit than not joining the preferred pharmacy network. Even if the pharmacy could improve its performance, the pharmacy would still lose substantial profit by joining the preferred pharmacy network. The sensitivity analysis showed that even if joining the Better Health preferred network resulted in a 25% increase in their Better Health prescription volume, the pharmacy still would have lower net profit under both performance scenarios than if they stayed out of the preferred network.

■ OTHER CONSIDERATIONS IN EVALUATING A THIRD-PARTY CONTRACT

Understanding the financial impact of a third-party contract clearly is important when making a decision about whether to accept or decline a third-party contract, but other factors also have a role in the decision. One factor that needs to be considered is the effect of the decision on pharmacy customers. If the decision is made to reject a third-party contract or not participate in a preferred pharmacy network, customers who have that third party will be forced to go elsewhere or pay more to obtain their prescriptions. This may mean angering, distressing, or inconveniencing some pharmacy customers. Many customers may not understand the pharmacy's decision and subsequently direct their anger toward the pharmacy staff. Pharmacists and pharmacy staff also may be distressed over losing customers with whom they have established relationships.

There also are pharmacy staffing considerations. Not joining a preferred network or refusing to participate in a third-party plan likely will result in reduced prescription volume. This may create a need to reduce labor costs by terminating employees or reducing their hours. Alternatively, pharmacy managers could maintain existing staffing levels and use the reduced prescription volume as an opportunity to expand pharmacist professional services or other sources of revenue. If pharmacies choose to participate in a new plan or join a preferred network, their prescription volume likely will increase. If the new reimbursement rates are not sufficient to increase staffing levels, pharmacists and other pharmacy staff may be asked to increase their hourly fill rates, potentially resulting in low staff morale and high turnover.

Pharmacy image is another concern. Some pharmacies want to avoid the reputation of being a pharmacy that overcharges for prescriptions and this image may occur if a pharmacy does not join a network. Conversely, a pharmacy may want to have an image as a high-quality service pharmacy and accepting a contract with a low reimbursement rate may jeopardize the pharmacy's ability to provide good service. If the low reimbursement rate means that pharmacists must dispense more prescriptions, therefore having less time for their patients, then the quality of patient care at the pharmacy may be affected.

Another critical factor to consider is the signal that the pharmacy's decision sends to other third parties. Accepting a low reimbursement rate from one

Table 23-6.   Conducting a Pro Forma Analysis

Step 1: Construct Do Not Join Preferred Network projected income statement

If the Good Service Pharmacy does not join the Better Health preferred network, assume that prescription volume for the Better Health plan will decrease by 10%. Recall that the pharmacy dispensed 62,920 prescriptions for 2018, and that 15% of these prescriptions (9,438) were Better Health prescriptions. To determine the decrease in prescription sales, first calculate the number of Better Health prescriptions that would be lost (9,438 × 0.1 = 943.8), multiply this by the average reimbursement for these prescriptions as calculated in Table 23-4 (943.8 × $41.53 = $39,196), and subtract this from the total prescription sales from the income statement in Table 23-3 ($2,679,334 − $39,196 = $2,640,138).

Second, calculate the decrease in COGS that would accompany this decrease in prescription volume. Multiply the average COGS by the number of Better Health prescriptions which are projected to be lost in 2019 ($33.65 × 943.8 = $31,759) and subtract this amount from the current COGS ($2,531,974 − $31,759 = $2,500,215).

Third, calculate changes in operating expenses that would accompany this decrease. Although the total prescriptions for Better Health are decreasing by 10%, Better Health only represents 15% of the total prescriptions dispensed at Good Service Pharmacy. Therefore, a 10% decrease in Better Health prescription volume translates to a 1.5% decrease in overall volume. Recall from Table 23-5 that some expenses are fixed and others are variable. A 1.5% decrease in prescription volume would result in a 1.5% reduction in prescription-related supplies, but assume for this scenario that the prospect of losing 1.5% of volume isn't necessarily enough to cause Natalie, the manager at Better Health Pharmacy, to cut back on technician labor. To calculate the reduction in expense for prescription-related supplies, multiply the total reduction in volume by the cost of supplies per prescription (943.8 × $0.18 = $170).

Step 2: Construct Join Preferred Network (Low Performance) projected income statement

This step is less complex because it only involves a decrease in revenue. Recall from Table 23-4 that the gross margin for the current contract is $7.88 and that gross margins for the contract if Better Health were to join the network as a low performing pharmacy with a 7% DIR fee is $3.93. Calculate the difference between these margins ($7.88 − $3.93 = $3.95), and multiply this figure by the total prescription volume for Better Health to produce the expected reduction in prescription sales which would result from this worse contract ($3.95 × 9,438 = $37,280). Finally, subtract this from the prescription sales form the income statement in Table 23-3 to calculate the expected prescription sales if Good Service Pharmacy joins the Better Health preferred network ($2,679,334 − $37,280 = $2,642,054).

Step 3: Construct Join Preferred Network (High Performance) projected income statement

This step is similar to Step 2, except that Natalie assumes Better Health Pharmacy can provide excellent care and reduce the DIR fee from 7% to 5%. By redoing the calculations in Table 23-3 and assuming a 5% DIR fee for the new formula, the reimbursement for brand name drugs by a high performing pharmacy is found to be $193.97 (vs. $189.89 for low performing) and $10.92 (vs. $10.70 for low performing). The weighted average reimbursement is therefore $38.38 ($193.97 × (1 − 0.85) + $10.92 × (0.85)) and the gross margin is $4.73. As in step 2, subtract this from the gross margin from the current contract gross margin ($7.88 − $4.73 = $3.15), multiply by the Better Health prescription volume ($3.15 × 9,438 = $29,729.70), and subtract this from the current prescription sales ($2,679,334 − $29,730 = $2,649,604).

(Continued)

Table 23-6. Conducting a Pro Forma Analysis (*Continued*)

Step 4: Compare net profit for the three projected income statements

The net profit under the "Do Not Join" scenario is $46,413, the net profit under the "Join (Low Performing)" scenario is $16,400, and the net profit under the "Join (High Performing)" scenario is $23,950 so the pharmacy would make between $22,463 and $30,013 less profit if they decide to join the preferred pharmacy network.

Step 5: Sensitivity analysis

Sensitivity analysis is a very important step in doing a pro forma analysis, and it involves changing one or more of the assumptions and seeing how that change affects the results. One possibility is that joining the network will result in an increase in prescription volume. The current share of prescription volume is 9,438 per year, a 25% increase would add 2,360 additional prescriptions. Using the previous gross margin calculations, this would add between $9,267.62 and $11,149.10 in additional revenue to the Join scenarios. However, the pharmacy would still make between $11,314 and $20,745 less than if the pharmacy didn't join the preferred network and had a 10% reduction in volume.

Results from the Pro Forma Analysis for Good Service Pharmacy

Sales	Do Not Join ($)	Join (Low Performing) ($)	Join (High Performing) ($)
Prescription sales	2,640,138	2,642,054	2,649,604
Other sales	592,317	592,317	592,317
Total sales	3,232,455	3,234,371	3,241,921
Cost of goods sold	2,500,215	2,531,974	2,531,974
Gross margin	732,240	702,397	709,947
Expenses			
Labor	517,335	517,335	517,335
Rent	58,059	58,059	58,059
Utilities	23,673	23,673	23,673
Prescription vials/labels	11,156	11,326	11,326
Computer	7,498	7,498	7,498
Advertising	25,781	25,781	25,781
All other expenses	42,325	42,325	42,325
Total expenses	685,827	685,997	685,997
Net profit (before taxes)	46,413	16,400	23,950

third party may encourage other third parties to lower their rates to comparable levels. As long as pharmacies continue to accept declining rates, the third parties are likely to continue offering progressively lower rates. Conversely, declining a low reimbursement-rate contract may send third-party payers a signal that the pharmacy is not willing to accept poor reimbursement rates.

One last factor to consider is the effect of the decision on other sources of revenue. In the pro forma analysis, it was assumed that other sales would not be affected if they declined to participate in the preferred network for Better Health. In reality, if the Better Health prescription volume decreased by 10%, it is likely that other sales would decrease as well. If there is less store traffic, there likely will be fewer over-the-counter (OTC) product sales and fewer sales of other products in the pharmacy. This loss of other sales may be more important for a store where other sales are a large percentage of total sales. OTC or other sales also sometimes are used as a justification to accept a third-party contract with a low reimbursement rate. The argument is that "even though we lose money on each prescription, we will make it up with other sales." While prescription customers may purchase some OTC or other products, managers need to be careful with this argument because only the profit on the OTCs will help to compensate for the prescription losses.

Third-Party Contract Terminology

It is important to understand the terminology commonly used in third-party contracts. For a more thorough discussion of this issue, see Fridy et al. (2002). Basic elements of a third-party contract include provider rights and responsibilities, transmission of claims process, requirements for pharmacy participation in the third-party network, and third-party rights and responsibilities. Some common provider rights and responsibilities relate to record-keeping, collecting patient copayments, complying with third-party formularies, and maintaining professional standards. The reimbursement rate and the timing of reimbursement are described in the section on requirements for pharmacy participation. It also will specify the procedure for changes in the contract. Most changes in the contract occur at the request of the third party. Pharmacies certainly can request changes in a contract, but often are not successful in getting the third party to accept the changes (Fridy et al., 2002). Third-party rights and responsibilities may include the right to inspect/audit pharmacy records and the provision of help-desk support. Pharmacy managers should pay

particular attention to the information on audits, since audits often result in the pharmacy needing to pay back money to the third party. Third parties may conduct *desk audits*, where third parties review pharmacy claims data but do not come to the pharmacy, and *field audits*, where a third-party representative visits the pharmacy and inspects pharmacy records and procedures. It is important to understand what information might be inspected in an audit and to make sure that your pharmacy has adequate record-keeping procedures in place. There have been reports that the frequency and intensity of third-party audits has increased, creating interest in pharmacy audit legislation (NCPA, 2013).

One thing to consider in a third-party contract is the length of time before the pharmacy will be reimbursed by the third party. If the third-party's reimbursement cycle is longer than the pharmacy's payment cycle with its vendors, this may create a cash-flow problem for the pharmacy (see Chapters 21 and 22). The length of time before the pharmacy receives payment will also be influenced by the percentage of claims rejected or challenged by the third party. Although electronic "real time" transmission of claims makes it possible to determine at the time of dispensing whether the prescription claim will be accepted, some rejected claims still will be identified during the claim reconciliation process. Having to resubmit rejected claims to the third party or having to try to obtain payment from the patient delays payment for the prescription.

A requirement of most third-party contracts with pharmacies is that the pharmacy *accepts assignment*. This clause means that the pharmacy agrees to charge the patient no more than the amount specified by the contract. In other words, a pharmacy that has accepted assignment cannot charge a third-party patient more to make up for a decrease in the third-party reimbursement rate. It is important to be careful that the assignment is confined to payment for prescription dispensing. The pharmacy manager should clarify that accepting assignment does not preclude the pharmacy from charging third-party patients for additional professional services.

Two clauses seen occasionally in pharmacy contracts are the *most favored nation clause* and the *all-products clause*. The most favored nation clause requires pharmacies to extend their lowest price or reimbursement rate to that third party. It is customary for third parties to require that the pharmacy charge the third party its U&C price if it is lower than the third-party's reimbursement formula price. However, having to give the third party the lowest reimbursement rate of all the other third-party rates is not customary. The all-products clause requires pharmacies to participate in all the third-party's plans if it wants to participate in any one plan. A pharmacy may want to participate in only some of a third-party's plans depending on the reimbursement rate and number of customers affected. Some states prohibit all-products clauses.

Two third-party contract issues that have received recent attention are *clawbacks* and *gag clauses*. Clawbacks occur when the patient's cost-sharing exceeds the third-party reimbursement amount and the pharmacy has to remit the difference back to the third-party payer. For example, if the patient paid a $15 copayment, but the third-party reimbursement rate to the pharmacy was only $3.50, the pharmacy would have to pay back $11.50 to the third party. This situation is most likely to occur in situations where the third-party plan requires high patient cost-sharing and the reimbursed price for the drug is low (e.g., generic drugs). In the above example, if the pharmacy had a $4 cash price for the prescription, both the pharmacy and the patient would have been better off if the patient paid cash for the prescription rather than filling it through their insurance. One study found that patient cost-sharing amounts were higher than the pharmacy's reimbursement for 23% of dispensed prescriptions (Van Nuys et al., 2018). Under a gag clause, the pharmacy is prohibited from telling the patient that their prescription would be cheaper if they purchased it without using their insurance. Gag clauses received considerable negative publicity and in 2018 federal legislation banning gag clauses was passed (Jaffe, 2018).

■ RESPONDING TO REDUCTIONS IN THIRD-PARTY REIMBURSEMENT

As was shown in the pro forma analysis, Good Service Pharmacy's faces lower net profits regardless of whether they choose to participate in the preferred pharmacy network for Better Health Part D plan. If they don't join the preferred network they will lose prescription volume, but if they join the preferred network they will earn less gross margin on each Better Health prescription. Pharmacies face many challenges with third-party reimbursement so pharmacies need to develop strategies to maintain their profit levels as reimbursement rates or prescription volume decrease. To accomplish this goal, pharmacy managers need to consider developing alternative sources of revenue or decreasing their expenses.

One source of revenue is to increase prescription volume by attracting new third-party or private-pay customers. As discussed earlier in this chapter, pharmacies tend to have a high percentage of fixed costs, so there usually are economies of scale to be achieved by dispensing more prescriptions. This strategy seems to have been used widely by pharmacies, and although it provides a short-term solution, it may not be a viable long-term strategy because the new private-pay patients may become third-party patients in the future, and the other third-party prescription reimbursement rates also likely will decline over time. As in the scenario, an added challenge is that it may be necessary to accept lower reimbursement rates to increase volume. A final challenge with large increases in prescription volume is that relatively fixed costs such as pharmacy salaries eventually must increase to accommodate the higher volume.

Another strategy for pharmacies to consider is diversifying their sources of revenue. A pharmacy that obtains most of its revenue from prescription drugs is more vulnerable to decreasing reimbursement rates than a pharmacy with other significant sources of revenue. One possible source of revenue is payment for professional and patient care services. Pharmacies may either directly charge patients for these services or bill third-party payers. MTM or other professional services are an opportunity (see Chapters 29 and 30). It should be noted that obtaining third-party payment for patient care services will likely result in many of the same concerns as obtaining third-party payment for prescriptions (Ganther, 2002). As long as the third-party contract does not prevent pharmacists from charging patients directly for their services, obtaining payment for patient care services is possible for both third-party and private-pay patients. The expansion of value-based payment in health care also is an opportunity for pharmacists who can improve health care outcomes for their patients. Another source of revenue is sales of items such as OTC products, durable medical equipment, and other health- or non–health-related products. Pharmacies that have the space for additional products may want to consider developing this source of revenue, but it is important to stay informed about ongoing reimbursement changes for these products, particularly in Medicare and Medicaid.

Another strategy to preserve net profit when reimbursement rates are decreased is to decrease expenses. The largest prescription department expense is labor, so labor costs are important to evaluate. The most expensive labor cost in most pharmacies is pharmacist labor, so pharmacies need to evaluate carefully how pharmacists are spending their time. Having pharmacists spend their time doing tasks that do not require a pharmacist's expertise is an inefficient use of resources. Pharmacy managers should consider using other pharmacy personnel such as pharmacy technicians and clerks to do some of the tasks associated with the dispensing of prescriptions, for example, counting tablets and reconciling third-party claims. Other pharmacy personnel costs and non-labor costs of the pharmacy department should also be evaluated.

■ REVISITING THE SCENARIO

In the scenario described at the beginning of the chapter, the pharmacy manager at Good Service Pharmacy (Natalie Hawkins) was faced with the decision to join or not join Better Health Medicare Part D plan's preferred pharmacy network. The reimbursement rates in the new contract had greater discounts off of AWP and higher DIR fees, but Natalie knew that if she didn't join the preferred network she'd probably lose more patients and wondered about the impact of the performance-based DIR fees in the preferred network contract.

1. Is it better for Good Service Pharmacy to accept a lower reimbursement rate in order to become a Better Health preferred pharmacy? How much will the net profit on an average Better Health prescription decrease under the contract terms for preferred pharmacies? Will the pharmacy lose money on each Better Health prescription it dispenses?

   The average net profit comparison showed that the preferred Better Health rate would results in an average net profit that is $3.95 less than the non-preferred Better Health rate. The pharmacy currently is losing money on each Better Health prescription they dispense, but under the new reimbursement rate, the pharmacy would lose even more, an average of $4.49 on each Better Health prescription.

2. If Good Service Pharmacy accepts the contract, what would be the difference in profit if the plan determines the pharmacy to be a high performer vs. low performer based on adherence scores and GDUR?

   If Good Service Pharmacy accepts the contract, maintains current prescription volume, and is a low performer, their net profit would be $16,400. If they were able to perform well, their profit would be $23,950, a difference of $7,550. Averaged over all Better Health prescriptions dispensed, the pharmacy would make an additional $0.80 per prescription by performing well as a preferred network pharmacy.

3. Overall, would Good Service Pharmacy be better off financially by joining the Better Health preferred pharmacy network?

   The pro forma analysis showed that Good Service Pharmacy would be better off financially by not accepting the contract, even with a 10% decrease in prescription volume for Better Health. The expected profit from the preferred network, even if performance is maximized, would still be $23,950 lower than the net profit if the pharmacy stayed out of the preferred network. The results from the differential analysis showed that Good Service Pharmacy might be better off accepting the contract if the contract can create additional prescription volume for the pharmacy. However, results from the sensitivity analysis that assumed a 25% increase in the number of Better Health prescriptions from joining the preferred network showed that the pharmacy still was better off not joining the preferred network.

4. What other factors need to be considered? Could the contract be renegotiated? What effect would signing or declining the contract have on its customers?

The pharmacy manager knows that if she joins the preferred network, the pharmacy risks sending a signal to other third parties that it will accept low reimbursement rates. The pharmacy may also have to raise its cash prices or decrease its level of service to decrease costs, but this may be necessary in either scenario. If she doesn't join the preferred network, the pharmacy will lose some long-term customers who are price-sensitive and may get a reputation for being a pharmacy that charges more for prescriptions. The pharmacy manager also knows that value-based reimbursement is increasing, so regardless of whether she joins the Better Health preferred network, she needs to start monitoring and trying to improve outcomes in order to be prepared for other contracts where reimbursement is based on pharmacy performance.

5. Good Service Pharmacy will likely lose revenue regardless of whether or not they join the Better Health preferred pharmacy network. Is there any way for Good Service Pharmacy to make up the lost revenue? Or decrease its expenses?

The pharmacy could try to attract new customers to generate new prescription volume. It also could try to generate revenue from pharmacist services or selling more products (e.g., OTC products or durable medical equipment). Its largest expenses are labor costs, so the best way to decrease its COD would be to decrease its staffing levels. The pharmacy also could think about expanding professional services.

In the end, Natalie decides not to join the Better Health Medicare Part D preferred pharmacy network. The financial impact of the lower reimbursement for preferred pharmacies was substantial. This is a tough decision, though, since it might mean that Mrs. Anderson and other Better Health customers who are highly sensitive to prescription drug costs might leave for a pharmacy which is in the preferred network. However, she is very worried that by joining the preferred pharmacy network she might not be able to make enough profit on prescriptions to stay in business. She decides that developing other sources of revenue is a better option for the pharmacy's future than joining the preferred network, so she decides to try to implement and obtain payment for some pharmacist services. This includes participating in any available Medicare Part D MTM service plans through a Community Pharmacy Enhanced Services Network (CPESN) (see Chapter 32). She also hopes to expand the pharmacy's sales of durable medical equipment. She hopes that these additional services might help retain some of the customers who are paying more at her non-preferred pharmacy. She also plans to closely monitor profit margins and pharmacy outcomes as other third-party plans continue to reduce pharmacy reimbursement and implement value-based reimbursement.

■ CONCLUSION AND FUTURE THIRD-PARTY REIMBURSEMENT ISSUES

It should be apparent that the decision to join a preferred pharmacy network is often very difficult. Even after the pharmacy manager answered the questions listed in the scenario, she still had to use her judgment about joining the new Better Health preferred network with its low reimbursement rate. It is important to understand and use the tools that were described in this chapter, but they do not necessarily yield an easy answer. Regardless of the manager's decision, Better Health pharmacy likely faces lower net profit unless it finds other sources of revenue or decreases its expenses.

Declining third-party reimbursement rates is likely to continue. There are some opportunities to obtain reimbursement for MTM or other professional services, but these reimbursement levels also need to be evaluated by managers. Another trend that should be monitored is value-based pharmacy reimbursement. This type of reimbursement may result in increased revenue for pharmacies that are able to demonstrate that they provide high quality care, and but even further reductions in reimbursement for those who do not.

It is crucial that pharmacy managers understand the impact of third-party payers on their pharmacies, as well as understand and use the decision-analysis tools described in this chapter to evaluate carefully third-party contracts. It is also important that pharmacy managers and owners manage expenses carefully and think creatively about developing new sources of revenue. Third-party payment for prescriptions will continue to be an important issue in pharmacy in the future, and pharmacy managers need to be aware continually of changing reimbursement levels and other third-party issues.

REFERENCES

Abelson R, Singer N. 2012. F.T.C. Approves Merger of 2 of the Biggest Pharmacy Benefit Managers. *The New York Times*. April 2, 2012.

Academy of Managed Care Pharmacy (AMCP) Task Force on Drug Payment Methodologies. 2007. *AMCP Guide to Pharmaceutical Payment Methods*, Version 1.0. Alexandria, VA: AMCP, October 2007.

Center for Medicare and Medicaid Services (CMS). 2015. *Medicaid Covered Outpatient Prescription Drug Reimbursement Information by State Quarter Ending June 2015*. Available at http://www.medicaid.gov/medicaid-chip-program-information/by-topics/benefits/prescription-drugs/downloads/xxxreimbursement-chart-current-qtr.pdf. Accessed July 18, 2015.

Center for Medicare and Medicaid Services (CMS). 2018a. *Medicaid Covered Outpatient Prescription Drug Reimbursement Information by State Quarter Ending September 2018*. Available at https://www.medicaid.gov/medicaid/prescription-drugs/state-prescription-drug-resources/drug-reimbursement-information/index.html. Accessed December 30, 2018.

Center for Medicare and Medicaid Services (CMS). 2018b. Contract Year (CY) 2020 Medicare Advantage and Part D drug pricing proposed rule (CMS-4180-P). CMS Fact Sheet. Available at https://www.cms.gov/newsroom/fact-sheets/contract-year-cy-2020-medicare-advantage-and-part-d-drug-pricing-proposed-rule-cms-4180-p. Accessed January 2, 2019.

Deninger M. 2016. Luck and the Narrow Network Contract. Available at http://www.thethrivingpharmacist.com/2016/02/02/luck-and-the-narrow-network-contract/. Accessed December 31, 2018.

Fein A. 2017. Preferred pharmacy networks will dominate 2018 Medicare Part D plans. Drug Channels blog. Available at https://www.drugchannels.net/2017/10/exclusive-preferred-pharmacy-networks.html. Accessed December 19, 2018.

Fein A. 2018a. McKesson leads another rounds of PSAO consolidation. Drug Channels Blog. April 17, 2018. Available at https://www.drugchannels.net/2018/04/mckesson-leads-another-round-of-psao.html. Accessed December 31, 2018.

Fein A. 2018b. CMS considers point-of-sale pharmacy DIR: Another prelude to a world without rebates? Drug Channels Blog. December 4, 2018. Available at https://www.drugchannels.net/2018/12/cms-considers-point-of-sale-pharmacy.html#more. Accessed January 1, 2019.

Fridy K, DeHart RM, Monk-Tutor MR. 2002. Negotiating with third-party payers: One community pharmacy's experience. *J Am Pharm Assoc* 42:780.

Ganther JM. 2002. Third-party reimbursement for pharmacist services: Why has it been so difficult to obtain and is it really the answer for pharmacy? *J Am Pharm Assoc* 42:875.

Jaffe S. 2018. No more secrets: Congress bans pharmacist 'gag orders' on drug prices. Kaiser Health News. October 10, 2018. Available at https://khn.org/news/no-more-secrets-congress-bans-pharmacist-gag-orders-on-drug-prices/. Accessed December 31, 2018.

Livingston S. 2018. CVS Health and Aetna close $70 billion merger. Modern Healthcare. November 28, 2018. Available at https://www.modernhealthcare

.com/article/20181128/NEWS/181129943. Accessed December 31, 2018.

Martin AB, Hartman M, Washington B, Catlin A. 2019. National health care spending in 2017: Growth slows to post-great recession rates; share of GDP stabilizes. *Health Affairs* 38(1):1–11.

Medicaid and CHIP Payment and Access Commission, MACStats: Medicaid and CHIP Data Book (Washington, DC: Medicaid and CHIP Payment and Access Commission, December 2017).

Murry L, Gerleman B, Urick B, Urmie J. 2018. Third-party reimbursement for generic prescription drugs: The prevalence of below-cost reimbursement in an environment of maximum allowable cost-based reimbursement. *J Am Pharm Assoc* 58(4):421–425.

Myers and Stauffer. 2018. *Survey of the Average Cost of Dispensing a Medicaid Prescription in the State of Iowa.* Available at http://www.mslc.com/uploadedFiles/Iowa/COD/IA_2018_COD_Report_FINAL.pd. Accessed December 19, 2018.

National Association of State Medicaid Directors (NASMD). 2010. Post AWP Pharmacy Pricing and Reimbursement. Washington, DC.

National Community Pharmacists Association (NCPA). 2013. Available at http://www.ncpanet.org/newsroom/news-releases/news-releases—2013/2013/05/07/ncpa-endorses-bipartisan-bill-to-address-egregious-pharmacy-audit-reimbursement-tactics-in-medicare. Accessed July 30, 2015.

National Community Pharmacists Association (NCPA). 2018. *NCPA Digest.* Alexandria, VA.

PBMI. 2018. Trends in Drug Benefit Design. Pharmacy Benefit Management Institute and Takeda Pharmaceuticals, Inc.

Pear R. 2015. House Hearing on Insurer's Mergers Exposes Health Care Industry Divide. *The New York Times.* September 10.

Pringle J, Rucker N, Domann D, Chan C, Tice B, Burns A. 2016. Applying value-based incentive models within community pharmacy practice. *Am J Pharm Benefits.* 8(1):22–29.

Sega T. 2018. Medicare 2019 Star Ratings Update. Presented at: Quality Forum Webinar; November 6th, 2018. Available at https://vimeo.com/299946946. Accessed December 10, 2018.

Urick B, Ferreri S, Shasky C, Pfeiffenberger T, Trygstad T, Farley J. 2018. Lessons learned from using global outcome measures to assess community pharmacy performance. *J Manag Care Spec Pharm.* 24(12):1278–1283.

Urick B and Urmie J. 2019. Framework for assessing pharmacy value. Research in Social and Administrative Pharmacy. 12(1):91–103. Available at https://doi.org/10.1016/j.sapharm.2018.12.008. Accessed July 22, 2019.

Van Nuys S, Joyce G, Ribero R, Goldman D. 2018. Overpaying for prescription drugs: The copay clawback phenomenon. White paper from the USC Schaffer Center. Available at https://healthpolicy.usc.edu/wp-content/uploads/2018/03/2018.03_Overpaying-20for20Prescription20Drugs_White20Paper_v.1-4.pdf. Accessed December 31, 2018.

Wilde Mathews A, Walker J. 2015. UnitedHealth to Buy Catamaran for $12.8 Billion in Cash. *The Wall Street Journal.* March 30.

SECTION V

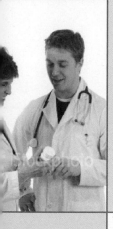

MANAGING TRADITIONAL

GOODS AND SERVICES

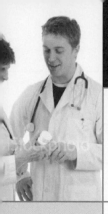

24

MARKETING FUNDAMENTALS

John P. Bentley and Meagen Rosenthal

About the Authors:. Dr. Bentley is a professor in the Department of Pharmacy Administration at the University of Mississippi, School of Pharmacy, with a joint appointment in the Department of Marketing in the School of Business Administration. He serves as the Chair of the Department of Pharmacy Administration and Program Coordinator for the University's Graduate Minor in Applied Statistics. He received his BS in pharmacy and MBA from Drake University, MS and PhD in pharmacy administration from the University of Mississippi, and MS and PhD in biostatistics from the University of Alabama at Birmingham (UAB). In the professional pharmacy curriculum, Dr. Bentley teaches elements of research design, biostatistics, epidemiology, and drug literature evaluation. At the graduate level, he teaches several applied statistics courses. He has conducted research in a variety of areas including pharmaceutical marketing and patient behavior; patients' evaluation of health care providers; direct-to-consumer advertising; practice management; quality of life; medication adherence; medication use, misuse, and outcomes; and ethics and professionalism. His statistics research interests include statistical mediation analysis and longitudinal data analysis. Dr. Bentley was named a fellow of the American Pharmacists Association in 2009 and the National Academies of Practice in 2019.

Dr. Rosenthal is an assistant professor in the Department of Pharmacy Administration, and a research assistant professor in the Center for Pharmaceutical Marketing and Management, Research Institute of Pharmaceutical Sciences at the University of Mississippi, School of Pharmacy. She is also a research associate with the Center for Population Studies, in the Department of Sociology and Anthropology, and a co-lead in the Community Wellbeing Constellation of the University of Mississippi's Flagship Constellation Initiative. She received her BA and MA in sociology from the University of Alberta, Canada. She also received her PhD in experimental medicine from the University of Alberta, Canada. In the professional pharmacy curriculum, she teaches pharmacy management and business methods. At the graduate level, she teaches primary research techniques. She has conducted research in community pharmacy practice, change management, practice management, and implementation science.

■ LEARNING OBJECTIVES

After completing this chapter, readers should be able to

1. Define marketing and describe its societal contributions.
2. Discuss the purpose of marketing within a business.
3. Define the concept of exchange and state its importance to marketing.
4. Differentiate among the concepts of needs, wants, and demands.
5. Identify orientations toward the marketplace that organizations might take when conducting marketing activities.
6. Describe and apply the marketing mix and the four Ps of modern marketing management.
7. Describe different types of product offerings, and define the distinguishing characteristics of a service.
8. Define expectations, satisfaction, quality, value, and loyalty and describe their role in purchase behavior and the profitability of organizations.
9. Explain the concept of relationship marketing and apply it to pharmacy management.

■ SCENARIO

Jim Smyth and Sue Davidson co-own and manage West Side Pharmacy. While looking over the books for the last year, both pharmacists begin to recognize that their pharmacy is struggling to meet its financial objectives. Jim and Sue decide to ask the staff pharmacist and the technicians to help brainstorm ideas for improving the pharmacy's financial performance. During the after-hours impromptu staff meeting, the following questions were asked: "What other services can we provide that people in our community need or want?" "What types of services can we develop given our resources?" "Should we provide the services in our pharmacy or at some other location?" "How will our services be different from Corner Pharmacy on the other side of town?" "What will be the impact of new competitors, such as PillPack Pharmacy, now owned by Amazon, with its incredible size and understanding of consumer markets?" "How should we respond to such new market entrants?" "What should we charge for our services?" "How do we let people know that we are offering these services?" "Are there any health-related goods that we should add to the line of products we sell?" "How will we know if our patients value the goods and services we provide?" "What kinds of relationships do we need to establish with our patients to be successful?" "Should we start a customer loyalty program?"

These are all marketing-related questions. This chapter will describe and discuss some of the basic building blocks of marketing that are essential for developing and implementing a successful marketing plan. Chapter 25 will provide practical tools for marketing pharmacy goods and services.

■ CHAPTER QUESTIONS

1. What is marketing, and what is its purpose in a business setting and in a pharmacy setting?
2. What are the differences among needs, wants, and demands?
3. What are the different philosophies that may be used to guide marketing efforts?
4. What is the marketing mix and what are the four Ps of modern marketing management?

5. What characterizes the different types of offerings that a business makes to its customers?

6. How do the concepts of expectations, satisfaction, quality, value, and loyalty relate to each other, and what is their importance to marketing?

7. What is relationship marketing, and how can it be used to enhance pharmacy practice?

■ INTRODUCTION: WHY MARKETING?

Marketing has received a "bad rap" (Smith, 1996), despite its contributions to society (Wilkie & Moore, 1999) and to our high standard of living (Smith, 1996). Some of these criticisms stem from the common misunderstanding that marketing is defined solely as the "art of selling products" (Kotler & Keller, 2016), while other criticisms stem from misperceptions that many marketers are unethical. The bottom line is that marketing is an activity that is misunderstood by many, including pharmacists and health care professionals. In the opinion of some, marketing is an often-overlooked activity that is critical to the success of any organization (Smith, 2002).

It is important to recognize that marketing is not just an activity performed by large, multinational corporations. Indeed, the principles of marketing are just as applicable to small, independently owned pharmacies, as well as to the profession of pharmacy more generally.[1] Marketing and pharmacy have been practiced together for a long time. Marketing tools have been used to help pharmacists address what to charge for a prescription drug, whether to add a pharmacokinetic monitoring service or a new clinical specialist at a hospital, which over-the-counter (OTC) products to carry, and how to best utilize wholesalers to purchase products.

As pharmacy continues to evolve, marketing's role grows in importance. Since the articulation of the concept of pharmaceutical care (Hepler & Strand, 1990), many innovative pharmacy services have been described and implemented, ranging from comprehensive medication therapy management (MTM) services, to specific disease management services, such as diabetes care, lipid management, tobacco cessation, and anticoagulation management. However, concurrent with the development and implementation of these services has been a continued growth in the literature documenting inappropriate use of medications, suggesting that a significant need still exists for services that are directed at enhancing the positive and reducing the negative consequences associated with drug therapy.

So why are these needs not being met? Concerns regarding prescriber, patient, and payer demand are often considered significant barriers to the provision of patient-centered pharmacy services (McDonough et al., 1998b). Understanding customers'[2] needs and using that understanding to create, deliver, and communicate the value of pharmacists' services are key components of marketing. While many pharmacists are interested in obtaining the necessary clinical knowledge and skills to deliver MTM services, many would argue that marketing knowledge and skills are equally important. Rovers et al. (1998, p. 136) note, "Pharmacists must build the demand and supply for pharmaceutical care services simultaneously." The importance of understanding the nuances of marketing to the success of pharmaceutical care is recognized by Hepler and Strand (1990, p. 541), who noted that "a pharmaceutical-care marketing strategy ... would differ fundamentally from the usual strategy developed for selling drug products." For innovative pharmacy services to help patients achieve optimal

---

[1]Marketing principles can also be applied at the personal level: for example, marketing your clinical services as a pharmacist to consult with a physician on drug therapy, or in the development of friendships, and even romantic relationships!

[2]While some authors appropriately argue that the terms *consumer, customer, patient,* and *client* have fundamentally different meanings, they are, for the most part, used interchangeably in this chapter. A discussion of the meaning and symbolism of these terms is best handled in another setting.

therapeutic outcomes, pharmacy practitioners must understand the important role of marketing. This chapter will define many of the terms and concepts that are critical to understanding how to incorporate marketing effectively and efficiently into management of the pharmacy enterprise.

■ MARKETING: DEFINITIONS AND CONCEPTS

Because the goal of this chapter is to introduce the basic building blocks of marketing, it becomes necessary to first define what *marketing* is. Prior to the 1960s, marketing was recognized as a set of *business* activities that existed to consummate *market transactions* between producers of goods and services and consumers (Hunt, 2010). However, beginning in the 1960s, others suggested that (1) the term should be broadened to include nonbusiness organizations and (2) the societal implications of marketing activities should be included in the domain of marketing (Hunt, 2010). After considerable debate, in 1985, the American Marketing Association (AMA) adopted the following definition of marketing (Keefe, 2004, p. 17): "Marketing is the process of planning and executing the conception, pricing, promotion, and distribution of ideas, goods, and services to create exchanges that satisfy individual and organizational objectives." The emphasis on *exchange* and the inclusion of *ideas* clearly demonstrate that marketing has been broadened to include nonbusiness organizations. The most recent AMA definition of marketing adopted in 2007 (Gundlach & Wilkie, 2009, p. 260) takes this idea a step further by making no reference to marketing as a business function, implying that nonbusiness organizations (and other entities) can implement marketing activities and processes:

"Marketing is the activity, set of institutions, and processes for creating, communicating, delivering, and exchanging offerings that have value for customers, clients, partners, and society at large."

The literature is replete with examples of how the principles of marketing have been used by charitable organizations, academic institutions, social issues groups, political candidates, and health care institutions. Hunt (2010, p. 10) remarked, "Today it is noncontroversial that marketing has an important role to play in nonbusiness organizations." The 2007 definition also explicitly recognizes the social role of marketing as well as the societal implications of marketing activities by focusing on offerings that have value not only for customers, clients, and partners but also for society at large.

Kotler and Keller (2016) further distinguished between social and managerial definitions of marketing. Kotler and Keller's (2016, p. 5) social definition reads: "Marketing is a *societal process* (emphasis added) by which individuals and groups obtain what they need and want through creating, offering, and freely exchanging products and services of value with others." There is little question that marketing fulfills a social role. Several authors have suggested that marketing exists to create a higher standard of living (Kotler & Keller, 2016; Smith, 2002).[3] From a managerial perspective, Kotler and Keller (2016, p. 5) defined marketing as "the art and science of choosing target markets and getting, keeping, and growing customers through creating, delivering, and communicating superior customer value." Marketing plays a demand management function within the organization, focusing partially on methods to stimulate demand but also, more important, on methods for how to control demand to meet the objectives of the organization.

Although each of these definitions sheds additional light on the domain of marketing, they also serve to introduce several additional explicit concepts that will be explored later in this chapter, namely, exchange and value (Gundlach & Wilkie, 2009), and needs and wants (Kotler & Keller, 2016). These

---

[3]While an in-depth discussion of this issue is beyond the scope of this chapter, the reader is referred to an article by Wilkie and Moore (1999) for an intriguing and insightful discussion of marketing's contribution to society.

definitions also imply several other important concepts including the four Ps of the marketing mix (i.e., product,[4] price, place [distribution], and promotion) and the concept of relationships, which will also be covered in greater detail in the remainder of this chapter.

■ MARKETING SCIENCE

Given that this chapter is entitled "Marketing Fundamentals," it is important to note that marketing also exists as an academic and scientific discipline, implying that at least some aspects of marketing can be fitted with the label of science. For this reason, it is worthwhile to briefly explore the question as to whether marketing is a science.

Like the broadening of the marketing debate, the debate as to whether marketing is a science has a rich history. Some authors have argued that marketing is a science, whereas others have argued that marketing is an art (e.g., see Hunt, 1976, 1983; Peter & Olson, 1983). One's view of the scope of marketing is critical to answering this question. While an understanding of the nature of science is also critical, it is beyond the scope of this chapter, and the reader is referred to an excellent discussion by Hunt (2010). With respect to the scope of marketing, Hunt (1976) has proposed that all marketing content can be classified into one of eight classes or cells. One criterion that is used to define these cells is whether the marketing content is positive or normative. *Positive* marketing attempts to describe, explain, predict, and understand marketing phenomena; the focus of the analysis is descriptive—what is. *Normative* marketing attempts to prescribe what an organization, individual, or society should do; the focus is prescriptive—what ought to be done.

If one defines the scope of marketing as only normative efforts designed to assist marketing decision makers (e.g., What methods can we use to sell more product? How much should we charge for this product or service?), then marketing is not a science. However, if one considers an expanded scope of marketing to also include the positive dimensions, then marketing can be considered to be a science. As a science, what does marketing purport to do? The concept of exchange becomes critical because "marketing science is the behavioral science that seeks to explain exchange relationships" (Hunt, 1983, p. 13). Marketing as an academic discipline has undergone significant transformation over the years (e.g., see Wilkie & Moore, 2003), and researchers in the field have become increasingly specialized.[5]

Because this chapter is more interested in the application of marketing principles to pharmacy, little more will be mentioned of the science side of marketing. The focus for the remainder of this chapter will be on the technology of marketing, or its applied side. However, it is important to remember that just as the "practice" of medicine and the "practice" of pharmacy are steeply rooted in a scientific knowledge base, so too is the "practice" of marketing. While the sheer quantity of the "product" of marketing science (i.e., the laws, principles, and theories that serve to unify, explain, and predict marketing phenomena) may be less than the quantity of the "product" of the sciences underlying medicine and pharmacy, this should not suggest that marketing is any less of a science. The scientific method is not any less appropriate to marketing than it is to other disciplines (Hunt, 2010).

■ EXCHANGE: THE CORE CONCEPT OF MARKETING

The core concept of marketing is *exchange* (Kotler, 2003). It is the unifying concept in marketing not only for marketing practice but also for marketing

---

[4]As will be discussed later in this chapter, the concept of product in marketing can refer to any item of value offered by an organization, including tangible goods, services, and even intangible concepts or ideas.

[5]Readers interested in the science of marketing are referred to the work of McAlister et al. (2010), who have developed a compilation of scholarly articles published in marketing-related journals.

science. In marketing thought, an *exchange* is a process of obtaining a desired product from someone by offering something in return. When two parties in an exchange process reach an agreement, a transaction takes place. A *transaction* is a trade of values between two or more parties. Although the items of value are often money and a tangible good, this does not have to be the case. The items of value can also be services, ideas, experiences, events, places, material, organizations, effort, and information (Kotler, 2003).

The idea of exchange can also be extended beyond a transaction. For instance, in a *transfer*, one party gives an item of value to another party while receiving nothing tangible in return. A charitable contribution is an example of a transfer. At first glance, transfers appear fundamentally different from transactions. However, in most cases, the giving party often expects something in return, such as gratitude, a change in the recipient, a positive feeling, or even a tax deduction. When observed in this light, transfers, like transactions, can be understood through the core concept of exchange. Indeed, marketers have included transfer behavior in their domain of study (e.g., see Mathur, 1996).

■ NEEDS, WANTS, AND DEMANDS

The previous definitions of marketing also suggest that marketers must attempt to understand the needs, wants, and demands of their target markets. While some may feel that these three words have similar meanings and use them interchangeably, understanding the fundamentals of marketing requires recognizing that each term conveys a distinctly different concept. Briefly, a *need* is a state of felt deprivation. Needs are basic human requirements. People have physical needs (e.g., food, clothing, and shelter), social needs (e.g., the need for affection and the need to belong), and individual needs (e.g., the need for self-expression). A *want* is a desire for a specific satisfier of a need. Thus, needs become wants, and these wants are shaped by culture and individual personality. A

need for food can translate into wanting pizza; a need for affection may result in wanting a hug. A *demand* is a want that is backed by an ability to pay. Many people may want a luxury car, a vacation at an exotic resort, or tickets to the World Series or Super Bowl, but the demand for these items is limited because only a relative few are able and willing to make such a purchase.

From the health economics literature, *need* is defined as "the amount of medical care that medical experts believe a person should have to remain or become as healthy as possible, based on current medical knowledge" (Feldstein, 1999, p. 83). Economists are quick to point out that need is only one factor affecting the demand for care; demand for medical care is determined by a set of patient and provider factors, including a patient's need for care (Feldstein, 1999). Thus, demand for care can be *greater than* the need; likewise, demand for care can be *less than* the need. Some might argue that certain lifestyle drugs such as Viagra are good examples of the former; immunizations and MTM services are good examples of the latter.

Some have argued that the traditional perspective that a marketer's responsibility is primarily about meeting or responding to people's stated needs is too limited a view of a marketer's role (Kotler & Keller, 2016). Frequently, customers do not know what they want or need in a good or service. Think about the many goods and services available today, such as smartphones, tablet computers, 24-hour discount brokerage accounts, and Internet service providers. Did most consumers want (or need) these things *before* they were available? For health care providers, this situation is all too common because most patients do not have the skills and knowledge that health care professionals have. Thus, health care providers often recognize a patient's need for a health-related good or service that the individual patient does not recognize.

The job of a marketer (and the job of a health care professional as well) is not only to understand and respond to people's *expressed* needs but also to help customers learn more about what they need and want. In essence, marketers also must understand and respond to people's *latent* needs. Narver et al. (2004) call the former a *responsive* market orientation and the latter a *proactive* market orientation. Marketers do not create needs, but they do help consumers to understand their latent needs and to translate needs into wants. An understanding of this issue is helpful in explaining pharmacy's current experiences with patient-centered services.

For example, assume that Mary Cooper enters a pharmacy wanting to purchase St. John's wort because her friend told her it would help her feel better. After talking briefly with Mary, the pharmacist realizes that her symptoms are more significant than communicated initially. Given this additional information, the pharmacist refers Mary to a mental health care provider for further evaluation and treatment. In this case, the customer (Mary) stated a solution (St. John's wort), not a need (her mental state of well-being). The pharmacist appropriately recognized Mary's need and was able to help her by appropriately influencing her wants and demands.

A problem faced particularly by health care providers is that people often do not want their goods or services. This situation is called *negative demand* (Kotler & Keller, 2016). Importantly for pharmacists, pharmaceutical products are often labeled as *negative goods* (Smith & Kolassa, 2001). Negative demand occurs when a major part of the market dislikes the service or product, and may even pay a price to avoid it. Other examples of negative services and goods include automobile repair services, legal services, and dental work.

One way to manage negative demand is to try to better understand people's true motivations for purchasing a product. For example, do people purchase drill bits because they want drill bits? Or do they purchase drill bits because they want holes? Considered in this light, it is clear that people purchase drill bits because they want holes (Smith, 1996). In the same way, most people use medications not for the sake of having and taking medications, but because appropriate use of medications provides benefits by alleviating, eliminating, or preventing a disease or its symptoms.

It is important to talk to patients to find out why they are using a product, what needs or wants they expect to meet by using a product, and what concerns they have about using the product. Thus, applying good marketing techniques to manage negative demand is consistent with good pharmacy practice.

There is little question as to the need for patient-centered pharmacy services given the well-documented negative outcomes associated with drug therapy. McDonough et al. (1998b, p. 89) noted that a common misconception among pharmacists is that "patients neither want nor will be willing to pay for pharmaceutical care." While this may be true of *some* patients, this certainly is not true of *all* patients. Part of the problem lies in the fact that many patients are unaware of their needs and possible solutions (i.e., their needs are latent). McDonough (2003, p. 275) argues that "a key reason why patients do not demand pharmaceutical care is that they do not understand the concept." Patients have to see the value of the service. It is up to the profession to help translate latent needs into wants and demands.

■ COMPANY ORIENTATIONS TOWARD THE MARKET PLACE

Given marketing's crucial role in the exchange of offerings of value to fulfill needs and wants, for many years, marketing authors have sought to clarify the role of marketing in an organization. In essence, questions have arisen as to the type of philosophy that should guide the marketing efforts of a company. Kotler (2003) has described six competing concepts that organizations use as guides in the conduct of marketing activities: the production concept, the product concept, the selling concept, the marketing concept, the customer concept, and the societal marketing concept.

The emphasis of the *production concept* is efficiency in the production and distribution of goods and services. The key assumption about consumers underlying this concept is that they are primarily interested in product availability and low prices. A production concept can also guide the efforts of service organizations, where the goal might be to handle as many cases as possible in a given period of time. A pharmacy dedicated to dispensing as many prescriptions as possible, often without regard to providing patient education or even to reviewing medication appropriateness, is practicing the production concept. As Kotler observes, such an orientation may lead to customer comments concerning the impersonal nature of the service delivery.

The emphasis of the *product concept* is on making good products, often as defined in the eyes of the producer, and improving them over time. The key assumptions about buyers in this concept are that they appreciate well-made products and that they can evaluate product quality. A company guided by the product concept is often focused on designing a great product (or service) and often gets little or no input from those who will benefit from its product. Kotler (2003) acknowledges that managers following this philosophical orientation might commit the "better mousetrap" fallacy. For example, consider a smoking-cessation program that has as its sole focus the use of a technologically advanced reminder system for patients who are using nicotine-replacement therapy. A pharmacist being guided by the product concept would assume that patients would enroll in the program and pay for the services with little other effort to educate the patient or provide other complementary services on his or her part.

The *selling concept* emphasizes actions directed at stimulating consumers' interest through aggressive sales and promotion efforts. Managers guided by the selling concept assume that consumers must be coaxed into buying products. The focus is on hard selling, and little concern is given to customers' needs, wants, and postpurchase satisfaction. This is a common approach and is cited as a reason why the public often identifies marketing with selling and advertising (Kotler, 2003). A pharmacy that engages in an overly aggressive campaign, including the use of advertising, sales discounts, and high-pressure personal selling, is practicing the selling concept.

The *marketing concept* was proposed as a challenge to the previous concepts.[6] Rather than focus on the needs of the organization or the seller, the marketing concept suggests that the needs of the buyer are paramount. The marketing concept holds that "the key to achieving its organizational goals consists of the company being more effective than competitors in creating, delivering, and communicating superior customer value to its chosen target markets" (Kotler, 2003, p. 19). Smith (2002, p. 9) succinctly summarizes the meaning of the marketing concept from the perspective of the pharmaceutical manufacturer: "The marketing concept states what seems obvious now but was not always practiced: It is easier to change the products and activities of the individual manufacturer to fit the market than it is to convince the entire market to use the products and services as the individual marketer prefers them."

A company guided by the marketing concept takes care to select appropriate target markets (i.e., distinct groups of buyers who may benefit from a given product or service mix), is focused on the needs of its customers, attempts to integrate a marketing orientation into all segments of the company, and does these activities with an eye toward achieving organizational goals and objectives, notably generating profits through the creation of customer value (Kotler, 2003). The last point regarding profitability through creating customer value is not specific to for-profit firms. This precept is also important for not-for-profit organizations, which instead may strive to generate funds through creating, delivering, and communicating value to their stakeholders to continue their useful work.

Increases in market diversity, changes in technology, and the need for enhanced marketing productivity have led some marketing scholars and practitioners to propose a fifth concept that moves beyond the more traditional marketing concept (Sheth et al., 2000).

---

[6]For an excellent review of the marketing concept and its implementation, referred to as market orientation, see Kohli and Jaworski (1990).

While companies guided by the marketing concept focus on segments of consumers known as target markets, the *customer concept* suggests that companies direct separate offers, services, and messages to individual customers (Kotler, 2003). The Internet (including social media), database software, and factory customization all have enabled such an approach to marketing. The customer concept calls for a focus on individual customer needs, sometimes leading to customization of the product or other elements of the marketing mix. The functions of the company should be integrated around customer value-added activities, and profitable growth is achieved through enhancement of customer loyalty and by focusing on the creation of lifetime value for individual customers (Kotler, 2003; Sheth et al., 2000). An example of the customer concept in pharmacy may be the delivery of tailored health information to customers based on health-related Internet searches or the use of pharmacogenetic testing as a tool to better customize drug therapy to individual patients.

A sixth orientation with respect to marketing thought and organizational philosophy has been proposed because of changes in our surroundings, such as deterioration of the environment, resource shortages, poverty, and neglected social services (Kotler, 2003). The previously discussed orientations give considerable weight to the interests of either the organization itself or its customers, but companies guided by these concepts still often act in ways that may not be in the best interests of society. Kotler (2003, pp. 26–27) has labeled this sixth orientation, the *societal marketing concept*, which "holds that the organization's task is to determine the needs, wants, and interests of target markets and to deliver the desired satisfactions more effectively and efficiently than competitors in a way that preserves or enhances the consumer's and the society's wellbeing." Thus, social and ethical considerations also must guide marketers' decisions. This means that company profits, satisfaction of consumers' wants and needs, and the public interest (each often having conflicting endpoints) must be balanced. Patient assistance programs offered by pharmaceutical manufacturers, recycling programs for customers'

empty vials, and prescription drug take-back programs offered by community pharmacies are examples of efforts guided by the societal marketing concept.

Recognizing marketing's central role in the organization and the many forces that have shaped marketing and business practices in the past decade, Kotler and Keller (2016) recently proposed a seventh overarching concept called *holistic marketing*. In essence, this philosophical orientation combines many of the features of the marketing concept, the customer concept, and the societal marketing concept (and even some elements of the production, product, and selling concepts). This term is intended to convey the importance of taking both a broad and integrated view of marketing. The term *holistic* communicates both the importance and complexity of marketing activities within an organization. Several of the broad components of holistic marketing, including relationship marketing and internal marketing with its focus on selecting, training, and motivating people (i.e., employees) to serve customers to help them achieve their goals, will be discussed later in this chapter.

■ THE FOUR P's OF MARKETING AND MORE

Explicit in the 1985 AMA definition of marketing, and implicit in the other definitions mentioned earlier, are several concepts that have come to be labeled as the *marketing mix*. A marketing mix is a set of tools an organization uses to pursue its objectives with respect to its target market. Although it has received criticism (e.g., Day & Montgomery, 1999) and other frameworks and classifications have been proposed (e.g., Van Waterschoot & Van den Bulte, 1992), McCarthy's (1960) schema has stood the test of time. He proposed that the tools of the marketing mix be classified into four broad groups: product, price, place, and promotion. These concepts have come to be called the *four Ps of marketing*, or simply the marketing mix, and represent variables within a company's control that can influence customer responses. Depending on whom one reads, other Ps, including positioning, have been added to the marketing mix (the fifth P). Kotler and Keller (2016) have taken this one step further, arguing that these four Ps are insufficient given the breadth and depth of marketing in today's environment. Using the holistic marketing concept as a guide, they suggest what they have called the *modern marketing management four Ps*, which include people, processes, programs, and performance, to complement the four Ps of the marketing mix. In the remainder of this section, a brief overview of each of these Ps will be offered; however, read Chapter 25 for insights into how marketing-mix decisions can be made.

Product

Product refers to an organization's offering. To a marketer, the term *product* means more than just a physical good. In pharmacy, physical goods (e.g., drugs and durable medical equipment) usually are combined with a service. Indeed, Shepherd (1995, p. 53) observed, "pharmaceutical products require a service component." However, in pharmacy, it is not uncommon for a service to be provided without a physical good. Kotler and Keller (2016) described five categories of offerings that are distinguished based on how much the service component is part of the offering:

- *Pure tangible good.* The offering consists primarily of a tangible good, such as toothpaste, toilet paper, or napkins.
- *Tangible good with accompanying services.* The offering consists of a tangible good accompanied by one or more services; as the sophistication for use of the good increases, the more dependent its sale is on services.
- *Hybrid.* The offering consists of equal parts of goods and services, such as the purchase of a meal at a restaurant (consists of food and service).
- *Major service with accompanying minor goods and services.* The offering consists of a major service accompanied by other services and supporting goods, such as the purchase of airplane transportation (primarily a service accompanied by some tangibles such as food and drinks).

- *Pure service.* The offering consists primarily of a service, such as attending an orchestra performance or psychotherapy.

Christensen et al. (1993) differentiated among three types of services associated with patient care provided by pharmacists. Although there are some differences, their classification scheme in many respects resembles Kotler and Keller's (2016) categories, which are applicable to all goods and services, not just those related to pharmacy.

- *Dispensing services.* These are services associated with dispensing a prescription that are obligatory under board of pharmacy regulations. These services include accurately filling a prescription order, clarifying orders, not dispensing an order that contains obvious errors that would be identified by a "reasonable and prudent" pharmacist, and communicating drug-use instructions as required by state statutes and regulations.
- *Dispensing-related value-added pharmaceutical services.* These are services that extend beyond *routine* dispensing activities. These services include activities such as selecting appropriate drug products, monitoring refill behaviors, and consulting with other health providers about a patient's drug regimen (beyond routine clarification questions).
- *Nondispensing-related value-added pharmaceutical services.* These are services that are not associated with the dispensing of a prescription nor inherent in the dispensing fee charged for a prescription. These services include screening programs (e.g., osteoporosis, lipids, and blood pressure), weight-management programs, in-service training provided to health care providers, and discharge counseling in an inpatient setting.

The preceding discussion may lead one to ask: What is the difference between a physical good and a service? Several authors have attempted to define characteristics that distinguish goods from services. Although there is some debate as to which characteristics best represent the fundamental differences, it is important to recognize that any list represents generalizations that may not be applicable to all services (Lovelock & Wright, 2002). The following list contains nine basic differences that can help to distinguish services from physical goods (Lovelock & Wright, 2002)[7]:

- Customers do not obtain ownership of services.
- Service products are intangible performances.
- There is greater involvement of customers in the production process.
- People may form part of the product, including other patrons.
- There is greater variability in operational inputs and outputs, making it more difficult to standardize and control.
- Many services are difficult for customers to evaluate.
- There is typically an absence of inventories.
- The time factor is relatively more important.
- Delivery systems may involve both electronic and physical channels.

Although establishing the differences between goods and services may seem trivial, this distinction has important implications for the design of a marketing program.[8] For example, a major consideration in service delivery is matching demand levels and capacity. This is so because services are perishable and cannot be inventoried. One mechanism that can be used to better match supply and demand is the use of reservations (e.g., hotel and airline industries) or appointments (e.g., for MTM services). As another

example, because of the greater variability inherent in the production of a service, service organizations need to pay special attention to the standardization of the service-performance process or risk damaging the quality of the service provided. One mechanism that can be used is a *service blueprint*, similar to a protocol or practice guideline in health care parlance, which is "a visual map of the sequence of activities required for service delivery" that specifies not only the elements of service operations that are both visible and hidden from the customer, but also the linkages between these elements (Lovelock & Wright, 2002, p. 153). Such a blueprint can be particularly helpful in evaluating the success of a service and its implementation by identifying fail-points or points in the process where there are significant risks for problems. See Chapter 30 for an example of how service blueprints have been used in the development of clinical pharmacy services.

Problems can emerge when organizations narrowly define their product (or business). Theodore Levitt (1960) labeled this as *marketing myopia*. Marketing myopia often results from the single-minded application of the product concept as a philosophical guide to marketing activities. This is common when a firm defines its business by a product rather than in terms of what customer needs are filled by its activities. Common examples include the railroad and movie industries. These industries nearly disappeared because they assumed that they were in the railroad and movie businesses, respectively, rather than the transportation and entertainment businesses. As other businesses emerged (e.g., the airline and automobile industries and the television and theme park industries), those in the railroad and movie businesses faced a fight for the consumer's dollar against competition generated by unanticipated sources. Given the fast-paced changes taking place within the larger health care system, to simply say that pharmacists are in the business of dispensing medications prescribed by physicians is too myopic. Pharmacists and pharmacies need to determine why people use their goods and services.

Another problem related to marketing myopia occurs when a single product becomes an organization's

---

[7]For an alternative view regarding the meaning and importance of these differences, see Vargo and Lusch (2004a).

[8]Services marketing, coupled with other streams of marketing literature, such as relationship marketing, resource management, and market orientation, have led some (e.g., see Vargo and Lusch, 2004b) to argue that marketing, as an academic discipline and as a business practice, has shifted from a goods-dominant view, largely based on discrete transactions, to a service-dominant view, where relationships play a central role. One could argue that pharmacy has experienced a similar evolution.

reason for being. If a company becomes too wrapped up in its product, it may miss the opportunity to fulfill the needs of the market. Pharmacist-delivered MTM services are a type of product that has the potential to fall victim to such a problem. Although MTM services are valuable for patients, for the profession, and for society, this does not imply that such services should be and will be a success. Just because pharmacists have the requisite clinical knowledge and skills to provide these services is not enough. Pharmacists must understand that these services represent an offering with a set of benefits that helps to meet the needs of customers and society. Pharmacists (and the profession) must be able to create, deliver, and communicate the value of what they do. Keep in mind that others (e.g., physicians, nurses, and information from the Internet) can also provide the benefits that pharmacists are purporting with MTM services. So the question then becomes what can pharmacists add? Although the answer to this question may be readily apparent to pharmacists, it is often not so apparent to patients, health care professionals, and other consumers of pharmacy goods and services. Understanding consumer needs and wants and effectively communicating how pharmacists can meet those needs is the key to more widespread acceptance of MTM and other pharmacist-delivered services.

Price

A producer should set a *price* after considering several variables, including the cost function (i.e., the cost of producing, distributing, and selling the product, including a reasonable return for effort and risk), competitors' prices, and the demand for the product (including the target market's perception of the benefits) (Kotler & Keller, 2016). Some researchers have distinguished between an *objective* price (the actual price of a product) and a *perceived* price (what is encoded by the consumer, e.g., "expensive" or "cheap") (Zeithaml, 1988). To a consumer, price is what is given up or sacrificed to obtain a product (Zeithaml, 1988). It is also important to recognize that from the perspective of the consumer, the monetary price is not the only cost associated with buying

a product (Lovelock & Wright, 2002; Zeithaml, 1988). Nonmonetary outlays include the costs associated with the time, effort, and discomfort related to the processes of searching for, purchasing, and using the product. For example, if a consumer has to travel a long distance to purchase a product, a sacrifice has been made that adds to what the consumer has given up to acquire that product.

The pricing of patient care service raises additional considerations, and perhaps, the most significant issue that must be addressed is the reluctance of pharmacists to request compensation for the services they provide (McDonough & Sobotka, 2003). When consumers obtain a prescription drug from a pharmacy, they are provided one price that has not been broken down into a "good" and a "service" component. This causes consumers to assume that either (1) there are no services that accompany prescription drug products or (2) the services that come with these products are included with the price of the drug.

Furthermore, some pharmacists feel that they must give their services away initially to develop demand for them in the future. However, consumers are generally reluctant to start paying for something that they have been able to obtain for free in the past. Most consumers are willing to pay lawyers for legal advice and auto mechanics for service primarily because (1) these professionals have expertise that most consumers do not have and (2) they have a tradition of charging for their services exclusive of charging for the goods they also might sell.

Place

Place, or *distribution,* refers to any activity designed to create utility by having the product available when and where targeted customers want to buy it. Many companies are considered successful because of their ability to deliver value in the distribution of products and services. Indeed, companies such as FedEx have made significant contributions to the success of many other companies that rely on prompt, efficient, and affordable delivery of goods (Siecker, 2002). In today's world of overnight delivery, telecommunications, and the Internet, speed and convenience are important elements in determining the distribution strategies of many firms (Lovelock & Wright, 2002). For a pharmacy, *place* may refer to providing a private area for counseling and providing other professional services (McDonough et al., 2003) or evaluating whether providing services at the work site for an employer group is feasible.

Although *physical location* has historically been the focus of this element of the marketing mix for traditional or brick-and-mortar pharmacies, the entrance of app-and-delivery businesses into the pharmacy marketplace, such as Amazon with PillPack Pharmacy, has the potential to redefine the meaning of *place* in the pharmacy environment. Many traditional pharmacies also have developed apps which enable simplified purchase and delivering to one's home or office. Although texting and chatting with a pharmacist working in an app-and-delivery pharmacy maybe convenient for many patients, it is also likely that other patients prefer face-to-face interactions with live pharmacists, and some interactions, such as immunizations, require in-person visits (Panda, 2018). Pharmacists' understanding of consumer needs and wants is not only important for product development; adapting and innovating based on understanding consumer needs and wants is critical for other aspects of the marketing mix, including place.

Promotion

Promotion activities seek to inform, remind, and persuade the target market about an organization and its offerings. Promotion activities also encourage members of the target market to take action at specific times. While advertising may be an important promotional tool, other tools in the promotion mix include sales promotion, public relations (including publicity), direct marketing, and personal selling.

Many pharmacies have used these tools successfully to spread the word about new and existing goods and services. Newspaper, radio, and television advertisements are used commonly by pharmacies. Pharmacies also employ promotional tools, such as websites and social media apps, coupons, newsletters, brochures, prescriber and patient mailings, health screenings, and presentations to civic groups or at community meetings. Some pharmacies have worked with the media to inform the public about their participation in public health events such as the many opportunities associated with the Million Hearts™ campaign, a national public–private initiative led by the U.S. Department of Health and Human Services (US DHHS, 2019). The Internet and social media provide powerful promotional tools to disseminate information (including time-sensitive information), foster relationships, and encourage others to take action. For example, pharmacies can use social networking services to connect with referring physicians and those with whom pharmacists have formed collaborative working relationships.

With respect to MTM services, promotion plays an essential role in the translation of needs into wants and demands. Depending on the individual situation, all elements of the promotion mix may have a role in communicating the value of a patient care service, and pharmacists should evaluate each of them for implementation and use. McDonough and Doucette (2003) provide an excellent discussion of the use of personal selling, a practice that can be very effective but is often not considered by pharmacists for a variety of reasons, including pharmacists' discomfort with this role.

Positioning

Positioning is "the act of designing the company's offering and image to occupy a distinctive place in the minds of the target market" (Kotler & Keller, 2016, p. 275). Positioning is about what a marketer can do to the mind of the target consumer; it is not about what marketers do to the product attributes per se. For example, Volvo's core positioning is safety and durability; this is what the company hopes its target market will think of when they think of a Volvo automobile. Because the target markets for many pharmacies (patients, other health care providers, third-party payers) do not understand what MTM services are, pharmacists have a great opportunity to position these services in the minds of consumers. These pharmacists can position themselves as innovators, medication experts, caring practitioners, and as partners in meeting health-related needs (McDonough et al., 1998a; McDonough et al., 2003).

People

People provide most services; thus, the selection, training, and motivation of employees are critical tasks for firms. Interactions with employees can have a significant impact on perceptions of service quality. Pharmacy managers need to pay special attention to all members of the pharmacy staff, not just pharmacists and technicians. Clerks, maintenance staff, volunteers, students, and anyone else who has contact with customers need sufficient training. See Chapter 17 to learn more about the critical role of human resources management in hiring and developing people to provide goods and services.

Customers are people too, with their own values, motivations, and behaviors. Pharmacists need to think of their patients not just as consumers of medications and their advice. They must try to understand the lives of their patients in a broader context. In addition, other patrons may form part of the service experience, and firms often need to take these individuals into consideration. For example, the behavior of other patrons at an amusement park may have a dramatic effect on the quality of one's experience and one's level of satisfaction. In pharmacy, the behavior or presence of a caregiver who is not supportive of a patient's need to make lifestyle adjustments may negatively alter the service experience during an MTM session. Chapter 26 describes important customer service constructs that pharmacists can apply to better serve those who could use and benefit from their goods and services.

Processes

The creation and delivery of product elements require that special attention be given to the design, implementation, and evaluation of processes. A *process* is the method and sequence in which a service is created, produced, and delivered. A service blueprint can be useful in understanding and designing processes. For example in a pharmacy, the focus may be on the entire process of dispensing a prescription starting with presentation of the prescription by a patient (or the receipt of an online order from a prescriber) through verifying patient understanding of the medication as they are picking up the prescription (Holdford & Kennedy, 1999). Alternatively, a pharmacy may focus on a specific component of the process, such as what steps will be taken if one learns during a patient history that he or she smokes cigarettes.

Poorly designed processes lead to ineffective service delivery, causing customers' and employees' frustration and dissatisfaction. For example, long waits at checkout lines in a retail environment caused by poorly designed systems that fail to anticipate customer flow are troublesome for customers in line as well as for employees who are running registers.

Programs

Programs encompass a company's activities directed to consumers. Beyond the traditional four Ps, marketers need to consider a variety of other issues that may be related to their programs. For traditional companies and brick-and-click organizations, the appearance of the physical environment (including buildings, landscape, employees, and furnishings), signs, printed materials, and other visible cues can provide evidence to customers concerning the quality of an organization and its offerings. Consistency of message in a company's Internet activities may also shape customers' impressions. Pharmacy managers should ask the following questions: Do we have adequate parking? Is the appearance of the pharmacy neat, and does it imply a professional image? Is our signage consistent and does it match what we are trying to convey via our website and in our social media apps? Is our equipment up to date?

Performance

Performance refers to a wide range of outcome measures, both financial and nonfinancial. Productivity focuses on the efficiency in the transformation of inputs into outputs, whereas quality, in this context, refers to the degree to which a product meets the needs, wants, and expectations of customers. Firms must attempt to balance these elements. Improving productivity may help to keep costs down, but cuts in service levels may adversely affect perceptions of quality. Similarly, while service quality may be critical for building customer loyalty, investing in quality improvement without understanding the impact on incremental costs and revenues can have negative consequences for profitability. From a managed-care pharmacy perspective, efforts to increase efficiency by limiting the use of certain medications may lead to a significant decrease in quality perceptions not only by patients but also by network providers. Performance also includes outcome measures that have implications beyond the company itself, such as social responsibility and ethical behavior, critical to the societal marketing concept.

■ EXPECTATIONS, SATISFACTION, QUALITY, VALUE, AND LOYALTY

Several terms have been used repeatedly in the preceding sections of this chapter. Although exchange is considered the core concept in marketing, these other concepts (i.e., expectations, satisfaction, quality, value, and loyalty) also play a critical role in understanding what marketing is all about.

Expectations

Expectations are internal standards used by customers when evaluating a product or service. In addition to influencing initial decisions concerning whether or not to purchase a product and from whom, they also play a critical role in consumers' judgments of service quality and satisfaction. Conceptual models have suggested that expectations consist of several different elements: desired service level, adequate service level, predicted service level, and a zone of tolerance (see also Parasuraman et al., 1994a; Zeithaml et al., 1993).

The *desired service level* is defined as what customers hope to receive and reflects a combination of what customers believe can and should be delivered. As customers realize that they cannot always get what they desire, they hold another, lower level of expectation

that reflects the minimum level of service they are willing to accept, called the *adequate service level*. The desired service level can be elevated or lowered based on personal needs and enduring beliefs about what is possible. The adequate service level can be influenced by a number of factors, including the perceptions of service alternatives and situational factors (e.g., emergencies and catastrophes). Explicit and implicit promises made by the service provider, past experiences, and word-of-mouth communications are proposed to influence the desired service level directly and affect the adequate service level indirectly through the predicted service level (Zeithaml et al., 1993).

The *zone of tolerance* represents the difference between adequate and desired levels and recognizes that customers are willing to accept some variation in service delivery. The range they are willing to accept is the zone of tolerance, suggesting that expectations are best characterized by a range of levels bounded by desired and adequate service levels. If a performance falls outside the range and below adequate levels, customers will likely be frustrated and dissatisfied. If performance exceeds desired levels, it will likely surprise and please the customer, leading to customer delight (Lovelock & Wright, 2002). Finally, there is a *predicted service level*, which reflects the level of service customers believe that they are most likely to get. This predicted service level directly affects how the adequate service level is defined for that occasion.

Marketers can have a significant role in influencing consumer expectations. Setting expectations in the mind of the consumer that are too high can create significant problems, such as possibly setting up the customer for frustration, disappointment, and dissatisfaction. This often occurs in pharmacies when they set expectations that prescriptions will be filled quickly, but then when circumstances dictate that the pharmacist and staff need to take additional steps to safely dispense the prescription, consumers are frustrated when they have to wait. On the other hand, setting expectations too low may lead to difficulties in attracting new customers. Indeed, a significant problem facing the profession of pharmacy is that many patients do not expect to receive MTM services. In planning their marketing communications effort and promotion mix, organizations (including pharmacies) must attempt to set a balance with respect to customer expectations.

Satisfaction and Quality

Some authors use the terms *quality* and *satisfaction* interchangeably. However, there are some notable differences. While there are different conceptualizations of satisfaction (Schommer & Kucukarslan, 1997), in marketing the most common approach is based on the confirmation/disconfirmation of expectations model.[9] Thus, Kotler and Keller (2016, p. 131) define *satisfaction* as "a person's feelings of pleasure or disappointment that result from comparing a product or service's perceived performance (or outcome) to expectations." Thus, if performance is worse than expected (negative disconfirmation), the customer will be dissatisfied. If performance matches expectations (confirmation), satisfaction will result. If performance exceeds expectations (positive disconfirmation), the customer will be highly satisfied and possibly delighted.[10] There are vast differences between merely satisfied and highly or completely satisfied customers (e.g., see Lovelock & Wright, 2002). For example, completely or highly satisfied customers are much more likely to remain loyal to a business and spread positive word of mouth about the company.

As with satisfaction, there is a rich history concerning the concept of *quality*. A broad definition of *quality* is superiority or excellence. Researchers note a difference between *objective quality* (i.e., measurable and verifiable superiority on some predetermined ideal standard) and *perceived quality* (i.e., a global assessment made by a consumer that is posited to exist at a higher level of abstraction from a consumer's perceptions of a product's specific attributes) (Zeithaml,

1988). *Service quality* is defined as "customers' long-term cognitive evaluation of a firm's service delivery" (Lovelock & Wright, 2002, p. 87) and results from a comparison of expectations and perceptions of service performance (Parasuraman et al., 1988). Because service quality represents a global impression rather than an encounter-specific evaluation, consumers are posited to update their perceptions of service quality following their interactions with service providers.

Service quality has been conceptualized to contain multiple dimensions (Parasuraman et al., 1985). One measure of service quality, the SERVQUAL scale (Parasuraman et al., 1988), identifies five such dimensions:

- *Tangibles*—the appearance of a firm's physical facilities, equipment, personnel, and communication materials
- *Reliability*—the ability of the firm to perform the promised service dependably and accurately
- *Responsiveness*—the willingness of the firm to help customers and provide prompt service
- *Assurance*—the knowledge and courtesy of employees and their ability to convey trust and confidence
- *Empathy*—the caring, individualized attention the firm provides to its customers

Another useful distinction made by service quality researchers is between technical quality and functional quality. *Technical quality* refers to customer perceptions about what is received from a service (e.g., Was the outcome of the service successful?), and *functional quality* refers to customer perceptions about how a service was performed (e.g., Did the service provider demonstrate concern and inspire confidence?) (Kotler, 2003). Perceptions of both functional and technical quality are important determinants of service quality, suggesting that service providers need to focus on being "high touch" as well as "high tech." In pharmacy, there is some evidence that functional quality has a greater impact on consumer perceptions of service quality than technical quality (Holdford & Schulz, 1999).

Both service quality and customer satisfaction are based on comparisons of expectations and

---

[9]For an interesting and somewhat alternative view of the concept of satisfaction, see Fournier and Mick (1999).

[10]For a provocative discussion of customer delight, see Oliver et al. (1997) and Rust and Oliver (2000).

performance. Are these really different constructs? There has been considerable debate in the marketing literature concerning this issue. One way that these two concepts have been distinguished is by examining the type of expectations that are used as the comparison. For service quality assessments, the focus is on desired and adequate service levels. For satisfactory evaluations, the focus has been on predicted service levels (Parasuraman et al., 1988; Spreng et al., 1996; Zeithaml et al., 1993). Another way these concepts have been distinguished is that service quality is a global judgment or assessment, whereas satisfaction is transaction specific (Parasuraman et al., 1988). This suggests that customer satisfaction leads to service quality. However, others have suggested that service quality leads to customer satisfaction. In an effort to work around this debate, Parasuraman et al. (1994b), building on the work of Teas (1993), suggested that both service quality and customer satisfaction can be examined meaningfully at the individual transaction level and be thought of as global (or overall) assessments that are formed following numerous transactions.

Regardless of this theoretical debate, there is considerable evidence that enhancing customer satisfaction and service quality can lead to positive outcomes for the organization and the consumer. As mentioned earlier, highly satisfied customers are more likely to exhibit loyalty, which means a consistent stream of revenues over a period of years for the firm (Lovelock & Wright, 2002). These customers may also be more forgiving when there is a service failure (see Chapter 26) and may make fewer demands and fewer mistakes as they gain experience as consumers of a company's products or services, thus reducing the firm's operating costs (Lovelock & Wright, 2002).

Positive word of mouth is also a key effect of high levels of satisfaction and perceived service quality. This outcome is extremely important to providers of professional services such as pharmacists. Satisfied customers also means less negative word of mouth, which can travel faster (and farther) than positive comments. Increasing reliance by consumers on the Internet for information seeking and ultimately purchase behaviors, as well as the growth in the use of social media by both consumers and firms, has created an electronic element to traditional word-of-mouth behavior. This element, termed electronic word of mouth, or eWOM, creates many additional considerations for firms as they attempt to navigate this rapidly evolving area.[11] Consumers' assessments via social media can be both immediate and widely available (Vogus & McClelland, 2016). Some marketers, including those in health care, have successfully employed the principles of *influencer marketing* using social media tools (Weiss, 2014). All these behavioral impacts can help to improve the bottom line of the company, namely, profitability (Zeithaml et al., 2001).

Given the potential consequences associated with health care services as well as the longer time horizon often associated with service encounters in health care, achieving high levels of satisfaction and service quality in health care can be challenging (Vogus & McClelland, 2016). Nevertheless, enhanced satisfaction and service quality can lead to greater patient willingness to participate in care as well as adherence to treatment, with subsequent effects on economic, clinical, and humanistic health outcomes (Vogus & McClelland, 2016). As in the general business environment, these effects have implications not only for the patient (consumer) but also for the organization in today's health care environment with its emphasis on pay-for-performance and value-based purchasing.

Value

Many marketers believe that the fundamental role of marketing is to create value for customers (Lovelock & Wright, 2002). But what is *value,* and how is it different from perceived quality? To begin, value and quality are not the same things. *Value* is conceptualized as either the ratio (Kotler, 2003) or the difference

---

[11]For a review of eWOM, including a discussion of what we know and what we need to know regarding antecedents of and consequents for eWOM senders and receivers, see King et al. (2014).

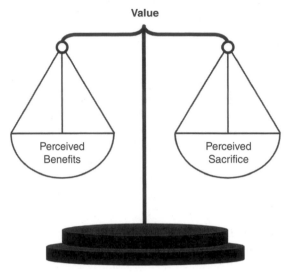

Value

Perceived Benefits

Perceived Sacrifice

Figure 24-1. A conceptualization of value.

(Lovelock & Wright, 2002) between the perceived benefits and the perceived costs (i.e., perceived sacrifice). Figure 24-1 is a useful approach to visualizing how a customer may conceptualize value. Moreover, the concept of value is more individualistic and personal than quality, thus it is theorized to exist at a higher level of abstraction in the mind of the consumer. Quality is usually conceptualized as part of the "get" component, whereas value involves a trade-off of both "get" and "give" components (Zeithaml, 1988). Because they are related, it is not surprising that efforts directed at increasing quality (or customer satisfaction for that matter) can also lead to increases in perceived value, which can contribute to increased consumer intentions and behaviors and ultimately to improved profitability.

An important consideration is that perceptions of value and quality exist after as well as prior to service delivery or product use. It is also important to recognize that a consumer's perception of the value of a product may be different before and after consumption. These pre-use perceptions may be based on word-of-mouth messages (e.g., what acquaintances have said) or may be based on the promotional message of the firm. For pharmacists, this suggests

that both effective provision of MTM services and appropriate use of the promotion mix are necessary for communicating value to prospective members of the target market. Pharmacists must understand how to use both sides of the value equation if they want to both attract and retain customers.

When customers evaluate a product or a service, they consider the benefits it offers (i.e., what they get) relative to the costs (i.e., what they give up). The benefits of a product or service include fulfilling a functional need, making a process more convenient, and providing an emotional payout such as prestige or a boost to self-esteem. As outlined in the previous section on the element of price in the marketing mix, costs to a consumer include not only monetary costs but also the nonmonetary outlays associated with the time, effort, and discomfort related to the processes of searching for, purchasing, and using the product (including costs associated with a product or service failure).

To increase the value for a customer, marketers can increase the benefits derived from the core product, enhance or provide supplementary services, or reduce the monetary costs or nonmonetary outlays associated with acquiring and using the product (Lovelock & Wright, 2002). Alternatively, a marketer can increase costs to the customer as long as there is a corresponding greater increase in benefits or an offset to some other outlay. Consumers paying a premium price to save time or gain greater comfort are an example of the latter. Marketers can also enhance value for customers by reducing benefits, as long as there is a corresponding greater decrease in costs.

Loyalty

Loyalty has received a considerable amount of attention from both marketing theorists and practitioners. It also has been the subject of investigation by pharmacy researchers (e.g., see Athavale et al., 2015). Most would agree that there are positive consequences associated with a loyal customer base. However, there are some areas of disagreement with respect to customer loyalty. Part of the debate has been with respect to how loyalty should be conceptualized and subsequently measured. Historically, the concept has been thought of as a behavioral outcome, namely, repurchase or switching intentions and behaviors (Oliver, 1999). Others have argued that loyalty has psychological meaning. For example, firm adoration, identification with the firm, and willingness to assist the service provider and other customers are thought to be part of the loyalty construct (Jones & Taylor, 2007; Oliver, 1999). To better understand the concept, some have suggested viewing loyalty in service provider–consumer relationships in the same manner as pro-relationship behaviors that develop in friendships and even romantic relationships (Jones & Taylor, 2007).

In addition to issues of conceptualization and measurement, marketers also have debated the antecedents of loyalty. The role of satisfaction in the development of loyalty has received the most attention. While there is most likely a relationship between these two variables (satisfaction begets loyalty), the relationship is not perfect; many customers may be satisfied or even highly satisfied yet fail to display repurchase behaviors (Oliver, 1999). A classic example of this in pharmacy is when antibiotics are dispensed to patients to treat infections. A patient may achieve a high level of satisfaction with the medication and level of service from the pharmacist and staff. And with that, the goal of this level of patient satisfaction is for the patient NOT to have to repurchase these goods and services to treat their infection! Others have demonstrated that it is not just the level of satisfaction that plays a role in determining loyalty but the strength (degree of certainty) with which a customer expresses his or her satisfaction (Chandrashekaran et al., 2007).

Oliver (1999, p. 41) states that ultimate loyalty requires that "the consumable must be subject to adoration." Or thought of in another way, the object or service must be lovable. The negative demand associated with most pharmaceutical products and services suggests that ultimate loyalty toward pharmacy may be an elusive goal. This should not suggest that pharmacy cannot learn from the growing body of knowledge regarding loyalty. Rather, because of its known relationship to firm performance, at the very least, pharmacy should be concerned with customer retention and repurchase intentions, even if such conceptualizations fail to recognize the psychological dimensions of loyalty. Reichheld (2003) suggests that firms need to be aware of only a single-item measure when thinking about the concept of loyalty: "How likely is it that you would recommend [Company X] to a friend or colleague?" This single-item measure is related to the revenue growth rate of firms in several industries. In the example from above, the patient who experiences high levels of satisfaction with their antibiotic treatment at a pharmacy may not have to repurchase the treatment itself, but hopefully would recommend the pharmacy to their friends and colleagues who have similar needs.

The recipient of loyalty attitudes and behaviors should also be considered. As mentioned earlier, some have conceptualized service loyalty to be similar to loyalty in interpersonal relationships like friendships. This suggests that the pharmacist, rather than the pharmacy, may be the subject of loyalty attitudes and behaviors (pharmacist-owned loyalty).[12] Such loyalty can be beneficial to the firm if the specific pharmacist continues his or her tenure with the pharmacy. Pharmacy employers need to understand this concept and the importance of good human resources management; management and marketing do not exist in isolation.

Collecting Customer Data

To create, deliver, and communicate superior customer value requires that a company understands its target market's expectations as well as its customers' assessments of satisfaction, quality, and value. Relying on customer complaints (or a lack of them) as evidence that a business is satisfying needs and meeting expectations is notoriously flawed. Studies show that most dissatisfied customers never complain to the company; rather, they buy less or switch to another

---

[12]For an interesting application to sales representatives, see Palmatier et al. (2007).

company (Lovelock & Wright, 2002). Therefore, companies need to take a more active approach in gathering data about improving their products or services. Some examples of how such an effort can be implemented include the following (Lovelock & Wright, 2002):

- *Post-transaction surveys.* The goal of this approach is to collect data concerning customer satisfaction and perceptions about the service experience immediately after (or within a few days of) the encounter. Questions are usually specific to the immediate past transaction or experience, although some more global questions may be included. You probably have been asked to fill out such a questionnaire after a visit to a restaurant, hotel, or a shopping experience at a retailer. In today's environment, many of these surveys are conducted via the Internet. Doucette and McDonough (2002) provide an example of a survey used for a weight control and wellness program at a pharmacy.

- *Overall evaluation surveys.* The focus when conducting an overall evaluation survey is on global impressions of a firm. This can include "customers" overall satisfaction with the firm, as well as "their overall impressions of the firm's service quality, product quality, and price" (Parasuraman et al., 1994b, p. 122). These evaluations should reflect customers' accumulated experiences over time. For this reason, as well as the costs associated with conducting these studies, Lovelock and Wright (2002) recommend that these surveys be administered less frequently than post-transaction surveys. Larson and MacKeigan's work regarding a measure of patient satisfaction with pharmacy services (Larson & MacKeigan, 1994; MacKeigan & Larson, 1989) and with pharmaceutical care (Larson et al., 2002) are examples of this approach. An example outside of pharmacy is the SERVQUAL scale (Parasuraman et al., 1988).

- *Mystery shopping.* This technique involves sending individuals posing as ordinary customers to gather information and provide feedback about service experiences. This technique allows for gathering information on individual employees and can be used to award superior performance or as an indication of the need for additional training. This approach may not be as useful for pharmacies that have few new customers because employees may be able to identify the mystery shopper. Consideration should be given to how employees might react to this deceptive practice. Suggestions include informing employees that this may be happening at some time, informing them on the criteria on which they will be assessed, and evaluating performance over a series of encounters rather than a single visit (Lovelock & Wright, 2002).

- *Noncustomer, new customer, and declining/former customer surveys.* Surveys of these groups may be useful for identifying unmet needs, expectations and image (e.g., noncustomer surveys), reasons for patronage (i.e., new customers), and information about a firm's deficiencies (i.e., declining and former customers).

- *Focus groups.* A qualitative approach to gathering customer data is the use of focus groups, which are groups of customers who are assembled by a researcher for an in-depth discussion on a specific topic. A trained moderator who is responsible for keeping the group on task leads the focus group. Focus groups can be useful in learning about customers' needs and expectations, determining how customers evaluate a firm's performance, gathering in-depth information about service problems, or obtaining feedback about a proposed product or service. Pharmacists should be cautioned about projecting results from a focus group to an entire market segment. Bislew and Sorensen (2003) provide an example of how focus groups might be used in a pharmacy setting.

- *Employee data.* Companies should not discount the value of the information that can be obtained from talking and *listening to* their employees. Employees have first-hand experience with customers that may lead to improvements in the product or service delivery. Surveys, focus groups, and one-on-one interviews all can be used to collect data from employees.

■ RELATIONSHIP MARKETING

While the concepts inherent in relationship marketing are not new, it is only in the past 35 years that the practice and science of marketing have grown aware of the relevance of relational exchanges. An understanding of the many concepts, such as expectations, satisfaction, perceived quality, value, and loyalty explored throughout this chapter so far, may be even more critical in a relationship-marketing paradigm because they are key to maintaining long-term collaborations and retaining customers. So what is relationship marketing? There has been considerable debate in the marketing literature concerning an appropriate definition of relationship marketing (e.g., see Parvatiyar & Sheth, 2000). Lovelock and Wright (2002, p. 102) define *relationship marketing* as "activities aimed at developing long-term, cost-effective links between an organization and its customers for the mutual benefit of both parties." The basic concepts of relationship marketing have historical roots dating back to the earliest merchants (Berry, 1995; Sheth & Parvatiyar, 1995). However, the concept of relationship marketing as we know it today gained popularity beginning in the early 1980s (Sheth, 2002).

Key to understanding relationship marketing is appreciating the distinction between relational exchanges and discrete transaction-based exchanges. Weitz and Jap (1995, p. 305) note that "… the growing interest in relationship marketing suggests a shift in the nature of general marketplace transactions from discrete to relational exchanges—from exchanges between parties with no past history and no future to exchanges between parties who have an exchange history and plans for future interactions." Thus, in the traditional practice of transactional marketing, each transaction is viewed as a separate event, or a one-shot deal. The fact that one transaction occurred does not predict that a future transaction will occur (Gummesson, 2002); the focus of both parties is to make the most of each individual transaction. However, a customer may use the same supplier repeatedly, possibly because of high switching costs, not because he or she is committed to that individual supplier (Gummesson, 2002).

While purely discrete transactions are rare, and while there are numerous benefits to both customers and producers who operate in a relationship-marketing paradigm, this should not imply that all forms of transactional marketing are inherently bad or wrong. Indeed, several authors have noted that transactional marketing can be a functional option for some marketers and customers based on the characteristics of the situation and the players involved (Gummesson, 2002; Kotler, 2003; Sheth et al., 2000). These characteristics include the time horizon of the customer, the level of customer involvement, the costs associated with switching to another organization, the level of customer interest in establishing a relationship, and the ability of an organization to implement such an approach efficiently (i.e., the cost and revenue implications must be understood).[13] Other authors have also noted that transactional marketing can be customer-centric, focusing on the needs, wants, and resources of individual consumers and customers rather than on those of mass markets or segments (Sheth et al., 2000).

In their synthesis of the relationship-marketing literature, Palmatier et al. (2006) find that relationship marketing is more effective when relationships are more important to customers, such as in the context of service offerings and business-to-business relationships, and when relationships are established with individuals rather than with the firm as a whole. Sheth (2002) has argued that the future of relationship marketing includes the selective and targeted use of relationship marketing coupled with transactional marketing efforts depending on the characteristics of the customer segment.

What Does Relationship Marketing Entail?

Gummesson (2002) outlines four fundamental values of relationship marketing:

- *Marketing management should be broadened into marketing-oriented company management.* This value

---

[13]For insight into why consumers in general may choose not to engage in relationships with retailers and service providers, see Noble and Phillips (2004) and Ashley et al. (2011).

is similar to the marketing concept's call for an integrated marketing orientation throughout an organization. Firms practicing relationship marketing must have an understanding of the importance of marketing throughout the whole organization, *not just for the marketing department.* This is consistent with the 2007 AMA definition of marketing as well as the holistic marketing concept of Kotler and Keller (2016). Effective relationship marketing requires a customer-centric focus (Sheth et al., 2000).

- *Long-term collaborations and win-win.* A key to relationship marketing is a focus on collaboration, viewing suppliers, customers, and others as partners rather than as combatants. This belief implies that relationships will create mutual value, leading to an extension of the duration of the relationship. This also implies that relationship marketing encourages retention marketing over attraction marketing.
- *All parties should be active and take responsibility.* The producer is not the only player in a relationship. Indeed, in many business-to-business relationships, the customers initiate innovation and force suppliers to change their products or services. With respect to services, customers are often involved in the production of the service, suggesting a critical interactive role, depending on the situation. See Table 24-1 for further discussion.
- *Relationship and service values instead of bureaucratic-legal values.* This value does not suggest that laws should be broken but instead implies that flexibility rather than rigidity should guide the management of customer relationships. Customers are individuals and should be treated as such.

Service firms and other businesses use a variety of approaches to maintain and enhance customer relationships, such as treating customers fairly, offering service augmentations, and treating each customer as if he or she were a segment of one (Lovelock & Wright, 2002). Significant to maintaining relationships in the delivery of services is the fulfillment of promises made to customers. Bitner (1995) outlined three essential activities to attracting, building, and maintaining service relationships:

- *Make realistic promises in the first place.* Through the Ps of the marketing mix and modern marketing management, an organization makes promises to its target market regarding what they can expect. As discussed previously, companies must strike a balance between setting expectations too high (possibly setting up the customer to be disappointed) and setting expectations too low (which may lead to a failure to attract customers). McDonough et al. (2003, p. 217) suggest that "it is better to over-perform than to over-promise."
- *Enable employees and systems to deliver on promises.* Processes and people, two of the Ps, are critical to the fulfillment of promises. Promises are easy to make, but without the right people using the right processes and tools, they are difficult to keep. Resources must be available, and people must have the training and motivation to serve customers.
- *Keep promises to customers when delivering services.* Every time a customer interacts with the organization (through its employees or a technological interface), an opportunity exists to keep or break a promise. These encounters, called *moments of truth,* form the basis for how a service relationship is built. Depending on the service and the situation, a single negative encounter (failure to meet a promise) can be enough to sever a relationship or at least cause a weakening of the relationship, even a long-lasting relationship. The provider's response to a service failure (i.e., service recovery effort) may be critical in maintaining satisfaction and repurchase intentions (Bunniran et al., 2011). Pharmacies should have a service-recovery plan for dealing with these situations (see Chapter 26). On the other hand, a series of positive encounters (repeatedly meeting promises and exceeding expectations) can lead to customer trust in the organization and a feeling of commitment to the relationship with the organization (Morgan & Hunt, 1994).

Table 24-1.   Coproduction, Cocreation of Value, and Shared Decision Making

A fundamental value of relationship marketing is the involvement of the customer in the production process. Coproduction has also been labeled as one of the hallmarks of the service-centered view of the discipline of marketing (Vargo & Lusch, 2004b). Coproduction means the involvement of the customer in the creation of value (i.e., cocreation). Examples of consumers as coproducers abound outside of health care. Some of these examples are considered somewhat firm centric (e.g., self-service applications such as ATMs and supermarket self-checkouts), while others are truly value cocreation experiences (e.g., certain video games, General Motors' OnStar service, and communication networks that allow for customer-to-customer [C-to-C] interaction) (Prahalad & Ramaswamy, 2004). The Internet, including social media, has fostered the growth of C-to-C communication and other innovations (e.g., online auctions and "price-naming" applications) that allow customers to personalize experiences.

In medicine and pharmacy, coproduction and cocreation of value are associated with patient-centered care and patient empowerment (Palumbo, 2016); these concepts are reflected by a patient relationship rooted in shared decision making (Prahalad & Ramaswamy, 2004). Involvement, information sharing, expression of preferences, and mutually agreeable treatment plans by providers and patients are key traits of a shared decision-making model (Charles et al., 1997). Joint development of treatment plans by patients and providers should lead to improved satisfaction and also enhance adherence to the treatment plan (Guadagnoli & Ward, 1998; Mead & Bower, 2002). The shared decision-making model is also central to several emerging practice models, such as the patient-centered medical home (Epperly, 2011). Pharmacists are educated to seek and use patient input when making treatment recommendations and also to help patients learn to manage treatment plans with respect to unique needs, situations, lifestyles, and behaviors. Relationship marketing and the process of coproduction are not only consistent with these practices but require them!

What Are the Consequences of Relationship Marketing?

The definition of relationship marketing stresses that its practice is mutually beneficial for an organization and its customers. Benefits to the organization, such as customer loyalty, referrals, and profitability (Palmatier et al., 2006), are manifested through improvements in marketing productivity and by making marketing more effective and more efficient (Sheth & Parvatiyar, 1995). As an example, loyalty programs are a common relationship-marketing tactic (see Table 24-2).

By focusing on individual customers (rather than on mass markets or market segments), and by increasing the involvement of the customer in the marketing effort, relationship marketing should be *more effective* in meeting customer needs and wants. Furthermore, focusing on customer retention, reducing some of the wasteful practices associated with mass marketing,

and letting the customer become a more active participant in the production process (i.e., letting customers perform some of the tasks historically performed by marketers—think ATMs) may lead to increases in *marketing efficiency*.

The point with respect to customer retention may need some elaboration. Estimates suggest that at least 65% of the average company's business comes from its present satisfied customers (Schoell & Guiltinan, 1990). Other evidence indicates that attracting new customers is significantly more expensive than retaining existing ones (Kotler & Keller, 2016). There is empirical evidence that shows that as customers remain in relationships for longer periods, they are more profitable to the firm (Sheth & Parvatiyar, 1995). These findings lead to the conclusion that focusing on customer retention rather than customer acquisition should be a less expensive (and more profitable) way to conduct business.

Table 24-2.   Loyalty Programs and Relationship Marketing

Loyalty programs have been used in many different industries, including pharmacy, for a number of reasons. These reasons include retaining customers, prompting purchases that would not otherwise be made, encouraging the consolidation of purchases (i.e., sometimes referred to as increasing the "share of wallet," which means buying more products from a single seller that would normally be purchased from multiple, competing sellers), and collecting and using data about consumers' purchases and behaviors (Nunes & Drèze, 2006). This often includes data about individual customers' preferences and their profitability to the firm. Airline frequent flyer programs, hotel preferred guest programs, and supermarket reward programs are prominent examples. Such programs have been shown to increase customer share of wallet and lifetime duration (Meyer-Waarden, 2007) as well as accelerate the customer relationship life cycle with a firm for those customers who are light-to-moderate buyers at the beginning of a loyalty program (Liu, 2007). Attaining success in loyalty programs appears to contribute to increased efforts at subsequent goal attainment (Drèze & Nunes, 2011).

Loyalty programs are common in the chain drugstore industry (Blank, 2009) and have increased in use by independent pharmacies as point-of-sale systems have grown in sophistication in this setting (Lockwood, 2014). There is evidence of their effectiveness in the pharmacy environment (Marques et al., 2017) and some have advocated for their use in other segments of the health care industry (McMahon et al., 2016). In addition to the potential benefits listed earlier, loyalty programs in pharmacy practice also have the advantage of encouraging patients to use a single pharmacy for their prescription medications, which may enhance the delivery of MTM services. However, pharmacy managers need to carefully consider the goals of a loyalty program as well as their specific situations when deciding to initiate such a program. In some industries, larger firms may benefit more from loyalty programs than smaller firms, and in some markets the degree of loyalty program saturation may limit the contribution of such program to the bottom line (Liu & Yang, 2009). Common mistakes made when initiating and managing a loyalty program include focusing on purchase quantity rather than profitability, overpromising and underdelivering, simply paying people to buy your product, giving away too much, and encouraging one-time use rather than the use of a program over time (Nunes & Drèze, 2006). Poorly designed and implemented loyalty programs might even create "disloyal" customers. Pharmacy managers also need to consider that pharmacy and health care are different from other services (Berry & Bendapudi, 2007), and thus loyalty programs may have different meanings for patients and other health care stakeholders. In addition, there are several legal issues surrounding certain aspects of these programs in pharmacy and health care (NACDS, 2016; Piacentino & Williams, 2014).

Relationship marketing also has significant benefits to the customer (Berry, 1995; Bitner, 1995). Certainly customers benefit economically (e.g., pricing incentives) when engaged in a relational activity and typically receive higher value when a company consistently fulfills promises. Long-term relationships can also reduce both stress and risk for customers as the relationship becomes more predictable and trust in the service provider increases. Such relationships also reduce the need to change, an act that most humans prefer to avoid. Remaining in a relationship simplifies one's life, saving time and effort by lessening the need for information search and decision-making. Finally, relationship marketing offers social benefits, such as being made to feel important and having a customer–service provider relationship developed into a friendship or part of a social support system. For years, pharmacists have recognized the importance of this last consumer benefit.

How Does Relationship Marketing Apply to Pharmacy?

Many of the applications of relationship marketing to pharmacy practice and health care are fairly self-evident. In many pharmacy settings, and particularly in community pharmacies, pharmaceutical goods and patient care services are provided to individuals who require attention and treatment over a long period of time because of their chronic conditions. The establishment of a provider–patient relationship is critical to the successful treatment of patients. Indeed, the nature of the therapeutic relationship between pharmacist and patient has been labeled as *foundational* to the conceptualization of pharmaceutical care (Cipolle et al., 1998). Interestingly, the definition of a therapeutic relationship (Cipolle et al., 1998, p. 344), "a partnership or alliance between the practitioner and the patient formed for the purpose of identifying the patient's drug-related needs," refers to several of the elements discussed throughout this chapter. In addition, the discussion of a therapeutic relationship explicitly recognizes that not only does the practitioner have responsibilities but also the patient—a concept not inconsistent with relationship marketing. While the nature of the patient–provider relationship takes on additional ethical meaning within the context of health care, many of the concepts discussed in this section (and throughout this chapter) have direct applications to the delivery of health care and pharmaceutical services.

A few additional points concerning relationship marketing and pharmacy practice are warranted. First, practitioners need to recognize that most pharmacies (and their computer systems) are full of data that can be used for one-to-one marketing and satisfying the unique needs of individual customers. When used to the extent allowed by current laws (e.g., HIPAA) and ethical business practices, these data can be used not only as part of the production and the delivery of the service but also to communicate with customers, prescribers, and other stakeholders. Second, it is important to consider individuals and organizations other than patients when implementing a relationship-marketing program within a pharmacy. These same principles can be applied to interactions with physicians and other providers, employer groups, third-party payers, computer vendors, wholesalers, and even others within your own firm. Establishing, developing, and maintaining relationships with these stakeholders have the potential to enhance or facilitate relationships with the ultimate customer, the patient. Third, building relationships does not happen overnight; relationships take time to establish and develop. However, practitioners should be encouraged to consider every service encounter as a relationship-building opportunity (Doucette & McDonough, 2002).

■ REVISITING THE SCENARIO: A SUMMARY

At the beginning of this chapter, we met Jim Smyth and Sue Davidson, who recognized that something needed to be done to enhance the financial position of their pharmacy. Many questions were raised during their impromptu brainstorming session with their employees, and most were related to marketing. To be effective (and efficient), health care providers and pharmacists (including Drs. Smyth and Davidson) need to wear a marketing hat as well as a clinical hat. They must understand how to integrate a marketing philosophy throughout their organizations. They must realize that focusing on customers' needs and learning how to translate those needs into wants and demands are critical steps. They must master the tools of the marketing mix and the four Ps of modern marketing management. The fundamentals of marketing can help them explain and predict their future environment and evaluate the potential impact of disruptive competitors like Amazon. To stay in business, and to continue to reap the intrinsic benefits from helping patients, requires that pharmacists keep an eye on the bottom line, namely, the profitability of the organization (or at least its financial success measured in other terms when considering not-for-profit firms). This means that pharmacists must understand the concepts of expectations, satisfaction, quality, value, and loyalty. Finally, while patient-centered pharmacy services already call for the establishment of a therapeutic relationship with patients, the practice of relationship marketing can help to enhance the level of service provided by pharmacists, potentially leading to improved outcomes for patients, improved financial performance for organizations, and rewarding practices for pharmacists.

■ QUESTIONS FOR FURTHER DISCUSSION

1. What philosophical approach to marketing is most common in today's pharmacy practice environment? Do you think one is more appropriate than the others?

2. What role does marketing play in ensuring the success of pharmacist-delivered MTM services? How can and should the profession (rather than individual pharmacists and businesses) use marketing principles and practices?

3. How can the expectations of patients be changed regarding the delivery of pharmacist-delivered MTM services?

4. How have your perceptions of marketing changed after reading this chapter?

5. Should the application of marketing principles be different for health professionals (compared with other service providers)?

6. Are loyalty programs appropriate for all types of pharmacies?

REFERENCES

Athavale AS, Banahan BF III, Bentley JP, West-Strum DS. 2015. Antecedents and consequences of pharmacy loyalty behavior. *Int J Pharm Healthcare Market* 9:36.

Ashley C, Noble SM, Donthu N, Lemon KN. 2011. Why customers won't relate: Obstacles to relationship marketing engagement. *J Bus Res* 64:749.

Berry LL. 1995. Relationship marketing of services: Growing interest, emerging perspectives. *J Acad Market Sci* 23:236.

Berry LL, Bendapudi N. 2007. Health care: A fertile field for service research. *J Serv Res US* 10:111.

Bislew HD, Sorensen TD. 2003. Use of focus groups as a tool to enhance a pharmaceutical care practice. *J Am Pharm Assoc* 43:424.

Bitner MJ. 1995. Building service relationships: It's all about promises. *J Acad Market Sci* 23:246.

Blank C. 2009. Pharmacy loyalty programs spur sales. *Drug Top* 153(8):21.

Bunniran S, McCaffrey D, Bentley J, et al. 2011. Patient service experiences in community pharmacy: An examination of health criticality, service failure incidents, and service recovery efforts and their influence on patronage outcomes (abstract). *J Am Pharm Assoc* 51:244.

Chandrashekaran M, Rotte K, Tax SS, Grewal R. 2007. Satisfaction strength and customer loyalty. *J Market Res* 44:153.

Charles C, Gafni A, Whelan T. 1997. Shared decision-making in the medical encounter: What does it mean? (or it takes at least two to tango). *Soc Sci Med* 44:681.

Christensen DB, Fassett WE, Andrews GA. 1993. A practical billing and payment plan for cognitive services. *Am Pharm* NS33:34.

Cipolle RJ, Strand LM, Morley PC. 1998. *Pharmaceutical Care Practice*. New York, NY: McGraw-Hill.

Day GS, Montgomery DB. 1999. Charting new directions for marketing. *J Market* 63:3.

Doucette WR, McDonough RP. 2002. Beyond the 4 P's: Using relationship marketing to build value and demand for pharmacy services. *J Am Pharm Assoc* 42:183.

Drèze X, Nunes JC. 2011. Recurring goals and learning: The impact of successful reward attainment on purchase behavior. *J Market Res* 48:268.

Epperly T. 2011. The patient-centred medical home in the USA. *J Eval Clin Prac* 17:373.

Feldstein PJ. 1999. *Health Care Economics*, 5th ed. Albany, NY: Delmar Publishers.

Fournier S, Mick DG. 1999. Rediscovering satisfaction. *J Market* 63:5.

Guadagnoli E, Ward P. 1998. Patient participation in decision-making. *Soc Sci Med* 47:329.

Gummesson E. 2002. *Total Relationship Marketing*, 2nd ed. Oxford, England: Butterworth-Heinemann.

Gundlach GT, Wilkie WL. 2009. The American Marketing Association's new definition of marketing: Perspective and commentary on the 2007 revision. *J Public Policy Mark* 28:259.

Hepler CD, Strand LM. 1990. Opportunities and responsibilities in pharmaceutical care. *Am J Hosp Pharm* 47:533.

Holdford D, Schulz R. 1999. Effect of technical and functional quality on patient perceptions of pharmaceutical service quality. *Pharm Res* 16:1344.

Holdford DA, Kennedy DT. 1999. The service blueprint as a tool for designing innovative pharmaceutical services. *J Am Pharm Assoc* 39:545.

Hunt SD. 1976. The nature and scope of marketing. *J Market* 40:17.

Hunt SD. 1983. General theories and the fundamental explananda of marketing. *J Market* 47:9.

Hunt SD. 2010. *Marketing Theory: Foundations, Controversy, Strategy, and Resource-Advantage Theory.* Armonk, NY: ME Sharpe.

Jones T, Taylor SF. 2007. The conceptual domain of service loyalty: How many dimensions? *J Serv Market* 21:36.

Keefe LS. 2004. What is the meaning of "marketing"? *Marketing News* 38:17.

King RA, Racherla P, Bush VD. 2014. What we know and don't know about online word-of-mouth: A review and synthesis of the literature. *J Interact Mark* 28:167.

Kohli AK, Jaworski BJ. 1990. Market orientiation: The construct, research propositions, and managerial implications. *J Market* 54(2):1-18.

Kotler P. 2003. *Marketing Management*, 11th ed. Upper Saddle River, NJ: Prentice-Hall.

Kotler P, Keller KL. 2016. *Marketing Management*, 15th ed. Boston, MA: Pearson.

Larson LN, MacKeigan LD. 1994. Further validation of an instrument to measure patient satisfaction with pharmacy services. *J Pharm Market Manage* 8:125.

Larson LN, Rovers JP, MacKeigan LD. 2002. Patient satisfaction with pharmaceutical care: Update of a validated instrument. *J Am Pharm Assoc* 42:44.

Levitt T. 1960. Marketing myopia. *Harvard Bus Rev* 38:45.

Liu Y. 2007. The long-term impact of loyalty programs on consumer purchase behavior and loyalty. *J Market* 71:19.

Liu Y, Yang R. 2009. Competing loyalty programs: Impact of market saturation, market share, and category expandability. *J Market* 73:93.

Lockwood W. 2014. Point-of-sale systems: The impact on customer loyalty. *ComputerTalk Pharmacist* 34(3):17.

Lovelock C, Wright L. 2002. *Principles of Service Marketing and Management*, 2nd ed. Upper Saddle River, NJ: Prentice-Hall.

MacKeigan LD, Larson LN. 1989. Development and validation of an instrument to measure patient satisfaction with pharmacy services. *Med Care* 27:522.

Marques SH, Cardoso MGMS, Lindeza ACA. 2017. Do loyalty cards enhance loyalty in the pharmaceutical sector? *Journal of Relationship Marketing* 16:143.

Mathur A. 1996. Older adults' motivations for gift giving to charitable organizations: An exchange theory perspective. *Psychol Market* 13:107.

McAlister L, Bolton RN, Rizley R (eds.). 2010. *Essential Readings in Marketing with 2006–2010 Update.* Cambridge, MA: Marketing Science Institute.

McCarthy EJ. 1960. *Basic Marketing: A Managerial Approach.* Homewood, IL: Irwin.

McDonough RP. 2003. Obstacles to pharmaceutical care. In Rovers JP, Currie JD, Hagel HP, et al. (eds.) *A Practical Guide to Pharmaceutical Care*, 2nd ed. Washington, DC: American Pharmaceutical Association, p. 267.

McDonough RP, Doucette WR. 2003. Using personal selling skills to promote pharmacy services. *J Am Pharm Assoc* 43:363.

McDonough RP, Pithan ES, Doucette WR, Brownlee MJ. 1998a. Marketing pharmaceutical care services. *J Am Pharm Assoc* 38:667.

McDonough RP, Rovers JP, Currie JD, et al. 1998b. Obstacles to the implementation of pharmaceutical care in the community setting. *J Am Pharm Assoc* 38:87.

McDonough RP, Sobotka JL. 2003. Reimbursement. In Rovers JP, Currie JD, Hagel HP, et al. (eds.) *A Practical Guide to Pharmaceutical Care*, 2nd ed. Washington, DC: American Pharmaceutical Association, p. 222.

McDonough RP, Sobotka JL, Doucette WR. 2003. Marketing pharmaceutical care. In Rovers JP, Currie JD, Hagel HP, et al. (eds.) *A Practical Guide to Pharmaceutical Care*, 2nd ed. Washington, DC: American Pharmaceutical Association, p. 203.

McMahon LF Jr, Tipirneni R, Chopra V. 2016. Health system loyalty programs: An innovation in customer care and service. *JAMA* 315:863.

Mead N, Bower P. 2002. Patient-centered consultations and outcomes in primary care: A review of the literature. *Patient Educ Couns* 48:51.

Meyer-Waarden L. 2007. The effects of loyalty programs on customer lifetime duration and share of wallet. *J Retail* 83:223.

Morgan RM, Hunt SD. 1994. The commitment-trust theory of relationship marketing. *J Market* 58:20.

Narver JC, Slater SF, MacLachlan DL. 2004. Responsive and proactive market orientation and new-product success. *J Prod Innov Manage* 21:334.

National Association of Chain Drug Stores (NACDS). 2016. NACDS Welcomes HHS-OIG Final Rule That Allows Medicare, Medicaid Patients to Access

Pharmacy Reward Programs. Available at https://www. nacds.org/news/nacds-welcomes-hhs-oig-final-rule-that-allows-medicare-medicaid-patients-to-access-pharmacy-reward-programs/. Accessed January 14, 2019.

Noble SM, Phillips J. 2004. Relationship hindrance: Why would consumers not want a relationship with a retailer? *J Retail* 80:289.

Nunes JC, Drèze X. 2006. Your loyalty program is betraying you. *Harvard Bus Rev* 84:124.

Oliver RL. 1999. Whence consumer loyalty? *J Market* 63:33.

Oliver RL, Rust RT, Varki S. 1997. Customer delight: Foundations, findings, and managerial insight. *J Retail* 73:311.

Palmatier RW, Dant RP, Grewal D, Evans KR. 2006. Factors influencing the effectiveness of relationship marketing: A meta-analysis. *J Market* 70:136.

Palmatier RW, Scheer LK, Steenkamp JE. 2007. Customer loyalty to whom? Managing the benefits and risks of salesperson-owned loyalty. *J Market Res* 44:185.

Palumbo R. 2016. Contextualizing co-production of health care: A systematic literature review. *International Journal of Public Sector Management* 29:72.

Panda V. 2018. How traditional pharmacies can survive the Amazon threat. Available at https://www.statnews.com/2018/12/13/how-traditional-pharmacies-survive-amazon-threat/. Accessed March 12, 2019.

Parasuraman A, Zeithaml VA, Berry LL. 1985. A conceptual model of service quality and its implications for future research. *J Market* 49:41.

Parasuraman A, Zeithaml VA, Berry LL. 1988. SERVQUAL: A multiple-item scale for measuring consumer perceptions of service quality. *J Retail* 64:12.

Parasuraman A, Zeithaml VA, Berry LL. 1994a. Alternative scales for measuring service quality: A comparative assessment based on psychometric and diagnostic criteria. *J Retail* 70:201.

Parasuraman A, Zeithaml VA, Berry LL. 1994b. Reassessment of expectations as a comparison standard in measuring service quality: Implications for further research. *J Market* 58:111.

Parvatiyar A, Sheth JN. 2000. The domain and conceptual foundations of relationship marketing. In Sheth JN, Parvatiyar A (eds.) *Handbook of Relationship Marketing*. Thousand Oaks, CA: Sage, p. 3.

Peter JP, Olson JC. 1983. Is science marketing? *J Market* 47:111.

Piacentino JJ, Williams KG. 2014. The Affordable Care Act on loyalty programs for federal beneficiaries. *J Pharm Pract* 27:106.

Prahalad CK, Ramaswamy. 2004. Co-creation experiences: The next practice in value creation. *J Interact Mark* 18:5.

Reichheld FF. 2003. The one number you need to grow. *Harvard Bus Rev* 81:46.

Rovers JP, Currie JD, Hagel HP, et al. 1998. *A Practical Guide to Pharmaceutical Care*. Washington, DC: American Pharmaceutical Association.

Rust RT, Oliver RL. 2000. Should we delight the customer? *J Acad Market Sci* 28:86.

Schoell WF, Guiltinan JP. 1990. *Marketing: Contemporary Concepts and Practices*, 4th ed. Reading, MA: Allyn and Bacon.

Schommer JC, Kucukarslan SN. 1997. Measuring patient satisfaction with pharmaceutical services. *Am J Health Syst Pharm* 54:2721.

Shepherd MD. 1995. Defining and marketing value added services. *Am Pharm* NS35:46.

Sheth JN. 2002. The future of relationship marketing. *J Serv Market* 16:590.

Sheth JN, Parvatiyar A. 1995. Relationship marketing in consumer markets: Antecedents and consequences. *J Acad Market Sci* 23:255.

Sheth JN, Sisodia RS, Sharma A. 2000. The antecedents and consequences of customer-centric marketing. *J Acad Market Sci* 28:55.

Siecker B. 2002. Principles of place, channel systems, and channel specialists. In Smith MC, Kolassa EM, Perkins G, Siecker B (eds.) *Pharmaceutical Marketing: Principles, Environment, and Practice*. New York, NY: Pharmaceutical Products Press, p. 219.

Smith MC. 1996. Pharmacy marketing. In *Effective Pharmacy Management*, 8th ed. Alexandria, VA: NARD, p. 423.

Smith MC. 2002. General principles. In Smith MC, Kolassa EM, Perkins G, Siecker B (eds.) *Pharmaceutical Marketing: Principles, Environment, and Practice*. New York, NY: Pharmaceutical Products Press, p. 3.

Smith MC, Kolassa EM. 2001. Nobody wants your products: They are negative goods. *Product Management Today* 12:22.

Spreng RA, MacKenzie SB, Olshavsky RW. 1996. A reexamination of the determinants of consumer satisfaction. *J Market* 60:15.

Teas RK. 1993. Expectations, performance evaluation, and consumers: Perceptions of quality. *J Market* 57:18.

United States Department of Health and Human Services (US DHHS). 2019. Partner Opportunities. Available at https://millionhearts.hhs.gov/partners-progress/partners/partner-opportunities.html. Accessed January 14, 2019.

Van Waterschoot W, Van den Bulte C. 1992. The 4P classification of the marketing mix revisited. *J Market* 56:83.

Vargo SL, Lusch RF. 2004a. The four service marketing myths: Remnants of a goods-based, manufacturing model. *J Serv Res* 6:324.

Vargo SL, Lusch RF. 2004b. Evolving to a new dominant logic for marketing. *J Market* 68:1.

Vogus TJ, McClelland LE. 2016. When the customer is the patient: Lessons from healthcare research on patient satisfaction and service quality ratings. *Hum Resour Manage R* 26:37.

Weiss R. 2014. Influencer marketing. How word-of-mouth marketing can strengthen your organization's brand. *Mark Health Serv* 34:16.

Weitz BA, Jap SD. 1995. Relationship marketing and distribution channels. *J Acad Market Sci* 23:305.

Wilkie WL, Moore ES. 1999. Marketing's contributions to society. *J Market* 63:198.

Wilkie WL, Moore ES. 2003. Scholarly research in marketing: Exploring the "4 eras" of thought development. *J Public Policy Market* 22:116.

Zeithaml VA. 1988. Consumer perceptions of price, quality, and value: A means-end model and synthesis of evidence. *J Market* 52:2.

Zeithaml VA, Berry LL, Parasuraman A. 1993. The nature and determinants of customer expectations of service. *J Acad Market Sci* 21:1.

Zeithaml VA, Rust RT, Lemon KN. 2001. The customer pyramid: Creating and serving profitable customers. *Calif Manage Rev* 43:118.

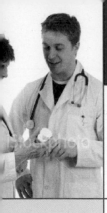

25

MARKETING APPLICATIONS

Benjamin S. Teeter and Jacob T. Painter

About the Authors: Dr. Teeter is an assistant professor of Pharmacy Practice and investigator in the Center for Implementation Research at the University of Arkansas for Medical Sciences in Little Rock, AR. He received his Bachelor of Science degree in Public Health from Indiana University, and his Master of Science and Doctor of Philosophy degrees in Pharmaceutical Sciences from Auburn University. His teaching interests include pharmacy management, managing organizational change, and the US health care system. His main research interest is how best to implement evidence-based interventions in community pharmacies. Specifically, his research focuses on adoption, implementation, and sustainability of innovations, effects of social and behavioral factors on participation in organizational quality improvement, and how community pharmacies implement and market patient care services to their clients.

Dr. Painter is an associate professor in the Division of Pharmaceutical Evaluation & Policy at the University of Arkansas for Medical Sciences. He received his Doctor of Pharmacy, Master of Business Administration, and Doctor of Philosophy in Pharmaceutical Sciences degrees from the University of Kentucky. His primary research interest is the improvement of health services especially as this concerns the management of pain and mental health disorders.

■ LEARNING OBJECTIVES

After completing this chapter, readers should be able to

1. Describe the role of marketing and its importance in the practice of pharmacy.
2. Describe the essential steps when preparing to market goods or services in a pharmacy.
3. Distinguish between the micro- and macroenvironment of an organization.
4. Conduct a situation analysis for a given organization.
5. Differentiate between mass marketing and market segmentation.
6. Analyze a target market.
7. Apply the marketing-mix components to various scenarios.
8. Describe the increasing importance of having a positive online presence.
9. Describe the importance of marketing control.

■ SCENARIO

Murray Rockefeller earned his PharmD degree 7 years ago. Upon graduation, he was presented with the opportunity to become a junior partner of Community Care Pharmacy in Weagle, AL. This pharmacy fills prescriptions, provides compounding services, offers a full line of durable medical equipment, and prepares unit dose blister packages of medications for residents of a local nursing home. For the first 5 years of Dr. Rockefeller's employment, he worked closely with the senior partner and learned about running a pharmacy business. Working side-by-side with the senior partner ensured the smooth transition of the pharmacy ownership when Dr. Rockefeller became the sole owner of Community Care Pharmacy 2 years ago. Since Dr. Rockefeller assumed ownership of the pharmacy, he has reflected that much of his effort has been focused on maintaining existing services provided by the pharmacy rather than planning for goods and services they might offer in the future.

During the past year, Dr. Rockefeller has realized a significant increase in competition from community pharmacies in the area, as well as lower profit margins from dispensing prescriptions. He has also noticed that consumers are eschewing "brick and mortar" stores in communities like Weagle and are making more purchases from on-line competitors like Amazon.com and Wal-Mart.com, even for health items that they would often purchase in pharmacies. He knows that he must investigate options to seek additional revenue sources for his pharmacy and integrate appropriate marketing channels into his business strategy. A few of the options he is considering include offering new goods and services that are in demand by his patients. He also knows that before launching any new good or service, he must do extensive planning and evaluate marketing options to ensure success.

■ CHAPTER QUESTIONS

1. Why is conducting a *Strengths, Weaknesses, Opportunities, Threats* (SWOT) analysis important, and how can it be used to help shape a pharmacy's marketing efforts?

2. How does setting goals and objectives benefit a pharmacy?
3. What are the characteristics of a good target market?
4. How are the Four Ps applied to a specific marketing effort?
5. Describe why monitoring the performance of marketing activities is important to a pharmacy's success?

■ INTRODUCTION

For more than 30 years, health care costs have increased faster than the costs of other goods and services. This has forced those who pay for health care services (e.g., patients, insurance companies, employers, government agencies) to seek ways to control the costs of health care. These cost control measures have had a direct impact on the practice of pharmacy, as pharmacy benefit managers have been aggressive in reducing their reimbursement rates for prescription drugs (see Chapter 23). Because of reduced reimbursement rates, profit margins generated from dispensing prescriptions, and hence, profit margins for the entire pharmacy's operations, have decreased over time. The reduction in profitability from dispensing, increased competition from other pharmacies and types of businesses, as well as increases in costs of drugs, salaries, and other operating expenses have forced pharmacies to seek alternative revenue sources. Pharmacies have generated additional revenues in a variety of ways, including selling different lines of goods and establishing patient care services such as immunizations, health and wellness screenings, medication reconciliation, point-of-care testing, and medication therapy management (MTM) services.

Marketing is a necessary and essential function in a highly competitive and resource-constrained environment. To successfully launch any new good or service, a thorough understanding of the organization, environment, and market is crucial. This chapter describes how marketing principles (see Chapter 24) can be applied in pharmacy practice, as illustrated through Dr. Rockefeller's scenario. Specifically, this chapter discusses several marketing concepts including situational analysis, market segments, target markets, and the marketing mix, and illustrates how these concepts are applicable in pharmacy practice.

■ STRATEGIC PLANNING AND EVALUATING BUSINESS OPPORTUNITIES

Strategic planning in pharmacy operations is crucial as it maximizes the organization's future success. Chapter 6 describes the strategic planning process and emphasizes the importance of an organization's vision and mission statement, as they create a sense of purpose and direction for the employees. Also, as previously stated in Chapter 7, a vital step in the development of a business plan is to create a marketing strategy. Therefore, pharmacists should consider what their organization is striving for, as well as the organization's values and overall purpose when preparing to market a good or service.

The following steps should be taken when preparing to market a good or service in a pharmacy (Hillestad & Berkowitz, 2013; Holdford, 2015). These steps are illustrated in Figure 25-1. First, the micro- and macroenvironment are analyzed to identify strengths and limitations of the organization's capacity, as well as opportunities and threats in the environment. Second, goals and objectives are formulated using the information compiled in the previous step. The goals and objectives must be consistent with the organization's vision and mission statements. It is possible that the first two steps have already been conducted as part of the strategic plan and business plan development processes. Third, market segments and the target market are identified. At this point, having the organization's goals, objectives, and possible target markets identified, a specific product or service can be developed. Fourth, the organization proceeds to formulate and design the marketing mix for each target market. The last step is to evaluate the extent to which marketing strategies are successful. Information gathered during this final step is crucial as it helps inform the organization and identifies if changes in any components of the marketing process are needed.

■ REVISITING THE SCENARIO

Dr. Rockefeller now knows that before he can develop new goods and services, he must consider the vision and the mission of Community Care Pharmacy and ensure that these goods and services are consistent with the organization's overall strategic plan. After reviewing the existing mission and vision statements, he realizes that they do not reflect the direction he

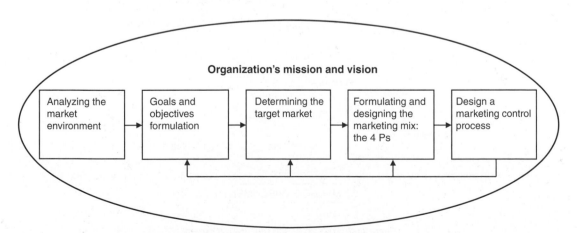

Figure 25-1. Steps in marketing a pharmacy good or service.

would like to take the pharmacy under his ownership. He has also come to realize that the pharmacy does not have a strategic plan in place. Dr. Rockefeller schedules a meeting with all of the pharmacy's employees to develop a strategic plan. Soon afterward, Community Care Pharmacy has the strategic plan in place, including updated mission and vision statements.

■ ANALYZING THE MARKET ENVIRONMENT

Situational Analysis

Before making a decision regarding what goods and services to offer and how to offer them, it is important for managers to analyze their organization's market environment. In essence, organizations interact with two areas of the market environment: the *microenvironment* and the *macroenvironment* (see Figure 25-2) (Kotler & Armstrong, 2018). Specifically, the microenvironment consists of the organization's internal and external environment. The organizational structure, culture, personnel, and resources make up the internal environment whereas the organization's suppliers, customers, and competitors make up the external environment. The characteristics of the microenvironment affect the organization's ability to serve its customers.

The macroenvironment consists of forces that influence the entire microenvironment. These forces can be categorized as demographic, economic, natural, technological, political, or cultural (Kotler & Armstrong, 2018). An aging population creates demand for chronic care services such as anticoagulation management, this is an example of a demographic force. Negative economic forces such as a recession increase the need for pharmacists to help patients reduce their health care costs. Technological forces affect how patients interact with health care providers and how patients manage their conditions and illnesses, pharmacists should be aware of both opportunities and threats presented by new technologies.

The situational analysis is an assessment of the organization's environment and of the organization itself (Berkowitz, 2017). This process starts with an assessment of the *S*trengths and *W*eaknesses of the organization, followed by the *O*pportunities and *T*hreats relevant to the organization's future strategy. This process is referred to as SWOT analysis. Similar to how SWOT analysis can be used in the strategic and business planning processes (see Chapters 6 and 7), SWOT analysis may also be used to develop new

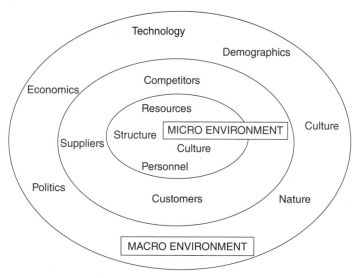

Figure 25-2. The micro- and macroenvironment.

goods and services that respond to the opportunities and threats of the organization's environment while recognizing their inherent strengths and weaknesses (Ferrell & Hartline, 2016).

■ REVISITING THE SCENARIO

Dr. Rockefeller and the employees of Community Care Pharmacy took some time to evaluate the pharmacy's microenvironment and macroenvironment. Community Care Pharmacy is located in the city of Weagle, which is located in Monet County, Alabama. Weagle is the principal city of this county. The county's economy is centered in Weagle as many employers, businesses, schools, and service organizations reside in the city. In fact, the city of Weagle is the largest city in Eastern Alabama. Approximately 15% of the population is elderly (>65-year old). Weagle is one of the fastest growing metropolitan areas in the South

and has recently been voted as one of the best retirement cities for active adults. The results of their environmental scan of the demographic characteristics of their communities are summarized in Table 25-1.

In reviewing the pharmacy's prescription records and health facts about Alabama (obtained from the Kaiser Family Foundation website [www.kff.org]), Dr. Rockefeller discovered that a wide variety of chronic diseases are prevalent among current pharmacy customers, and that state-level health statistics on some health risk factors are concerning (see Table 25-1).

Monet County has a total of 29 community pharmacies. Specifically, there are 10 independently owned pharmacies, 10 chain pharmacies, 5 grocery store pharmacies, and 4 mass merchandise pharmacies. Most of these pharmacies (22 of them) are located within the Weagle metropolitan area. Given the growing economy in the area, several chain pharmacies have expressed an interest in expanding their businesses in the area.

Table 25-1. Community Care Pharmacy's Community Profile

	Weagle, AL	Monet County, AL	Alabama	United States
Population	61,688	161,604	4,889,817	327,167,434
Median household income	$79,936	$59,656	$46,472	$57,652
Education				
High school education	94.1%	89.7%	85.3%	87.3%
4 years of college	61.1%	34.9%	24.5%	30.9%
Health insurance status				
Uninsured	–	9%	12%	10%
Medicaid	–	18%	26%	19%
Medicare	–	18%	18%	16%
Employer-sponsored insurance	–	55%	44%	55%
Prevalence of health conditions				
Diabetes	–	–	13.2%	9.5%
Smokers	–	–	20.9%	14.0%
Overweight adults	–	–	69.6%	65.4%
Overweight adolescents	–	–	33.1%	31.5%
Death per 100,000				
Deaths: stroke	–	38.5	55.5	41.2
Deaths: heart disease	–	196.2	228.4	169.8
Number of community pharmacies	15	26	–	–

Strengths and Weaknesses

To complete an assessment of an organization's strengths and weaknesses, the organization should consider both the current and potential capacity to compete in the market (Holdford, 2015). A *strength* is a resource or capacity of the organization that can be used to achieve its objectives, while a *weakness* is a limitation within the organization that hinders the organization from achieving its objectives. An organization must assess various factors internal to the organization, including resources (e.g., financial resources, intellectual resources, location, etc.), relationships with patients, reputation among patients, relationships with other health care providers, staff, workload, efficiency, management, and culture.

■ REVISITING THE SCENARIO

Table 25-2 describes the SWOT analysis for Community Care Pharmacy. Dr. Rockefeller and the pharmacy staff agreed on several strengths of the pharmacy. One is that the pharmacy has loyal customers.

Table 25-2.	A SWOT Analysis for Community Care Pharmacy
Strengths	The pharmacy has loyal customers.
	The pharmacy has a wide range of services including dispensing, compounding, long-term care, and durable medical equipment.
	The pharmacy has a professional image.
	All pharmacists have excellent clinical skills and knowledge; all are certified to administer vaccines.
	The pharmacy has positive relationships with prescribers in the community.
Weaknesses	Because the pharmacy has not established advanced pharmacy care services, most staff pharmacists have limited experience in delivering patient care services other than dispensing.
	Working relationships with pediatricians in the area have not yet been developed.
	Financial resources are somewhat limited and pharmacists' workload has increased.
Opportunities	A large number of people in the community are enrolled in Medicare.
	Elderly population is at risk for influenza, pneumonia, and shingles, but they have limited access to nontraditional vaccination services.
	A large number of people in the community are obese and at high risk for developing heart disease, hypertension, and diabetes.
	Opening of a technology park nearby has resulted in a recent influx of young residents with relatively high incomes.
	Several companies in the community are self-insured; self-insured employers have expressed their interest in reducing health care cost among their enrollees.
Threats	There has been an increase in competition among community pharmacies for the dispensing business.
	A large chain has recently purchased two independently owned pharmacies and plans to expand their stores to other locations within the community.
	One of the self-insured employers in the area has strongly encouraged its enrollees to obtain their chronic medications from an online pharmacy.
	Some members of a local physician group have expressed their concern about pharmacy-based disease state management services.

In fact, many new patients have been referred to the pharmacy by other patients. The pharmacy has been in business for more than 25 years, and every patient receives medication counseling when they pick up their medications. The pharmacy also has a large customer base and currently provides a wide range of services including medication dispensing, compounding, serving a local long-term care facility, and providing durable medical equipment. Another strength is that the pharmacy was remodeled 3 years ago; thus, it emanates a professional image. All five staff pharmacists at Community Care Pharmacy have excellent clinical skills and knowledge of pharmacotherapy. Their most recently hired pharmacist has completed a community pharmacy residency. All pharmacists are certified to administer vaccines. The excellent skills and knowledge of the pharmacists along with their dedication to patient care has led to positive relationships with physicians and nurse practitioners in the community.

Dr. Rockefeller and his colleagues also recognize the weaknesses of Community Care Pharmacy. Although a wide range of services are provided, dispensing medications takes up the bulk of the pharmacists' time and effort. The pharmacy does not currently offer any patient care services beyond medication counseling. Aside from the pharmacist who completed a residency, the rest of the staff has limited experience in the delivery of patient care services. Regarding relationships with prescribers, working relationships with pediatricians in the area have not yet been developed. Due to low profit margins on prescription dispensing, the pharmacy's financial resources are somewhat limited. Specifically, the pharmacy was forced to lower operating costs by reducing technicians' hours 6 months ago. This has increased the pharmacists' workload.

Opportunities and Threats

An organization must conduct an assessment of *opportunities* and *threats*. Opportunities are gaps between market demand and what is currently available, as well as changes in the market that enhance the demand for the organization's goods and services

(Holdford, 2015). In contrast, threats are factors that may prevent the organization from achieving its intended objectives, as well as changes in the market that may reduce the demand for the organization's goods or services. To help the organization identify opportunities and threats, the following questions should be asked (Berkowitz, 2017; Holdford, 2015):

1. What are changes and trends in the environment?
2. How will these changes affect the organization?
3. What opportunities do these changes present?
4. What needs are not being met in the current marketplace?
5. How is the environment changing to the organization's advantage or disadvantage?
6. What potential problems might threaten the success of the organization's plans?

■ REVISITING THE SCENARIO

Dr. Rockefeller and his colleagues analyzed the environment and have identified several opportunities for Community Care Pharmacy (Table 25-2). First, a large number of people are enrolled in a traditional Medicare program with Medicare Part D plans. Since the city of Weagle has been cited as one of the best cities to retire, there has been an influx of relatively healthy, active patients in their 60s and 70s to the area. This group of patients has chronic conditions and needs preventive care services (e.g., immunizations, health screening services). Given Community Care Pharmacy's strengths, they feel that there are opportunities to develop new goods and services that meet the demands of this population. Many people in the area are at risk for influenza, pneumococcal disease, and shingles. However, the ability of local physicians to provide immunizations is limited by their busy schedules, and access to other immunization providers is limited. The pharmacy staff has also recognized that more than 50% of local residents are overweight, and many are obese. This population is at high-risk for developing heart disease, hypertension, and diabetes and may be a good group to target with new pharmacy goods and services. A conversation with the local Chamber of Commerce indicated that many local businesses are self-insured employers and have expressed a strong interest in reducing their health care costs. Dr. Rockefeller and his colleagues agree that these businesses should be targeted, as new pharmacy services may help improve their enrollees' health, and therefore reduce health care costs in the long run. The threats to Community Care Pharmacy as they consider developing new services include declining reimbursement levels for prescriptions, increased competition from traditional, mail-order and on-line pharmacies, and concerns from local physicians regarding the pharmacy's potential development of disease management services.

Now that Dr. Rockefeller and his colleagues have completed the SWOT analysis, they realize that additional sources of revenue are needed. They are now ready to identify new goods and services to bring to the market.

Goals and Objectives Formulation

Results of the SWOT analysis should be used to inform the organization in the development of new goods and services. Plans to bring new goods and services to market are commonly described in business plans (see Chapter 7). Business plans should contain a set of goal statements that lead to objectives that an organization wants to accomplish. Goal statements are usually general and abstract (Rossi et al., 2004). They describe a desired state the organization strives to accomplish. Each goal statement may include several objectives. In contrast to goal statements, objectives are specific statements detailing the desired accomplishments of the plan (Rossi et al., 2004). In other words, objectives are quantitative measures of accomplishment by which the success of marketing strategies can be measured. Objectives might include retention, sales growth, and gains in the organization's share of their market (Berkowitz, 2017). It is important to formulate SMART objectives (Doran, 1981). That is, objectives should be *s*pecific, *m*easurable, *a*ttainable, *r*elevant, and *t*imely. A specific objective is one that describes exactly what the organization is going to do, with whom, and for

whom. A measurable objective is one that can be assessed to determine whether or not the objectives are being met. The objectives that are formulated for the pharmacy should be attainable, or realistic considering the pharmacy's available resources. Next, the objectives should specify outcomes that are relevant to the goals of the organization. Finally, the objectives should be time-specific, meaning that each objective has a deadline for achievement.

■ REVISITING THE SCENARIO

Dr. Rockefeller and his colleagues utilized the information gained from the SWOT analysis to formulate goals and objectives for Community Care Pharmacy (see Table 25-3 for an example). They agreed that given the degree of competition in the dispensing business, Community Care Pharmacy needs to capitalize on its strengths and offer a new service which will serve as a separate revenue source. The goals and objectives formulated by Dr. Rockefeller and his colleagues will be used to measure the success of the new service.

Determining the Target Market

After an organization's goals and objectives are identified, the next step is to determine the target market. The purpose of identifying the target market is to determine the population that will serve as the focus of the organization's marketing efforts (Berkowitz, 2017).

Table 25-3.	Goals and Objectives Formulated by Community Care Pharmacy
Goal 1	To increase pharmacy profitability from providing a new service
Objective 1.1	To attract 100 new patients to the pharmacy by the end of 12 months
Objective 1.2	To increase the pharmacy revenues by 5% within 12 months

Various factors can be used to identify target markets including the organization's capabilities, the competition within the market, the cost of capturing market share, and the potential financial gain from the targeted group (Berkowitz, 2017).

The process to identify target markets includes two steps: market segmentation and target marketing (Kotler & Clarke, 1986). *Market segmentation* is a process in which a market is divided into distinct and meaningful groups of consumers based on their profiles. For example, the market can be segmented by demographic variables such as income, age, disease categories, sex, health insurance coverage (e.g., cash payers, third-party payers), or buying behaviors. There is no single best way to segment a market, and a market can be segmented in a number of ways. The organization should segment the market in a way that makes the most sense and reveals the most market opportunities for the types of goods and services they plan to introduce. Once the organization identifies the market segments, they then can evaluate the attractiveness of each segment and choose one or more segments that are desirable (Holdford, 2015). Desirable market segments should be identifiable, accessible, of sufficient size, and responsive to targeted marketing mix strategies (Holdford, 2015). It is difficult to reach and appeal to all consumers for most goods and services; therefore, organizations often choose to focus on one or more market segments, known as the target markets, and develop strategies that are tailored to meet the needs of those specific consumers.

■ REVISITING THE SCENARIO

Dr. Rockefeller and his colleagues identify target markets for Community Care Pharmacy by reviewing the existing customer databases (e.g., patient profiles, insurance coverage). With the characteristics of desirable market segments in mind, two desired target markets were identified (Medicare enrollees and young, cash-paying customers). Table 25-4 describes characteristics of each group.

After selecting the target market(s), an organization must formulate and design elements of the marketing mix that position a good or service in the minds of targeted consumers. Positioning a good or service in this manner is achieved through use of each of the four elements of the marketing mix. Since Community Care Pharmacy ultimately aims at attracting two different target markets, elements of the marketing mix may have to be customized for each market to yield optimal benefits.

■ THE MARKETING MIX: USING THE FOUR Ps

After completion of an organizational SWOT analysis, creation of goals and objectives, and identification of two target markets, Community Care Pharmacy is ready to develop the details of their *marketing mix*. The marketing mix is defined as the set of controllable variables that an organization can manipulate and use to reach its goals and objectives (Berkowitz, 2017).

Table 25-4. Target Markets Identified by Community Care Pharmacy	
Medicare enrollees	This target market consists of elderly people (65 years or older). They have multiple chronic conditions and take multiple medications. Because they are likely to be at risk for preventable infectious diseases, they are candidates to receive influenza, pneumococcal, and zoster vaccines.
Young population who are cash-based payers	This target market is made up of people who are young and relatively healthy. They are employed, well educated, and have income above average. Even though they may have insurance coverage, they are willing to pay out of pocket for certain services. They are interested in prevention services such as immunization services.

These variables are often viewed as the *four Ps*: product, price, place, and promotion (see Chapter 24). The forthcoming sections explain how Community Care Pharmacy can apply each of the four Ps to position themselves in the eyes of their target markets and reach their goals and objectives.

Product

Products are defined as the goods, services, or ideas that are offered by an organization. Goods are tangible and can be touched or examined, while services are intangible and are seen as activities or processes that are offered to help patients solve problems. In pharmacy, over-the-counter pharmaceuticals and prescription medications are examples of goods that are normally sold to consumers. Being that they are tangible, consumers can easily understand many of their attributes. On the other hand, marketing plans for services often require additional effort because their attributes are not as easily examined or understood.

The five key components of services that differentiate them from goods are commonly referred to as the *five Is* (Berkowitz, 2017). Since a service is *intangible*, the marketing of a service needs to somehow portray the tangible benefits the patient will receive from the service. *Inconsistency* refers to the fact that services are delivered by individual providers to individual consumers, resulting in inherent variability each time that the service is delivered. *Inseparability* means that a service cannot be separated from its provider. Consumers who feel they are disrespected during the delivery of a service are likely to have a negative impression of the service even if the provider delivered the service correctly. Unlike physical goods, services cannot be *inventoried* and stored until they are ready to be delivered or received. Therefore, attention must be paid to scheduling service delivery at a time and in a manner that is consistent with an organization's operations and meets the consumer's needs and wants. Finally, consumers often evaluate a service based on the *interaction* they have with the person providing the service. Each person a consumer interacts with while receiving a service molds his or her overall satisfaction with the service.

Therefore, each person interacting with consumers has a responsibility to make these interactions as pleasant as possible.

■ REVISITING THE SCENARIO

Community Care Pharmacy has decided that they are going to address opportunities provided by the two target markets they previously identified. With their SWOT analysis, goals, and objectives in mind, Dr. Rockefeller and his colleagues have decided that a vaccination service is aligned with the strengths outlined in the SWOT analysis. For example, all pharmacists are already certified to administer vaccines, and a private area is available in the pharmacy. In addition, a vaccination service seems to be a good fit considering their limited financial resources and workload. The community offers tremendous market opportunities as the Medicare enrollees in the area has a need for influenza, pneumococcal, and zoster vaccines and the young, cash-paying population has an unmet need for influenza vaccinations. Hence, Dr. Rockefeller and his employees decide that Community Care Pharmacy will provide influenza, pneumococcal, and zoster vaccines for these patients. If the service is successful, Dr. Rockefeller believes they will be able to expand the types of vaccines they provide and may expand the service to different market segments.

Dr. Rockefeller realizes that this service is difficult to classify as purely tangible or intangible. Although the delivery of the service is intangible, the vaccine solution is tangible. Because of this, Dr. Rockefeller concludes that this service is a hybrid. He also realizes the risk of inconsistency in the delivery of a service; however, he believes the pharmacists are well-trained to provide a consistent, high-quality service in a polite and respectful manner that is representative of the pharmacy's image and, therefore, inconsistency should not be a major issue. His technicians and store employees are also kind and respectful, so he is not worried about interactions with patients. Dr. Rockefeller currently has optimal staffing levels but understands that this service may require him to hire another part-time pharmacist. As previously stated, elements of the marketing mix may differ among different market segments. In the case of Community Care Pharmacy, the young population market would desire a different product from the elderly market.

Price

The next step in marketing Community Care pharmacy's new vaccination service is to establish a *price* for the product. To ensure the success of any new good or service, organizations must offer them at an appropriate price. There are many factors to consider when setting a price, including the costs of providing the good or service, overall consumer demand for the good or service, competition from other organizations offering similar goods or services, and the use of pricing strategies that appeal to consumers.

Costs of Providing a Good or Service

The first thing to consider when pricing a new good or service is the costs the organization will incur to provide them. In the case of Community Care Pharmacy's new vaccination service, they must purchase vaccines, syringes, needles, a refrigerator, cotton swabs, alcohol wipes, bandages, and the proper medical waste disposal supplies to comply with state and federal disposal laws. Also included in the cost of providing the vaccination service is the salary and benefits they have to pay their pharmacists, technicians, and other employees involved in providing this service. A decision must be made that relates to how they will compensate their pharmacists. Will they offer their pharmacists and technicians additional monetary or nonmonetary rewards? Or will they require their staff to provide vaccination services in addition to their normal dispensing activities without additional compensation? These are important questions that will need to be addressed when pricing the service. Overhead expenses must also be considered when pricing the new vaccination service. The principles used to calculate a pharmacy's cost to dispense a prescription can also be applied to calculate their costs to provide any service, such as the costs to provide an immunization (see Chapter 23).

As seen in Community Care Pharmacy's SWOT analysis, consumer need for vaccination services appears to be high. The SWOT analysis also shows that there is little competition from other providers in the area when it comes to providing these vaccinations, especially for pneumococcal and herpes zoster vaccines. These two opportunities allow the pharmacy to consider the potential profit of providing vaccinations. To break-even from providing the service is not the goal, a sufficient profit should be built into the pricing strategy. However, pricing the service too high may result in failure due to low utilization and an increase in competitors who see the high price as an opportunity to provide the service at a lower cost.

Pricing Strategies

For many goods and services offered in pharmacies, reimbursement rates depend on contractual agreements between third-party payers and the pharmacy (see Chapter 23). For instance, pharmacies that provide medications and MTM services to Medicare Part D plan enrollees are reimbursed at levels stated in the contract. In this case, pharmacies have limited flexibility in determining prices for services they provide. On the other hand, pharmacists have greater flexibility setting prices for services offered to cash-paying customers or services offered through a contractual agreement with self-insured employers.

There are many pricing strategies to consider when determining an optimal price for a new good or service. One pricing strategy that is commonly used is known as *odd pricing* or *psychological pricing*. This pricing strategy is the practice of pricing a service just below whole dollar amounts (Berkowitz, 2017). In the case of Community Care Pharmacy, let us assume that their costs of providing an influenza vaccination (including overhead costs and the cost of the vaccine itself) are $20.00. Taking into consideration government regulations regarding the pricing of the service, the price for a similar service by competitors, and the profit desired, Community Care Pharmacy needs the price of influenza vaccination service for cash payers to be more than $20.00. Using the odd pricing strategy, the pharmacy can price this service for out-of-pocket payers at $24.99, just under $25.00. The rationale behind this strategy is that consumers believe products and services priced just under whole dollar amounts ($24.99) are priced at the lowest possible price or that the product or service has been discounted from a higher price.

A second pricing strategy is *bundled pricing*. Bundled pricing is the practice of selling several items or services together for one total price. This is becoming a common strategy in health care and can be appealing to consumers (Berkowitz, 2017). If Community Care Pharmacy chooses to do this, the amount of savings to the patient must be seen as a real advantage. For example, because their influenza vaccine is priced at $24.99 and their vitamin supplements are priced at $11.99, bundling them and selling them for $36.98 would not be beneficial. The pharmacy would need to bundle them and sell them at a discount while still covering their costs. A reasonable bundled price for both the good and the service at the pharmacy would be $29.29 (assuming that the acquisition cost of the vitamin supplement is under $10). Community Care Pharmacy can also apply a similar strategy by offering a bundled price for influenza and pneumococcal vaccines for those who need both vaccines.

Discounts are another strategy used in the pricing of goods and services in pharmacy. A *functional discount* can be given to a large organization by offering vaccination services to its employees for a lower price than the general public (Berkowitz, 2017; Kotler & Armstrong, 2018). As seen in Community Care Pharmacy's SWOT analysis, there are several large, self-insured organizations in Weagle to whom they could offer such a discount. By offering a functional discount to all employees and retirees of these self-insured employers, Community Care Pharmacy can increase the utilization of their vaccination service.

A *seasonal discount* is another pricing strategy commonly used to increase utilization of services. These discounts are given to consumers who purchase goods or services when they are out of season (Berkowitz, 2017; Kotler & Armstrong, 2018). For example, many people wait until the spring and summer months to purchase gym memberships and get in shape. A seasonal discount would offer the same gym membership during the off months for a discounted price. In the case of vaccination service, flu shots are usually offered between September and November and flu season generally starts in December and lasts through the spring. Even though it is ideal to get vaccinated early, a flu shot in January can still be helpful as there are still 2 or 3 months left in the flu season. To apply a seasonal discount strategy, Community Care Pharmacy may offer influenza vaccine at a discounted price in January or February, if they still have a supply.

Place

The third P in the marketing mix is *place*. This component refers to distribution of a good or service. In other words, place refers to how and where the product is accessed by the consumer. Consumers have traditionally accessed health goods and services by shopping at a community pharmacy. An independently-owned pharmacy will adjust the hours they are open to best meet the needs of their customers, while a chain community pharmacy often focuses on the convenience of accessing their goods and services by providing multiple locations in the area where they compete with the goal of customers not having to go out of their way to access what they offer. Chain pharmacies such as CVS and Walgreens are examples of organizations that employ this strategy. Community pharmacies have also extended their hours of operation and offered conveniences such as drive-throughs to increase access. Consumers also have options to obtain health goods and services in places that are not traditional community pharmacies. As the majority of prescription drugs have come to be paid for by someone other than the patient, third-party payers have developed alternative methods for patients to obtain drugs and related services, particularly through mail-order pharmacies. Enhancements in technologies which allow for the delivery of telepharmacy services (see Chapter 9) and the introduction of online vendors such as Amazon.com and Wal-Mart.com are certain to result in changes to how prescriptions drugs and other health goods and services reach consumers in the coming years.

Intensity of distribution refers to how available the service is to the consumer and varies along a continuum ranging from intensive distribution to selective distribution with exclusive serving as a midpoint between the extremes (Berkowitz, 2017). Deciding which form of distribution intensity to utilize with a new good or service is vital to its success. Intensive distribution is a strategy used when the good or service is available from a large number of locations. Everyday products that community pharmacies sell such as toothpaste, eye drops, aspirin, and ibuprofen are examples of products that are intensively distributed. These products can be found in many different locations and, therefore, consumers will not go out of their way to patronize a specific organization to purchase them. Exclusive distribution is the opposite of intensive distribution, and is the strategy used when a good or service is only offered in very few locations. In the Weagle community, most pharmacy goods and services are offered at multiple locations. This is not the case with Community Care Pharmacy's compounding service. Since other pharmacies in the area do not provide compounding services, consumers of this service are required to patronize Community Care Pharmacy to take advantage of this service. Selective distribution is the strategy used when a product or service is offered in multiple locations, but fewer locations than an intensive distribution approach. It is known as the selective approach because the consumer has the option to shop around and select the location where they purchase the product based on their expectations of customer service. Many community pharmacy retail items fall into this category, where pharmacies attempt to attract customers with over-the-counter or herbal products that may be difficult to find in other stores.

■ REVISITING THE SCENARIO

For a patient to receive vaccination services in the Weagle area, they have the option to be vaccinated at Community Care Pharmacy, their primary care physician's office, public health departments, or the local hospital. The patient has fewer options than an intensively distributed service, but more options than an exclusively distributed service, and therefore will choose the option that best fits their needs and budget. By offering this service in the evenings and on weekends (when physicians' offices are closed), and by offering this service on a walk-in basis (most physicians' offices require appointments), Community Care Pharmacy can increase access and utilization of their vaccination service. They also have the opportunity to increase access to this service by occasionally providing vaccinations at a public place such as the local mall, church, or at events like the Monet County Fair in October.

Promotion

The fourth P in the marketing mix and the next step in marketing Community Care Pharmacy's new vaccination service is *promotion* of the service. There are four primary methods used to promote any good or service to potential consumers. These are advertising, personal selling, publicity, and sales promotion (Berkowitz, 2017). These methods can be used individually or in combination to promote goods and services to target markets. In the following section, the four methods will be defined and applied to the marketing of Community Care Pharmacy's new vaccination service to better understand the use of promotion in the pharmacy setting.

Advertising

Advertising can be defined as any directly paid form of nonpersonal presentation of goods, services, and ideas (Kotler & Armstrong, 2018). Traditionally, there have been three primary outlets for advertisements: broadcast media, print media, and Internet marketing. Broadcast media consists of television and radio advertisements, while print media includes newspaper, magazine, direct mail, and outdoor advertisements. In recent years, Internet marketing has evolved with the emergence of social media applications (Constantinides et al., 2009) such as Facebook, Instagram, YouTube, and Twitter. This new venue has become increasingly popular among health care organizations. While many of these Internet applications are free to use as a way for organizations to promote themselves, organizations should plan for the personnel cost necessary to develop and regularly manage these applications. There are various outlets for advertisements. It is important to determine where to place advertisements for a new good or service based on the amount an organization plans to spend and what the organization plans to gain from each venue. Although many pharmacy managers often work with their corporate marketing departments or even an advertising agency to develop advertising materials, it is important to understand the benefits of each form of advertising and what makes an advertisement effective.

Broadcast Media

Television advertisements have the ability to incorporate both visual images and sounds with the potential to reach a vast number of consumers. In the United States, about 35% of all advertising dollars are spent on television advertising (Griner, 2017). While the costs of television advertising have begun to decrease, it is still considered an expensive form of promotion. The costs of producing television advertisements and purchasing airtime to show them are usually higher than that of other advertising mediums. Advances in technologies, particularly by local cable systems, have made the use of television advertising feasible for many community pharmacies. Community pharmacies now have the ability to select the channel and time of day when they would like their advertisements to air. This is the most difficult part of television advertising for many organizations because, to be effective, the organization must know the media habits of their target markets, including what times of day they watch television, and when they do watch, what channels and even programs they view. An advertisement run at 11:00 AM will most likely reach a different market than the same advertisement run at 11:00 PM. The same is true about an advertisement run on a sports network versus an advertisement run on a news network.

Radio advertisements are a popular form of promotion in community pharmacy because radio stations are highly segmented (i.e., the listeners to any particular station often share demographic characteristics) and the production of radio advertisements is relatively simple and inexpensive (Kotler & Armstrong, 2018). For example, if the goal is to reach the most working-age consumers, an organization may choose to place a radio advertisement on an early morning or early evening talk show because these are the peak listening times as people drive to and from work. The disadvantages of radio advertising are its lack of a visual component, and given the market segmentation among radio stations, the stations used for advertising must be carefully chosen to assure that the desired target markets are being reached (Berkowitz, 2017).

■ REVISITING THE SCENARIO

After discussing their options for broadcast media advertising, Dr. Rockefeller and his colleagues believe that a television advertisement is a good investment to promote their new vaccination service. Since one of their target markets is the local elderly population, they have decided to pay to have their advertisement aired during the 5:00 PM local news broadcast. Although this is one of the more expensive time slots, they believe that a large portion of the elderly population in the area views this program regularly.

Print Media

Despite the common misconception that "print is dead", newspapers reach 169 million adults or 69% of the US population in a given month (The Nielsen Company, 2016). Newspaper advertising is commonly used to promote pharmacy goods and services. Newspapers are a good source for health care advertisements because they are seen as highly credible sources of information (The Nielsen Company, 2016). Another advantage of newspaper advertising is the ability to geographically select who will see the advertisement. Even in metropolitan newspapers, the creation of zone editions allows advertisers to target specific geographic locations within a city. The cost associated with newspaper advertising is relatively inexpensive compared with broadcast media. A disadvantage of newspaper advertising is the lack of flexibility and creativity relative to other types of media. Many newspapers require that advertisements fit a particular template and format, limiting a marketer's ability to make their advertisements eye catching and unique.

Magazine advertisements are a popular medium for health care organizations. The number of specialized publications that allow organizations to target specific market segments has increased dramatically in recent years. Large chain pharmacies can target health-focused magazines, such as *Men's Health* and *Fitness* for national advertisements. Smaller community pharmacies can target regional magazines as well as national magazines that publish zone and geographic editions. An advantage of magazine advertisements is that they have a longer shelf life than other types of print media. Some consumers choose to keep magazines for weeks, months, or even years, meaning the advertisement may be seen and read multiple times before the magazine is discarded. Another advantage is that magazines produce high-quality, colorful advertisements that attract the reader's attention. As with other forms of advertising, magazine advertisements have their disadvantages. One major disadvantage is the amount of time before the advertisement is seen. Magazines may require that advertisements be received 4 to 6 weeks before the publication will be on the shelf for consumers to read. This makes magazine advertisements a good option for long-running goods and services, but not so viable for short-term offerings.

Direct mail advertising is one of the most utilized forms of print advertising in North America because of its ability to target specific markets, such as consumers who live in a specific neighborhood or patients who are known from pharmacy records to have a particular characteristic or condition (Clow & Baack, 2005). Direct mail advertising allows an organization to target potential consumers by age, income, prior purchasing habits, geographic location, and many other identifiers (Berkowitz, 2017). For direct mail advertising to be effective, the list of recipients must be both well-conceived (reaching people known to be part of a pharmacy's target markets) and accurate (a large percentage of direct mail never reaches the intended target due to inaccurate addresses). A disadvantage of direct mail is that many consumers view this type of advertising as junk mail. With multiple organizations using this method, it is hard to make one direct mail advertisement stand out among others. It also has a disadvantage because of the high costs associated with printing these advertisements with bright colors to attract attention, as well as the high costs of postage. Given the costs of both printing and postage, the costs per person reached can be higher than other forms of promotion.

Outdoor advertising, such as billboards and transit ads, is useful as a reminder or introduction to a new product or service. Health care organizations often use this medium to create awareness, but many consumers view this type of advertisement as visual pollution. There are many regulations that affect the availability of billboards in the United States and therefore this form of advertising is most used in metropolitan areas on public transportation.

There are five main components of an effective print advertisement (Ladd, 2010). The *headline* is the print in the largest font and usually bolded to grab the reader's attention. A headline should be short, direct, and clear so the reader knows exactly what is being advertised. The *copy* further elaborates the headline and explains important information such as price and benefits of the good or service. The *illustration* can be a photo or drawn image that gives the reader a visual portrayal of the good or service. The *sub-headline* can be used to explain specific information that may not be clear in the headline. A common example of a sub-headline is an offer of an item for free with the purchase of another item. Finally, the *signature* is the branding of the organization that produced the advertisement including logos, slogans, and trademarks. This helps the organization to build brand recognition and helps the reader to associate the advertisement with the organization.

■ REVISITING THE SCENARIO

Dr. Rockefeller and his colleagues at Community Care Pharmacy believe that a print advertisement in the local daily newspaper that is also available online is a good way to reach both target markets (elderly and young population). Further, a print advertisement can reach those who may not be existing customers of their pharmacy. The cost of the advertisement is low and there is a large percentage of the population that receives the daily newspaper and frequents the newspaper's website. The local newspaper does not require purchasers of ad space to use a specific template with the design of their advertisements, allowing

Community Care Pharmacy to design an advertisement that best fits their needs. Dr. Rockefeller and his colleagues have designed a print advertisement (Figure 25-3) to promote Community Care Pharmacy's new vaccination service.

Internet Marketing

With the increased use of the Internet and the emergence of social media, organizations have begun utilizing new methods of advertising. The Internet allows users to collaborate with colleagues, share information with others, and build new business and social relationships that were more difficult to create in the past. The use of social media outlets like Facebook, Twitter, Instagram, and YouTube have increased dramatically. Additionally, websites like Yelp, Angie's List, and Google Reviews allow pharmacy customers to write reviews based on their experiences and are being frequented regularly by savvy consumers.

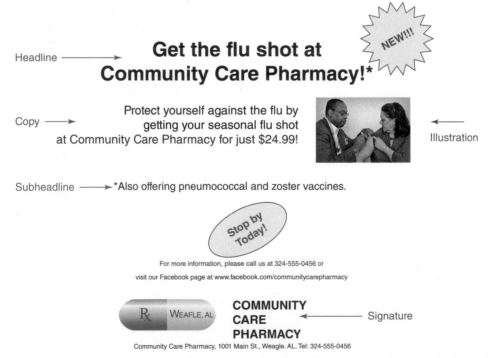

Figure 25-3. Print advertisement for vaccination services offered by Community Care Pharmacy. (Photo credit: James Gathany, Centers for Disease Control and Prevention; accessible at Public Health Image Library, www.cdc.gov. PHIL ID#9420.)

Health care organizations have begun to see increased use of the Internet and social media as an opportunity to get their message to target markets at a relatively low cost. Social media is not only used widely by large chain pharmacies, but is also a great opportunity for smaller pharmacies to level the playing field. Promotion of Community Care Pharmacy's new vaccination service through social media could be very beneficial as a supplemental advertising strategy. On their pharmacy's Facebook business page, they can post announcements about new goods and services, focusing on their new immunization services. Pharmacy customers can "Like" the page and "Follow" the business. By following the business' page, customers will see the announcement of their new vaccination service. Another strategy may be to conduct a promotion through their Facebook or Instagram page. For example, posting a comment that says, "Like and share this post and get a free $5 gift card with your flu shot today!" may be a good option. Twitter and Instagram can be used with hashtags like "#Pharmacy" or "#FluShot" to spread the news when influenza vaccines are being offered. YouTube is a video-sharing site that Community Care Pharmacy could use to create their own commercials explaining the benefits of getting vaccinated. These videos can then be shared through Facebook, Instagram, and Twitter. While the possibilities to use social media to advertise are endless and many social media applications are free for the pharmacy to use, it is vital to select the applications that are utilized most frequently by the selected market segments. The pharmacy must then ensure that these applications are monitored and updated regularly.

It is crucial for marketers to keep applications current and to generate interactions with their target markets. The Facebook "news feed" algorithm is complex and utilizes many signals to prioritize the feed, one of which is the interaction between the follower and the page. For some pharmacies, there is just not enough time to update their Facebook, Twitter, LinkedIn, Pinterest, Instagram, and YouTube accounts. One option for these pharmacies is to hire a social media marketing specialist who can craft targeted content to attract new customers. These specialists have the ability to measure the impact of their efforts and provide evidence of the power of social media on the pharmacy's bottom line. They ensure that customers are getting an enjoyable experience when visiting the pharmacy's social media pages by keeping the content fresh and appealing and can respond to negative reviews to try to address customer complaints. If hiring a social media marketing specialist is not an option, it is important to remember to build the online presence of the pharmacy through existing customers and not with the purpose of chasing after new customers. By taking pictures with customers and posting them on the pharmacy's social media accounts, or creating contests that get customers writing on the pharmacy's Facebook wall, a pharmacy can attract new customers *through* their current customers.

While social media can be used as a tool to positively promote pharmacies and their services to their target markets, some of these sites can hurt a pharmacy's image if pharmacy owners and managers are not careful and vigilant. Specifically, sites that allow individuals to review and rate their experience, such as Yelp, Angie's List, Trip Advisor, and Facebook, have done damage to the reputations of many organizations since becoming popular. In an investigation into the impact of negative reviews online found that a one-star increase in Yelp review rating led to a 5% to 9% increase in revenue among a sample of independently-owned restaurants (Luca, 2011). As more individuals review their experiences at pharmacies, it is important for pharmacy owners and managers to know where they stand in relation to other pharmacies in their area. The best way to avoid poor reviews is, of course, by providing a great experience for customers (see Chapter 26). The reason this is not a foolproof system is that the majority of review sites do not confirm that a reviewer actually visited the business before writing a review. In other words, some reviews may not be justified because almost anyone can write a review and say whatever they want. Because of this, it is important that pharmacies continuously monitor the review sites and have resources ready to respond to reviewers. As previously mentioned, social media marketing specialists can be hired to respond to reviews and help fix any unwarranted negative reviews. If the cost of hiring one of these firms is unaffordable, there are other options that can help manage a pharmacy's online presence. For example, reputation management software like Hootsuite® is available that compiles reviews from all review sites and places them in an easy-to-use dashboard so that time is not spent visiting each site individually. These software options are available for less than $50 per month and range up to more than $500 per month depending on the number of features an organization desires. Many of these software options include access to resources that will help improve responses to both negative and positive reviews.

■ REVISITING THE SCENARIO

Community Care Pharmacy decided to increase their social media presence through their Facebook business page, Instagram account, and Twitter account. While they have had these accounts for some time, they have not been regularly updated or used to market their products in the past. Until now, they have used these sites as a place for individuals to get basic information such as location, hours of operation, and telephone number. They believe use of these accounts to as Internet advertising venues will help to spread the word about their pharmacy and their new vaccination services to young cash-paying customers. Customers and patients of Community Care Pharmacy are invited to "Like" and "Follow" the Facebook page and to "Follow" the pharmacy's Instagram and Twitter accounts. Announcements of new goods and services offered will be made through these media outlets. Additionally, given how the Facebook News Feed algorithm works, Dr. Rockefeller realizes the importance of interactions with followers of the page. Dr. Rockefeller's plan is to highlight a pharmacy follower each week and a picture of Dr. Rockefeller with that individual will be featured on the pharmacy's Facebook page and Instagram account. When posted, the pharmacy's twitter account will tweet a link to the Facebook and Instagram photos to encourage followers to like, share, and comment on the photos.

Community Care Pharmacy will make their logo their profile picture for Facebook, Instagram, and Twitter pages to build brand recognition and help readers associate their posts on these sites with their organization. In addition to the creation of their Facebook, Instagram, and Twitter accounts, Community Care Pharmacy has purchased a software system that will help them to monitor and respond to reviews from their customers.

Personal Selling

Personal selling differs from advertising in that it is a direct, personal form of communication. Advertising is a form of mass communication and, therefore, it is more difficult to control who receives the message, while personal selling allows the organization to directly target the intended audience (Berkowitz, 2017). Community Care Pharmacy could use personal selling in the form of a salesperson who makes calls to referral physician offices or large self-employed insurers in Weagle to introduce and "sell" the new vaccination service. The advantage of this method is that any questions the receiver of the call may have can be answered immediately, and the service can be fully explained to avoid any confusion. It is also an opportunity to build relationships in the community. A disadvantage to personal selling is the cost as it is both time consuming and expensive. Employing a salesperson is costly, and if they can only make a few calls per day, the impact the calls have on developing the market may be small.

Pharmacists and other pharmacy personnel can also utilize personal selling when they interact with their patients. Any patient who has a prescription filled at Community Care Pharmacy presents an opportunity for the pharmacy staff to describe the benefits of the new vaccination service and answer any questions the patient may have. If the staff identifies a patient as someone who would benefit from the vaccination service, they can offer the service to the patient, schedule an appointment, or provide supplemental information that can be reviewed at the patient's convenience. If the patient elects not to utilize the service, the relationship that the staff and patient have built is still beneficial in that the pharmacy has learned something about why the patient is not interested in receiving the service. This information can be used when developing and marketing future goods and services.

■ REVISITING THE SCENARIO

After realizing the importance of personal selling, Dr. Rockefeller agrees to visit several physicians' offices (especially those who do not offer vaccination services) to introduce their new vaccination service and request that they refer their patients to Community Care Pharmacy. Further, pharmacy staff members will begin to provide patients with information about their vaccination services when they pick up their prescriptions.

Publicity

Publicity is a form of communication of goods, services, and ideas that is not paid for directly by the organization (Berkowitz, 2017). Dr. Rockefeller can encourage local newspapers, television, and radio stations to report stories about the importance of vaccinations and places to get vaccinated (such as Community Care Pharmacy). The benefit of publicity is that much of the audience that reads a newspaper article or watches a report on the local news does not realize that Dr. Rockefeller had to contact these outlets and ask for this coverage. This leads the consumer to believe that the message is coming from a credible source and is unbiased. The limitation of publicity is that there is very little control on who receives the message, or for that matter, of the message itself. There is no way to know when the local news will air the story about the pharmacy, what day the newspaper will print the article, or what the media will say about the pharmacy and their services in their coverage. Therefore, it is difficult to know if the target market is reached, and if they are reached, whether they will receive the message the pharmacy desires. There are costs of using publicity, as someone from the pharmacy typically has to reach out to media outlets to encourage them to produce these stories, requiring resources (especially time) that could be used elsewhere. Publicity can also work negatively against an organization. A customer who has a bad experience at Community Care Pharmacy can alert the press with negative information about the pharmacy.

Sales Promotion

Sales promotions are temporary efforts to encourage consumers to purchase a good or utilize a service. These promotions come in the form of coupons, sweepstakes, rebates, or samples. In health care, the use of promotions such as a free trial of a medication is common, but the use of promotions to influence consumers to utilize a service is not. Community Care Pharmacy may be able to use a sales promotion in the form of a rebate by offering patients who utilize their vaccination service some in-store credit to be applied to other purchases in the pharmacy. It is important to maintain the professional image of the pharmacy and to ensure the message that a sales promotion portrays does not negatively impact that image.

Marketing Control

It is important for an organization to put methods to evaluate the effectiveness of their marketing efforts in place, just as the organization would put methods to evaluate the outcomes of the service in place. Marketing control is defined as the process of measuring and evaluating the outcomes of marketing strategies and, if necessary, taking action to correct the four Ps to ensure that marketing objectives are met (Kotler & Keller, 2016). For a control process to be successful, it is necessary that the regular collection of marketing performance data (e.g., website hits, patient questionnaires) be a part of normal pharmacy operations. Specific indicators should be developed and used to track actual performance, such as tracking hits on a pharmacy's website and asking new patients where they heard about the pharmacy's services. By tracking actual performance, the pharmacy will be able to compare these measures with expected performance and make corrections to their marketing mix to reach its goals. If needed, corrections can be made to the goals to make them more attainable.

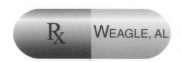

COMMUNITY CARE PHARMACY

1001 Main Street
Weagle, AL
(324)555-0456

Please take a moment to help us improve your experience with Community Care Pharmacy. We strive to provide the best possible patient care and want to make sure you are informed of our new patient services. When you are finished, please give this questionnaire to one of our staff.

How did you hear about our new vaccination service? (Please check all that apply)

☐ TV ad
☐ Newspaper
☐ Facebook
☐ Twitter
☐ Family member
☐ Friend
☐ Other (please list):_____

How would you rate our newspaper ad?

☐ Professional, High quality
☐ Average quality
☐ Poor quality
☐ Never saw it

Why did you choose Community Care Pharmacy to get vaccinated today? (Please check all that apply)

☐ Flu Season
☐ Inexpensive
☐ Open late
☐ Open on the weekend
☐ Just turned 65!
☐ Friendly staff

How would you rate our TV ad?

☐ Professional, High quality
☐ Average quality
☐ Poor quality
☐ Never saw it

Did you make an appointment today?

☐ Yes
☐ No, Walk-In
☐ No, Other

How would you rate our Facebook and Twitter presence?

☐ Frequently updated
☐ Adequately updated
☐ Poorly updated
☐ I don't use Facebook or Twitter

Interaction with our staff has been:

☐ Very Pleasant
☐ Pleasant
☐ Unpleasant
☐ Very Unpleasant (please explain):_____

How often do recommend our pharmacy to a friend?

☐ All the time
☐ Most of the time
☐ Some of the time
☐ Absolutely not

Additional Comments: _____

Thank You for Helping Us Provide the Best Care Possible!

Figure 25-4. Patient satisfaction questionnaire.

■ REVISITING THE SCENARIO

To evaluate the effectiveness of their marketing mix, Dr. Rockefeller and his colleagues at Community Care Pharmacy have put in place methods of collecting data on performance indicators to track the performance of their marketing effort. One of the methods they have chosen to employ is a brief questionnaire (see Figure 25-4) that they request their vaccination service patients to complete. Their plan is to analyze the responses to the questionnaire and evaluate the effectiveness of their marketing mix and determine if/how their marketing efforts should be modified.

■ CONCLUSIONS

Dr. Rockefeller and his colleagues at Community Care Pharmacy have developed a strategic plan, analyzed their market environment by conducting a SWOT analysis, formulated goals and measurable objectives, determined their target market, selected their service, prepared their marketing mix, and put controls in place to evaluate the success of their marketing efforts. Although this service is a good start and will put Community Care Pharmacy in a position to reach their additional revenue goals, the competition from other pharmacies in the area will not dwindle. Dr. Rockefeller and Community Care Pharmacy can use everything they have learned through this process to further expand their patient care services and address the additional market segments they have already identified.

In the ever-changing health care environment, it is vital for pharmacists to expand the scope of their professional services. Pharmacists are in a unique position to provide patient care services in a highly accessible venue and move toward a more influential position in the health care system. Those who choose not to embrace this shift from a dispenser role to a provider role will find it difficult to remain relevant and keep their businesses viable. Community Care Pharmacy has made an important first step in the continuous effort to stay ahead of the competition and be successful by integrating well-planned marketing strategies.

■ QUESTIONS FOR FURTHER DISCUSSION

1. To address the overweight and obese population in Weagle, would it be beneficial for Community Care Pharmacy to offer a weight management service? Why? Why not?
2. On the basis of the SWOT analysis presented, what are other viable target markets?
3. Some argue that the use of social media by health care organizations to advertise is unprofessional. Do you agree or disagree? Why?
4. Describe circumstances or examples when sales promotion or discount strategies may negatively impact the professional image of pharmacy.
5. Community Care Pharmacy used a questionnaire to evaluate their marketing effort. What are other ways that can be used to monitor the success of a marketing effort?

REFERENCES

Berkowitz EN. 2017. *Essentials of Health Care Marketing,* 4th ed. Burlington, MD: Jones and Bartlett Learning.

Clow KE, Baack D. 2005. *Concise Encyclopedia of Advertising.* New York, NY: Best Business Books: The Haworth Reference Press.

Constantinides E, Romero CL, Boria MAG. 2009. Social media: A new frontier for retailers? In Swoboda B, Morschett D, Rudolph T, Schnedlitz P, & Schramm-Klein H (eds.) *European Retail Research* Gabler Verlag, pp. 1–28.

Doran GT. 1981. There's a S.M.A.R.T. way to write management's goals and objectives. *Manage Rev* 70(11): 35–36.

Ferrell OC, Hartline MD. 2016. *Marketing Strategy: Text and Cases,* 7th ed. Boston, MA: Cengage Learning.

Griner D. 2017. *18 Bullish Stats About the State of U.S. Advertising.* Adweek. Available at https://www.adweek.com/agencies/18-bullish-stats-about-the-state-of-u-s-advertising. Accessed April 9, 2019.

Hillestad SG, Berkowitz EN. 2013. *Health Care Market Strategy: From Planning to Action*, 4th ed. Burlington, MA: Jones and Bartlett Learning.

Holdford DA. 2015. *Marketing for Pharmacists: Providing & Promoting Pharmacy Services*, 3rd ed. Washington, DC: American Pharmacists Association.

Kotler P, Armstrong G. 2018. *Principles of Marketing*, 17th ed. Hoboken, NJ: Pearson Higher Education.

Kotler P, Clarke RN. 1986. *Marketing for Health Care Organizations*. Englewood Cliffs, NJ: Prentice-Hall.

Kotler P, Keller KL. 2016. *Marketing Management,* 15th ed. Boston, MA: Pearson.

Ladd AD. 2010. *Developing Effective Marketing Materials: Newspaper and Magazine Print Advertising Design Considerations*. Knoxville, TN: University of Tennessee: Center for Profitable Agriculture.

Luca M. 2011. Reviews, Reputation, and Revenue: The Case of Yelp.Com. Harvard Business School NOM Unit Working Paper No. 12–016. Available at SSRN: http://ssrn.com/abstract=1928601 or http://dx.doi.org/10.2139/ssrn.1928601. Accessed September 7, 2015.

The Nielsen Company. 2016. *Newspapers Deliver Across the Ages.* Available at https://www.nielsen.com/us/en/insights/news/2016/newspapers-deliver-across-the-ages.html. Accessed April 3, 2019.

Rossi PH, Lipsey MW, Freeman HE. 2004. *Evaluation: A Systematic Approach*, 7th ed. Thousand Oaks, CA: Sage.

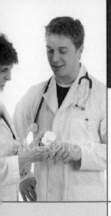

26

CUSTOMER SERVICE

Erin R. Holmes and Leigh Ann Bynum

About the Authors: Dr. Holmes is an associate professor with the School of Pharmacy and research associate professor of the Research Institute for Pharmaceutical Sciences, both at the University of Mississippi. Dr. Holmes received her PharmD degree and MS in pharmacy administration from Duquesne University and PhD in pharmacy administration from the University of Mississippi. She taught pharmacy management for 7 years and currently teaches pharmacy law, personal finance, and health care policy. Her research focuses on organizational behavior, human resource management, and service implementation in community pharmacy practice.

Dr. Bynum is an associate professor with the Belmont University College of Pharmacy. Dr. Bynum received a BA degree in psychology, an MS in wellness, and a PhD in pharmacy administration from the University of Mississippi. She teaches courses in pharmacy management, human resource management, the US health care system and communications. Dr. Bynum's research focuses on human resource management, the student pharmacist experience, and organization citizenship behaviors.

■ LEARNING OBJECTIVES

After completing this chapter, readers will be able to

1. List the principles for ensuring good customer service.
2. Provide ways of meeting each standard that patients use to evaluate services.
3. Define and describe the significance and implications of service failure, service recovery, service recovery paradox, and zone of tolerance.
4. Choose service recovery efforts for low-, mid-, and high-criticality service failures.
5. Explain the four perspectives of customer satisfaction assessment.
6. Identify ways to develop pharmacy staff members to provide good customer service.
7. Describe how an employee's work life can affect customer service.
8. Recommend steps for dealing with "difficult" patients.

■ SCENARIO

Sarah Laird, a 60-year-old woman, walked into the pharmacy in the morning with a prescription for promethazine 25-mg tablets. After suffering a back injury on an assembly line job at her workplace last week, she had been taking a pain medication as prescribed for a couple of days. While her pain has significantly reduced, the nausea from the pain medication has been difficult to deal with.

Upon presenting the prescription directly to the pharmacy manager and telling him that it should be covered by her workman's compensation insurance, he returned to her a clearly puzzled look. The look was not judgmental—just puzzled. He knew that promethazine is not a drug that is usually covered by workman's compensation insurance and that a prior authorization from the physician would be needed. She did not take his look as a puzzled one; rather, she took it as a judgmental one. "Um, ma'am, this promethazine is not a drug typically covered by your workman's comp. I need to get a prior authorization from your doctor. You'll have to come back tomorrow for it." The pharmacist said this to her pretty hastily, as he had quickly moved from his puzzled look to her on toward gazing at the computer to fill the next prescription. This morning was one of the busiest mornings that he could remember in a long time. Confused and still not quite sure what was going on, she left the pharmacy.

Sarah returned to the pharmacy later in the afternoon to pick up her prescription, but it still was not ready. She was steamed. On top of feeling bad from the nausea, now the pharmacist just will not fill the prescription. To be honest, she really believed that the pharmacist was discriminating against her because of the workman's compensation insurance. "You just don't want to fill my prescription, do you?" she angrily told him. Now, the pharmacy manager is agitated by and frustrated with Sarah because all he hears is, "What is taking so long?" "How many times have I heard *that* one," he thought to himself. "Didn't I tell you this morning that your prescription wasn't going to be ready until tomorrow?" he said in an impatient and very angry tone.

Sarah went home and immediately called the pharmacy back, asking the pharmacy manager for *his* manager. Not wanting to bring this to the attention of the pharmacy district manager, he forwarded the call to the general store manager. "I don't know why that pharmacist doesn't want to fill my prescription" she said. Sarah's daughter, a nurse, who was also on the line, repeated the question. "I want you to explain it to me," she said. Not knowing about the situation, the general manager took down Sarah's phone number and assured her that he would look into the situation and call her back within the next hour. He spoke with the pharmacy manager about the situation and called her back within 15 minutes. "It's not that he doesn't want to fill the prescription," the general manager told Sarah in a very slow and calming tone. "It's just that this is a medication that isn't usually covered by workman's comp. The pharmacist needs to call your doctor for a prior authorization. A prior authorization is a special permission for you to get the drug paid for by workman's comp. The doctor needs to fill out some paperwork and send it to the pharmacist, so that's why it is taking so long. The pharmacist wasn't trying to be mean or not want to fill your prescription. He was just confused about the promethazine being covered on workman's comp, and then had to go through some special procedures to get it covered for you." "Oh, well, is that all?" she asked. Well then, that's just fine!" The general manager assured Sarah he would call her in the morning when the prescription was ready so that she could come pick it up. He took no further action on the matter. After receiving the general manager's phone call the next morning Sarah returned to the pharmacy and picked up her prescription without any additional problems.

■ CHAPTER QUESTIONS

1. Why is the provision of service particularly challenging in the pharmacy setting?
2. What standards do patients use to evaluate the quality of services?

3. What should pharmacy managers do when customer service goes wrong?

4. How does an employee's quality of work life affect the quality of service they provide?

5. What are the potential outcomes of both good and bad customer service?

■ INTRODUCTION

While there is no one universal definition of "good" or "bad" customer service, most of us have probably experienced some of each and can distinctly remember the feelings that ensued from these experiences. Maybe a customer service agent went well above and beyond the call of duty to resolve a problem. Their efforts greatly surpassed your expectations, and you felt a huge sense of relief and gratitude after your experience. You left that interaction with a very positive impression of that company. You may also have encountered a store clerk with an "I couldn't care less" attitude and wondered; how could that person have so little regard for their job and for other people? Maybe the encounter left you feeling offended, invisible, angry, and with a bad taste in your mouth about the company.

Regardless of the type of pharmacy setting, there is no question that providing good customer service is intricately tied to patient care and gives an organization or business a competitive advantage. Providing good customer service, however, is sometimes easier said than done, especially in a busy pharmacy. Think of a time you have worked in a pharmacy and ask yourself the following questions. Did you give your patients your complete attention and use eye contact and avoid other activities like working on the computer when having a conversation with them? Did you sincerely apologize to a patient if a mistake was made by you or the pharmacy? When speaking to a patient over the phone, did you use inflection in your voice to convey interest and concern (Leland & Bailey, 2006)?

There is no question that unique characteristics of the pharmacy profession make the provision of good customer service challenging. First, the medications dispensed are typically viewed as "negative goods," which means that patients purchase them because they *have* to, not because they *want* to (Kolassa, 1997). In addition, patients may already come in with negative perceptions of the price of medicines, other health care professionals, or their insurance plan, which can sometimes be transferred (either intentionally or unintentionally) to the pharmacy staff. Patients may be experiencing symptoms from a condition or disease and not feeling well. At the same time, they likely have high expectations for pharmacy service given the very serious consequences of potential medication errors. Moreover, work in the pharmacy can be very hectic, making the provision of customer service especially challenging. In the scenario presented at the beginning of the chapter, Sarah was not feeling well, and the pharmacy manager was busy. The combination of these factors likely contributed to the misunderstanding and the resultant service failure.

With these unique characteristics of the pharmacy profession in mind, this chapter begins by providing ways that pharmacy managers can ensure good customer service and provides strategies for addressing service failures that can occur in the pharmacy setting. Then, satisfaction and other outcomes of a patient's experience in the pharmacy are discussed. Next, how employees' work life, as well as how the management of pharmacy employees affects the provision of customer service in a pharmacy will be addressed. Later, methods for collecting patients', customers', and employees' feedback about customer service will be discussed. Finally, techniques for dealing with "difficult" patients and patient complaints will be explored.

First, a few clarifications of terminology are warranted. Although the primary topic of this chapter is *customer* service, there is significant debate as to whether the term "patient," "client," "consumer," or "customer" is the most appropriate term to describe those who are served by pharmacists, especially in the community pharmacy setting. While often used interchangeably, these terms have different meanings. In fact, one study described the characteristics and needs of patients, clients, consumers, and customers of community pharmacies and outlined the best ways pharmacists can the meet the needs of each of these groups that they serve (Austin et al., 2006). For example, the authors describe a *patient* as being more reliant on a pharmacist and more desiring of a personal relationship with a pharmacist than a *customer*, who tends to be more autonomous, information driven, and self-confident. It follows, then, that a pharmacist may appropriately treat and communicate with a *patient* who is inquiring about the side effects of her infertility treatment differently than a *customer* who approaches the pharmacy counter to ask where they might find greeting cards or batteries. Regardless, both patients and customers are entitled to high-quality service in a pharmacy. Therefore, both the terms "customer" and "patient" will be used when appropriate in this chapter. In a few final notes of clarification, while many concepts of customer service in this chapter are presented in the context of the community pharmacy setting, the concepts very much can be applied to other pharmacy practice settings. Additionally, the concepts outlined in this chapter also apply to interactions with other health care professionals such as nurses and physicians, as well as other firms that we interact with such as health insurance companies and pharmacy benefit managers.

PRINCIPLES FOR ENSURING GOOD CUSTOMER SERVICE

Whether perusing the Internet, reading business publications, or evaluating research studies, there appears to be a consistent set of principles to which pharmacy managers can (and should) adhere to in providing good customer service. Table 26-1 provides a summary of these principles. This list of principles can be captured into an easy-to-remember concept known as the "golden rule of customer service." That is, treating your patients as you would want to be treated (Obarski, 2010).

Table 26-1.	Principles for Ensuring Good Customer Service

Anticipate patients' and customers' needs and wants

Solve patient and customer problems without hassle

Solve patient and customer problems promptly

Treat patients and customers with dignity, empathy, and respect

Correct mistakes when they are made

Apologize for mistakes when they are made

Underpromise and overdeliver

Do work right the first time

Actively listen to patients and customers

Make patients and customers feel important and appreciated

Help patients and customers understand how your pharmacy works

Always look for ways to help patients and customers

Data from Friedman, 2010; Tipton, 2009; Umiker, 1998.

STANDARDS PATIENTS USE TO EVALUATE SERVICES

While abiding by this list can be challenging, it is worth remembering that patients keep an "invisible report card" in their head, and they grade you on the basic needs (standards) that they require. They are not going to overtly ask for those standards. They are not going to approach the pharmacist and say, "Here is my prescription to be filled. Can you please make sure that you fill it accurately and treat me with empathy and fairness? Oh, and by the way, I have to be at my meeting in 10 minutes." However, they are going to evaluate you for accuracy, empathy, fairness, and responsiveness (Leland & Bailey, 2006). The literature suggests ten standards that patients and customers use to evaluate services: (1) reliability, (2) responsiveness, (3) assurance, (4) empathy, (5) tangibles, (6) friendliness, (7) fairness, (8) control, (9) options, and

(10) alternatives (Leland & Bailey, 2006; Parasuraman et al., 1988). Table 26-2 provides a description of each standard and an example of how each standard can be met in the pharmacy setting.

It should be noted here that the "responsiveness" standard should be interpreted with caution. There is no question that some patients who come to the pharmacy are in a hurry. And, indeed, pharmacies were known (and in some cases, still known) for advertising "15-minute prescription guarantees" for prescription fills (Gamble, 2011) (although these guarantees had exceptions for calling a prescriber or third party,

Table 26-2. Description of Standards that Patients and Customers Use to Evaluate Services

Standard	Description	How Standard Can Be Met
Reliability Parasuraman et al. (1988)	Receiving the promised service dependably and accurately	Accurate prescription filling and patient counseling
Responsiveness Parasuraman et al. (1988)	Receiving help and prompt service	Staff who are eager to help patients and customers any way they can
Assurance Parasuraman et al. (1988)	Knowledgeable and courteous employees who convey trust and confidence	Staff who are knowledgeable about the location of products in the store and help customers find products
Empathy Leland and Bailey (2006); Parasuraman et al. (1988)	Caring, individualized attention; appreciating a patient's or customer's circumstances and feelings without criticism or judgment	Acknowledging that patients may be sick, scared, confused, worried, and responding to their feelings
Tangibles Parasuraman et al. (1988)	The appearance of physical facilities, equipment, personnel, and communication materials	Using spare minutes in the day to wipe shelves or counters; providing medication information that is easy to understand and read
Friendliness Leland and Bailey (2006)	Polite and courteous treatment	Friendly and upbeat staff; calling patients by their name; having packages ready as patients and customers walk to the counter
Fairness Leland and Bailey (2006)	Fair treatment from service providers	Helping patients and customers in order of their arrival at the pharmacy
Control Leland and Bailey (2006)	The patient's or customer's need to have an impact on the way things turn out	Letting patients know that the remainder of a partial fill will not be available for 2 days
Options Leland and Bailey (2006)	The patients or customer's need to feel that other options are available	Ordering products for patients and customers when necessary
Information Leland and Bailey (2006)	The patient's or customer's need to be educated and informed about products, policies, and procedures	Patient counseling and patient information to take home

or before or during lunch break). Prescriptions cannot always be processed quickly. Sometimes the prescriber needs to be called for a drug-related problem or reauthorization. Sometimes the pharmacy benefits manager (PBM) needs to be called for a problem or prior authorization. Patient education takes time. Hastily filled prescriptions can result in a service failure that is much worse than waiting on a prescription—one that potentially can be very detrimental to the patient. As a result these prescription guarantees have received pushback from medication safety organizations and pharmacists (ConsumerMedSafety.org, 2012). Fortunately, it is not necessarily a long wait that is perceived as a service failure; but rather, it is a wait that was longer than *expected* or *promised*. This is known as *disconfirmation of expectations* (Oliver, 1980; Spreng et al., 1996), or the idea that patients evaluate the gap between their expectations and perceptions of a service (see "Outcomes of Service Failure and Service Recovery" for more information). So, pharmacists must provide honest and realistic expectations about the time needed to fill a prescription or provide other services. The pharmacist must clearly explain why there will be a delay (this also meets the standard of "control" in Table 26-2). If the pharmacist in the scenario at the beginning of the chapter clearly communicated in simple language the reason for delay, the ensuing confusion and inconvenience may have been avoided. Because this can be challenging in a busy pharmacy, it might be best to overestimate the time required to fill a prescription when communicating with a patient. As noted in Table 26-1, exceeding a patient's expectations can result in their satisfaction, or even delight, with the pharmacy.

■ PHARMACY ISSUES THAT ARE IMPORTANT TO PATIENTS

Providing quality customer service in a pharmacy requires understanding what pharmacy experiences are most important to patients, and working to improve those experiences. A 2016 survey of over 32,000 pharmacy patients identified issues most important to them. Not surprisingly, filling prescriptions accurately and efficiently, pharmacy staff, and overall convenience, were most important to patients, followed by additional medical services and prescription pricing (Boehringer Ingelheim, 2016).

An interesting observation to be made from these findings is that filling prescriptions accurately and efficiently and convenience are most important to patients, while additional medical services are less important to patients. This requires pharmacies and their staff to achieve a balance between ensuring customer satisfaction by being accurate, efficient, and convenient, and also focusing on patient care and expanding services to improve health outcomes. There is growing evidence, that pharmacies, particularly national chain pharmacies, are achieving that balance by ensuring patients are satisfied with the experiences most important to them, while also providing a growing list of services such as medication therapy management (MTM), medication adherence programs, and disease state management initiatives (Simone, 2014). While not every patient needs MTM or disease management programs from a pharmacy, it can be assumed that every patient who is getting a prescription filled expects that it will be filled accurately, efficiently and conveniently. The challenge to pharmacists is to identify their subset of patients who need and would benefit from MTM and other services, and then to provide those services in a manner that exceeds the patient's expectations. As these pharmacy services become more prevalent, patients may soon include these among the pharmacy experiences that are most important to them.

■ WHEN CUSTOMER SERVICE GOES WRONG

Even the best efforts to ensure customer service can result in failure to meet the expectations of a patient. Failing to meet the expectations of a patient is called *service failure*. Examples of service failures include patients not getting what they expected or were promised; having to wait longer than they expected or were promised; rude, patronizing, or indifferent treatment from a pharmacy staff member; and a "can't do" attitude or a "sorry, it's our policy" response from a pharmacy staff member (Umiker, 1998). A widespread example of service failures in pharmacies occurred with the implementation of the Medicare Part D program on January 1, 2006. Pharmacists struggled to dispense medications under the new drug benefit and required more time to sort out the new rules and regulations. Data suggest that overall satisfaction with pharmacies decreased during that time but recovered soon after (Boehringer Ingelheim, 2008).

By their very nature, service failures in the pharmacy can range from the inconvenient (a long wait for a prescription, or a partial fill due to limited stock) to the very serious (giving a patient the wrong drug or wrong dose). *Service criticality* refers to the magnitude of the consequences of a potential service failure to the patient or customer (Webster & Sundaram, 1998). For example, a car dealer forgetting to wash your car as promised during servicing has a low service criticality while a serious car accident due to fixing your brakes incorrectly during that servicing has a high service criticality. Obviously, the higher the service criticality, the more seriously the patient will perceive the service failure, and the more important it is for the pharmacy to address the failure. Service criticality is important; it has been shown that with increasing service failure criticality, satisfaction with, trust in, and commitment to the business by the customer is more likely to decrease, and negative word-of-mouth can become that much more problematic (Weun et al., 2004). It is important to keep in mind that patients will have varying perceptions of the severity of a failure. Just because the provider of the service may perceive a service failure as insignificant does not mean that the patient will perceive it, likewise.

■ RIGHTING THE WRONG

Given the negative consequences of service failures on patients and businesses, the way in which a service provider responds to a failure is critical. While it is well understood that service failures are sometimes inevitable, this does not mean that dissatisfied patients and customers are inevitable (Hart et al., 1990). That is the premise of service recovery. *Service recovery* is the attempt to correct the service failure and make things right for the patient (Tipton, 2000). Service recovery has been formally defined as an effort to "alter the negative perceptions of dissatisfied customers and to ultimately maintain a business relationship with these customers" (Schweikhart et al., 1993, p. 3). Service recovery requires more than correcting the error and making things right, but requires going above and beyond to satisfy the patient (Bell & Zemke, 1987). The way in which a provider responds to service errors can dictate patients' satisfaction and dissatisfaction (Bitner et al., 1990) and whether they will continue to patronize the pharmacy (Hoffman et al., 1995).

■ RECOVERING FROM LOW- AND MID-CRITICALITY SERVICE FAILURES IN THE PHARMACY

As previously mentioned, low-criticality service failures in the pharmacy can include a longer than expected wait for a prescription, a partial fill, and rude treatment from pharmacy staff, among others. Mid-criticality failures can include drug errors that are easily reversible or have resulted in little or no patient harm such as mislabeling a prescription bottle and providing the wrong dose to a patient, among others. Ideally these types of errors in the pharmacy are minimal; however, they do occur. Readers are referred to Chapters 10, 11, and 12 for a more detailed discussion about medication errors. For low- and mid-criticality service failures, similar recovery efforts can be applied. Suggested recovery efforts for these types of failures are provided in Table 26-3.

In one pharmacy service failure study, pharmacy students were asked to indicate the best way a pharmacist can handle the following hypothetical situation (Tipton, 2000, p. 75):

Table 26-3.	Suggested Recovery Efforts for Low- and Mid-criticality Service Failures
Bell and Zemke (1987)	Apology Urgent reinstatement Empathy Symbolic atonement Follow-up
Johnston (1995)	Provide information about the problem Provide information about what is being done Action in response to customer (but preferably without being asked) Staff appearing to go out of their way to help Involving the customer in decision-making
Kelley et al. (1993)	Discount Correction Manager/Employee intervention Correction plus (correction of problem and compensation to customer) Replacement Apology Refund
Tipton (2000)	Apology Compensation for substantial financial losses Assurance system is either not defective and this was a unique situation, of that system is defective and will be corrected Explanation of how the mistake was made Expression of sincerity and genuine concern

Having picked up your prescription, you do not notice that it is incorrect and take the medication for several days. This results in headaches and several days missed at work. You fully recover, and there are no permanent damages. You return to the pharmacy to discuss this situation with the pharmacist.

The most commonly mentioned "best way" that pharmacy students thought the pharmacist should respond to the situation was an apology, followed by compensation for financial losses, assurance about the system, explanation about how the mistake was made, and expression of sincerity and genuine concern (Table 26-3). Other qualitative studies of consumers' perceptions of pharmacy service failures have lent less credence to an apology by the pharmacist (Bunniran et al., 2010). This contradiction in findings may be a result of pharmacy students being more empathetic than a consumer with a pharmacist's mistake. In addition, the latter study also examined low-criticality service failures. It has been suggested that in low-criticality situations, an apology might be perceived as more trivial to a patient then actual correction of the problem (Tipton, 2000). Regardless of the criticality of the failure, an apology is called for in addition to correcting the problem and compensating the patient when necessary.

The importance of recovering from a service failure in a pharmacy is clear. It has been found that reducing customer loss by 5% can increase profits from anywhere between 25% and 100% (Reichheld, 2001, p. xi). In addition, it is estimated to cost five to 25 times more to recruit a new customer than it does to retain a current one (Gallo, 2014). The good news is that effective recovery from a service failure can potentially result in a more satisfied patient than if no service failure ever happened. This phenomenon is known as the *service recovery paradox* (Smith & Bolton, 1998).

One of the most landmark examples of the service recovery paradox in pharmacy occurred after the Chicago Tylenol Murders of 1982. In what still remains an unsolved mystery, seven people were killed by cyanide-laced Tylenol after someone tampered with capsules of Extra Strength Tylenol. After the crisis and subsequent recalls, McNeil Consumer Products responded quickly with numerous safety solutions for the product including new dosage forms and tamper-resistant packaging. McNeil's parent company, Johnson & Johnson, is still known for its "exemplar corporate responsibility" (Haberman, 2018).

Readers should be warned, however, that some research suggests that the service recovery paradox does not always occur, especially if the service failure is one of high criticality. It has been found that after a severe service failure, a customer may remain dissatisfied and engage in negative word-of-mouth about the pharmacy, even if the service recovery appears strong (Weun et al., 2004). A study of service failure and service recovery in community pharmacy also was unable to demonstrate that a service recovery paradox exists (Bunniran, 2010). It has been suggested that after a mistake in health care, it may be impossible to return to an "error-free state in the patient's mind" and that it may be "better not to fail than to have a great recovery from a service failure" (Bunniran, 2010, p. 86). *These findings, however, are not meant to imply that service recovery efforts should not be taken for every service failure, regardless of the level of criticality.* Even if a patient's satisfaction does not exceed the prefailure state after a service recovery, they still can potentially return to a level of satisfaction that exceeds postfailure levels. A study of service failure and service recovery in pharmacy suggests that assurance of correction of the problem and a $25 gift card can result in satisfaction ratings that are higher after the recovery than after the failure (Bunniran, 2010).

Another important consideration in the successful recovery of low- and mid-criticality service failures is empowering pharmacy employees to solve customer and patient problems. Empowering employees to do whatever it takes to make patients and customers happy with minimal oversight from managers and "red tape" requires training of employees, but can pay big dividends for customer service (Gonell, 2014). Readers should be cautioned that empowerment of pharmacy employees should be done with care and within state and federal regulations (e.g., pharmacy technicians should not be making decisions requiring clinical judgment).

Although she may feel differently, we can assume that the service failure that Sarah experienced in the chapter scenario was one of low criticality, and one that happens quite often in pharmacies. The general manager attempted to recover from the failure by explaining how the mistake was made. For Sarah, that was all that was needed. If this was not enough to remedy the situation, the manager could have used additional techniques to recover from the service failure, such as providing her with store credit. Every service failure is unique, and as such not all service recovery techniques are going to be effective for all patients and customers. Blanket policies for service recovery are not recommended. Rather, a variety of recovery efforts should be made available and staff empowered to utilize them as needed.

■ RECOVERING FROM HIGH-CRITICALITY SERVICE FAILURES IN THE PHARMACY

It should not be surprising that methods to recover from a high-criticality service failure in the pharmacy are different from recovering from low- and mid-criticality service failures. High-criticality service failures (also known as catastrophic prescription errors—see Chapters 10, 11, and 12 for more information about medication errors) in the pharmacy include those causing severe harm that is irreversible (Tipton et al., 2003). Relative to low- and mid-criticality service failures, high-criticality service failures are emotionally disturbing in addition to being potentially or actually life-threatening. The implications of a catastrophic error are without question, significant. Implications can include loss of trust in the pharmacist and/or pharmacy, injured public image, spread of negative word-of-mouth, legal action, board of pharmacy action, as well as loss of customers and profit. Not only are patients and their families affected, but so are a variety of other stakeholders such as employees, management, other patients, regulators, competitors, media, suppliers, accrediting bodies, the legal system, and stockholders/investors; making service recovery infinitely more complex (Pearson & Mitroff, 1993).

To the extent possible, victims of catastrophic medication errors are due just and equitable compensation for their suffering. Tipton (2009) outlines recommendations for response to a victim and his or her family after a catastrophic event:

- *Tell the truth* about what happened.
- Attempt to compensate for *emotional costs* with an apology.
- Attempt to compensate for *psychological costs* with assurances the system will be fixed.
- Attempt to compensate for costs related to *time, money,* and *inconvenience* through financial settlements.

Managing media relations after a catastrophic event requires thoughtful consideration due to audiences and stakeholders with different interests. For example, the general public will want to be informed because they are asking the question, "what if I went or had to go there?" They demand openness and forthrightness. Another group of stakeholders who have financial or other interests in the organization may be concerned about how their interests are affected and demand circumspection (Tipton et al., 2003). Six options have been detailed for dealing with the media, including (1) saying nothing at all, (2) denying or repudiating the charge, (3) claiming no responsibility for the event, (4) minimizing the impact of the event, (5) admitting the mistake and asking for forgiveness, and (6) any combination of the above (Benoit & Brinson, 1994).

It has been suggested that one way to deal with the media is to say nothing. However, the recommended approach is to be honest and open immediately while emphasizing the good your organization has done because this helps disarm the media. Doing the former puts you on the defensive and may further tarnish the organization's reputation (Tipton, 2009). In addition, the pharmacy organization should address how they are assuring that the same mistake will not happen again. One of the most poignant stories of a catastrophic medication error comes from the death of 7-year-old Ben Kolb in Martin Memorial Hospital in Stuart, Florida, in 1995. What makes this story impactful is the how the hospital administrators responded quickly and openly, providing compensation and assurances that this error would not happen again at their hospital or other hospitals who learned of their mistake (Belkin, 1997).

Then there is the question of whether or not to apologize. While apologies are good for the conscience, there may be concern that apologies may lead to legal consequences (Roberts, 2007). Some recommend ambiguity in announcements rather than an outright apology (Sellnow & Ulmer, 1995). For example, Jack in the Box in 1993 following reported deaths due to *Escherichia coli*–contaminated burgers stated: "Although it is unclear as to the source of an illness linked to undercooked beef, Jack in the Box announced today that it has taken measures to ensure [that] all menu items are prepared in accordance with an advisory issued yesterday by the Washington State Department of Health" (Sellnow & Ulmer, 1995, p. 142).

When it comes to consequences of a catastrophic service failure, there are four things to be considered; (1) a price cannot be put on human life, (2) no one can adequately compensate for the suffering that a catastrophic service failure causes, (3) no one can really understand the impact of the failure on the practitioners, and (4) the event cannot be undone (Tipton, 2009). However, Tipton (2009, p. 194) best summarizes what can (and should) be done as health care professionals:

The response can be open, caring, concerned, empathetic, and ethical. It is a test of character. The choice, ultimately, is between taking the high road and taking the expedient path of self-interest. As practitioners involved in the higher moral activity of health care as opposed to pure commerce, it is an obligation. The high road also will be good for business.

■ USING SOCIAL MEDIA TO RECOVER FROM SERVICE FAILURES IN PHARMACY

Social media (i.e., Facebook, Twitter, Instagram, You-Tube) are increasingly being used as a mechanism for not only providing customer service (particularly in the technology industries) but also recovering from service failures (Duris, 2018). Please see Chapter 25 to learn more about how pharmacies are using social media to market their goods and services and communicate with the public. Without question, the impact of social media on service failure incidents can be profound. First, social media facilitates how quickly news about a service failure can spread. Second, social media facilitates the ability of the general public to comment on matters, regardless of how much or little they may know about what actually took place. Both factors play a critical role in what the pharmacy will have to do to manage information and recover from the service failure. Pharmacies must use sound judgment when considering (1) whether to issue a public response via social media regarding a service failure, (2) how various social media outlets may best be used (i.e., should Twitter be used to enable more rapid patient feedback?), (3) what exactly will be communicated about the incident, and (4) when would be the best time to communicate.

While apologies (or, at least acknowledgment of a service failure) via social media are thought to be a sound practice and a good way to proactively deal with a service failure, it is important to decide whether it is more beneficial to only target those that experience the failure, or share what happened with a wider audience. While different situations may require different strategies and there is no one rule for how to handle an apology or service failure acknowledgment on social media, research findings suggest that social media apologies result in more positive outcomes for those affected by the service failure than those that are not. In other words, it is more likely that a company keeps a customer who experienced a service failure and receives a targeted apology than it is for the company to gain a customer who didn't experience a service failure, but yet still saw the apology (Manika et al., 2017).

The concern here is that general apologies may reach unintended audiences who are potential customers and thus possibly put a company's reputation at risk or negatively affect their market share, thus, "better targeting & audience control for a social media apology is necessary" (Manika et al., 2017).

■ OUTCOMES OF SERVICE FAILURE AND SERVICE RECOVERY

It should be no surprise that service failures can result in negative consequences for the pharmacy if not adequately addressed after they occur. Service failures and how well pharmacies recover from them have serious implications not only for patients and customers but also for the future of the business. The implications can be permanent. While many outcomes of service failure and recovery have been studied, including word-of-mouth communications (positive and negative), relationship quality, attitude toward the service provider, loyalty, repurchase intentions, service provide switching behaviors, and complaining behaviors, this section of the chapter focuses on satisfaction, word-of-mouth, trust, and customer retention.

Satisfaction

Satisfaction can be defined as the extent to which patients' needs and wants are met (Chui, 2012) or as meeting the expectations of the patient's or consumer's anticipation of how a service encounter should occur (Bunniran, 2010)*. In a study of hotel service

---

*A discussion of **patient satisfaction**, or the "degree to which a consumer perceives a health care good or service (or delivery of said good or service) to be valuable, beneficial, useful, appropriate, and effective" (von Waldner & Abel, 2011) is beyond the scope of this chapter. In the context of the economic, clinical, and humanistic outcomes (ECHO) model, patient satisfaction is a humanistic outcome. As a humanistic outcome, patient satisfaction is becoming an increasingly salient measure of pharmacy quality. However, patient satisfaction should be kept in mind during this discussion of customer service, as customer service is integral to patient satisfaction.

failures, it was found that a strong recovery can have a positive influence on satisfaction. However, satisfaction still remains negative after recovery if a more severe service failure occurs (Weun et al., 2004).

There are four perspectives of customer service including performance evaluation, affect-based assessment, equity-based assessment, and disconfirmation of expectations. *Performance evaluation* refers to determining satisfaction with characteristics of a particular service such as the physical environment of the pharmacy (e.g., convenient location, availability of parking, safety, cleanliness). *Affect-based assessment* refers to emotional reaction that a patient experiences as a result of the service (e.g., "I am delighted with this service"). *Equity-based assessment* refers to a patient's perceptions of fairness in the provision of service based on inputs and outputs and other individuals' service experiences (Schommer et al., 2002; von Waldner & Abel, 2011).

When assessing satisfaction, one of the most prevalent approaches is *disconfirmation of expectations* (Oliver, 1980; Spreng et al., 1996). With this approach, patients evaluate the gap between their expectations and perceptions of a service. If a patient perceives that a service outperforms their expectations, they will be satisfied (or delighted, if their expectations are significantly outperformed) with the service. Conversely, if the service does not meet their expectations, they will be dissatisfied. Their expectations may come from their own experiences with that particular service, other services like it, or the experiences of others (Oliver, 1980). The challenge from the service provider's perspective is that the expectations are dynamic—they can differ among patients and change constantly (Tipton, 2009). For example, if a patient enters the pharmacy with the expectation that their prescription will be filled in 20 minutes, and it is filled in 10 minutes, they will be satisfied (perhaps even delighted). However, if it takes 45 minutes to fill because the prescriber needs to be called about a problem, they may be dissatisfied. This is not unlike having one's satisfaction with a movie being governed to a large extent by the expectations of the movie they had before seeing it.

A similar theory, the *perceptions–expectations gap* conceptualization, suggests that patients also evaluate the gap between their expectations and perceptions of service *quality* (Parasuraman et al., 1985). An extension of this theory is the *zone of tolerance* (Zeithaml et al., 1993). This suggests that for patients, there is a level of service that is *desired* and a level of service that is *adequate*. For example, at the airport, a desired level of service would include on-time arrivals and departures, graciously helpful staff, and luggage that is never damaged or lost. Realistically, an adequate level of service might include 15-minute delays, staff that helps when asked, and the occasional lost bag (Tipton, 2009). The zone of tolerance includes any level of service between desired and adequate. Pharmacy managers should keep in mind that the zone of tolerance may be narrow or wide depending on the particular element of service. For example, the zone of tolerance for accurate prescription filling is likely narrow, and the zone of tolerance for pharmacy appearance may be wider (Tipton, 2009). Pharmacy managers also should be cognizant of the fact that patients can vary in their tolerance for service failure. In other words, some patients are less affected by, or more tolerant to service failures than others.

Word-of-Mouth

Word-of-mouth occurs when patients provide each other with information about products or services in a noncommercial way (Arndt, 1967). Word-of-mouth can be positive or negative. It has been suggested that unhappy customers may tell up to 20 people about a bad service experience (Mattila, 2001). The growth of web-based social networking through media such as Facebook and Twitter can result in an exponential dissemination of word-of-mouth by making it possible for one person to communicate their experience to hundreds, even thousands of people (Mangold & Faulds, 2009). This behavior is particularly notable among "millennials," or those born between 1980 and 2000, who are now thought to be the largest consumer demographic and the most digital-savvy (Zhang, 2017). In addition, in recent years, there has been an influx of websites and mobile applications or "apps" specializing in providing consumer reviews and ratings of products and services. For example, you may be familiar with websites such as "Zomato," "Yelp," and "Angie's List." Data suggest that negative word-of-mouth can be hard to mitigate even with strong service recovery. In a study of hotel service failures, it has been found that perceived severity of a service failure can increase negative word-of-mouth and negative effect on satisfaction. In cases of a severe service failure, even strong recovery efforts might not be enough to stop negative word-of-mouth (Weun et al., 2004). However, more recent research suggests that effective service recovery may actually create a sense of justice in the customer's mind. And, if the customer who experienced the service recovery is a loyal one, the manager can leverage this loyalty to impact positive word-of-mouth (Harun et al., 2018).

Trust

Just as with negative word-of-mouth, it similarly has been found that trust in the organization can be hard to regain even with strong recovery efforts in the event of severe service failures (Weun et al., 2004). In contrast, an encouraging finding was made with regard to service failures and service recovery in pharmacy. In the pharmacy setting, it appears that trust in the pharmacy and pharmacist remains relatively high, regardless of how severe a patient condition is (symptomatic cough or severe infection) or how serious the service failure is (partial fill or medication error); even before the service recovery is initiated (Bunniran, 2010).

Customer Retention

A single service failure is one of the primary reasons customers switch service providers (Keaveney, 1995). This is significant considering the aforementioned cost to recruit a new customer (Hart et al., 1990). Although previously cited research suggests that the *service recovery paradox* (exceeding pre-service failure satisfaction levels after a service recovery) may not exist, evidence suggests that service recovery efforts can be effective in retaining 75% of customers who

experience service failures (Hoffman et al., 1995). It should be noted here that the service recovery paradox does not necessarily have to exist to retain a customer. If a service recovery does not result in a service recovery paradox, it can likely result in satisfaction levels that exceed postfailure satisfaction. Consistent with other earlier findings (Hoffman et al., 1995; Weun et al., 2004), Bunniran (2010) found that in the case of more serious service failures, it is generally more difficult to execute an effective recovery.

■ COLLECTING FEEDBACK AND SATISFACTION RATINGS

Pharmacy satisfaction studies suggest that patients continue to raise the bar on their expectations, demanding higher levels of service and convenience. The good news is that pharmacies appear to be meeting or exceeding patients' expectations (Boehringer Ingelheim, 2016). Measuring patient satisfaction and feedback with the service they receive at the pharmacy requires time and effort, but is important for two reasons. First, it helps identify any gaps or deficits in service provision. Second, the pharmacy manager can implement strategies to improve customer service (von Waldner & Abel, 2011). However, one should not measure *only* patient satisfaction feedback. It is a good idea also to survey or interview staff to get their feedback about customer service in the pharmacy. They may see problems that the manager does not see, and they may even provide effective solutions (which, of course, boosts their own morale). When surveying patients, a variety of methods can be used, such as web-based surveys, written questionnaires, telephone surveys, focus groups, or face-to-face interviews. The best method chosen depends on the type of patients or customers being surveyed (young, elderly, low literacy, etc.) and the type of information, or data needed. A combination of methods might be required (Leland & Bailey, 2006).

Keep in mind that nearly every retailer (especially large retailers) is currently offering surveys with nearly all, or every transaction. This can result in a phenomenon known as "customer satisfaction survey fatigue" (Ryan, 2012). Therefore, be judicious in your surveying of patients, and remember that incentivizing patients for participation is important, if not necessary, to avoid survey pitfalls such as nonresponse bias. Nonresponse bias can be particularly problematic when you primarily receive survey responses from patients who had either exceptionally good or exceptionally bad experiences at your pharmacy (Brogle, 2013).

■ THE EMPLOYEE'S PERSPECTIVE

If you have ever wondered why a service associate in a retail establishment seems to care so little about their job, there may be good reason why they do not. Ideally, pharmacy employees should be enthusiastic and passionate about what they do. There is no question that employees who are passionate about what they do will take great care of patients; however, not all employees are going to display such enthusiasm. Table 26-4 outlines fifteen items that are critical for pharmacy managers to remember when wanting to create a climate for the provision of good customer service to patients by their employees. One of the most important points of the information in Table 26-4 is the idea of ensuring employees' quality of work life and job satisfaction. Researchers in customer service consistently have found that employee satisfaction and customer satisfaction are positively correlated (Harter et al., 2002; Wangenheim et al., 2007). The stressful environments of pharmacies have been found to be related to decreased job satisfaction in pharmacy technicians (Desselle & Holmes, 2007). However, job stress can be mitigated by supervisor support, which, along with employer support is related positively to job satisfaction (Desselle & Holmes, 2007). These findings lend credence to pharmacy managers providing a supportive and quality work environment for their employees for not only the provision of customer service, but for the good of their employees.

Table 26-4.	Developing a Staff That Provides Good Customer Service

Recommendation

Hire employees with a caring attitude

Hire employees who are problem solvers

Reinforce customer service in employee training and orientation

Monitor employees' customer service and coach deficiencies

Empower employees to solve patient and customer problems

Reward employees who make special efforts to please patients customers

Get feedback from employees

Support wide-ranging company knowledge

Make customer satisfaction a condition of satisfactory employee performance

Encourage active listening

Model good customer service as a manager

Model patience and empathy as a manager

Make customer service everybody's job

Ensure employees' quality of work life and job satisfaction

Treat employees fairly

Data from Bowen, 1999; Monych, 2019; Umiker, 1998; Wangenheim, 2007.

Another phenomenon that employees experience (and pharmacy managers should be aware of) is emotional labor. *Emotional labor* describes the process of modifying the emotions you *feel* or the emotions you *express* to meet the goals of your organization (Grandey, 2000). For example, a customer lashing out at a gate agent in an airport over a cancelled flight may induce an emotional response in the agent (such as yelling back at or insulting the customer). Because this would not be a desired response for his or her airline (and may result in disciplinary action or termination of the agent) the agent may choose to regulate her emotions (Holmes, 2008). There are two types of emotional labor. If the gate agent modifies the emotions she *feels* about the situation (e.g., feels empathy for the customer and the inconvenience the cancelled flight has caused) she is undergoing *deep acting*. If the gate agent does not really change her feelings about the situation, but rather, puts on a "mask" to simply change her expression, this is known as *surface acting* (Hochschild, 1983). The pharmacist in the chapter scenario is a good example of someone *not* undergoing emotional labor. He was agitated, frustrated, and angry. He did not modify what he felt or what he expressed to respond to Sarah more appropriately, and it certainly escalated the situation.

The phenomenon of emotional labor has been studied in pharmacists and pharmacy technicians, and a number of things have been observed. First, pharmacists and pharmacy technicians' perception that they have role overload (feeling that there is too much needed to accomplish at work), appears positively related to emotional labor (particularly, surface acting) (Holmes et al., 2009a; Holmes & Bunniran, 2011). In addition, surface acting appears to be related to negative outcomes in pharmacists, such as reduced job satisfaction, intentions to leave their pharmacy, and emotional exhaustion (in technicians, surface acting has been shown to predict intentions to leave their job) (Holmes et al., 2009b; Holmes & Bunniran, 2011). In these same studies, pharmacists and technicians did not seem to undergo deep acting, nor did deep acting seem to be related to other work variables. This is not surprising, as pharmacists may feel that deep acting requires more effort than surface acting and therefore not use it as much (Holmes, 2008).

There are important considerations for managers with regard to emotional labor. First, despite the seemingly negative consequences of emotional labor, it is not likely to go away and it most likely should not. While some employees will a have very high tolerance for difficult patients and never have to undergo emotional labor, not everyone does, and there always will be "difficult" patients. It is not acceptable to pharmacy organizations, or to the profession of pharmacy to act out negative feelings toward patients like the

pharmacist did in the scenario. What can pharmacy managers do about the negative consequences? It has been demonstrated that coworker social support (Abraham, 1998) and perceived organizational support (Duke et al., 2009) can mitigate the negative effect of emotional labor on job satisfaction (although, organizational support has not been shown to do this for pharmacy technicians [Holmes & Bunniran, 2011]). Pharmacy chain managers and administrators are encouraged to implement various support mechanisms to mitigate the negative effects of emotional labor (Holmes et al., 2009b).

How far can the way in which you manage your employees and ensure their quality of work life go when it comes to good customer service? Some companies' extraordinary reputations are a result of the legendary customer service they provide as a function of their employees. Probably the most prominent example is Southwest Airlines. Southwest is well known for keeping fares low, getting passengers and their baggage to their destinations on time, and ensuring that passengers enjoy their flight (and even have fun!) (Freiberg & Freiberg, 1996). How do they do it? It is Southwest's policy that employees are first, and customers are second. Their philosophy is that customers will always be treated well because employees are treated well and fairly. They hire only employees who are passionate about people and who fit Southwest's mission. They do their best to ensure that employees' quality of life is exceptional. They give employees the authority to solve customer problems on their own, thus resolving problems faster and providing those employees with a greater sense of autonomy (Freiberg & Freiberg, 1996).

Another company that is legendary for its customer service as a result of employee management is Nordstrom. Nordstrom has been described as having a cult-like culture among its employees (Collins & Porras, 1994). Employees emphatically claim that it is the best job they have ever had. At Nordstrom, employee empowerment (see recommendation 4 in Table 26-4) is job number one. Nordstrom one rule for employees is to "use your good judgment in all situations." There are no other rules for employees. As a result, employees at Nordstrom ("Nordies," as they are called) are said to have (Collins & Porras, 1994):

- Ironed a newly purchased shirt for a customer who needed it for a meeting that afternoon
- Cheerfully wrapped gifts a customer bought at Macy's
- Warmed customer's cars in the winter while they finished shopping
- Personally knitted a shawl for an elderly customer to be of a length that did not get caught in her wheel chair
- Delivered party clothes at the last minute to a frantic hostess
- Refunded money for a set of tire chains (which are not sold at Nordstrom)

Granted, the highly regulated nature of the pharmacy profession and its associated risk makes the Southwest Airlines and Nordstrom examples somewhat extreme and not necessarily appropriate for the pharmacy profession. However, it does speak to the influence employee treatment and development can have on the provision of customer service.

■ DEALING WITH PATIENT—COMPLAINTS

Customer complaints are a natural part of the service industry no matter how hard managers and employees try to ensure good customer service. Some patients will never complain no matter how poor the service they receive, while others will do nothing *but* complain. Regardless, few things irritate customers more than not having a venue to lodge complaints, or concerns (Leland & Bailey, 2006). Most likely they will find another venue for their complaints (like Facebook or Twitter) if they cannot use their pharmacy as a venue. While stressful and challenging, complaints should not be perceived negatively but rather as a way to improve the service the pharmacy provides (Leland & Bailey, 2006). It is important not to take a defensive approach to complaining patients, as this may hinder employees' and managers' ability to hear what they are

saying and think about ways to improve the provision of service in the pharmacy. Leland and Bailey (2006, p. 250) suggest that complaints can "prove to be a great source of information, innovation, and inspiration." That is because you can discover problems you did not know existed (which may be frustrating other customers) or get ideas for new products or services. Thus, the complaints ultimately help retain current customers, recover customers thought to have been lost, or even gain new ones (Leland & Bailey, 2006).

Leland and Bailey (2006) provide eight principles for constructively dealing with customer complaints.

- View complaints as gifts.
- Make it easy for customers to complain.
- Identify the elements of the complaint.
- Thank customers for complaining.
- Sincerely apologize.
- Fix the problem.
- Practice prevention.
- Follow-up.

■ DEALING WITH "DIFFICULT" PATIENTS

Working in a pharmacy or other service environment can present challenges, including having to deal with "difficult" patients. But rather than think of these patients as "difficult," it is more important to keep in mind *why* patients may be unhappy. As noted in the beginning of the chapter, (1) patients likely view their medications as "negative goods" (Kolassa, 1997), (2) patients may already come in with negative perceptions of the price of medicines, their other health care professionals, or their insurance plan, which can sometimes be translated to the pharmacy and to pharmacists, and (3) patients may be symptomatic and not feeling well. It is also important to reinforce that patients and customers will have varying perceptions of the severity of a failure, which may not coincide at all with employees' own perceptions of the severity of failure. Moreover, even after employing the principles of good customer service and ensuring that standards for customer service are met, there can still be the occasional patient who is not happy. While it is very rare, some patients may even become threatening or violent. If a patient's behavior appears to be escalating out of control, staff in your pharmacy should be trained to call security or dial 911. Such behavior can result in serious consequences and should never be tolerated in the pharmacy setting. For the rest of the dissatisfied patients and customers, Leland and Bailey (2006) suggest a six-step process.

Step 1: Let the customer vent. When patients and customers are upset, their priorities are to vent (not necessarily to the person who is at fault), and to solve their problem. Service providers are encouraged to let the patient or customer express his or her feelings without interruption. Trying to calm them down can anger them further.

Step 2: Avoid getting trapped in a negative filter. This occurs when employees' negative thoughts about a patient or customer bleed into their conversation with them. For example, a patient may come in for a refill not realizing that they do not have a refill authorization left. When a pharmacist informs the patient that he or she will need to call the doctor to get the refill authorization, they may respond with frustration toward the pharmacist because of the delay. A negative filter (perceptions that the patient for customer is being unreasonable) may result in a response by the pharmacist such as, "Look, you are the one who came in with no refills left." Leland and Bailey (2006) suggest replacing this "negative filter" with a "service filter." Pharmacy employees should ask themselves, "What does this customer need, and how can I provide it?" This will change an employee's focus from anger and frustration (and a possible argument) to that of problem solving.

Step 3: Express empathy to the customer. Expressing empathy allows employees to recognize and appreciate a patient's or customer's feelings. But, employees should not sympathize, or over-identify with the patient's or customer's feelings.

Step 4: Begin active problem solving. Once the patient or customer has aired their grievances, employees can begin active problem solving by gathering additional information and double-checking the facts of the situation.

Step 5: Mutually agree on the solution. In this stage, employees should work with the customer to come up with an acceptable solution to the problem. By doing this, employees are meeting the patient's or customer's requirement for control (see Table 26-2).

Step 6: Follow-up. Following up to make sure that the solution worked can go a long way with patients and customers. If the solution did not work, this is the employee's opportunity to try again.

Looking back at the scenario at the beginning of the chapter, how did the general manager approach Steps 1–6? How did the pharmacist approach Steps 1–3?

■ PREVENTING PATIENT CONFLICT AND COMPLAINTS

When it comes to dealing with "difficult" patients, sometimes prevention is the best medicine. Avoid using phrases and language that make patient or customer feel like an adversary or that express disinterest on your part. For example, phrases such as "I don't know," "no," "that's not my job," "you're right; this stinks," "that's not my fault," "you need to talk to my manager," "you want it by when?," "calm down," "I'm busy right now," and "call me back," can demonstrate to patients that you are not willing to help, and can sometimes be a catalyst to conflict (Leland & Bailey, 2006). However, phrases such as "I'll find out," "what I can do is…," "this is who can help you," "I understand your frustration," "let's see what we can do about this," "I can help you," "I'll try my best," "I'm sorry," "I'll be with you in just a moment," and "I will call you back," can demonstrate to the patient or customer that you are willing to go the extra mile, and create a positive image in the mind of the patient (Leland & Bailey, 2006).

In addition to avoiding certain phrases and language, also important, if not more important, is avoiding body language, tone of voice, and other nonverbal behaviors that can express similar negativity. Body language and tone of voice can say a lot, even if nothing is said at all. In fact, it has been shown that 55% of what is learned from others comes from body language, 33% comes from tone of voice, and 7% comes from actual spoken words (Leland & Bailey, 2006). For example, in a restaurant a customer might request from the server that their hamburger come without mayo or onion, with extra pickle, and no salt on the fries. The server might roll her eyes in exasperation. She is connoting that the customer has annoyed her with his request. Ways in which eye contact, facial expressions, nodding, hand gestures, and personal space are used can drastically affect the patient or customer encounter and communicate to them whether an employee is engaged in helping him or her, is uninterested in helping or sees them as an adversary (Leland & Bailey, 2006).

Body language might have played a significant role in the scenario presented at the beginning of the chapter. The pharmacy manager's look toward the patient was a puzzling one. He was simply confused and perplexed. However, Sarah did not interpret it that way. She interpreted his look to be judgmental. In addition, the pharmacy manager did not look at her directly while explaining the situation. This may have sent the message that he did not care about her situation, even if he did (Leland & Bailey, 2006).

Tone of voice also can send a message to the customer. A flat, monotone voice suggests boredom or disinterest in the patient or customer; a slow speed and low pitch suggests that an employee wants to be left alone; a high-pitched emphatic voice suggests enthusiasm; an abrupt speed and loud tone suggests an employee is too busy for the patient; and, high pitch and drawn out speed expresses disbelief in what the patient is saying. In addition, inflection (wave-like movement of highs and lows in the pitch of your voice), stress on words, breathing, volume, and pacing can influence communication to the patient (Leland & Bailey, 2006).

■ REVISITING THE SCENARIO

Sarah's experience at the pharmacy is probably not an unusual one. Pharmacies get hectic, and misunderstandings occur and escalate due to a patient's fragile state and the communication methods of the staff. The concepts from this chapter, such as the principles for ensuring good customer service, standards that customers use to evaluate services, how to help and motivate employees to provide good customer service, and how to prevent customer conflict are worth remembering. Despite a provider's best efforts, service failures likely will still occur. After they do, every effort should be made to genuinely compensate for a patient's loss, however, big or small. Sarah seemed satisfied with the information provided to her by the general manager. Will she return to the pharmacy? Will she still trust the pharmacist? Will she tell her friends about what happened? In the end, the high road will be good for business.

■ QUESTIONS FOR FURTHER DISCUSSION

1. Describe a time when you, as a customer, received great customer service, and bad customer service. Why was it great or bad, and how did it make you feel?
2. What kind of impact has social media like Facebook, Twitter, Instagram, and YouTube had on the provision and evaluation of customer service?
3. How do Leland and Bailey's (2006) steps 1 to 3 in dealing with difficult customers compare and contrast to the concept of emotional labor?

REFERENCES

Abraham R. 1998. Emotional dissonance in organizations: antecedents, consequents, and moderators. *Genet Soc and Gen Psych Mono* 124(2):229.

Arndt J. 1967. Role of product-related conversations in the diffusion of a new product. *J Market Res* 4:291.

Austin Z, Gregory PA, Martin JC. 2006. Characterizing the professional relationships of community pharmacists. *Res Soc Admin Pharm* 2:533.

Belkin L. 1997. The New York Times. How can we save the next victim? Available at http://www.nytimes.com/1997/06/15/magazine/how-can-we-save-the-next-victim.html? pagewanted = 1. Accessed January 2, 2019.

Bell CR, Zemke RE. 1987. Service breakdown, the road to recovery. *Manag Rev* 76(10):32.

Benoit W, Brinson S. 1994. Apologies are not enough. *Commun Q* 42(1):75.

Bitner MJ, Booms BH, Tetreault MS. 1990. The service encounter: Diagnosing favorable and unfavorable events. *J Mark* 54:71.

Boehringer Ingelheim. 2008. Pharmacy Satisfaction Digest (on-line). Available at http://www.rx-edge.com/research%20pdfs/PharmacySatisfactionDigest_2008.pdf. Accessed January 2, 2019.

Boehringer Ingelheim. 2016. Pharmacy Satisfaction Full Industry Report November 2016. Available at https://www.pharmacysatisfaction.com/sites/default/files/pdfs/Pharmacy_Satisfaction_2016_Report_Full_Report_0.pdf. Accessed January 2, 2019.

Bowen DE, Gilliland SW, Folger R. 1999. HRM and service fairness: How being fair with employees spills over to customers. *Organ Dyn* 27(3):7.

Brogle R. 2013. How to avoid the evils within customer satisfaction surveys. Available at http://www.isixsigma.com/methodology/voc-customer-focus/how-to-avoid-the-evils-within-customer-satisfaction-surveys/. Accessed January 2, 2019.

Bunniran S. 2010. *Patient Service Experiences in Community Pharmacy: An Examination of Health Criticality in Service Failures and Service Recovery Incidents and Its Influence on Trust, Satisfaction, Repurchase Intentions and Word-of-Mouth [doctoral dissertation]*. Oxford: The University of Mississippi.

Bunniran S, McCaffrey DJ, Bentley JP. 2010. Service failure and service recovery incidents in community pharmacy. *J Am Pharm Assoc* 50(2):261.

Chui MA. 2012. Outcomes evaluation of pharmacy operations. In Desselle S, Zgarrick D, Alston G (eds.) *Pharmacy Management*. New York: McGraw-Hill, p. 142.

Collins J, Porras J. 1994. *Built to Last*. New York: Harper-Business, pp. 115–121.

ConsumerMedSafety.org. 2012. Prescription speed-ups leading to errors. Available at https://www.consumermedsafety.org/medication-safety-articles/item/596-prescription-speed-ups-leading-to-errors. Accessed March 11, 2019.

Desselle SP, Holmes ER. 2007. Structural model of certified pharmacy technicians' job satisfaction. *J Am Pharm Assoc* 47:58.

Duke A, Goodman J, Treadway D, Breland J. 2009. Perceived organizational support as a moderator of emotional labor-outcomes relationships. *J Appl Soc Psychol* 39:1013.

Duris S. 2018. Is Your Social Media Customer Service Helping or Hurting Your Customer Experience? Available at: https://www.icmi.com/resources/2018/Is-Your-Social-Media-Customer-Service-Helping-CX. Accessed March 11, 2019.

Freiberg K, Freiberg J. 1996. *Nuts! Southwest Airlines' Crazy Recipe for Business and Personal Success*. New York: Broadway Books, pp. 282–295.

Friedman S. 2010. Customer Service Manager. At your service: The ten commandments of customer service. Available at https://www.customerservicemanager.com/at-your-service-the-ten-commandments-of-great-customer-service/. Accessed January 2, 2019.

Gallo A. 2014. Harvard Business Review. The value of keeping the right customers. Available at https://hbr.org/2014/10/the-value-of-keeping-the-right-customers. Accessed January 2, 2019.

Gamble KH. 2011. Pharmacy Times. Do speedy prescription guarantees compromise safety? Available at http://www.pharmacytimes.com/web-exclusives/Do-Speedy-Prescription-Guarantees-Compromise-Safety. Accessed January 2, 2019.

Gonell D. 2014. Empowering your employees to make decisions. Available at http://www.trainingmag.com/empowering-your-employees-make-decisions. Accessed January 2, 2019.

Grandey A. 2000. Emotion regulation in the workplace: A new way to conceptualize emotional labor. *J Occup Health Psychol* 5:95.

Haberman C. 2018. How an unsolved mystery changed the way we take pills. Available at https://www.nytimes.com/2018/09/16/us/tylenol-acetaminophen-deaths.html. Accessed March 11, 2019.

Hart CW, Heskett JL, Sasser WE. 1990. The profitable art of service recovery. *Harv Bus Rev* 68:148.

Harter JK, Schmidt FL, Hayes TL. 2002. Business-unit-level relationship between employee satisfaction, employee engagement, and business outcomes: A meta-analysis. *J Appl Psychol* 87(2):268.

Harun A, Rokonuzzaman M, Prybutok G, Prybutok V. 2018. How to influence consumer mind set: A perspective from service recovery. *J Retailing Consum Serv* 42:65.

Hochschild A. 1983. *The Managed Heart: Commercialization of Human Feeling*. Berkley, CA: University of California Press, pp. 48–49.

Hoffman KD, Kelley SW, Rotalsky HM. 1995. Tracking service failures and employee recovery efforts. *J Serv Market* 9(2):49.

Holmes E. 2008. *The Role of Emotional Dissonance as an Affective State on the Emotional Labor Process of Retail Chain Pharmacists [doctoral dissertation]*. Oxford: The University of Mississippi.

Holmes E, Bentley, Bouldin A, Garner D. 2009a. The role of affective emotional dissonance as an affective state on the emotional labor process of retail chain pharmacists. *Am Pharm Assoc* 49(2):284.

Holmes E, Bentley, Bouldin A, Garner D. 2009b. The impact of emotional labor on retail chain pharmacists work life outcomes. *J Am Pharm Assoc* 49(2):277–278.

Holmes E, Bunniran S. 2011. Community pharmacy technicians' emotional labor and resultant work life outcomes. *J Am Pharm Assoc* 51(2):300.

Johnston R. 1995. Service failure and recovery: Impact, attributes, and process. *Adv Ser Mark Manage* 4:211.

Keaveney S. 1995. Customer switching behavior in service industries: An exploratory study. *J Mark* 59:71.

Kelley SW, Hoffman KD, Davis MA. 1993. A typology of retail failures and recoveries. *J Retail* 69(4):429.

Kolassa EM. 1997. Pricing, politics, and problems-a pricing philosophy. In Kolassa EM (ed.) *Elements of Pharmaceutical Pricing*. Binghamton, NY: Pharmaceutical Products Press, pp. 28–31.

Leland K, Bailey K. 2006. *Customer Service for Dummies*. Hoboken, NJ: Wiley Publishing, Inc.

Mangold W, Faulds D. 2009. Social media: The new hybrid element of the promotion mix. *Bus Horiz* 52:357.

Manika D, Papagiannidis S, Bourlakis M. 2017. Understanding the effects of a social media service failure apology: A comparative study of customers vs. potential customers. *Int J Info Manage* 37(3):214–228.

Mattila A. 2001. The effectiveness of service recovery in a multi-industry setting. *J Serv Mark* 15:583.

Monych B. 2019. 8 ways to coach employees to better customer service. Available at https://www.insperity.com/blog/better-customer-service/. Accessed March 11, 2019.

Obarski AM. 2010. Customer Service Manager. Customers are us! The golden rule of customer service. Available at http://www.customerservicemanager.com/customers-are-us-the-golden-rule-of-customer-service/. Accessed January 2, 2019.

Oliver R. 1980. A cognitive model of the antecedents and consequences of satisfaction decisions. *J Mark Res* 17(4):460.

Parasuraman A, Zeithaml VA, Berry LL. 1985. A conceptual model of service quality and its implications for future research. *J Mark* 49:41.

Parasuraman A, Zeithaml VA, Berry LL. 1988. SERVQUAL: A multiple-item scale for measuring consumer perceptions of service quality. *J Retail* 64(1):12.

Pearson CM, Mitroff II. 1993. From crisis prone to crisis pre-pared: A framework for crisis management. *Acad Manage Exec* 7(1):48.

Reichheld F. 2001. *The Loyalty Effect: The Hidden Force Behind Growth, Profits, and Lasting Value*. Brighton: Harvard Business School Press:xi.

Roberts RG. 2007. The art of apology; When and how to seek forgiveness. *Fam Pract Manage* 14(7):44.

Ryan T. 2012. Consumer Satisfaction Survey Fatigue? Available at http://www.retailwire.com/discussion/15841/consumer-satisfaction-survey-fatigue. Accessed January 2, 2019.

Schommer JC, Wenzel RG, Kucukarslan SN. 2002. Evaluation of pharmacists' services for hospital inpatients. *Am J Health Syst Pharm* 59:1632.

Schweikhart SB, Strasser S, Kennedy MR. 1993. Service recovery in health service organizations. *Hosp Health Serv Admin* 38(1):3.

Sellnow T, Ulmer R. 1995. Ambiguous argument as advocacy in organizational crisis communication. *Arg Advoc* 31:138.

Simone A. 2014. National chain pharmacies: Expanding community care. Available at http://www.pharmacytimes.com/publications/career/2014/pharmacycareers_fall2014/national-chain-pharmacies-expanding-community-care/P-1. Accessed January 2, 2019.

Smith A, Bolton R. 1998. An experimental investigation of customer reactions to service failure and recovery encounters: Paradox or peril. *J Serv Res* 1(1):65.

Spreng R, MacKenzie S, Olshavsky R. 1996. A reexamination of the determinants of consumer satisfaction. *J Mark* 60:15.

Tipton DJ. 2000. Service recovery in pharmacies. *J Pharm Mark Manage* 13(3):71.

Tipton DJ. 2009. Customer service. In: Desselle S, Zgarrick D (eds.) *Pharmacy Management*. New York: McGraw-Hill.

Tipton DJ, Giannetti VJ, Kristofik JM. 2003. Managing the aftermath of medication errors: Managed care's role. *J Am Pharm Assoc* 43:662.

Umiker W. 1998. *Management Skills for the New Health Care Supervisor*. Gaithersburg, MD: Aspen Publishers, Inc.

von Waldner TK, Abel SR. 2011. Achieving and measuring patient satisfaction. In: Chisholm-Burns M, Vaillancourt A, Shepherd M (eds.) *Pharmacy Management, Leadership, Marketing, and Finance*. Sudbury, MA: Jones and Bartlett.

Wangenheim F, Evanschitzky H, Wunderlich M. 2007. Does the employee-customer satisfaction link hold for all employee groups? *J Bus Res* 60:690.

Webster C, Sundaram DS. 1998. Service consumption criticality in failure recovery. *J Bus Res* 41:153.

Weun S, Beatty SE, Jones MA. 2004. The impact of service failure severity on service recovery evaluations and post-recovery relationships. *J Serv Market* 18(2):133.

Zeithaml VA, Berry LL, Parasuraman A. 1993. The nature and determinants of customer expectations of service. *J Acad Market Sci* 21(1):1.

Zhang V. 2017. Salesforce Blog. 6 ways millennials are redefining customer service. Available at https://www.salesforce.com/blog/2017/08/how-millennials-are-redefining-customer-service. Accessed January 3, 2018.

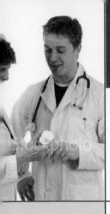

27

SUPPLY CHAIN MANAGEMENT

Perry L. Fri, Susan E. Higgins, and Rachel Sullivan

About the Authors: Perry L. Fri is the Healthcare Distribution Alliance's (HDA) executive vice president of Industry Relations, Membership & Education and chief operating officer of the HDA Research Foundation. At HDA, Fri is responsible for the direction, supervision, and development of industry initiatives that facilitate improved business processes and operational efficiencies in the health care supply chain. Fri currently serves on the Board of Directors for Healthcare Ready, a 501(c)(3) organization established to help public and private sector stakeholders across the pharmaceutical supply chain prepare for (and maintain operations during) disasters. Prior to joining HDA, Fri served as vice president of Industry Relations and Program Development for the Health Industry Distributors Association (HIDA). He holds a BA in history from the University of Maryland.

Susan E. Higgins is an independent management and strategy consultant who serves clients in the pharmaceutical industry, including pharmaceutical companies, federal public health agencies, hospitals, consumer health companies, and health care industry associations. Higgins specializes in supply chain and operations strategy, helping clients design and implement end-to-end supply chain strategies which enable profitable growth. Prior to her independent consulting work, Higgins was a principal with Strategy & based in New York. She holds an MBA in finance and entrepreneurship from New York University's Stern School of Business, and a BS in logistics and marketing from The Ohio State University.

Rachel Sullivan is a project manager for the HDA Research Foundation. She is responsible for managing all research projects and events within the Foundation. She holds a BS from Miami University.

■ LEARNING OBJECTIVES

After completing this chapter, readers should be able to

1. Explain the importance, both financially and operationally, of supply chain management: demand planning, procurement, and inventory management to a pharmacy.
2. List demand management, inventory management, and procurement objectives for a pharmacy.

557

3. Describe procurement and carrying costs for a pharmacy.
4. Calculate inventory turnover rates (ITORs) and use this information to make purchasing and inventory control decisions.
5. Describe three methods of inventory management.
6. Describe the role of technology in improving inventory management in pharmacies.
7. Describe the importance of supply chain integrity, and a pharmacy's role in ensuring that its supply chain has integrity.

■ SCENARIO

Marie Rodriguez, PharmD, recently stepped into a new role as the pharmacist-in-charge (PIC) of the Springfield location of Community Pharmacy, a chain pharmacy with 25 stores. Marie was successful as a pharmacist at another pharmacy in the Community Pharmacy network for 3 years. After a couple of weeks at the new location, she is preparing for a business review meeting with the Community Pharmacy district manager. Her new pharmacy has been underperforming financially, and customer satisfaction levels are lower relative to the other pharmacies in the chain. Marie has been tasked with identifying the causes and creating a plan to improve the pharmacy's performance. After reviewing the pharmacy's reports, and meeting with the other pharmacists at the pharmacy, Marie has identified the following challenges:

- The pharmacy has experienced stock outs on several products in the last couple of weeks. While the products can be available as soon as the next day, Marie is concerned about losing customers who may become frustrated with the delays and making multiple trips to the pharmacy.
- Community Pharmacy is currently in compliance with the Drug Supply Chain Security Act (DSCSA). The pharmacy only orders drugs from an authorized trading partner and is checking that the transaction information received from their distributor matches the drugs that are received. However, the pharmacists have expressed concerns about future DSCSA requirements for data serialization, and are uncertain of Community Pharmacy's plan to support these requirements.

As the Community Pharmacy corporate office management team prepares for the upcoming fiscal year, it is also in the middle of renewing its contract with its current distributor. Marie has been asked to help the management team with the proposal review and negotiation process, and is in the process of reviewing proposal information from Vendor XYZ and the Current Distributor (see Table 27-1).

■ CHAPTER QUESTIONS

1. What are the three key components of the supply chain, and how do they interact to balance supply and demand? Why is this important?
2. How does inventory management affect a pharmacy's profit margins and cash flow?
3. How does the ITOR indicate how efficient a pharmacy is at managing their inventory investment?
4. What are the advantages of joining a group purchasing organization (GPO)?
5. How has technology improved a pharmacy's ability to manage the pharmacy's supply chain?
6. What is supply chain integrity? What role does a pharmacy's pharmaceutical distributor play in ensuring this integrity? What role do the pharmacy and pharmacists play in ensuring this integrity?
7. What is the DSCSA? In what way will it impact pharmacy operations in the future? What are the assumed benefits to patients?

Table 27-1.   Scenario Wholesaler Comparisons

I. Price on Two Drug Products	XYZ Distributor Drug		Current Distributor	
Product (No. of Bottles per Month)	Unit Price	Ext. Price	Unit Price	Ext. Price
Zyprexa 5 mg 30s (9)	$359	$3,231	$370	$3,330
Atacand 8 mg 30s (19)	$95	$1,805	$105	$1,995
Total		$5,036		$5,325
II. Cash discounts	Weekly EFT: 1.25% Weekly prepay EFT: 1.50%		EFT every 7 days: 1.25% EFT every 15 days: 1.00%	
III. Inventory management systems	Perpetual inventory system; provide inventory management reports		Perpetual inventory system, internet accessible; provide inventory management reports	
IV. Return-goods policy	If the merchandise is saleable and returned within 180 days of purchase date, wholesaler will provide a 100% credit. If it is returned after 180 days, only 85% credit will be given. Partial bottles, products that are 3 months after date of expiration, and other selected products are nonreturnable.		Merchandise that is returned within 30 days of invoice date will be credited 100% of original invoice amount (assuming it is in saleable condition). If the merchandise is returned after 30 days and is in saleable condition, 75% of the original invoice amount will be credited. Partial bottles, controlled/schedule II products, and other selected merchandise cannot be returned.	

■ INTRODUCTION TO THE PHARMACEUTICAL SUPPLY CHAIN

The pharmaceutical supply chain is a large, complex global network of manufacturers, distributors, and health care providers, each of whom performs a unique and vital role in the health care system. These entities collaborate in a global supply chain to ensure that life-saving pharmaceutical products are manufactured and distributed to providers to meet patient needs. While pharmacists may not interact with all tiers in the supply chain at a global level, it is important to understand the pharmaceutical supply chain

and how it works because issues and events at a global level can and do impact practicing pharmacists and their patients at a local level.

The pharmaceutical supply chain begins with *manufacturers*, who produce the drugs after long periods of research and development, testing, and eventually product launches. The majority of these products flow through either *traditional distributors*, the high-volume supply chain that handles traditional prescription pharmaceuticals, or through *specialty distributors*, a part of the supply chain that addresses many of the unique needs of specialty pharmaceutical products. *Health care providers*—from large hospitals to smaller clinics, physician practices, and pharmacies—order and receive drugs from distributors, or in some cases, directly from the manufacturer.

The core function of the pharmaceutical supply chain is to provide efficient, safe, and reliable access to pharmaceutical drugs. But supply chain partners also offer additional value-added services. Manufacturers offer health care providers product education, patient support programs, and support with navigating insurance reimbursement. Distributors offer health care providers financing, inventory management, patient education, and many other value-added services. This supply chain is a network of relationships and interactions that support the increasingly complex environment of today's health care system. Figure 27-1 shows the flow of goods and exchanges of value in the US pharmaceutical supply chain from manufacturers, through distributors, providers, and ultimately to patients.

A pharmacist's level of interaction with the other supply chain partners will depend on their role and the type of health care organization in which they work.

■ UNDERSTANDING KEY SUPPLY CHAIN FUNCTIONS

The pharmacy manager must understand how three key supply chain management functions work to properly manage the demand side and supply side of the pharmacy. An effective pharmacy supply chain management program balances demand and supply with inventory. The pharmacy manager will understand consumer demand for goods and services and ensure that there is inventory on hand to meet the demand at the time of need. At the same time, the pharmacy manager will be mindful of the various costs of inventories and maintain inventory levels that are aligned with both the revenue and the cost targets of the pharmacy (Table 27-2).

From a financial perspective, effective supply chain management decreases the cost of goods sold (COGS) and operational expenses, resulting in increased gross margins and net profits. For example, saving $100 on the purchase of unneeded prescription drugs will increase the gross margin and net profit by

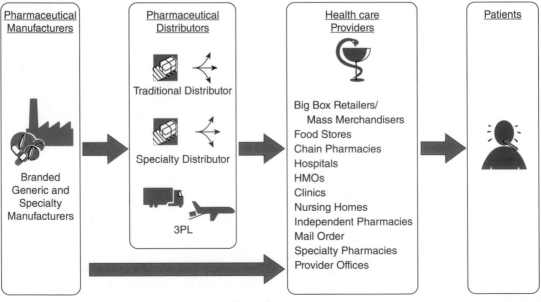

Figure 27-1. The pharmaceutical supply chain in the United States. (Data from 2018 Speciality Pharmaceutical Distribution Facts, Figures and Trends. Copyright © 2018 by the Healthcare Distribution Alliance (HDA) Research Foundation.)

Table 27-2.   Supply Chain Management Functions

Demand Management	• Methodology used to generate, revise, and improve a demand forecast of the products and services that the organization will provide to customers.
Inventory Management	• Methodology used to control inventory and stock, including controlling inventory levels and overseeing ordering and storage of inventory. The objective is to meet sales and customer service levels at an optimal cost.
Procurement: Sourcing and Purchasing	• *Procurement* includes the functions of buying products and services for a specific business purpose. • *Sourcing* is the methodology used to identify and manage the right product suppliers, considering vendor capabilities, pricing, and service levels. • *Purchasing* is the process used to finalize order quantities, order and receive the products.

$100 (assuming that operational expenses remain constant). Moreover, having less money invested in inventory improves cash flow (West, 2001). A pharmacy that has merchandise that is not selling or an oversupply of product sitting on the shelf has less cash available to pay expenses and/or invest in other business operations. A pharmacy that is able to align demand and supply and reduce its inventory by $100 has that much more cash to spend on day-to-day operations, invest in new services, or place in a savings or checking account.

From an operational perspective, effective supply chain management is important in meeting consumer demands for both goods and services (Carroll, 1998). Not having a product when needed may cause the pharmacy to lose a sale and potentially a customer. Furthermore, not having a needed product at the right time may cause physical harm to a patient, especially in settings (e.g., hospitals) where lifesaving emergency drugs are routinely needed at a moment's notice.

People use supply chain management in their everyday lives. For example, when people shop for groceries, they think about what they would like to eat (i.e., needs and wants—which ultimately drive the demand for specific foods and services which they purchase) and what items they have on hand (i.e., current inventory). From this, they create a grocery list. This list is revised depending on how much money they have, grocery store specials, storage space, and

how quickly the food will spoil. They may compare products and shop at various grocery stores. They eventually make purchases and evaluate how well those purchases satisfy their needs and wants. The process is repeated and reevaluated on a continuous basis. This is similar to how pharmacies purchase their inventory. Pharmacists or their staff create lists of products they need, revise the lists based on current inventory, determine how much money they have to purchase these goods, evaluate any specials from their vendors and their available storage space, and then finally make and evaluate their purchases.

■ DEMAND PLANNING

The goal of demand planning is to produce a reliable projection of future customer demand—a forecast for the items that the pharmacy expects to dispense to patients and sell to customers. The demand forecast reflects what (1) what products will be needed (the product mix), (2) in which amounts, and (3) when they will be needed.

Product Mix

There are many factors that will influence the specific variety of different products that will be needed or wanted by a pharmacy's customers. It is important for the pharmacy manager to understand these factors so that the demand forecast reflects the needs of the pharmacy's patients, patrons, and prescribers and the subsequent inventory management and procurement decisions are properly aligned with customer needs. The pharmacy manager should consider the following factors when deciding what products to include in the demand plan:

- *Pharmacy mission or specialization:* The product mix should be aligned with the pharmacy's mission, type of specialization, and business goals. For example, a pharmacy that is attempting to establish itself as a diabetes care center will include more specialty diabetes products in its demand plan. Today, many community pharmacies want to be known as a vaccine provider and, therefore, they will include vaccines in the forecast.
- *Patient population demographics:* The area where the pharmacy is located and the patient populations it serves will affect product mix. A pharmacy located in a children's hospital will need different products than a pharmacy located in a mental health facility. Likewise, a community pharmacy located next to a pediatric clinic likely will need more liquid antibiotics than other pharmacies. Prescribing behaviors of area physicians can provide insight into what drug products are needed.
- *Sales history:* Reviewing historical sales at a monthly, quarterly, or seasonal level provides an understanding of historical demand patterns for specific products. Historical sales and dispensing reports are a good starting point for building the demand forecast, as historical demand and patterns can be used as the baseline forecast. The exact mix of products sold in a given year will of course vary, so it is important to understand if there are any anomalies or outliers in the historical data that may not occur in present or future years. For example, formulary changes, patent expiries, new drug launches, and drug shortages will occur each year, and the demand forecast will need to be updated to reflect the anticipated changes where possible.
- *Drug formularies:* Formularies often drive the decision of what goods to include in the demand plan.

A formulary is essentially a list of preferred drugs for use in that institution that are selected based on a combination of clinical and economic benefits (ASHP, 2019b). Pharmaceutical products that are placed on a formulary are an important part of the product mix because these are the products that prescribers will be encouraged to use. In general, nonformulary items may not be a part of the demand forecast as they can be specially ordered, if and when needed. Pharmacy managers also must consider intravenous tubing, needles, and other supplies that may be needed at their institutions. Formularies may also influence drug-purchasing decisions in the community pharmacy setting. Products that are more prominent on third-party payer formularies may comprise a greater part of the product mix than products that are not paid for by third-party payers in the area.

- *Industry data:* Pharmacy journals and magazines contain a wealth of information that can be used to provide insight into what drug products should be selected. In addition, these publications commonly alert pharmacy managers to new products or product changes that may affect patron and prescriber needs in the future.
- *Patent Expiries:* Pharmacists will need to adjust plans when a branded product is going off patent and becoming generic. Less of brand name drug will be needed, and the pharmacy will need to begin the transition to the generic version. The impact of the patent expiry will depend on whether or not the drug is a non-biologic drug or a biologic drug. If the drug is not a biologic, in general, bioequivalent generic drugs usually bring immediate generic competition when the patent expires. If the drug is a biologic drug, a biosimilar drug may enter the market when the patent expires, but the pace of adoption of the new drug will be slower due to provider preferences, formulary management, and current US and state regulations which do not allow for automatic substitution of the biosimilar when a prescription is written. In late 2018, Eli Lilly's Cialis drug lost patent protection, and Teva was first to file with a generic version of the drug (tadalafil)

(Fierce Pharma, 2018a). Ongoing patent extension litigation often means that a branded drug will not lose its protection on the original patent expiry date. For example, Pfizer's Lyrica (pregabalin) was expected to expire in late 2018 but won an extension and is now expected to expire in June of 2019 (Fierce Pharma, 2018b).

- *New product launches:* When a new product is launched, the plan may need to be adjusted to account for both demand for the new product and similar substitute products. The new plan should reflect anticipated demand for the new product, and reduced demand for substitutes. New product launches can be difficult to forecast, so the pharmacy manager should understand product lead times and expiry dates to ensure that unanticipated demand can be quickly ordered and received from vendors, and that over-forecasted demand does not result in spoilage or wasted inventory.

- *Drug shortages/substitutions:* Drug shortages occur due to unforeseen increases in demand, manufacturing issues, product recalls, natural disasters, raw material supply gaps, and product discontinuations. Pharmacy managers can access information on drug shortages on the FDA's Drug Shortage website (FDA, 2019a) and the American Society of Health-System Pharmacists (ASHP) Drug Shortage website (ASHP, 2019a).

- *Manufacturer/distributor representative data:* Both drug company and wholesaler representatives can provide valuable information about available products. These representatives often have industry trend data and are familiar with prescribing habits in the local geographic area. Moreover, industry representatives have information about new and soon-to-be-released products.

- *Consumer information:* Asking patrons, prescribers, and employees is another way to determine what to include in the plan. Monitoring consumer requests for products is also helpful.

Quantity and Timing

In addition to understanding the specific products that will be needed, the pharmacy manager also must understand the expected quantities of product that will be needed, and when they will be required. Historical sales information provides a good baseline for understanding trends including the quantity and timing of demand. By reviewing several years of history, the pharmacy manager can develop an understanding of the demand trends and patterns that repeat consistently, year after year, and this "normal" demand can be used as a baseline demand forecast. This baseline forecast must be adjusted to reflect the product mix factors discussed above.

The manager must also seek to understand additional factors that may have created unusual changes in sales volume and timing, such as disease outbreaks (both their severity and timing), weather events, and promotions. For example, if influenza is more severe in the current year than in prior years, it is possible that more people will seek out flu vaccines later in the flu season, so additional demand may occur, and this additional demand will appear later in the season than the normal demand history suggests. A severe weather event may create additional demand in prior to the event, as patients seek to ensure they have their necessary medicines, and then less demand following the event due to post event road accessibility and travel difficulties. Finally, if the pharmacy begins running a promotional campaign for a good or service earlier or later than in prior years, the timing demand for said good or service will shift accordingly, and the demand forecast timing must be adjusted.

Creating the Demand Forecast

The people responsible for creating the demand forecast, as well as the process for generating and adjusting the demand forecast, will vary depending upon the size and complexity of the pharmacy organization, as well as the technical capabilities and tools the pharmacy uses. Large pharmacy chains may have a robust multi-layered Sales and Operations Planning process (S&OP) where the demand forecast is generated at a central, company-wide level using sophisticated forecasting modeling tools, then adjusted with input from sales, marketing, and operations teams. The adjusted demand forecast is then pushed out to the chain's pharmacy stores. A small independent pharmacy may leverage forecasting and planning tools provided by a third-party entity (often their distributor), to allowing the pharmacy owner or a designate to generate their demand forecast.

■ INVENTORY MANAGEMENT

Inventory refers to the stock of products held to meet future demand. Pharmacies hold inventory to guard against fluctuations in demand, to take advantage of bulk discounts, and to withstand fluctuations in supply (e.g., late deliveries) (West, 2003). Inventory usually represents a pharmacy's largest current asset. Inventory is also the least liquid current asset, given that it generally cannot be turned to cash until it is sold to a consumer. The value of inventory to all pharmacies continues to rise owing to the increased variety and expense of pharmaceutical products. Therefore, proper management of inventory has a significant impact on both the financial and the operational aspects of any pharmacy (Huffman, 1996; West, 2003).

Inventory management is the practice of planning, organizing, and controlling inventory so that it contributes to the profitability of the business (Huffman, 1996; West, 2003). The goals of inventory management are to *minimize* the financial amount invested in inventory and hold procurement and carrying costs at the *lowest possible amounts*, all while *balancing supply and demand* (Huffman, 1996; Tootelian & Gaedeke, 1993; West, 2003). Inventory management is a key factor to success in a pharmacy because efficient inventory management can keep costs down, improve cash flow, and improve customer service. Alternatively, inventory mismanagement results in increased operating and opportunity costs.

Costs Associated with Inventory

Acquisition, procurement, carrying, and stock-out or shortage costs are the four general "costs" associated with inventory. The *acquisition cost* is the price the pharmacy pays for the product. *Procurement costs* are the costs associated with purchasing the product:

checking inventory, placing orders, receiving orders, stocking the product, and paying the invoices. *Carrying costs* refer to the storage, handling, insurance, cost of capital to finance the inventory, and opportunity costs. Another carrying cost is the cost of loss through theft, deterioration, and damage. Procurement and carrying costs must be balanced. For example, increasing the average order size and decreasing the number of orders placed decrease procurement costs but at the expense of increased carrying costs (e.g., more space needed to store inventory, higher costs of capital to finance larger purchases, greater risk for losses from theft, deterioration or damage). The fourth cost is the *stock-out cost,* which is the cost of not having a product on the shelf when a patient needs or wants it. This is frustrating to the pharmacist who has to explain why the product is not available and is an inconvenience to the patient and prescriber (Carroll, 1998).

Acquisition, procurement, and carrying costs can be calculated accurately and are an important financial consideration in pharmacy management. These three types of inventory costs generally place little direct stress on busy pharmacy staff but can depress the organization's operating margins if not monitored appropriately. Shortage costs represent failures in customer service and therefore lost sales. These costs may be difficult to quantify but definitely have an impact on any pharmacy.

Measuring the Effectiveness of Inventory Management

The most common ratio used to determine how well a pharmacy is managing its inventory is the Inventory Turnover Ratio (ITOR). It can be calculated for the entire pharmacy, for departments (e.g., prescriptions or over-the-counter [OTC] products), and even for individual products. The ITOR is expressed as a ratio and is calculated by using the following formula (Tootelian & Gaedeke, 1993; West, 2003, 2010):

ITOR = COGS ÷ average inventory value (at cost)

ITOR = COGS ÷ [(beginning inventory value
+ ending inventory value) ÷ 2]

The Cost of Goods Sold (COGS) can be found on the pharmacy's income (profit-and-loss) statement for a given period of time (see Chapter 21). The average inventory value can be found by obtaining the pharmacy's balance sheets for both the beginning and the end of the period represented on the income statement. The balance sheets should contain the value of the pharmacy's inventory at each point in time. The ITOR indicates the efficiency with which inventory is used. It measures how quickly inventory is purchased, sold, and replaced. Two advantages of increasing the ITOR are that reducing the investment in inventory frees capital for other business activities and increases the return on investment in inventory.

Table 27-3 provides an example of how to calculate ITOR. In this example, the pharmacy's overall annual ITOR is 10. This means that this pharmacy, on average, sells all the inventory that is typically kept in the pharmacy a total of 10 times over the course of a year. This is similar to the national average for independent pharmacies which was 10.6 in 2017 (NCPA, 2018), indicating that the pharmacy manager is probably managing inventory efficiently. Comparing the current year's ratio with last year's ratio also indicates that the manager is improving her efficiency in managing inventory because the ITOR has increased over time. Note that if the COGS remained constant for the year and the average inventory increased, the ITOR would have decreased. This would have indicated that inventory was sitting on the shelf and not selling. The pharmacy manager then would want to determine if she was ordering too much product or the wrong products.

Overall, pharmacy managers need to assess their ITOR. Deciding what is too high or too low is pharmacy-dependent. Overall a high ITOR is desirable, as long as the pharmacy is not running out of stock at a level inconsistent with its desired level of service. If out-of-stocks are occurring too frequently, one may interpret the ITOR as being too high. Alternatively, if the pharmacy is carrying too much inventory that is not selling and is not being used, one may interpret the ITOR as too low. Hence cash is being spent to purchase the product, but cash is not flowing in from the sale of the product. The pharmacy manager should consider national or regional benchmarks, as well as the pharmacy's trends, when interpreting the ITOR. The ITOR is one indicator that should be considered when managing inventory, but it must be interpreted given the context of the pharmacy. For example, an ITOR of 30 may be acceptable if the pharmacy can order and receive items quickly from the vendor and there have not been complaints of shortages. It may also be helpful for the pharmacy manager to look at the ITOR within product lines or departments to facilitate decision-making.

As gross margins have continued to shrink in community pharmacies and drug budgets have gotten tighter in hospital pharmacies, pharmacy managers have been forced to become more efficient in their operations. One way to increase efficiency is to manage inventory properly. Trends have shown that pharmacy managers in various practice settings are making efforts to manage their inventories more efficiently. For example, independent pharmacy owners have increased their overall ITOR from 6.3 in 1995 (West, 2010), to 9.8 in 2009 to 10.6 in 2017 (NCPA, 2018). Just-in-time (JIT) deliveries and computerized inventory systems have facilitated this increased efficiency in inventory management, especially prescription

Table 27-3.	Inventory Turnover Ratio (ITOR) Example
ITOR for Smith Pharmacy for FY 2017 = 8.2	
ITOR for Smith Pharmacy for FY 2018 = 9.5	
Data for Smith Pharmacy for FY 2019	
Sales:	$4,000,000
Cost of goods sold:	$3,000,000
Gross margin:	$1,000,000
Total expenses:	$900,000
Net profit:	$100,000
Average inventory: $300,000	
ITOR = cost of goods sold/average inventory	
ITOR = $3,000,000/$300,000	
ITOR = 10	

inventory. Hospital pharmacy ITORs vary by hospital size, with smaller hospitals having ITORs of 8 to 10 turns per year, and larger hospitals having ITORs of 12 to 18 or higher (ASHP, 2008).

Another indicator of a pharmacy manager's ability to manage the investment in inventory efficiently is the net-profit-to-average-inventory ratio. This ratio indicates whether the inventory is being used efficiently to make a profit. Pharmacy managers desire to have a ratio greater than 20%.

Factors to Consider in Inventory Management

Pharmacy managers must consider multiple factors when evaluating their inventory:

- *Selection of generic products.* Generic drug products usually have a lower acquisition cost, and therefore, by stocking generic products, the amount of money invested in inventory is reduced (Carroll, 1998). For example, a pharmacist may decide not to stock brand name Lasix because generic furosemide is less expensive, thereby reducing the amount of money invested in inventory.
- *Reduction of inventory size.* A pharmacist may decide to have a small front end in his or her store to reduce the amount invested in inventory. He or she may carry only basic product lines (i.e., a smaller numbers of brands and items) as opposed to full product lines (i.e., every brand and every item).
- *Returned-goods policies.* One critical component is the evaluation of returned-goods policies. Many manufacturers and wholesalers have established policies regarding merchandise that may be returned. In exchange for returning unsalable goods, these vendors may provide credit on future purchases, replacement goods, or even cash back to the pharmacy. An example of wholesaler returned-goods policies is provided in Table 27-1. Pharmacy managers should monitor products closely that qualify for the various returned-goods policies, making certain that such returns are made on a regular, periodic basis before time limitations take effect. It is advised to have a staff member responsible for checking the shelves periodically for out-of-date items or items that are not selling. Because the management of return goods is critical, some pharmacies use returned-goods service companies to assist them with managing their returned goods. These companies will evaluate the pharmacy's inventory, return the appropriate products, and often return money from the returned products within 30 to 60 days. These companies charge a fee based on the amount of returns. One major advantage to these companies is that they are aware of each manufacturer's and wholesaler's specific policies and can quickly identify product to be returned.

- *Management of unclaimed prescriptions.* Approximately, one-in-eight (12%) new prescriptions for chronic medications received in community pharmacies remain unclaimed (Jackson et al., 2014). A pharmacist must be aware of the amount of inventory that has been used to fill these unclaimed prescriptions. It is important for pharmacists to monitor these unclaimed prescriptions and after a specified period (e.g., 10–12 days) return the stock to the shelf so that it can be used to fill prescriptions for other patients.
- *Monitoring shrinkage.* Inventory shrinkage includes losses owing to shoplifting, employee theft, and robbery. In 2018, it was estimated that approximately 2.0% of drugstore and pharmacy annual sales were lost to shrinkage (Planet Retail Limited, 2018). The largest source of shrinkage for most retailers is employee theft. It is important to recruit honest personnel and monitor their activities, especially those working in the prescription area of a pharmacy, because theft of medications, and in particular controlled substances such as opiates, is increasingly problematic. Equally important, however, is for the pharmacy staff to be observant, say hello to customers, keep displays neat, install security mirrors and cameras, and remove high fixtures to minimize shoplifting. Some pharmacies use technologies, such as inventory-control bars, cameras and remote monitoring, and electronic article surveillance, to prevent loss of product from theft.

- *Use of formularies.* As stated previously, institutional pharmacies commonly use formularies to facilitate inventory management, and the American Society of Health-Systems Pharmacists (ASHP) maintains a reference page on their website which includes links to their educational materials and policy statements on formulary management (ASHP, 2019b). A formulary allows the pharmacy manager to carry one therapeutic equivalent within a class of drugs instead of each drug product within the class. This allows pharmacy managers to lower their overall investment in inventory.

Methods of Inventory Management

Three methods are used commonly in pharmacy to manage inventory: the visual method, the periodic method, and the perpetual method (Carroll, 1998; Tootelian & Gaedeke, 1993; West, 2003). The *visual method* requires the pharmacist or designated person to look at the number of units in inventory and compare them with a listing of how many should be carried. When the number falls below the desired amount, an order is placed. The *periodic method* requires the pharmacist or designated person to count the stock in hand at predetermined intervals and compare it with minimum desired levels. If the quantity is below the minimum, the product is ordered.

Usually, a designated person is responsible for checking the shelves and placing orders. The pharmacy manager may have a specific checklist, indicating that the person should conduct a stock review weekly or look for expired products monthly, in addition to placing orders and keeping inventory orders to a specific level. This purchasing person will learn the turnover rates for specific products and will develop a skill for purchasing for the pharmacy. This method allows the purchasing person to account for fluctuations in supply and demand. Today, the purchasing person is likely to use a handheld electronic device into which item numbers and quantities are entered or a handheld scanning device that scans the bar codes on the product packaging or shelf labels (Carroll, 1998; West, 2003). These devices then can be used to submit an order electronically.

Although the visual and periodic methods are still used today, *perpetual inventory systems* are common in all pharmacy settings. These perpetual systems are computerized inventory management systems. Perpetual inventory management systems are the most efficient method to manage inventory. This method allows the inventory to be monitored at all times. The entire inventory may be entered into the computer, and with the filling of each prescription, the appropriate inventory can be reduced automatically. A perpetual system can tell precisely the amount of inventory in hand for any product at any time. Moreover, the pharmacy manager can quickly assess the value of current inventory.

Computer systems can be used to calculate the Economic Order Quantity (EOQ) and reorder point so that a product is reordered automatically when the inventory falls below a minimum standard (West, 2003). Computer systems can also be programmed to use the pharmacy's demand forecast (as discussed in the demand management section) and automatically order product based on these forecasts. These types of systems reduce procurement costs significantly, particularly by reducing the amount of time pharmacists and other pharmacy personnel must spend monitoring and ordering their inventory. Although the computer can be programmed to order products automatically, it is important for pharmacy staff to monitor inventory daily and to make corrections for variances owing to fluctuations in supply and demand.

To maintain a perpetual inventory system, all purchases and sales must be entered into the computer system (Carroll, 1998; West, 2003). A clerk can enter data from purchases, use a point-of-sale (POS) device to scan the products upon receipt, or the computer dispensing system can be interfaced with the computer order system. A POS system or interfaces between different systems allow for the inventory to be reduced when a product is dispensed. The sales data can also be entered at the POS by devices that use optical scanning and bar code technology. POS devices are advantageous in that they improve the accuracy of pricing and inventory data. They eliminate the need for price stickers, reduce the frequency of pricing errors, and automatically track inventory.

Regardless of which method is used, most pharmacies also conduct a physical inventory at least annually. This encompasses counting or scanning every item in the pharmacy. Pharmacy staff then can compare the product on-hand quantities in the computer or the value of inventory on the financial statements with what is actually on the shelves. It is important to conduct a physical inventory check periodically to verify the accuracy of the pharmacy's financial records. In addition, pharmacy managers should follow state board of pharmacy regulations with respect to inventory counts of controlled substances, especially narcotics.

Role of Technology

Based on the preceding description of the purchasing process and perpetual inventory systems, one can recognize the value of technology in inventory management. Thus, computerized inventory management systems are common today in pharmacies in all practice settings. Technology enables pharmacists to manage inventory faster and more accurately.

These computer systems can integrate the management of inventory, information, and costs. The ability to integrate inventory and cost data allows for the generation of a wide array of reports and analyses. Pharmacists use these management reports to identify high- and low-turnover items and determine stock levels for better allocation of shelf space. Examples of inventory management reports include the following:

- *Purchase-trend report*—describes the quantity purchased of OTC products or prescription drug products by month or by quarter.
- *Sales-analysis report*—features a rolling 12-month statement that includes order quantity, shipped quantity, unavailable quantity, returns, credits, and dollars spent.
- *Item-movement report*—lists which items are selling the best, and which inventory items are "slow moving."

As discussed in the Demand Management section, the types of systems used by different types of pharmacies vary depending on the type, size, and complexity of the pharmacy organization. Large chain retailers may have POS and inventory management systems that are integrated with the parent company's corporate enterprise technology systems. Chain store pharmacies may upload sales and inventory data from the pharmacy on a daily basis, and pharmacies may also receive updated demand forecast projections from the parent organization.

For independent pharmacies, pharmaceutical distributors may provide the hardware and software for the inventory management system. Today, web-based systems prevail. These allow pharmacy managers to view in real time the quantity in hand at the distributor, the list price, the manufacturer backorder status, and the online catalog. These web-based systems also enable pharmacy staff to check purchase orders, invoices, and account information in real time. Another advantage is that the pharmacy staff can place orders and view account information from other locations besides the pharmacy. POS systems can integrate with many pharmacy systems. As previously mentioned, POS systems allow product to be deducted from inventory as it is sold or dispensed, thereby, improving inventory management in the pharmacy. POS systems also provide other management efficiencies, such as speeding up checkout times with credit card processing and reducing pricing errors.

Pharmacy staff can also order inventory via the Internet, which is termed *e-procurement*. E-procurement allows the pharmacy to receive immediate item allocation and order confirmation. These sophisticated systems drastically reduce the time and effort spent on procurement. Prices can be updated daily or weekly by using electronic invoice transmission, and returns and credits can be completed electronically. Invoices are then paid by electronic funds transfer (EFT).

Note that Class II (C-II) controlled substances now can be ordered electronically. Pharmacies must be registered with the US Drug Enforcement Agency (DEA) and obtain a DEA Controlled Substance Ordering System (CSOS) digital certificate. The C-II orders are created using a computerized inventory system, electronically signed using a password-protected digital certificate, and then submitted electronically to the wholesaler.

Radiofrequency identification (RFID) microchips or "tags" may be attached to product packages to improve product distribution within the supply chain. RFID tags are different from bar codes in that they have larger memory capacity, allow for data to be added and changed, and do not have to be physically swiped on a scanner to access the stored information. The sensors can track when products arrive at and depart from a defined physical location, and the RFID reader or sensor can update the store inventory. Hence RFID tags can provide a chain of custody and may help protect against counterfeiting and theft.

At the present time, RFID is an emerging technology in pharmacies. The use of barcodes is mandated by the Drug Supply Chain Security Act (DSCSA), and 2-D barcode scanning is the primary technology used to scan in product information in pharmacies. There is some limited RFID deployment in hospital pharmacies, where pharmacists are using RFID to track medical kits and trays which include prescription items. Amerisource Bergen's Cubixx system uses RFID technology to manage consignment inventory, and while is presently primarily used in hospital settings, has also been used at small number of community pharmacies (Amerisource Bergen, 2019b).

■ PROCUREMENT: PURCHASING AND STRATEGIC SOURCING

Some pharmacists perceive that procurement is just a routine function necessary to keep inventory on the shelf. However, since most pharmacies literally spend millions of dollars every year to acquire medications and other goods, purchasing is actually a substantial investment process.

Procurement includes the functions of buying products and services for a specific business purpose. Two aspects of the procurement function are purchasing and sourcing. *Purchasing* is the process used to determine the right order quantities, place orders, and receive the products. *Sourcing* is the methodology used to identify and manage the right product suppliers, considering vendor capabilities, pricing, and service levels.

Purchasing

Purchasing involves buying the *right products* (as determined in the Demand Forecasting process) in the *right quantity* at the *right price* at the *right time*. Many pharmacies, especially in hospitals and other health care facilities, have a designated person or purchasing agent whose responsibility is to order and receive products.

Right Quantity at the Right Time[1]

As stated previously, having too much product ties up a pharmacy's money without providing an adequate return on investment. On the other hand, having too little product may result in lost sales and profits when the product is not available when consumers want to make a purchase. Not having enough products available also inconveniences pharmacy staff and customers, and may result in the loss of customers in the future. Thus, not only having the right product is critical to inventory management but also having the right quantity at the right time is essential.

The right quantity means having just enough product on hand to cover consumer demand at any given time. Determining the right quantity for any given product is difficult, if not impossible, given that demand may fluctuate unexpectedly. However, it is still important for pharmacy managers to track consumer demand for their products and monitor trends that may affect their use. While managers may not always have the right quantity on hand, use of this information helps them to anticipate fluctuations in demand (e.g., increasing the supply of antibiotics and certain OTC medications during winter months).

---

[1]Parts of this section are excerpted, with permission, from West DS. 2003. Purchasing and inventory control. In: Jackson R (ed), *Effective Pharmacy Management CD-ROM*, 9th ed, Sec. 17. Alexandria, VA: National Community Pharmacists Association Foundation.

For example, the pharmacy manager may use last year's numbers plus some expected growth in sales to determine the number of flu vaccines to order initially for the upcoming flu season. Then more vaccines can be ordered as needed.

In general, there are three types of stock to consider. *Cycle stock* is the regular inventory that is needed to fulfill orders. *Buffer,* or *safety, stock* is additional inventory that is needed in case of a supply or demand fluctuation. *Anticipatory,* or *speculative, stock* is inventory that is kept on hand because of expected future demand or expected price increase (e.g., flu vaccine in the fall and winter months). Buying anticipatory stock is risky and, therefore, pharmacists usually do not carry much anticipatory stock and place higher mark-ups on such anticipatory stock. These types of stock are important to consider when deciding how much to order and when to order (Silbiger, 1999).

To estimate the minimum quantity of goods needed to meet demand, the pharmacy manager or purchasing agent should know the following information for each item stocked:

1. How much is on hand?
2. At what point to reorder?
3. How much to order?

How do pharmacy managers determine *stock depth* (i.e., the point where it is reasonably certain that the item will be available on demand)? Establishing stock depth (product quantity) involves consideration of

1. An item's rate of sale (average demand)
2. The length of time between stock checks (review time)
3. The period of time between placing and receiving an order (lead time)
4. A safety stock to account for variations in average demand during the buying time (review time plus lead time)

Thus, the formula to set the *reorder point* is as follows:

Reorder point = [(review time + lead time)
               × average demand] + safety stock

This basic formula has been used to develop an *EOQ* model (Carroll, 1998; Huffman, 1996; Silbiger, 1999; Tootelian & Gaedeke, 1993). While the EOQ model may be difficult to derive and calculate, it is often incorporated into computer software used by many pharmacies to manage their inventory and make purchasing decisions. The EOQ model describes the level of inventory and reorder quantity at which the combined costs of purchasing and carrying inventory are at a minimum. The formula is as follows:

$$Q = \sqrt{\frac{2(c)(D)}{(I)(UC)}}$$

where

Q = economic order quantity
c = procurement cost per order
D = demand for the product expressed either in dollars or physical units
I = inventory carrying costs
UC = unit cost of the item

Another factor determining how much to order is the budget. Hospital pharmacy directors may estimate this year's budget by increasing last year's budget by a certain percent (e.g., 5% or 10%). This budget estimate will provide a guide for how much money can be spent each month to order product. Community pharmacy managers also evaluate profit-and-loss statements to determine whether too much product is being bought compared with the amount of sales.

Using an *open-to-buy budget* helps to control the total dollar investment in inventory (Carroll, 1998; West, 2003). It limits the manager to a set predetermined dollar amount of purchases during a given time period. The basic steps of this purchasing technique are listed below (Huffman, 1996; West, 2003). This procedure is repeated on a monthly basis.

Step 1. Forecast purchasing budget for each month in the next fiscal year using the demand planning process described in the last section
Step 2. Each month's forecasted sales are then multiplied by the COGS percent to calculate the monthly unadjusted purchasing budget.

Step 3. At the end of each month, the month's actual sales and purchases are recorded. Next month's purchases are then adjusted based on the past month's actual sales and purchases. If sales were greater than predicted, then next month's purchasing budget may be increased to accommodate for the increased sales. Alternatively, if the sales were lower than expected, then the purchasing budget for the next month would be decreased.

Right Price

Once the right product is selected, it is important to acquire it at the right price. Purchasing pharmacy products (especially prescription drugs) is not unlike purchasing a car in that the "list" or "sticker" price is often different from the final price that pharmacies actually pay. For pharmacy products, the list price and the terms of sale have an impact on the overall acquisition cost. *Terms of sale* pertain to discounts and dating (Huffman, 1996; West, 2003).

DISCOUNTS *Discounts* describe the reduction(s) in price, whereas *dating* pertains to the period of time allowed for taking the discounts and the date when the invoice becomes payable. Although there are a number of discounts, three main discounts are described below.

Quantity discounts: Quantity discounts have traditionally been offered as an incentive for purchasing large quantities of single products or a special grouping of specific products offered by a manufacturer (West, 2003). For example, a distributor may sell one bottle of a drug for $100. A quantity discount may apply so that if the pharmacy orders a dozen bottles at one time, a 2% discount is given. Thus, the pharmacy that orders 12 bottles will pay a total of $1,176 (or $98 per bottle), resulting in a total saving of $24 than if these 12 bottles had each been purchased separately. These discounts, based on a quantity of the same product being purchased on the same order, are described as *noncumulative quantity discounts* (Huffman, 1996; Tootelian & Gaedeke, 1993; West, 2003).

The purchasing agent or pharmacy manager should be aware of these special discounts and adjust ordering to take advantage of them. Assuming that

the product purchased is saleable in the pharmacy, quantity discounts can decrease the actual acquisition cost of the drug product. However, managers should also balance the savings generated by quantity discounts with the costs of storing and carrying excess inventory, the risks of not being able to sell the extra products, and the opportunity costs that come with spending money on inventory that could have been used in other ways.

Some vendors offer quantity discounts to pharmacies if their total purchases reach a target monetary amount during a specific time period. These discounts involving a variety of products on separate orders over a period of time are termed *cumulative quantity discounts* or *deferred discounts* (Huffman, 1996; Tootelian & Gaedeke, 1993; West, 2003). For example, generic drug manufacturers often offer rebates to pharmacies based on the amount of generic product purchased during a given time period (e.g., quarterly or yearly). Similarly, hospital pharmacies, community pharmacies, and others negotiate discounts based on volume purchasing. The pharmacy receives a discount based on the volume purchased in a specified time period. A hospital or institutional pharmacy may be able to negotiate lower prices because a pharmaceutical product is placed on its formulary. The pharmacy can estimate that a certain amount of volume will be purchased or the product will get a percent of the market share. In exchange for this market share or volume purchasing, a discounted price is negotiated.

Cash Discounts: Cash discounts are small discounts offered for the prompt payment of invoices (Huffman, 1996; Tootelian & Gaedeke, 1993; West, 2003). The discount is stated as a percentage of the amount remaining after all other discounts have been deducted from the bill. A common discount is "2/10, net 30," which translates into a 2% discount if the invoice is paid within 10 days of the date of the invoice, otherwise, the net amount is due in 30 days.

Pharmacy managers should be aware of these discounts and take advantage of them, especially because they are not required to purchase excess inventory to do so. Many managers state that they do not take advantage of cash discounts because they do not have enough cash on hand to pay their invoices quickly. One thing that these managers could do is to take out a short-term loan or line of credit to obtain the cash needed to take advantage of the discount. In most cases, the savings provided by the cash discount more than makes up for the interest expense on the borrowed money.

Electronic Funds Transfer (EFT) is now being used by pharmacies to take advantage of cash discounts and even prepay for purchases. An example of this is displayed in Table 27-1 (West, 2003). Prepayment requires the pharmacy to pay a week or month ahead of actual purchases based on its average weekly or monthly purchases over the last 3 to 6 months. In exchange for prepayments, vendors offer additional cash discounts to pharmacy managers, allowing them to reduce their COGS further. Vendors offer web-based systems that allow pharmacy managers to view their account information and invoices online in real time. This allows accounts payable to be monitored closely and invoices to be paid quickly online in real time. In addition, these systems reduce procurement costs for the pharmacy by decreasing personnel time and bookkeeping expenses.

Serial Discounts: Serial discounts occur when multiple discounts are applied at the same time. Serial discounts accumulate as shown in Table 27-4. In this example, the pharmacy manager is able to obtain the product at approximately $12 less than the original list price by taking advantage of both quantity and cash discounts.

DATING The other purchase term that needs to be considered is the dating of the invoice. *Dating* refers both to the time before the specified amount of

discount may be taken and to the time at which payment becomes due (Huffman, 1996; West, 2003). There are three general types of dating: (1) *prepayment,* where the pharmacy pays for the merchandise before it is ordered and delivered, (2) *collect on delivery* (COD), where there is no time before a discount may be taken and payment becomes due, and (3) *delayed* or *future dating,* where the invoice is due sometime in the future (West, 2003). When no specific dating has been placed on the invoice, it is usually assumed that payment is due 10 days from the last day of the month in which the purchase was made. This is often specified by the term EOM (end of month) in the invoice. Two other terms related to the dating of invoices and statements for merchandise include *AOG,* meaning "arrival of goods," and *ROG,* meaning "receipt of goods." For example, "2/10 ROG, net 30" means deduct 2% within 10 days after ROG or otherwise pay net within 30 days after ROG.

Sourcing

Being able to obtain the right product at the right time, price, and place depends on selecting the right vendor. Selecting the right vendor for pharmaceutical products is an important decision for the pharmacy manager: the vendor's capabilities, product and service offerings, pricing, and service levels must be a good strategic fit with the needs of the pharmacy. Additionally, the DSCSA requires that pharmacies do business with an authorized trading partner.

Although a pharmacy can select a single vendor or multiple vendors, it is advised that pharmacies have a primary vendor and a secondary vendor. Establishing a positive relationship with a primary vendor can be helpful because it is a close working relationship, and may lead to prompt delivery, special buying opportunities, special pricing information, and prompt resolution of problems. A secondary vendor is advised for times when product is not available from the primary vendor owing to drug product shortages and to obtain special pricing opportunities.

Among the many effective mechanisms used by vendors to market their products to pharmacies are salespersons, service representatives, and account representatives. These individuals try diligently to

Table 27-4.	Example of Serial Discount
Invoice price	$100
10% Quantity discount	$100.00 × 0.1 = $10.00 $100.00 − $10.00 = $90.00
2% Cash discount	$90.00 × 0.02 = $1.80 $90.00 − $1.80 = $88.20

maintain good communications with their clients. Many pharmaceutical distributor representatives, for example, visit or telephone major purchasers every 2 to 4 weeks. The salesperson or representative serves as an important source of market information; consequently, many pharmacy managers make it a practice to talk with salespersons and representatives who call on them. In addition, talking with the representative keeps them aware of new programs and services offered by the vendor.

While favorable pricing and purchase terms are important considerations when selecting vendors, additional criteria should also be used (Tootelian & Gaedeke, 1993; West, 2003) (Table 27-5). Selecting a

---

Table 27-5. Criteria to Select Vendors

- Are they reliable and dependable? What is their order accuracy? Do they have a good reputation?
- Will they provide the information and documents needed to meet the Drug Supply Chain Security Act (e.g., drug pedigree information, transaction history, transaction information, and statement that the drug is not stolen, diverted, or counterfeit)?
- Will they negotiate price and purchase terms with the pharmacy? Will they help to ensure contract compliance when ordering?
- What is their delivery schedule?
- Are they innovative?
- Do they provide financing and credit options?
- Do they have good customer relations? How often will a representative call on the pharmacy? Can I develop a positive business relationship with this supplier?
- Do they offer any value-added services? Will they help with advertising and promotion, provide inventory reports and analyses, or assist with pharmacy layout and design? Do they offer a private-label line of products?
- What technology do they offer to help with purchasing and inventory management?

---

vendor with a good reputation is desirable. Accuracy and fill rates are also important considerations. Pharmacy managers should select vendors that provide quality products and services and have few out-of-stock situations. It is important to select vendors with prompt and reliable delivery schedules. Inconsistent deliveries will likely result in the pharmacy not having the right products at the right times. Moreover, it is suggested that pharmacy managers evaluate their vendors periodically to ensure that they are receiving competitive prices and discounts. Many pharmacies seek bids from wholesalers periodically (e.g., every 3 years) to ensure competitive pricing and quality service.

Types of Vendor

The most common type of vendor for pharmacies is the pharmaceutical distributor. There are two types of pharmaceutical distributors that carry slightly different product lines and serve different types of health care providers and pharmacies:

Traditional pharmaceutical distributors (also known as pharmaceutical wholesalers) carry a broad line of pharmaceutical drugs, including specialty drugs. These distributors' customer base typically includes hospitals, community pharmacies (both chains and independents), specialty pharmacies, mail-order pharmacies, and home health care providers.

Specialty pharmaceutical distributors primarily carry specialty pharmaceutical drugs. These distributors' customer base typically includes independent specialist physician offices, physician-owned clinics, hospital-owned clinics, specialty pharmacies, home health care providers, and to a lesser extent, hospital pharmacies.

Pharmaceutical distributors provide many vital services to support health care providers, including pharmacies. These services ensure that pharmaceutical products are readily available to health care providers, pharmacies, and the patients who need these drugs. These services include core, foundational services that ensure the pharmaceutical supply chain is safe and secure, highly efficient, and responsive. Foundational services include supply chain, financial, information,

Supply Chain

- Order management and fulfillment
- Inventory management
- Reverse logistics and returns
- Recalls
- Security
- Special handling services
- Disaster preparedness
- Business continuity risk management
- Packaging and repackaging services
- New product launch support

 Regulatory

- Support compliance with federal/state regulations
- REMS support
- Product compliance support services

 Financial Services

- Ownership of credit risk (receivables)
- Chargeback administration
- Payer economic modeling and negotiation support
- Financial management and access to credit

 Data/Information

- Web-based portal solutions
- Basic data services (e.g., sales, inventory, returns)
- Enhanced data services (e.g., clinical performance)
- Pharmacy management systems and services

Figure 27-2. Core distribution services offered by pharmaceutical distributors. (Reprinted with permission from 2018 Speciality Pharmaceutical Distribution Facts, Figures and Trends. Copyright © 2018 by the Healthcare Distribution Alliance (HDA) Research Foundation.)

and regulatory compliance services. Figure 27-2 illustrates the core services provided by distributors.

The pharmaceutical distributor anticipates the pharmacy's needs, goes into the market to obtain the necessary goods from manufacturers, and ensures that they are available at the appropriate time (West, 2003). This assembling of merchandise is a gigantic task involving thousands of different items that pharmaceutical wholesalers store until the goods are wanted by a pharmacy. From a pharmacy manager's standpoint, it is much more efficient to do business with a full-service pharmaceutical distributor that carries many products from many different vendors than to have to purchase products from each vendor separately. Most pharmaceutical distributors offer JIT delivery that allows for next-day or even same-day delivery, thereby reducing the pharmacy's risk and improving the pharmacy's cash flow.

In addition to these core services, specialty distributors offer providers and patients many additional valuable support services that may be offered either complementarily or for a fee. These services include patient and provider support services, reimbursement support services, marketing services, and hub services (Figure 27-3). These services are generally offered by affiliate businesses that are owned and operated by the specialty distributor.

The account representative may provide information on marketing and merchandising techniques, assist with pharmacy layout and design, and provide customized inventory management reports and information on the availability of new products.

Programs offered by wholesalers include offering private-label products, repackaging services, and backorder programs to improve inventory management for the pharmacy. A backorder program means that the pharmacy can order a product on backorder, and as soon as the wholesaler receives the product, the pharmacy's backorders get top-priority filling status and are shipped before the day's regular orders. Some wholesalers offer programs where products are delivered on consignment, meaning that the pharmacy does not have to pay until the product is sold. This reduces the amount of money the pharmacy has invested in inventory. Some wholesalers also offer pharmacy ownership programs and third-party assistance services. Ownership programs assist people with buying a pharmacy by providing special financing for the initial inventory, store layout design consulting, and other services. Third-party assistance services include

Patient and Provider Support

- Adherence management programs
- Provide third-party support services (contract review, reimbursement support)
- Utilization management
- Patient counseling
- Refill reminders
- Disease management
- Disease state advocacy
- Provider advocacy
- Treatment initiation and education

 Reimbursement Support

- Reimbursement services/consulting
- Medication preauthorization
- Patient assistant program management
- Claims/co-pay collection

 Marketing

- Promotional material distribution
- Provider access and information

 Hub Services

- Customer call centers

Figure 27-3. Other specialty distribution support services. (Reprinted with permission from 2018 Speciality Pharmaceutical Distribution Facts, Figures and Trends. Copyright © 2018 by the Healthcare Distribution Alliance (HDA) Research Foundation.)

third-party contracting, pharmacy benefit management audit assistance, and tools to help with other third-party reimbursement issues. It is important to note that one of the reasons wholesalers offer these services to pharmacies, often at no cost, is that the success of the wholesaler is predicated on the success of the pharmacy. Programs and services that wholesalers can offer to help pharmacies sell more items will ultimately benefit the wholesalers themselves.

Some large pharmacy chains perform many of the wholesaler's service functions within their own organizations. These chains must assume wholesaler functions, such as purchasing, storing, financing, and delivering products to each of their units. While these chains serve as their own primary "vendor," they often still use full-line wholesalers as secondary vendors to obtain selected products or in special circumstances.

Pharmacies in practically every practice setting participate in some type of Group Puchasing Organization (GPO) or central purchasing organization (Carroll, 1998; West, 2003). The purpose of a GPO is to pool the buying power of pharmacies together to obtain better prices and discounts from vendors. With profit margins being squeezed and drug budgets being scrutinized, pharmacies are looking for ways to decrease the cost of goods. A GPO negotiates with wholesalers and manufacturers for better pricing. One caveat to remember is that participating pharmacies must order products according to the terms of their GPO contract to receive special pricing and drug cost savings. If the pharmacists or technicians are not cognizant of the contract when they order, they may select the needed product at random from the list of potential sources. If the selection is not compliant with the contract, the pharmacy will not receive any negotiated prices.

Hospitals and hospital pharmacies are commonly members of GPOs, using the purchasing power of hundreds of hospitals to negotiate the best acquisition costs through competitive bidding. These hospital GPOs typically "bid out" almost every type of good used within the hospital, including equipment, supplies, and drugs. GPOs may also contract wholesaler services to select the wholesaler with the best combination of services, dependability, and costs. The GPO's central office organizes these bids and contracts through formal processes. Highly skilled representatives and professionals within these member hospitals represent the buying groups in the bidding and selection process. For example, GPOs commonly seek the advice of clinical pharmacists regarding comparative drug efficacy and future trends in drug therapy.

A *pharmacy buying group* is defined as a pharmacy organization whose purpose is to seek better drug prices for its members (e.g., community pharmacies, hospital pharmacies, and long-term care facilities) based on their collective buying power. Most, if not all, wholesalers are connected with one or more buying groups. The wholesaler will work with the pharmacy to find the best buying groups to join. Also, the pharmacist may identify a buying group with competitive pricing and then select a wholesaler that has a relationship with that buying group. Most buying groups charge a monthly or annual fee to members.

Another option used by pharmacies is to purchase directly from a pharmaceutical manufacturer. However, many manufacturers have substantial minimum purchase requirements, making it less favorable to buy from the manufacturer. Pharmacies may be receiving discounts based on volume purchased from the wholesaler, thereby giving an incentive to the pharmacy to buy most of its products from one wholesaler. Wholesalers also offer next-day delivery and other value-added services that help pharmacy managers minimize inventory costs. Thus, most pharmacies do not purchase products from manufacturers very often.

Pharmacies, particularly those with formularies (e.g., hospital pharmacies) that purchase large volumes of select drug products, may negotiate prices directly with manufacturers. Bids for these products are sought from manufacturers, and then a contracted price is agreed upon between the pharmacy and the manufacturer. While the contract involves a pharmacy and a manufacturer, distribution of the product usually involves a wholesaler (Carroll, 1998). The pharmacy will order the product from the wholesaler and receive the price that has been negotiated with the manufacturer. The wholesaler then bills the manufacturer the difference between the list price and the negotiated price (often called a *chargeback*), and in return, the manufacturer credits the wholesaler's account.

■ PURCHASING PROCESSES

Usually, a designated person (e.g., purchasing agent or pharmacy technician) will submit an order via telephone, fax, or computer and receive order confirmation. It may seem that the purchasing function ends when the order is made and the merchandise arrives at the pharmacy; however, this is not the case. The products need to be counted, checked for damage, and stocked on the shelves (West, 2003). When an order arrives, a pharmacy technician or other designated individual should physically count each item in the shipment and compare it with the invoice. Handheld devices that use bar coding technology are being used to facilitate this process. The designated person can scan the bar codes of all items in the tote to create a list of exactly what is in the tote. This list then can be compared to the invoice. The products should also be checked for any damage or short expiration dates. The vendor should be notified immediately if there is any discrepancy or any damaged products.

On receipt, the products need to be moved to a temporary storage area or stocked on the shelves. Proper storage of inventory is vital. Improper storage can result in product that no longer can be sold, resulting in losses of inventory, sales, and profits. When new products are added to the shelves, the technician should rotate the stock, placing the newest stock behind the older stock bottles. This will ensure that the oldest stock is used first, hopefully before it becomes outdated. Within most community and hospital pharmacy software systems, options are available for the software to count incoming and outgoing products and automatically order product to replenish stock based on models such as the EOQ. However, it is important to remember that these systems only work if all inventory information is recorded in the system, including the changes in of inventory levels through all channels including theft and obsolescence.

■ CURRENT TOPICS IN SUPPLY CHAIN MANAGEMENT

Risk Evaluation and Mitigation Strategies

The Food and Drug Administration Amendments Act (FDAAA) of 2007 gave the Food and Drug Administration (FDA) new authorities and responsibilities to enhance drug safety. This act gave the FDA the authority to require that manufacturers develop and implement a *Risk Evaluation and Mitigation Strategy* (REMS) for certain medications with serious safety concerns to ensure that the benefits of the drug do not outweigh the risks. The FDA may require a REMS during the new drug approval process, or for an already-approved product if new safety information becomes available.

REMS are a safety strategy intended to manage known or potential risks associated with a drug product. REMS may include several different components. Most REMS include a communication component about the specific safety risk or risks that the REMS is intended to mitigate. Some REMS include additional requirements such as clinical activities that the health care providers may need to perform prior to prescribing or dispensing a medication to the patient (FDA, 2019b).

REMS are defined and tailored for specific drug products, and the requirements and key risk messages are specific to each medication, its risks, and the setting in which the drug is likely to be used. Manufacturers, distributors, health care providers, and pharmacists all play different roles in ensuring compliance with REMS.

REMS may require that a pharmacy become certified to dispense a medication. Certification can involve having the pharmacy or health care setting enroll in the certification program, ensure that REMS policies and procedures are implemented and executed, and ensuring that staff is trained on the REMS requirements. For example, a pharmacist may be required to complete REMS training, ensure that "safe use conditions are met prior to dispensing a drug (e.g., verifying results of required laboratory tests for a patient, or ensuring that a patient or prescriber is enrolled in the REMS), and provide patients with required counseling, educational materials, or a medication guide.

Three examples of REMS programs with protocol impacting pharmacists include the following:

- OxyContin® (controlled-release oral formulation of oxycodone hydrochloride) is used to treat pain and is associated with potentially life-threatening risks. Thus, the FDA and the manufacturer developed a REMS program that requires health care providers who prescribe the product to receive training. Dispensers will have to be trained and authorized as well and will be required to provide a medication guide about the product to each patient.
- Jynarque® (tablet) is used to slow kidney function decline in adults who are at risk for rapidly progressing autosomal dominant polycystic kidney disease. There is the risk of serious and potentially fatal liver injury associated with the use of Jynarque. The REMS program requires that only certified pharmacies dispense the drug, and that the pharmacists verify that the prescriber is certified to prescribe the drug, and the patient is enrolled in the REMS program and authorized to receive the drug.
- Palynziq® (medication used to lower blood levels of phenylalanine in adults with phenylketonuria) can cause a severe allergic reaction (anaphylaxis) that may be life threatening. The REMS program for this product requires that pharmacies be certified before they are able to prescribe and/or dispense the product. Additionally, the pharmacist must verify and document that the patient has auto-injectable epinephrine and must obtain authorization to dispense each prescription by contacting the REMS program to verify prescriber certification and patient enrolment.

Distributors have positioned themselves to be a specialty supplier for products with REMS, and have capabilities to support REMS requirements. Pharmacies, both institutional and retail, are also reengineering to manage these requirements. Pharmacies are reevaluating their purchasing and inventory management processes for drug products with REMS. It is important for pharmacists to consider the administrative and logistical issues associated with dispensing drug products with REMS requirements. It will be important for pharmacists to stay abreast of the development and implementation of REMS programs for various products.

Specialty Pharmacy

Specialty pharmaceutical drugs are a growing and increasingly important part of the global and United States pharmaceutical market. The HDA Research Foundation (2018b), in collaboration with its specialty pharmaceutical task force and industry thought leaders from IQVIA (formerly QuintilesIMS), defines specialty pharmaceuticals as products that treat chronic, complex, and rare diseases; and have a minimum of four out of seven additional characteristics related to the distribution, care, delivery, and/or cost of the medicines (see Table 27-6).

Between 2013 and 2017, spending on specialty pharmaceuticals in the United States increased by more than 87%, from $105 billion to $196 billion (IQVIA, 2018). Specialty pharmacies have expanded and evolved to support this growth, developing the unique capabilities required to dispense specialty pharmaceutical products. Specialty pharmaceutical products typically have special handling or storage requirements and may require administration at time of dispensing or other more involved patient support.

They also have high costs to the pharmacy and the patient, presenting unique payment and reimbursement challenges.

Community pharmacies often may not have the capabilities to support the dispensing of specialty pharmaceuticals, which can include supplies or personnel to provide injections or infusions, special storage and handling expertise and infrastructure, the ability to bear inventory-carrying costs for expensive drug products, and the ability to navigate the reimbursement requirements of major medical insurance carriers (Suchanek, 2005). Specialty pharmacies have developed to fill this need in the marketplace. Payers often contract with a specialty pharmacy and require beneficiaries to obtain certain products through the specialty pharmacy.

It is important to mention that all pharmacies face challenges with respect to purchasing, inventory management, and dispensing as products become

---

Table 27-6   Definition of Specialty Pharmaceutical Drugs

Specialty Medicines Treat Diseases With the Following Characteristics:

Chronic	• Disease is long-lasting and often without direct cure • Treatments for disease are intended to be used for more than 6 months
Complex	• Diseases have both environmental and genetic components, meaning they may be hereditary and/or exacerbated by environmental factors (obesity, diet, etc.) • Complex diseases can affect multiple organ systems and may be caused or be the cause of secondary diseases
Rare	• Defined as those with fewer than 200,000 new cases annually • Equivalent to the US definition of orphan diseases but not exclusively linked to the granting of an FDA orphan drug designation

Medicines Must Exhibit Four of These Seven Criteria to be Considered Specialty:

1) Are high in cost (~$6000 or more per year)
2) Treatment initiated/maintained by a specialist
3) Require administration by another individual or health care professional (i.e., not self-administered)
4) Require special handling in the supply chain (e.g., refrigerated, frozen, chemo precautions, biohazard)
5) Require patient payment assistance
6) Distributed through non-traditional channels
7) Medication has significant side effects that require additional monitoring/counseling (including, but not limited to REMS programs) and/or disease requires additional monitoring of therapy (e.g., monitoring of blood/cell counts to assess effectiveness/side effects of therapy)

Reprinted with permission from 2018 Speciality Pharmaceutical Distribution Facts, Figures and Trends. Copyright © 2018 by the Healthcare Distribution Alliance (HDA) Research Foundation.

more expensive, have REMS requirements, or require other "special" considerations (e.g., storage, administration). For example, hospitals are challenged when a patient is hospitalized and his insurance company requires a drug product to be purchased through a specialty pharmacy or the patient has already purchased the product and needs it to be administered while in the hospital (Kirschenbaum, 2009). If the hospital has to purchase it through the specialty pharmacy, they may not get as good a price as if they had purchased it through their distributor. The hospital may allow the patient to bring the specialty product into the hospital; however, there are concerns about product integrity (e.g., how the product has been stored while in possession of patient). Pharmacies need to continue to evaluate their policies and procedures with respect to drug distribution systems.

340B Drug Pricing Program

The federal government's 340B Drug Pricing Program has played a modest but increasingly important role in the US health care market since its inception. The 340B program was introduced in 1992 and allows certain types of "safety-net" providers to buy prescription drugs at reduced prices, which are usually less than the net cost of drugs paid by state Medicaid programs (US Government Accountability Office, 2011). Hospitals, clinics, and health centers, which meet certain eligibility requirements, are known as 340B covered entities, and qualify to purchase drugs

at the discounted rate (HRSA, 2019). Covered entities may access 340B drug pricing for all of their eligible patients, including those with Medicare and commercial insurance.

The 340B program has expanded significantly over time and evolved to include family planning centers (1998) and children's hospitals to participate as covered entities. The most significant expansion came in 2010, when the Affordable Care Act (ACA) extended eligibility to include children's' hospitals, critical access hospitals, sole community hospitals, rural referral centers, and cancer centers (see Table 27-7). Pharmacy services provided by a 340B-covered entity may be provided through either an in-house pharmacy or with a contract with an outside pharmacy.

Growth of different 340B entity types continues to expand. In the year of program inception, there were 51 340B entities. As of January 2017, there were 2,357 hospital organizations participating in the 340B program (HRSA, 2017). The number of 340B covered entities has increased, and the number of 340B pharmacies and contract pharmacies has expanded as well. Prior to 2010, covered entities were limited to one pharmacy per site, which could either be operated in-house, or with a single external contract pharmacy unless they applied to the Office of Pharmacy Affairs (OPA) for an alternative arrangement (Federal Register, 2010). In April of 2010, OPA guidance was revised to allow covered entities to enter into contract pharmacy arrangements with more than

Table 27-7. 340B Eligible Entities	
Federal Grantees	**Hospital Types**
• Comprehensive hemophilia treatment centers	• Disproportionate share hospitals
• Federally qualified health centers/lookalikes	• Children's hospitals*
• Urban/638 health center	• Critical Access hospitals*
• Ryan White programs	• Free-standing cancer hospitals*
• Sexually transmitted disease/tuberculosis	• Rural referral centers*
• Title X family planning	• Sole community hospitals*

*340 B Eligible via Section 7101 of the Affordable Care Act (ACA).
Data from Health Resources and Services Administration (HRSA), 340B Eligibility. Available at https://www.hrsa.gov/opa/eligibility-and-registration/index.html.

one external contract pharmacy. Since this time, contract pharmacy growth has expanded significantly. As of January 2017, there over 12,000 unique locations acting as 340B contract pharmacies (HRSA, 2017).

A 340B pharmacy or contract pharmacy must operate in a way that fits the needs of the 340B covered entity. The pharmacy must ensure that it has sufficient inventory required by the covered entity, should participate in the insurance plans required by the covered entity's patient population, and comply with 340B program requirements including ensuring that there is no diversion of drugs bought at 340B prices to anyone other than the covered entity patients, and collaborating with Medicaid to ensure that there is no opportunity for potential duplicate discount/rebates (NCPA, 2014).

Supply Chain Integrity: The Importance of an Authorized Distributor

This chapter has focused mainly on supply chain management from the pharmacy's internal business perspective—understanding the demand for products and having the right products available to sell while reducing the investment in inventory. Yet the flow of pharmaceuticals from the manufacturer to the pharmacy is of critical importance to ensure product integrity and safety: Pharmacy staff must also focus on ensuring supply-chain integrity. It is estimated that worldwide drug counterfeiting is a multibillion-dollar business, and 1% to 2% of drugs in North America are fraudulent (National Association of Boards of Pharmacy Foundation, 2015).

Pharmacy staff must be aware of the potential for purchasing and dispensing counterfeit products. To ensure that drug products are authentic, pharmacists should choose a reputable vendor with a reliable delivery system. There are large national and regional pharmaceutical distributors that are "authorized distributors" which purchase prescription medicines and other medical products directly from pharmaceutical manufacturers—which ensures the products they supply to health care providers and pharmacies are safe, reliable, and secure.

In addition to DSCSA requirements, some also look to accreditation programs such as National Association of Boards of Pharmacy wholesaler Verified-Accredited Wholesaler Distributors program. There are thousands of secondary wholesalers that purchase products from other wholesalers or repackagers that may or may not be legitimate. If a lesser known vendor calls with a special deal on a product that appears to be too good to be true, that probably is the case. When a package arrives, the staff person should look for problems, such as old or worn packaging, a faded label around the expiration date, missing overt packaging marks, or product or packaging appearance that is different from normal. Pharmacists who suspect that they have purchased counterfeit drugs should contact the FDA Medwatch program, the manufacturer of the drug product, their state board of pharmacy, and their local law enforcement authorities.

Supply Chain Integrity: The Drug Supply Chain Security Act

The DSCSA is Title II of Public Law No. 113-54, the Drug Quality and Security Act, which was signed into law on November 27, 2013 (FDA, 2013). This law outlined critical steps that must be implemented by 2023 to identify and trace prescription drugs in the United States. In the years leading up to its passage, U.S. state legislatures had enacted various laws related to the pedigree (a document that provides a transaction history) of pharmaceutical products. The DSCSA pre-empted this 50-state "patchwork" of pedigree requirements with one federal solution to trace prescription medicines in the supply chain (Drug Supply Chain Security Act, 2019). Leading up to full implementation in 2023, the law mandates specific requirements for manufacturers, repackagers, distributors, and dispensers/pharmacies. This law:

- **Required product tracing requirements, increasing the efficiency and safety of the supply chain.** Beginning in January 2015, manufacturers and distributors were required to adhere to enhanced product tracing requirements, with pharmaceutical dispensers following later that year. Over a

10-year horizon, product tracing information will be exchanged in a secure, electronic interoperable manner that will allow for the electronic tracing of drug products at the package level throughout the U.S. pharmaceutical supply chain.

- **Pharmaceuticals can only be bought and sold between entities that are authorized.** All trading partners (manufacturers, repackagers, wholesale distributors, dispensers, and third-party logistics providers) must "authorized," that is, hold an appropriate registration or license. An authorized trading partner may only sell products to and buy products from other another authorized trading partner.
- **Strengthened distributor and third-party logistics provider licensure standards across the United States.** Through the DSCSA, the FDA must issue national standards for the licensure of wholesale distributors and third-party logistics providers. Once finalized, states have 2 years to adopt these standards. This approach is intended to create greater uniformity across states and enhance federal authority, while enabling states to maintain their authority to issue licenses and partner with FDA in enforcement efforts.
- **Established new processes for identifying suspicious and illegitimate products in the supply chain.** Trading partners (manufacturers, repackagers, wholesale distributors, dispensers) must have systems to quarantine and conduct investigations of suspect products; to notify FDA and immediate trading partners within 24 hours, if a product is illegitimate; and to terminate notifications about illegitimate product in consultation with FDA.

The requirements, development of standards, and the system for product tracing have been ongoing since November 27, 2013, and will continue to be phased in until 2023.

The DSCSA requires that pharmacies take the following specific actions to protect patients from harmful counterfeit or illegitimate drugs (FDA, 2018).

- **Confirm partner licenses:** Pharmacies may only buy from authorized trading partners and so must confirm that their trading partners are licensed or registered. This means checking the registrations of manufacturers or repackagers, and the licensing of distributors, third-party logistics providers, and other pharmacies.
- **Receive, store, and provide product-tracing documentation:** Pharmacies may only accept prescription drugs that are accompanied by the DSCSA-required product tracing documentation. This documentation must be stored either electronically or on paper for 6 years.
- **Investigate and properly handle suspect and illegitimate drugs:** Pharmacies must have a process for investigating and managing drugs that are suspect or illegitimate, that is, counterfeit, diverted, stolen, intentionally adulterated, or unfit for distribution. This process should include steps to quarantine and investigate suspect prescription drugs to determine if they are illegitimate; and if they are determined to be illegitimate ensure that patients do not receive them. The pharmacy must also work with manufacturer, notify the FDA, and notify the trading partners from whom they bought the drug.

■ REVISITING THE SCENARIO

Referring back to Marie's predicament, it is easy to see that a number of factors may be influencing her pharmacy's purchasing and inventory control mechanisms. It is apparent that the pharmacy had minimized its investment in inventory to an extent that it may be hurting sales. The pharmacy appears to be having frequent out-of-stock situations, resulting in decreased sales, loss of goodwill, loss of patrons, and possibly harm to patients. Marie should evaluate the pharmacy's supply chain processes, inventory targeting, and purchasing policies and decisions. She should evaluate the inventory management reports to determine which products have a high turnover rate and which products have a low turnover rate. Knowing this should facilitate ordering decisions.

Marie should take the opportunity to participate in the distributor contract negotiation process.

Reviewing the two bids and collaborating with the distributors to understand their capabilities during the bidding process should help Community Pharmacy negotiate a good agreement and ensure competitive pricing and quality service. Marie should develop a relationship with the selected distributor's customer representative and examine the services and programs offered by the wholesaler. Marie may also want to select a secondary wholesaler.

Buying goods at the lowest price is another concern. It is difficult to compare prices because price often depends on (1) purchasing volume, (2) rebates and discounts earned, and (3) membership in a GPO. In addition, certain pharmacies, such as disproportionate share (DPS) hospital pharmacies, qualify for other pricing considerations. (*Note:* DPS hospitals qualify for special pricing because they provide a significant amount of care to low-income patients.) Marie should also work with her purchasing and accounting personnel to ensure that appropriate discounts are earned. Taking advantage of discounts is one way to reduce costs and improve cash flow for the pharmacy. Marie should also consider participating in a GPO. One of the most significant factors that affect pharmaceutical costs, other than discounts and rebates, is participation in a GPO or a buying group.

These are just a few of the parameters that Marie should consider. There are other purchasing and inventory management activities that Marie could evaluate. For example, she may want to contract with a return-goods company to assist with the return of goods. Another example would be to purchase and dispense more generic drugs because these products reduce the amount of money invested in inventory. Marie should enhance her awareness of the formularies established by the payers and health plans most frequently used by her patients. Knowing the drug products which are and are not on their formularies will help her plan her pharmacy's purchasing accordingly. Overall, Marie constantly must be aware of the purchasing and inventory management activities. These activities can have a significant impact on both the financial and the operational health of the pharmacy.

With regards to the DSCSA, many changes are just around the corner, and the Community Pharmacy is not completely prepared at this point. Under the DSCSA, all prescription products covered under the law that are packaged after November 27, 2018, are serialized, which means they contain a 2D Data-Matrix bar code encoded with the product identifier (NDC embedded in a GTIN-14, serial number, lot, and expiry). As of November 27, 2020, pharmacies may only transact (i.e., purchase and sell) serialized products unless the product is "grandfathered" (packaged before November 27, 2018) or exempt from serialization requirements. Verification requirements in suspect and product investigations will also go into effect, and the pharmacy will need to be able to verify the unique product identifier back to the manufacturer of at least three packages or 10% of the suspect product, whichever is greater. Currently, pharmacies have up to 2 days to provide transaction data in response to certain requests in suspect and illegitimate product investigations and in the event of a recall.

By 2023, there is a requirement for electronic-only data exchange across the pharmaceutical supply chain. The pharmacy must be able to securely receive electronic transaction data with each sale of a drug product, maintain them electronically for 6 years, and provide transaction data in response to appropriate requests in suspect and illegitimate drug product investigations and recalls. To support and meet these requirements, the Community Pharmacy's computer systems will need to be upgraded and enhanced, and the management team will need to ensure that the pharmacy managers and staff are prepared to implement these changes.

REFERENCES

American Society of Health-System Pharmacists (ASHP). 2019a. Current Drug Shortages. Available at https://www.ashp.org/drug-shortages/current-shortages. Accessed February 19, 2019.

Amerisource Bergen. 2019a. ABC Order. Available at https://www.amerisourcebergen.com/abcnew/-/

media/assets/gnp/pdf/abc-order-sell-sheet.pdf?la=en&hash=3BA479BAF5B2620EC66DB7869260E17AF6E392AB. Accessed February 19, 2019.

Amerisource Bergen. 2019b. Cubixx System: Increase Cost Efficiency and Improve Health System Pharmacy Workflow. Available at https://www.cubixxsolutions.com/-/media/assets/cubixx/documents/2019-pdf-brochures/cubixx-consignment.pdf?la=en&hash=3E4C825BEE0F94E76FF4BBEFA3ABB8BFD0445D7A. Accessed March 1, 2019.

ASHP. 2008. ASHP guidelines on medication cost management strategies for hospitals and health systems. *Am J Health-Syst Pharm* 65:1368–1384.

ASHP. 2019b. Formulary Management. Available at https://www.ashp.org/pharmacy-practice/policy-positions-and-guidelines/browse-by-topic/formulary-management. Accessed February 19, 2019.

Cardinal Health. 2019. Cardinal Health™ Inventory Manager (CIM) for Pharmacies. Available at https://www.cardinalhealth.com/en/services/retail-pharmacy/business-solutions/business-advantage/cardinal-health-inventory-manager.html. Accessed February 19, 2019.

Carroll NV. 1998. *Financial Management for Pharmacists*, 2nd ed. Baltimore, MD: Williams & Wilkins.

Drug Supply Chain Security Act. 2019. *Title II of the Drug Quality and Security Act*. Available at https://www.fda.gov/drugs/drugsafety/drugintegrityandsupplychainsecurity/drugsupplychainsecurityact/ucm376829.htm. Accessed April 1, 2019.

Federal Register. 2010. Notice Regarding 340B Drug Pricing Program—Contract Pharmacy Services, 75 Fed. Reg. 10272 (March 5, 2010).

Fierce Pharma. 2018a. Teva launches first U.S. generic Cialis as Eli Lilly braces for loss of its ED blockbuster. Available at https://www.fiercepharma.com/pharma/teva-launches-first-us-generic-cialis-as-lilly-investors-brace-for-loss-ed-blockbuster. Accessed March 2, 2019.

Fierce Pharma. 2018b. Pfizer wins blockbuster Lyrica patent extension to safeguard sales till June. Available at https://www.fiercepharma.com/pharma/pfizer-wins-blockbuster-patent-extension-for-lyrica-exclusivity-now-stretches-until-june. Accessed March 2, 2019.

Food and Drug Administration (FDA). 2013. Drug Supply Chain Security Act. Available at http://www.fda.gov/Drugs/DrugSafety/DrugIntegrityandSupplyChainSecurity/DrugSupplyChainSecurityAct/default.htm. Accessed February 19, 2019.

Food and Drug Administration. (FDA) 2018. Drug Supply Chain Security Act (DSCSA) pharmacy requirements flyer. Available at https://www.fda.gov/downloads/Drugs/DrugSafety/DrugIntegrityandSupplyChainSecurity/DrugSupplyChainSecurityAct/UCM607076.pdf. Accessed February 19, 2019.

Food and Drug Administration (FDA). 2019a. FDA Drug Shortages. Available at https://www.accessdata.fda.gov/scripts/drugshortages/default.cfm. Accessed February 9, 2019.

Food and Drug Administration. (FDA) 2019b. FDA.gov, "What's in a REMS? Types of REMS requirements." Available at https://www.fda.gov/Drugs/DrugSafety/REMS/ucm592636.htm. Accessed January 10, 2019.

Heathcare Distribution Alliance (HDA) Research Foundation. 2019. Understanding Pharmaceutical Distribution Presentation. Available at https://www.hda.org/resources/2019-understanding-pharmaceutical-distribution-presentation. Accessed February 19, 2019.

Heathcare Distribution Alliance (HDA) Research Foundation, 2018. Specialty Pharmaceutical Distribution Facts Figures and Trends. Available at https://www.hda.org/resources/2018-specialty-pharmaceutical-distribution. Accessed January 10, 2019.

Healthcare Distribution Alliance (HDA) Research Foundation. 2019. 340B Whitepaper Available at https://www.hda.org/resources?cat={19D63219-6FC1-4749-BCBE-880B932D70B2}. Accessed July 22, 2019.

Health Resources and Services Administration. (HRSA). 2017. Office of Pharmacy Affairs 340B Database, January 2017.

Health Resources and Services Administration (HRSA). 2019. 340B Eligibility. Available at http://www.hrsa.gov/opa/eligibility-and-registration/index.html. Accessed January 10, 2019.

Huffman DC (ed.). 1996. Purchasing and inventory control. In: *Effective Pharmacy Management*, 8th ed. Alexandria, VA: National Association of Retail Druggists: 355.

IQVIA, 2018. National Sales Perspectives, April 2018.

Jackson T, Bentley J, McCaffrey D, et al. 2014. Store and Prescription characteristics associated with primary medication non-adherence. *J Manag Care Spec Pharm* 20(8):824–832.

Kirschenbaum BE. 2009. Specialty pharmacies and other restricted drug distribution systems: Financial and safety considerations for patients and health-system pharmacists. *Am J Health Syst Pharm* 66 (Suppl 7): S13–S20.

McKesson. 2019. McKesson Pharmacy Management Software. Available at https://www.mckesson.com/Pharmacy-Management/Software/. Accessed February 19, 2019.

National Association of Boards of Pharmacy Foundation. 2015. AWARxE: Counterfeit Medications. Available at http://www.awarerx.org/get-informed/safe-acquisition/counterfeit-medications. Accessed September 15, 2015.

National Community Pharmacists Association (NCPA). 2014. NCPA Pharmacy's Guide to 340B Contract Pharmacy. Alexandria, VA: National Community Pharmacists Association.

National Community Pharmacists Association. 2018. Private communication regarding inventory turnover in independent pharmacies. December 2018.

Planet Retail Limited. 2018. The Sensormatic Global Shrink Index, http://shrinkindex.sensormatic.com/wp-content/uploads/2018/05/Sensormatic-Global-Shrink-Index.pdf. Accessed February 7, 2019.

Silbiger S. 1999. The Ten-Day MBA, revised edn. New York: Quill William Morrow.

Suchanek D. 2005. The rise and role of specialty pharmacy. *Biotechnol Healthc* 2(5):31–35.

Tootelian DH, Gaedeke RM. 1993. *Essentials of Pharmacy Management*. St. Louis, MO: Mosby.

US Government Accountability Office. 2011. *Manufacturer Discounts in the 340B Program Offer Benefits, but Federal Oversight Needs Improvement*, GAO-11-836, 2011.

West DS. 2001. *Managing Efficiencies in Pharmacy Cash Flow*, vol. 6. Birmingham, AL: Mylan Institute of Pharmacy, Continuing Education Series.

West DS. 2003. Purchasing and inventory control. In: Jackson R (ed.) *Effective Pharmacy Management CDROM*, 9th ed. Sec. 17. Alexandria, VA: National Community Pharmacists Association Foundation.

West DS (ed.). 2010. *2010 NCPA Digest sponsored by Cardinal Health*. Alexandria, VA: National Community Pharmacists Association.

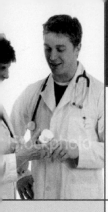

28

MERCHANDISING

Edward Cohen and Erna Mesic

About the Authors: Dr. Cohen received a BS in pharmacy from the University of Illinois at Chicago (UIC) and a PharmD from Midwestern University Chicago College of Pharmacy (MWU). After owning an independent pharmacy for many years, he moved into the corporate sector as Director of Pharmacy for Dominick's Finer Foods (a division of Safeway). He has served as Senior Director, Clinical Services, for Walgreens. Today, he serves as Executive Vice President of Pharmacy Advocacy at MJH Associates, a health care communications company. Dr. Cohen has been recognized nationally for his role in bringing patient care to the forefront of community pharmacy practice. He holds adjunct faculty positions at UIC and MWU, as well as serving on both colleges' advisory committees. Dr. Cohen has served as Chair of the Administration Section of the American Pharmacists Association—Academy of Pharmacy Practice and Management and on the Board of Directors of the Illinois Pharmacists Association.

Erna Mesic received a BS in biology from the UIC and Masters in Public Health from Benedictine University. She has worked for Walgreens, first as a pharmacy technician and later moving into the corporate sector serving pharmacy services programs such as immunizations, health system transitions of care, and most recently as Director of Pharmacy Operations (Market Access).

■ LEARNING OBJECTIVES

After completing this chapter, readers should be able to

1. Describe the evolution of merchandising in pharmacy from the beginning of the 20th century to current practices used today.
2. Identify merchandising techniques that enhance the awareness and use of the pharmacy department as a health care destination for patients.
3. Explain omnichannel merchandising challenges to changes in the way patients access pharmacy health care services.
4. Identify and discuss the implications of ineffective omnichannel pharmacy merchandising.
5. Evaluate the impact of merchandising on the financial success of a pharmacy.

■ SCENARIO

Jerry Western, a third-year Doctor of Pharmacy student, was home recently to attend a family gathering. There was much ado about Jerry's progress in pharmacy school. His family was asking questions about school, his classes, his job, and his future. As the conversation continued, Jerry found the family involved in a discussion about how they search for and access pharmacy goods and services. The family had a full range of opinions that addressed everything from the ability to easily access a pharmacy, the range of goods and services they offer (including delivery services), and even a pharmacy's online offerings. They discussed the pharmacists and staff, convenience, and the store hours.

Jerry was impressed with the conversation. He had never thought much about the issues being discussed by his family. It seemed that the pharmacy where he works as an intern, Middletown South Pharmacy, is the least liked by his family. Middleton South Pharmacy is perceived to be an "old standard" in the community. It is a traditional drugstore, built on a corner in the center of town. They have limited parking, a smaller front of the store where nonprescription items are sold, a nice prescription department, and an old-fashioned soda fountain that is still a busy part of the business. While Jerry's family spoke highly of their memories of Middleton South Pharmacy (and particularly of the treats at their soda fountain), they also said that it is "just an old fashioned drugstore" and doesn't offer many of the conveniences and new pharmacy services the other pharmacies are providing.

His family's favorite pharmacy in town is Healthway Pharmacy, which was remodeled last year. Healthway Pharmacy is bright and open, making it easy to find items. The staff is friendly and is always doing something to make the store look nice. As people shop, they often find and buy items that they need, as well as items that they had not even planned on purchasing that day. Healthway Pharmacy uses technology to enhance their product offerings and information. Many of the services offered by the pharmacy, such as prescription delivery or an "ask a pharmacist" service,

can be accessed on-line or through the pharmacy's smartphone app. Healthway Pharmacy has many new products, making it enjoyable to shop in the store. The prescription department is large and open with a comfortable waiting area, as well as a private room to meet with the pharmacist. Healthway's pharmacists' offer many patient care services, including health screenings, immunizations, and classes to teach people about how to make the most of their medicines. There is a kiosk that allows patients to pick up their prescriptions 24 hours a day and access a pharmacist via the Internet at any time. The store is easy to access from the major streets in the area and has a large parking area. The store also has a drive-through window by the pharmacy, and in-store medical clinic staffed by a nurse practitioner. Healthway Pharmacy is open 24 hours a day, 7 days a week. Everyone encouraged Jerry to visit Healthway Pharmacy and inquire about getting a job there.

■ CHAPTER QUESTIONS

1. What are the most prominent merchandising features that drive customers to shop in a pharmacy?
2. How does merchandising affect customer choices while shopping online or in the store?
3. What is the impact of merchandising on the overall operation and profitability of a pharmacy?
4. What are the goals of effective merchandising methods for a pharmacy?
5. Which factors should be considered in the design of the digital site of a pharmacy? In the design and layout of the physical store?

■ INTRODUCTION

The scenario demonstrates the effects of some "invisible" principles of merchandising. The lack of effective merchandising at Middletown South Pharmacy was enough to send Jerry's family to Healthway Pharmacy. Many of the physical features of community pharmacies are frequently taken for granted. The exterior design is important to create an identity and connection with customers. The colors and shapes of the outdoor signage add to the pharmacy's identity. Pharmacy managers can plan the ease of entry into the store and everything seen and felt by consumers inside the pharmacy. Merchandising activities used by pharmacy managers can attract customers and make their shopping experience more enjoyable.

Almost every retail store (including community pharmacies) is designed for selling merchandise (Hilditch, 1981). Given the decline in profit margins in the prescription department, the success of a pharmacy's "front end" is crucial to the total financial success of the business.

Community pharmacies have traditionally been retail establishments where customers can find staple items, basic health care needs, and prescription medications. Today, in addition to the traditional offerings, pharmacies are a destination where a wide variety of health care services can be obtained. Immunizations, health screenings, primary care clinics, hearing, vision, dental, and many other services are now available in community pharmacies. Pharmacies today offer an omnichannel shopping experience, allowing patients and customers to shop online, coordinate in-store shopping with online purchases, track their purchases, and make appointments for services offered in the store as well as online (Fiorletta, 2014).

Larger chain pharmacies have expanded the definition of a traditional pharmacy by promoting and selling large varieties of merchandise that often are well beyond the basic mixture of products found in a traditional drugstore (Francke, 1974). Today, pharmacies are also found in hospitals, clinics, grocery stores, and even large discount stores. The location of the pharmacy within these often very large buildings, as well as the mix, location, and types of the goods and services offered, is important to the pharmacy's success.

Attracting customers into a retail business and inviting them to make purchases while they are there are the main objectives of all merchandising efforts. However, merely relying on having what people need is not going to produce sales. Pharmacies must consider many different factors such as design, layout, and the mix of merchandise offered to ensure customers can find what they are looking for, as well as to entice them to make unplanned purchases that may meet their latent needs. It is important to keep in mind that most of the items sold in a pharmacy can also be purchased in other retail outlets or on the Internet. The proper mix of convenience, price, and service will add to the appeal of the pharmacy.

Today's community pharmacy strives to be viewed as a health care destination in the eyes of their customers. The pharmacy of the future may follow several business models. One model centers on a retail merchandising operation, while another centers on providing health care services. Pharmacies that focus on providing health care services generally still sell merchandise, but they focus more on offering health-related products and provide fewer nonhealth related items such as greeting cards and cosmetics. As pharmacies expand their offerings of professional goods and services, some have stopped the sale of tobacco products (O'Donnell & Ungar, 2014) and increased offerings of healthier foods. These pharmacies carry more lines of health-related products such as durable medical equipment, blood glucose, and other diabetes specialty items as well as an expanded vitamin and herbal offerings. Most community pharmacies today provide immunizations and have developed services to help patients better understand their health conditions and become more adherent to their medications (Japsen, 2014). Some pharmacies have even added in-store medical clinics for treatment of minor ailments.

Today's community pharmacies continue to strive to differentiate themselves and offer an inviting mix of goods and services. Increased competition from online retailers, with the convenience of ordering and delivery, is stressing tradition retail locations. Community pharmacies continue their transformation through formation of alliances and partnerships to enhance and offer delivery services, informational kiosk placements, grocery offering with a focus on nutrition, and private label differentiation. Collaborating with other businesses can expand a pharmacy's reach and build additional awareness of their business. Collaborations can also be a good source of new business tactics (see Figure 28-1). For example,

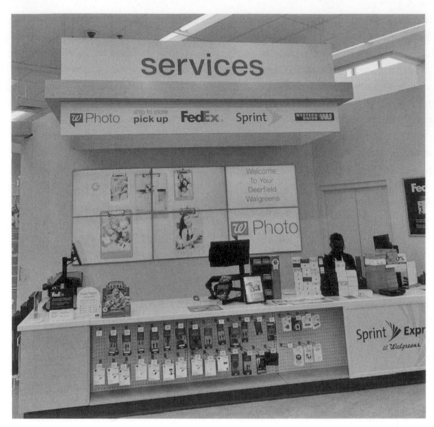

Figure 28-1. Community pharmacy partnerships with other businesses.

a collaboration between FedEx and Walgreens has resulted in benefits for both partners. Consumers can drop off their FedEx packages at any one of thousands of Walgreens locations, which not only enhances convenience for FedEx customers but also increases foot traffic in Walgreens stores. Walgreens then utilizes the FedEx shipping network to enable overnight delivery of prescriptions and other health goods almost anywhere in the United States (Japsen, 2018).

Customers respond to what they see, hear, and feel. Offering customers choice, allowing them to get what they want, when they want it, and how they want creates customer loyalty and is key to the success of any business, including pharmacies and other health care providers. Many pharmacies utilize technology to assist and support the customer in their shopping. Designing a pharmacy to address the everyday needs of our on-the-go society makes the in-store experience successful. Coordinating the in-store and on-line experience enhances that experience. Merchandising tools are used in every aspect of the pharmacy business. By drawing customers to the online and in-store locations, and making it easy and comfortable for consumers to purchase what they need and want, customer loyalty is enhanced.

■ PHARMACY MERCHANDISING TRENDS THROUGH THE 1900s

Early in the last century, people came to drugstores for relief from their ailments. Pharmacists had a handful of drugs, sold mostly in compounded mixtures, and did what they could to ease their patients' discomfort. Drugstores were not merchandised as they are today. Drugstores contained low-cost traditional items that people used every day. Some of the traditional items found in drugstores were cosmetics, magazines, tobacco, stationery, and candy. Preparing and dispensing medications from a prescription, often compounded on site at the pharmacy, was a small portion of the total sales of the store. Each pharmacy owner built his or her reputation on individual relationships with his or her customers.

When the 18th Amendment to the US Constitution was enacted in 1920, the sale, production, and distribution of alcoholic beverages in most traditional establishments (e.g., bars, restaurants, liquor stores) was outlawed (Encyclopedia Britannica, 2019). During the period from 1920 to 1933, otherwise known as "Prohibition," the drugstore fountain replaced the tavern as the new socially acceptable gathering place. Pharmacists and their clerks were busy making milkshakes and other soda fountain creations. During Prohibition, pharmacies became the only legitimate place to purchase alcohol products because they were only available with a doctor's prescription. When Prohibition was lifted in the 1930s, many pharmacies continued to sell liquor, having developed a reputation as legitimate outlets (Higby, 1997).

After World War II, many new medications came to the market. Pharmacies began filling more prescriptions using prefabricated dosage forms, and thus spent less time compounding medications. Pharmacists began to spend most of their time dispensing prefabricated prescription drug products, making sure the patient received the medication in an efficient manner, with the focus on providing drug products, not drug information. The front end of the store took on a new look and feel as well. Pharmacies began to stock many prefabricated staple items. As a result of filling an increasing number of prescriptions, pharmacists had less time to manage the front ends of their pharmacies. Prescriptions were becoming another commodity in the store, much to the dismay of pharmacists. Pharmacists were looking to transition their practices to have patient safety as their primary

concern. By the late 1960s, the profession had taken a firm stand to change and regain the professional stature of the pharmacy (Higby, 1997).

■ PHARMACY DESIGN, LAYOUT, AND MERCHANDISING

While some purchases made in pharmacies are planned by consumers in advance (e.g., picking up a new or refilled prescription), many purchases made in pharmacies are not. For example, while many people may come to a pharmacy planning to purchase a prescription for a particular disease or condition (e.g., an antiviral drug to treat the flu), while they are in the pharmacy they often pick up additional items, some related to their prescription or condition (e.g., acetaminophen, a box of tissues), some that help them care for others (e.g., a bottle of cough medicine for a child), and some just because they are conveniently offered and available to meet a latent need (e.g., the magazine or box of chocolates at the check-out counter). Pharmacy managers use store design, layout, and merchandising strategies to affect the purchasing behaviors of their customers. Studies have shown that more than 80% of all purchases made in pharmacies are made by people who less than a week before were not planning to buy these particular items (Eisenpreis, 1983). The primary reasons why consumers make unplanned purchases are emergencies (running out of a needed item), latent buying interests brought on by a good price or a new product, and impulse purchases (buying on a whim to try something new or different).

An important contribution to sales success in a pharmacy is the store design and layout of merchandise. Getting people into a pharmacy, making it easy to find and purchase both needed and wanted items, and increasing the number of return visits consumers make to a pharmacy all can be influenced by store design and layout factors. The store design and layout of a pharmacy must allow for customer convenience, ease of shopping, and an exciting atmosphere that will promote the purchase of both goods and services.

Consumer shopping behavior is quickly changing. Much of this change in behavior can be attributed to improvements in technology, especially smartphones and other devices that enable consumers to obtain information about goods and services in a manner that was not available previously. Technological improvements not only affect consumer shopping behaviors, it also affects how pharmacies merchandise and conduct business with their customers. As patients and customers utilize the convenience brought through digital devices, the need for face-to-face interaction, particularly when shopping or purchasing, is decreasing. Researchers have found that people have developed such a strong bond with digital devices that the term "nomophobia" has been coined to describe the anxiety brought on by being separated from one's smartphone (Slawsky, 2015). Consumer access to real time data equips and empowers them to know what they want and when they want it. When consumers shop online, they have the same expectations and look to have the same experiences regardless of if they are visiting a pharmacy website or Amazon.com. Patients and customers can search for pharmacy goods and services over the Internet using a web browser or a smartphone app. Pharmacy customers may now search, review, and order products that can be picked up in the store the same or next day or can have their orders delivered to their home or office (see Figure 28-2). Services provided in the pharmacy can be reviewed online and appointments can be made to have a set day and time to obtain the desired services in the store. Having an online site for customers is important to pharmacy success and brand loyalty.

Pharmacy Design

Today's consumers demand convenience, great service, and ambience. While pharmacies have not always been known for these attributes, consumers have come to expect a certain atmosphere and comfort level from any retail establishment.

From the 1940s to the 1960s, pharmacy store design and decor did not highlight merchandise or professional activities. Most pharmacies carried a mix of staple items, tobacco, and liquor; had soda

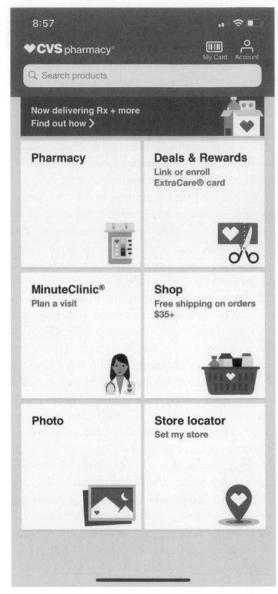

Figure 28-2. Screen shot of CVS mobile app.

fountains; and gave little thought to where the best place might be to locate these items in the store. During the 1970s and 1980s, pharmacy designs transitioned to highlight the products to be sold, resulting in simpler decor and allowing the merchandise to become part of the pharmacy's design.

It is important to select the most appropriate design aspects for a pharmacy without becoming too trendy or rapidly outdated. To determine a pharmacy design, managers first must determine the characteristics and needs of the customers to be served. Customers want pharmacies that are convenient to home or work, are clean and well organized, and are in supply of the goods and services they need, when they need them. Even though most consumers will conduct research online before making a purchase, many still desire the connection with either the physical goods, or the people involved in producing or selling that good, when they make the actual purchase (PBA Health, 2018). Pharmacies, where the pharmacist and staff are an important component of the product offerings, need to be effective in both their online presence as well as their physical ("brick and mortar") presence.

Women are the key decision makers for the family and make most pharmacy purchase decisions (Hamacher Resource Group, 2013). Today, families must be efficient with their time. They often have so many competing demands on their time that they have little to no time to plan shopping trips. Because of this, consumers are choosing to purchase some goods and services online as it is more convenient for their lifestyle. Retailers, including community pharmacies, are adjusting the physical layout of their stores to allow people to get in and out quicker as well as the ability to pick-up in store items that have been ordered online. For example, CVS has an online service where certain items can be ordered online and then picked up in the store within 1 hour (CVS, 2019).

The size of a pharmacy or pharmacy department commonly is determined by industry averages or by evaluating the sales per square foot of various pharmacy departments. Store managers can obtain industry information on the ideal size for their pharmacies from wholesalers and other vendors, as well as from their professional associations (e.g., National Community Pharmacists Association or National Association of Chain Drug Stores).

Managers can calculate the ideal size of a department (an area within a pharmacy that contains related goods or services) by estimating the total dollar amount of sales from that department and dividing by their expected sales per square foot. While this method is simple to use, it should be applied with care and common sense. Estimates of sales are not always accurate indicators of the need for space for types of goods and services. The characteristics of space inside the store (e.g., walls, lighting, and fixtures) and the physical characteristics of the goods and services to be sold in a department both should be considered when allocating space within a pharmacy (Rodowskas, 1996).

Another key point when designing a pharmacy is to make sure that prescription dispensing, and counseling sections meet the legal, technical, and professional standards of modern pharmacy practice. Most state boards of pharmacy have regulations with pertain to the physical aspects of the pharmacy, and in particular the security and safety of prescription medications and controlled substances, which must be incorporated into the design of a pharmacy before the pharmacy will be issued a license (NABP, 2018). Advances in technology have impacted both dispensing of medication and the provision of related services. Prescription departments should be designed to incorporate automated dispensing technologies, sterile and nonsterile compounding, and other technologies that make dispensing and service provision more efficient and effective. And with pharmacists providing an array of counseling, education, and patient care services, additional space for pharmacists and other health professionals to meet privately with patients is needed. Setting aside and designing an appropriate consultation area and a patient waiting area are important. As community pharmacies begin to incorporate primary care services, patient examination rooms, laboratory, and vision and hearing facilities are now being added into pharmacy store designs (see Figure 28-3). Finally, pharmacies sell many items that do not require a prescription, but often sell better if a pharmacist is available to explain their use to patients (e.g., durable medical equipment, diabetes supplies, point-of-care devices, vitamins and minerals, other drugs and goods that are best used with a pharmacist's advice). These items often are placed near the

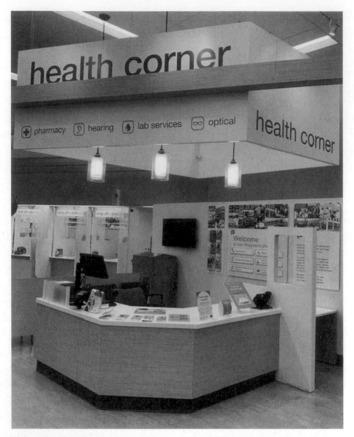

Figure 28-3. Vision, hearing, and lab services inside community pharmacy.

pharmacy department for the convenience of both the patient and the pharmacist.

The Americans with Disabilities Act (ADA) of 1990 has affected almost all businesses, including pharmacies. This federal mandate prohibits discrimination based on any form of disability. To comply with the ADA, pharmacies may be required to adjust counter heights, aisle widths, telephone equipment, doorways, and almost any other physical aspect of their operations. The act allows for reasonableness in designing stores without undue hardship on daily operations. The design goal is to have a store that offers equal access to all products and services for all customers (Laskoski, 1992).

The Heath Insurance Portability and Accountability Act (HIPAA) is a federal mandate designed to protect the confidentiality of patient information. HIPAA considerations in the design and layout of a pharmacy are to ensure that disclosure of protected health information is minimized. Pharmacy managers are to make reasonable efforts to protect the privacy of their patients. Some of the efforts made by pharmacy managers include installation of a partition extending the height of the pharmacy counter, redesigned storage areas for prescriptions that are waiting to be picked up by customers, designated staging areas for patients waiting to be served by pharmacy staff, and private patient consultation areas (see Figure 28-4).

Internal and external environmental factors play a major role in the design and layout of a pharmacy. The age, race, sex, and income levels of consumers are important characteristics that should be addressed.

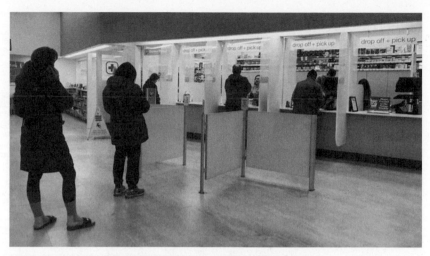

Figure 28-4. HIPAA compliant pharmacy design.

Addressing the needs of a predominant ethnic or age group is beneficial in attracting these potential patrons to a pharmacy. For example, elderly people may be more likely to patronize a pharmacy that has a large section of durable medical equipment.

Designing the exterior of a pharmacy is just as important as design and layout of the interior. When designing the exterior of a pharmacy, one must consider legal requirements, local codes, or ordinances that govern materials, the number and sizes of windows, external signage, and the number and placement of doorways.

The exterior design of a pharmacy may need to complement other stores in a shopping center. Many shopping centers place restrictions on the exterior designs of their stores. Pharmacies commonly will try to add defining features (e.g., signage and lighting) that allow their stores to be recognized easily. Today, pharmacies across the world use the "green cross" as a universal pharmacy symbol. In North America, an image of a mortar and pestle can often be seen on a pharmacy's exterior signage, along with the symbol "Rx" (Nix, 2014).

The placement of entrances and exits to the shopping center is key to the ease of getting to the pharmacy. The traffic patterns and placement of traffic signals on the roads adjacent to the shopping center affect the convenience of shopping in the pharmacy. Pharmacy managers often negotiate with local officials to have traffic signals at or near the entrance and exit of the center.

The traffic pattern of a shopping center will influence the placement of entrances and exits of the pharmacy. Pharmacy managers wish to maximize the number of patrons that find their store once they are in the shopping center. Pharmacies often desire to be located next to a grocery store or other high-traffic stores to attract cross-shoppers.

Pharmacy Layout

A pharmacy's layout contains numerous cues, messages, and suggestions that communicate to shoppers. A pharmacy manager's goal is to create a mood that welcomes customer traffic, increases time spent browsing (yet not wasting time searching for needed items), encourages customers to make more purchases than originally planned, and invites them to return to the pharmacy in the future.

The layout or arrangement of in-store fixtures should be designed to move patrons around the pharmacy to obtain the items they need or desire. Ideally, customers should visit as many areas of the pharmacy as possible to increase the probability of impulse purchases.

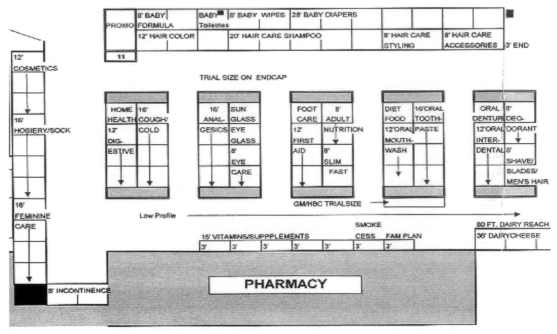

Figure 28-5. Pharmacy design.

Pharmacy layout should capitalize on the strengths of the prescription department and pharmacist because they are what make pharmacies unique from other retail outlets. Pharmacy layout should have the prescription department very prominent and visible to patrons in any part of the store (see Figure 28-5). Ideally, consumers should travel past a variety of merchandise on their way to the prescription department. This explains why prescription departments are often located in the rear of a pharmacy. While this layout is popular with pharmacy managers, it is not always popular with consumers. For example, some elderly patrons may find it difficult to walk through the entire store to get to the prescription counter. They may choose to use the drive-through window or frequent a pharmacy that has the prescription counter in the front of the store. The demographics of the population that shops the pharmacy will be very influential to the design of a pharmacy and prescription counter (Walker, 1996).

Gaedeke and Tootelian (1993) discussed two types of store layouts: grid and free flow. In a *grid*

layout, all the counters and fixtures are at right angles to one another. Merchandise is displayed in straight, parallel lines, encouraging maximum travel time in the aisles and maximum product exposure. The *free-flow layout* groups merchandise and fixtures into patterns that allow for an unstructured flow of customers. Many of the fixtures are irregularly shaped circles, arches, and triangles. This design is used often in gift and specialty stores, mostly encouraging browsing and impulse buying.

Grid layouts are more common in community pharmacies than free-flow layouts. Aisles are set in straight-line grid arrangements with key departments or service areas located to encourage shoppers to visit the four corners of the store. Departments are arranged to place high-demand items in the rear of the store, promoting traffic past lower-demand and impulse-purchase items. In grid layouts, the prescription department is often located in the back of the store, adjacent to high-demand over-the-counter (OTC) items and other items that may sell better if accompanied by a recommendation from a pharmacist (e.g., durable medical equipment or vitamins and supplements).

Department placement is done with the intent to entice customers to purchase more than they had intended originally. Some locations in a pharmacy tend to attract more traffic. High-traffic areas are good places to generate additional sales with placement of new product displays or impulse items. In pharmacies, placement of impulse items near or on the prescription counter may increase sales of these items owing to the increased traffic in that area of the store.

In almost any retail business, the risk of theft of merchandise (both by shoppers and by employees) is always present. Pharmacy managers can use store design and layout to minimize losses from theft. High-cost and other items that may be liable to theft are generally placed in areas where store personnel can observe both the items and the shoppers easily. Pharmacies are increasingly using locked cabinets to store items that are liable to theft (e.g., smoking-cessation products and weight-control products). States have also enacted laws that require products containing pseudoephedrine be kept behind the pharmacy counter. This has been done to decrease the theft and inappropriate use of pseudoephedrine, particularly in the production of methamphetamine. Efforts should be taken not to place high-cost and high-theft items in corners (which are more difficult for personnel to see) or near exits (where it would be easier for shoppers to steal an item leave without being noticed). Many pharmacies use store security personnel, video surveillance equipment, one-way mirrors, and even sensors embedded in products to detect and prevent losses of merchandise. Experts note that in order to have real impact on loss prevention, surveillance cameras may not be enough and a "top-down, strategic focus on loss prevention" is a must (Abbamonte, 2018).

Pharmacy Merchandising

Merchandising involves the proper placement of goods on pharmacy shelves. The space a pharmacy has for goods to be displayed is limited by the size and design of the store. Pharmacies commonly separate their space into departments or sections that contain major categories of products (e.g., prescription area, cough and cold, headache, and first aid).

Pharmacies tend to be arranged by placing related products next to or near each other. For example, OTC cough and cold products are commonly placed near the over the counter analgesics, which in turn are placed near the first-aid items. This placement makes it easier for consumers to find not only the item they have come to the pharmacy to purchase, but also purchase related items they may not of thought of when planning their visit. This enables the pharmacy manager to manage the flow of consumers through the pharmacy, directing them to the areas where they can find needed items, receive advice they may need, and efficiently make their purchases. *Cross-selling* is the process of selling across departments to facilitate customers purchasing more items than they may have intended originally. Arranging departments in a logical transition from the front to the back of the store will guide shoppers to areas where they may find additional items to purchase. Cosmetics, hair-care products, and health and beauty aids commonly are located near toiletries and feminine hygiene products because consumers who come to a pharmacy to purchase the former products also tend to need the latter (see Figure 28-6).

Pharmacy aisles are of various lengths and heights. For the convenience of shoppers, aisles tend not be more than 50 feet in length (Raven, 1984). If an aisle is longer, cross aisles should be provided. Cross aisles are a break in a long run of shelving creating an aisle that allows customers to move easily across the store. Cross aisles provide for smooth traffic flow and increase visible space for item placement.

Many pharmacies use the space at the beginnings and ends of the aisle runs. These spaces often are referred to as *end caps*. End caps often feature displays of promotional and seasonal items, bulk items, impulse items, and new products designed to gain shoppers' attention (see Figure 28-7).

Aisle heights also vary among pharmacies (Raven, 1984). Some smaller pharmacies use a lower aisle height of 54 in. This allows store personnel to see

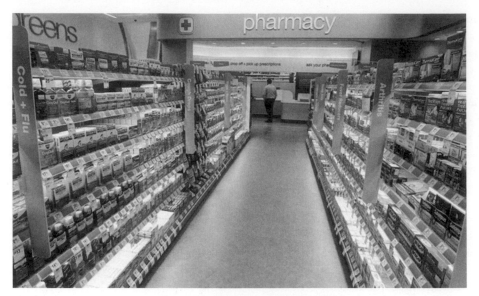

Figure 28-6. Pharmacy aisle design.

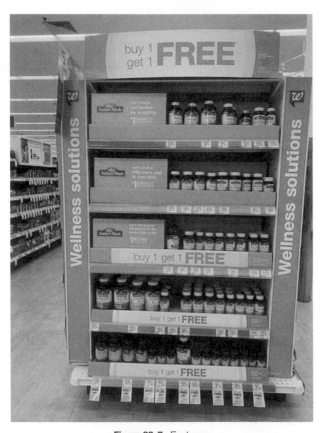

Figure 28-7. End cap.

across the entire pharmacy. Larger pharmacies often use fixtures with heights of 60 to 72 in. Higher shelves provide additional space for merchandise and storage. Higher shelves also help consumers to maintain eye contact with products in the aisles. Not allowing visibility across aisles is a tool used by retailers to keep the shopper's eye on the items in that section.

When deciding what items and how many of each item to place in a section or a department, pharmacy managers strive for balance between variety and duplication. This balance will vary by and within categories of merchandise. The two considerations to be addressed in achieving such a balance are an understanding of the customers and an analysis of current market trends. Both of these considerations address the placement of merchandise to respond to demographics, the type of customer and his or her needs, or market trends, responding to a new or very popular item.

To assist with proper placement of items on shelves, many pharmacy managers use *plan-o-grams*. Plan-o-grams are diagrams that show the placement, space, and management of each item in a particular section of shelves. Plan-o-grams may be produced by manufacturers, wholesalers, corporate pharmacy offices, or the pharmacy staff itself. Plan-o-grams should be based on current sales and market information, as well as on the size and physical characteristics of the items themselves. A properly planned and executed plan-o-gram enables pharmacies to maximize sales and profit opportunities for a given section of space (see Figure 28-8).

Plan-o-grams should arrange products to increase their visibility to consumers. Manufacturers strive to make the fronts and tops of their packaging clearly visible to consumers. A product *facing* is the arrangement of a product one package wide on a shelf. Placement of items on shelves, so that these package facings

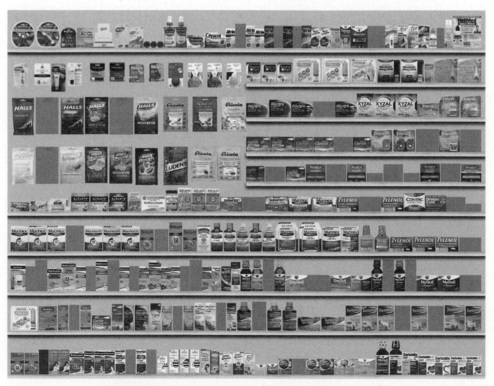

Figure 28-8. Pharmacy merchandising plan-o-gram example.

are visible to consumers, allows for maximum exposure and increases the likelihood of sales. By increasing the facings of a single product from two to four, pharmacies have found that sales of that product will increase (Portner, 1996).

When viewing a section in a pharmacy, the most popular items will be placed at eye level for the majority of shoppers (approximately 60 in high). Items placed very high or very low in a section traditionally will be slower-selling items. Customers in North American pharmacies typically scan from left to right when looking at items on a shelf. Items on the shelf should be set vertically, from top to bottom, allowing the customer's eye to scan the shelf across as he or she goes from top to bottom (Burks, 2019). Pharmacy managers use this concept to cross-merchandise and add items for impulse purchasing. In addition, most customers are right-handed and will grab the item to the right. Consumers commonly find larger-sized products (which generate higher sales and profit margins) kept to the right of smaller-sized products followed by the private label brand (Burks, 2019).

Pharmacy managers will place some items in more than one department. Fast-moving, high-profit items can be displayed in various departments throughout the pharmacy using a technique known as *cross-merchandising*. For example, displaying facial tissues not only with the paper products but also in the cough and cold section will increase impulse sales of these items.

In addition to placing items in designated sections or departments, pharmacy managers commonly use displays throughout a pharmacy to highlight specific products. Displays often are set in an aisle in front of a shelf to showcase new items or those with special pricing. Floor-stand displays are used to place large quantities of an item on display, making the products easily accessible to consumers. Manufacturers often supply these displays and other promotional materials to pharmacies to highlight their products (see Figure 28-9).

Point-of-purchase materials (signage) also are used to highlight items. Header cards, banners, and price signs are all examples of point-of-purchase

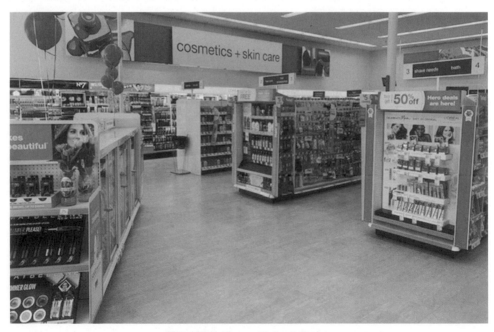

Figure 28-9. Floor end stand display.

materials. These sales aids give product information, demonstrate features, reinforce a sale or special price, and can generate sales. Other methods used to highlight products are shelf extenders. These are small trays that are attached to a shelf and extend out several inches to highlight an item. Shelf talkers are signs that extend outward from the shelving and "speak" to customers about items or services found in the store.

Retail stores, including pharmacies, often use *private label* (also known as a *store brand*) offerings to create a unique brand strategy and differentiation. Brands that are owned and marketed by pharmacies and other stores are referred to by various names, such as "private-label," "store brands," "proprietary brands," "owned-brand," and others. Examples of private label brands in pharmacies include *Well at Walgreens*™, *Equate*™ (offered at Wal-Mart), and *Skin+Pharmacy*® (offered at CVS). Provided the sales volume is sufficient, a private-label strategy can provide the retailer with several advantages unavailable to them by carrying national or manufacturer brands only. In fact, the vast majority of chain retailers, regardless of the category, carry some mix of national brands versus private-label brands, some carry private-label brands exclusively (Friederichsen, 2018).

Pharmacies that use private label products are looking to create a brand strategy that is not interchangeable with other retailers. Differentiation for the retailer in the marketplace, more freedom and flexibility in pricing, greater control over product attributes and quality, the ability to fill gaps not filled by national brands, as well as keeping national brands competitively priced are distinct advantages to a successful private label strategy. Simply having a lower cost brand available to purchase is not enough today. Self-care, for many shoppers, is more than a cure for an occasional ailment; it includes healthy living and preventative care. Having a unique and differentiating private label offering, merchandised throughout the store can create a draw for customers to frequent the pharmacy.

Pharmacies have started to focus more on beauty and expand their beauty categories such as make-up, skin care product, naturals, therapeutics and clinically-proven products with the objective of bringing health and beauty together (Thulin, 2015). Customers known as "savvy beauty shoppers" look to purchase beauty products at pharmacies while also looking to save on items such as skin care items, cosmetics, and health essentials without compromising on quality (The Information Daily, 2013). Pharmacies are capitalizing on this opportunity by focusing on women, being the key decision makers for their family, and making most of pharmacy purchases. Appropriate placement of these items in the beauty section and throughout the store is crucial.

Merchandising the Prescription Department

The prescription department is the one area that distinguishes a pharmacy from other retail stores that sell similar merchandise. The prescription department should be given a position of prominence in the store. This department usually takes up 300 to 600 square feet of space, having 18 to 24 feet across the front of the department. The prescription department is usually identified with prominent signage or decor to make it easily identifiable to customers to see and use (see Figure 28-10).

Consumers typically view the prescription department as a professional area. When they are able to view the interior of the pharmacy, they should see that this department is clean and well organized. Pharmacy personnel need to exhibit a friendly and professional demeanor because individual attention can distinguish one pharmacy from another.

The front of the prescription department traditionally is used to highlight vitamins and herbal remedies, products that commonly require the advice of a pharmacist for proper use (e.g., diabetes supplies), or high-priced specialty items that may be at risk for theft if stocked in a less visible section (e.g., smoking-cessation products). The areas where prescriptions are dropped off or picked up are good places to display new products or impulse-purchase items (e.g., Chap-Stick™ or pill reminders). These areas are also natural spots for small displays of new OTC items that previously were prescription items (e.g., Xyzal™ or Differin

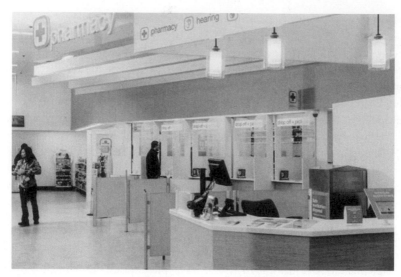

Figure 28-10. Prescription department.

Gel™). The pharmacist's recommendation is one way to increase purchases of these items.

Designing prescription departments with the pharmacist–patient relationship in mind is a merchandising technique intended to have an impact on prescription sales, OTC purchases, and purchases of professional services (e.g., patient education programs, screenings, or immunizations). When pharmacies design prescription departments to be open, patrons feel more comfortable approaching pharmacy staff with questions. Some pharmacies have designed the prescription department with the pharmacist out in front where patients have easy access to the pharmacist for assistance. Having the prescription department, with the pharmacist out front, near other health care items makes the pharmacist's recommendation more likely to result in increased sales of these goods.

Some prescription departments are built elevated from the rest of the pharmacy, giving the department an appearance of prominence to the customer. Special lighting may also be used to highlight the pharmacy. The use of brighter lighting in and around the department highlights the pharmacy and draws customers to that area of the store.

Pharmacy design should also include a patient waiting area, a patient consultation area, and in many locations a drive-through window. The patient waiting area provides patients with space away from the sales floor to wait comfortably for their prescriptions. As prescriptions are being filled, customers have an opportunity to view health information or learn more about specific goods or services the pharmacy may offer (see Figure 28-11).

The patient consultation center of the prescription department provides an area for patients and the pharmacist to discuss medications and related patient questions. The consultation center may be as small as window built into the prescription counter or as large as a freestanding patient care center. Patient care centers provide pharmacy staff with a place to offer counseling and medical information. Screenings for various disease states, therapeutic drug monitoring, and immunizations are usually in a private area near the prescription department but away from other customers and store activities.

Drive-through windows are seen today in many pharmacies. Patients are able to purchase prescriptions and limited OTC items without having to leave their cars. Industry measurements have shown that drive-through windows are viewed by customers as an added convenience, as it saves people time and effort, and is very useful for those that cannot get out of the

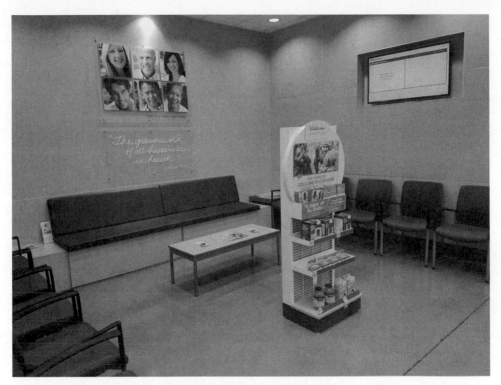

Figure 28-11. Patient waiting area.

car easily such as mothers with children and elderly (Barker, 2018) (see Figure 28-12).

Pharmacies are continually looking for new and better ideas to differentiate themselves from other retail outlets and to offer additional health care services to their customers. Expanding the front end of the store with health-related items and services helps to differentiate pharmacies from other general merchandisers. Finding a niche area such as compounding, immunizations, or consultative services will develop a different business model based on the needs of their unique customer base. Health-focused pharmacies use merchandising practices to place these niche services prominently in their stores.

The expansion of health-related products and services will attract patients referred to the pharmacy from physicians, hospitals, and health plans. By developing this health care focused model, the pharmacy will develop a greater relationship with the patient and capture more of their health care dollars.

The Impact on Technology on Pharmacy Design and Merchandising

Today's consumers are becoming more accustomed to utilizing self-service devices to accomplish tasks quickly and with convenience. For example, think about the last time you were at a store that had the option of self-service check out. Chances are that you opted for that option because waiting in the cashier line took longer. A similar concept now applies in the health care industry, including pharmacies, as self-service kiosks are now being used to check-in patients, fill prescriptions, and provide consultations to health care professionals (Slawsky, 2015). One of the most common ways that the self-service kiosks are being utilized in health care is for self-check in. The check-in process can be time consuming, not only for the patient but also for health care staff. For example, once the patient manually completes all of the necessary forms, the staff member has to manually enter

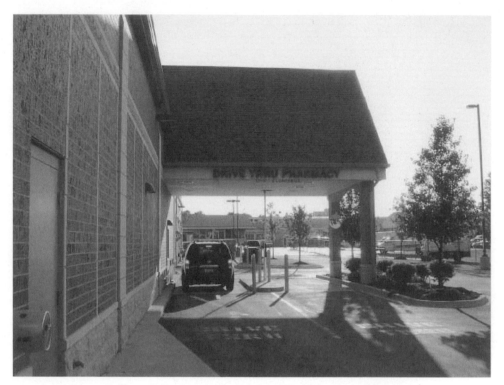

Figure 28-12. Community pharmacy drive-through window.

the information into the computer. With self-service check in this two-step process is now a single step, reducing time, cost, and potentially errors. Self-service kiosks are also enabling telepharmacy and telehealth services. Telehealth is a way to connect patients with health care professionals who normally would not be able to interact due to time or distance constraints using technology (Siwicki, 2018). Telehealth may reduce health care costs and provide more convenient ways to access care for those living in rural and underserved areas. Telepharmacy is the delivery of pharmaceutical care via telecommunications to patients in locations where they may not have direct contact with a pharmacist. Telepharmacy services include drug therapy monitoring, patient counseling, prior authorization and refill authorization for prescription drugs, and monitoring of formulary compliance with the aid of teleconferencing or videoconferencing. Remote dispensing of medications by automated

packaging and labeling systems can also be thought of as an instance of telepharmacy. Telepharmacy services can be delivered at community pharmacy sites or through hospitals, nursing homes, or other medical care facilities.

Self-service kiosks can now be used to dispense prescription drugs. These kiosks provide the patient with the convenience to fill their prescription through a live, two-way audiovisual conversation with a pharmacist 24 hours a day, 7 days a week. These kiosks accept various prescription insurance carriers and are "staffed" with a trained health care professional whose role is to assist the patient and answer any questions (Slawsky, 2015).

As the pharmacy is evolving from a place where patients can pick-up their medications and miscellaneous items to a health care destination where patients can receive an array of health care services, placing the primary care clinic adjacent to the pharmacy allows for a convenient collaboration between the health care

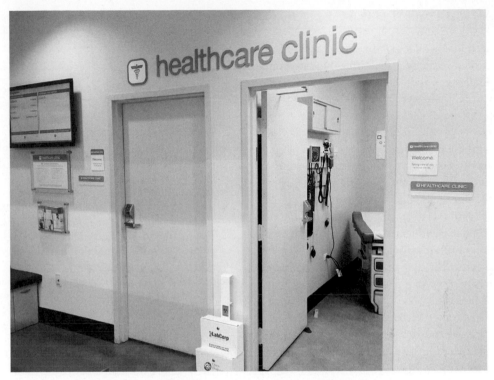

Figure 28-13. In-store health care clinic.

professions and an additional point to access care for the patients. Retail clinics (see Figure 28-13) are an extension of care service through which patients can be triaged to appropriate site of care, reducing unnecessary hospital and ER visits, while driving chronic disease management, medication adherence, and providing patients with the ability to receive lower cost alternative care in their community, close to work or home. Pharmacists can interact and support the retail clinics and patients by triaging patients to the retail clinic (when appropriate) and recommending additional health care services to the patient (i.e., annual wellness visit or school physicals).

Pharmacies and retail health clinics provide greater access to medical care for common problems, providing increased access to primary care in their communities, helping to ease the burden of the shortage of primary care providers in other health care settings (Rand Corporation, 2019; Robert Wood

Johnson Foundation, 2015; Sarasohn-Kahn, 2016). With millions of people visit pharmacies daily, making pharmacies the ideal location for health clinics. Retail clinics are open in the evenings and on weekends, allowing patients more convenient and easier access to care close to their home and work.

Patients can walk in without appointments and receive care for acute and chronic health issues from nurse practitioners and physician assistants who specialize in family health care. Many retail clinics take walk-ins patients, and the visits tend to be shorter than in traditional primary care settings. Clinics can provide easier access to immunizations, treatment for minor illnesses and injuries, travel health, skin conditions, women's services, preventive health screenings and monitoring, and general wellness care. Clinics are not intended to replace primary care, and patients who need a higher level of medical attention would be referred to doctors in a timely manner.

■ REVISITING THE SCENARIO

Jerry, our third-year Doctor of Pharmacy student, recently visited Healthway Pharmacy. He took some time to understand the factors that made his family so happy to shop there. The pharmacy manager indicated that the store's goal is to create an environment for shoppers that will make the pharmacy easy, fun to shop, and the health care destination of choice for its customers. He explained that the store attempts to satisfy customers' needs by appealing to their senses both in the store and online.

What customers see and hear throughout the store and online is influential to their shopping experience. Customers are assisted by merchandising techniques to find what they need and experience items and services they may not have thought of purchasing. The location is easily accessible to the wide variety of consumers who shop there. All this made Jerry think about his future and the role he may have in community pharmacy.

■ QUESTIONS FOR FURTHER DISCUSSION

1. Given that the female head of household makes the majority of health care decisions for her family, how would you design a pharmacy around the needs of women with families?
2. While customers like the convenience of pharmacies with a drive-through window, what are some potential drawbacks of including them in a pharmacy?
3. How may technology (i.e., smartphones, tablet computers) impact the merchandising practices of community pharmacies?

REFERENCES

Abbamonte K. 2018. How to put together a loss prevention plan for your store. Available at https://www.shopify.com/retail/retail-loss-prevention. Accessed April 16, 2019.

Barker A. 2018. A brief history of the drive-thru pharmacy: Who created it and how it spread. Available at https://opmed.doximity.com/articles/a-brief-history-of-the-drive-thru-pharmacy-who-created-it-and-how-it-spread. Accessed April 16, 2019.

Burks F. 2019. Visual Merchandising Placement Process. Available at https://smallbusiness.chron.com/visual-merchandising-placement-process-12616.html. Accessed April 16, 2019.

CVS. 2019. CVSpharmacy Store Pickup. Available at https://www.cvs.com/content/storepickup. Accessed April 16, 2019.

Eisenpreis A. 1983. How today's customers shop: What it means to drugstores. *American Druggist* 188:92.

Encyclopedia Britannica. 2019. United States Constitution: Eighteenth Amendment. Available at https://www.britannica.com/topic/Eighteenth-Amendment. Accessed April 16, 2019.

Fiorletta A. 2014. CVS/pharmacy revs up omnichannel strategies for holiday season. Available at http://www.retailtouchpoints.com/features/retail-success-stories/cvs-pharmacy-revs-up-omnichannel-strategies-for-holiday-season. Accessed September 24, 2015.

Francke DE. 1974. Accepting things as they are. *Drug Intell Clin Pharm* 8:221.

Friederichsen P. 2018. How manufacturer and private-label brands differ. *Branding Strategy Insider*. Available at https://www.brandingstrategyinsider.com/2018/11/how-manufacturer-and-private-label-brands-differ.html#.XKUZqHdFzIV. Accessed April 9, 2019.

Gaedeke R, Tootelian D. 1993. *Essentials of Pharmacy Management*. St. Louis: Mosby–Year Book.

Hamacher Resource Group. 2013. Independent pharmacy shoppers: Who, what, and why? Available at https://hamacher.com/wp-content/uploads/2016/05/Independent-Phcy-Shoppers-Who-What-Why-FINAL-2013-01-30.pdf. Accessed April 9, 2019.

Higby GJ. 1997. Pharmacy in the American century: 100 years of change. *Pharm Times* 63:16.

Hilditch J. 1981. Maximizing the value of the sales area. *Pharm J* 227:638.

The Information Daily 2013. Savvy beauty shoppers ditch big-name products. http://www.theinformationdaily.com/2013/11/25/savvy-beauty-shoppers-ditch-big-name-products. Accessed August 29, 2015.

Japsen B. 2014. Why Walgreens won't stop selling tobacco like CVS. Available at http://www.forbes.com/sites/brucejapsen/2014/09/04/why-walgreen-wont-stop-selling-tobacco-like-cvs-health. Accessed September 28, 2015.

Japsen B. 2018. Bracing for Amazon, Walgreens launches next-day drug delivery with Fed Ex/. Available at https://www.forbes.com/sites/brucejapsen/2018/12/06/bracing-for-amazon-walgreens-launches-next-day-drug-delivery-with-fedex/#48b0b09a50e6. Accessed April 9, 2019.

Laskoski G. 1992. Design: Good, the bad, and the ugly. *American Druggist* 205:38.

National Association of Boards of Pharmacy (NABP). 2018. *Survey of Pharmacy Law.* Mount Prospect, IL: National Association of Boards of Pharmacy.

Nix E. 2014. Where did the Rx symbol come from? Available at https://www.history.com/news/where-did-the-rx-symbol-come-from. Accessed April 16, 2019.

O'Donnell J, Ungar L. 2014. CVS stops selling tobacco, offers quit-smoking programs. Available at http://www.usatoday.com/story/news/nation/2014/09/03/cvs-steps-selling-tobacco-changes-name/14967821. Accessed September 28, 2015.

PBA Health. 2018. *Five Consumer Trends Your Pharmacy Should Know.* Available at https://www.pbahealth.com/5-consumer-trends-pharmacy-know/. Accessed April 16, 2019.

Portner T. 1996. *Effective Pharmacy Management: A Comprehensive Presentation of Practical Management Techniques for Pharmacy*, 8th ed. Alexandria, VA: National Community Pharmacists Association.

Rand Corporation. 2019. Retail health care clinics. Available at https://www.rand.org/topics/retail-health-care-clinics.html. Accessed April 9, 2019.

Raven M. 1984. Drugstore design and layout: Looking at the right angles. *Drug Top* 128:44.

Rodowskas C. 1996. Space allocation and profit maximization. *Pharm Times* 62:70.

Sarasohn-Khan J. 2016. Retail Clinics continue to share local healthcare markets. *Healthcare IT News.* Available at https://www.healthcareitnews.com/blog/retail-clinics-continue-shape-local-healthcare-markets. Accessed April 9, 2019.

Siwicki B. 2018. Telepharmacy at rural hospitals provides big savings, quality improvements. Healthcare IT News. Available at https://www.healthcareitnews.com/news/telepharmacy-rural-hospitals-provides-big-savings-quality-improvements. Accessed April 9, 2019.

Slawsky R. 2015. Kiosks in health care 101. Available at http://www.kioskmarketplace.com/static_media/filer_public/c9/3f/c93f6759-35f8-4b0a-9ecb-29117741db01/guide_frankmayer_kiosks_in_health_care_101.pdf. Accessed August 29, 2015.

Thulin L. 2015. CVS/pharmacy to release products that focus on health-beauty connection. Available at http://www.drugstorenews.com/article/cvspharmacy-release-products-focus-health-beauty-connection. Accessed July 30, 2019.

SECTION VI

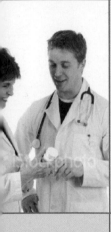

MANAGING VALUE-ADDED SERVICES

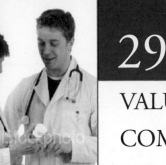

29

VALUE-ADDED SERVICES AS A COMPONENT OF ENHANCING PHARMACISTS' ROLES IN PUBLIC HEALTH

Leticia R. Moczygemba and Antoinette B. Coe

About the Authors: Dr. Moczygemba is an associate professor and associate director of the Texas Center for Health Outcomes Research and Education at The University of Texas College of Pharmacy. Her research program focuses on working with communities and health systems to mitigate health disparities by developing patient-centered interventions to optimize medication-related health outcomes. She has worked to advance the health care of homeless individuals, older adults, and those living in rural areas through the development, implementation, and evaluation of care models that integrate pharmacists with health care teams. She teaches in the health care systems course in the PharmD program and is engaged in interprofessional education initiatives with a focus on quality improvement and patient safety.

Dr. Coe is an assistant professor at the University of Michigan College of Pharmacy. As a health services researcher-pharmacist she is devoted to improving medication-related outcomes and ensuring safe and effective medication use in vulnerable populations, particularly in older adults. Her research focuses on improving medication use through pharmacist-provided comprehensive medication reviews, preventing medication-related problems during care transitions, and examining the impact of pharmacists' care on health outcomes. She teaches in the communications and health care systems course in the PharmD program and is engaged in interprofessional education initiatives focusing on academic-community partnerships providing care to low-income housing residents.

■ LEARNING OBJECTIVES

After completing this chapter, readers should be able to

1. Describe ways that the development of value-added pharmacist services can enhance pharmacists' roles in public health.
2. Identify factors that should drive the development of value-added public health pharmacist services.

3. Describe how the business planning process applies to value-added pharmacist services.
4. Evaluate the market for value-added pharmacist services:
   a. Consumer characteristics and needs
   b. Impact of the internal and external environments
   c. Services already available in the market
   d. Market potential
   e. Consumer willingness and ability to pay for services
5. Evaluate the ability of a pharmacist to provide public health services that meet consumer needs.

■ SCENARIO

Sarah Smith, PharmD, MPH, is a community pharmacist with training in public health. She graduated at the top of her pharmacy class with a joint PharmD/MPH degree and then completed a Postgraduate Year One Community-based Pharmacy Practice Residency. After completing her residency, she started a career with an independent pharmacy in suburban Chicago. As part of her position, she has dedicated time each week for designing, implementing, and providing clinical pharmacist services.

As a pharmacy student and as a resident, Dr. Smith volunteered at several health fairs. The activity she enjoyed the most was taking advantage of her certification as an immunizing pharmacist. She was able to provide influenza (flu) vaccinations to her fellow students, faculty members, and patients to help prevent the flu. Her independent pharmacy currently provides medication synchronization and adherence packaging for their patients. When deciding which clinical service she wanted to start, she thought that building an immunization program was a good fit. Her pharmacy did not offer any vaccines to their patients. She was the first pharmacist with immunization certification among a team of three additional pharmacists, including her pharmacy manager. She convinced her pharmacy manager of the benefit of providing flu vaccines to the pharmacy's patients for the upcoming flu season, to remodel the pharmacy to include a private counseling area for administering vaccines and patient care, and to spend money promoting these new clinical services in the pharmacy.

■ CHAPTER QUESTIONS

1. How can value-added pharmacist services address a population's public health needs, in addition to those of individual patients?
2. How does an organization's strategic plan affect the kinds of goods and services it offers?
3. In what ways is business planning useful in the development of value-added pharmacist public health services?
4. In addition to patients, who else should be considered consumers of value-added public health pharmacist services?
5. What information should be gathered before making a decision to offer a value-added pharmacist service? Where and how can this information be gathered?

■ VALUE-ADDED PHARMACIST SERVICES AND PUBLIC HEALTH

According to the Institute of Medicine (IOM), *public health* is simply "what we, as a society do collectively to assure the condition for people to be healthy"

(Institute of Medicine [IOM], 2003a). The primary public health role that many associate with pharmacists is assuring the safe and effective use of medications. For many years, this was done primarily through safeguarding the preparation and distribution of drug products. However, as pharmacist's roles have moved beyond traditional dispensing and national organizations such as the American Public Health Association have recognized a role for pharmacists in advancing public health (American Public Health Association, 2015), pharmacists have become increasingly engaged in a number of public health activities ranging from health and wellness screenings to immunization education and administration to emergency response and emergency preparedness. Further, more than 90% of Americans live within five miles of a community pharmacy and community pharmacies accept walk-ins with little to no waiting and may offer extended hours (Bach et al., 2015). The accessibility of a pharmacist combined with enhanced clinical skills and training has led to pharmacists being able to impact the health of individuals in diverse groups and settings.

The Centers for Disease Control and Prevention's list of ten essential public health services (Centers for Disease Control and Prevention [CDC], 1994) has been used as a framework for implementing and categorizing public health activities of pharmacists (Strand et al., 2016; Truong et al., 2012):

1. "Monitor health status to identify and solve community health problems.
2. Diagnose and investigate health problems and health hazards in the community.
3. Inform, educate, and empower individuals about health concerns.
4. Mobilize community partnerships and action to identify and solve health problems.
5. Develop policies and plans that support individual and community health efforts.
6. Enforce laws and regulations that protect health and ensure safety.
7. Link people to needed personal health services and assure the provision of health care when otherwise unavailable.

8. Assure competent public and personal health care workforce.
9. Evaluate effectiveness, accessibility, and quality of personal and population-based health services.
10. Research for new insights and innovative solutions to health problems (CDC, 1994)."

Some of these services, such as Numbers 6 and 8, are inherent to a pharmacist's roles and responsibilities which ensure safe and appropriate medication use for patients and continuing education to maintain licensure. Likewise, pharmacists are required to counsel on new medications and often assist walk-in patrons with over-the-counter medications or help triage or refer an individual to a community resource to address a health concern (Numbers 3 and 7). A number of pharmacists have expanded the scope of public health service offerings by implementing activities such as immunization delivery or health screenings as part of a pharmacy's business model. A recent review examined literature related to pharmacist public health services and found evidence that pharmacists are contributing to all ten essential areas to varying degrees, with the most common public health activities categorized by Numbers 9, 7, and 3 (Strand et al., 2016).

Pharmacists commonly join forces with other health care professionals and health researchers to determine ideal treatment regimens given clinical, epidemiologic, and economic data. Pharmacists also work to identify adverse drug events and medications errors (IOM, 2003b; Trinkley et al., 2017). This and other medication-related research improves health outcomes for individual patients and for society at large. Pharmacists help assure the health of their communities through activities at a macro level to plan for needs of a population (e.g., administering medication use systems, designing drug benefit plans, creating policies for health programs), as well as at the micro level which focuses on implementing public health activities (e.g., speaking to community groups, developing health education materials, conducting health-screening programs) (American Society of Health-System Pharmacists, 2008).

Perhaps the most significant impact pharmacists have had on public health has been in immunization delivery. From 2007 to 2017, the total number of pharmacists trained in immunization delivery increased from 40,000 to 320,000 and pharmacists in all 50 states now have the legal authority to immunize under protocols developed with physicians (American Pharmacists Association [APhA], 2017; National Association of Boards of Pharmacy [NABP], 2015). A national survey of community pharmacies, reported that, in 2016, 80% of pharmacies offered immunization services with the most common immunizations provided being influenza, herpes zoster, and pneumococcal (Westrick et al., 2018). More importantly, pharmacists stepping forward to provide immunizations have increased the number of Americans receiving immunizations. Indeed, it has been estimated that pharmacist immunization delivery results in an additional 6.3 million adult influenza immunizations and 3.3 million pneumococcal immunizations each year (Patel et al., 2018).

In addition to immunizations, pharmacists play a role in increasing the health knowledge of people in their communities on topics ranging from the importance of vaccines to disease-specific education about chronic conditions such as diabetes (Gonzalvo & Lantaff, 2018; Queeno, 2017). Given their accessibility, pharmacists can play a valuable role in enhancing the health literacy in underserved and ethnically diverse communities (Gerber et al., 2010; Vargas et al., 2011). Pharmacists can play an active role in disease prevention and health promotion, particularly through their efforts in health education, screening, and wellness programs (Darin et al., 2015; Eades et al., 2011). Further, pharmacists' accessibility in communities makes them ideally situated to be responsive to public health epidemics and emergencies. One example is how pharmacists have actively contributed at local and state levels to combat the US opioid epidemic (Cochran et al., 2016). Pharmacists are using prescription drug monitoring program data as a tool to assess appropriateness of opioid use at the point-of-care (Cochran et al., 2016) and screening for opioid misuse in community pharmacies (Strand et al.,

2018). They are educating law enforcement and lay groups about how to use naloxone (Hill et al., 2018) and contributing to state-wide implementation of standing naloxone orders (SAMHSA, 2018). Pharmacists have also had increasing roles in emergency preparedness planning and responding to natural disasters such as serving on local boards to plan for pandemics and assisting with relief efforts for hurricanes (Fitzgerald et al., 2016; Melin & Rodriguez-Diaz, 2018). And pharmacists have stepped forward to take the lead in efforts to protect the environment by offering medication and syringe disposal services (Athern et al., 2016; Perry et al., 2014).

As pharmacists' roles in public health have expanded, formal training in public health has also increased. Curricular guidelines used by schools and colleges of pharmacy now emphasize preparation of pharmacy students to provide both patient-specific and population-based care (Medina et al., 2013). Accreditation standards for Doctor of Pharmacy programs also state that the graduates must possess a set of minimum skills and attributes to practice, including the ability to provide population-based care (Accreditation Council for Pharmacy Education [ACPE], 2015). Schools and colleges of pharmacy have responded by integrating public health concepts into the curriculum. Many colleges have developed courses or introductory pharmacy practice experiences designed specifically to teach public health concepts to pharmacy students (Hannings et al., 2016; Westrick, 2009) and a number of co-curricular activities focus on health screenings, health promotion, and promoting pharmacist's roles to legislators in local communities. Many universities have developed joint degree programs, allowing graduates to obtain both the Doctor of Pharmacy (PharmD) and Master of Public Health (MPH) degrees (American Association of Colleges of Pharmacy [AACP], 2005; Gortney et al., 2013).

■ REVISITING THE SCENARIO

Dr. Smith was pleased that the pharmacy was being remodeled and that there would be a private space she could utilize for administering vaccines. However, this remodeling took far longer than expected. Her pharmacy manager felt that starting this immunization program would be difficult during the ongoing construction and they agreed to delay the marketing for this service. While the pharmacy was being remodeled, she worked to make sure that the new area had all of the necessary supplies on hand to provide this service. She collaborated with a local physician to develop a standing order protocol and developed a process to report her pharmacy's administered vaccines to her state immunization registry. Once the remodeling was complete, Dr. Smith started offering flu vaccines to patients. She had been able to administer flu shots to some of her patients; but, the uptake was not as high as she had hoped.

■ APPLYING THE BUSINESS PLANNING PROCESS TO PHARMACIST SERVICES

No doubt, there are a number of services that a pharmacist or pharmacy *could* implement to impact public health and one might say that a pharmacist *should* deliver some of these services in the interest of serving the public. Yet, without careful planning, valuable pharmacist resources may not be used efficiently and ultimately lead to frustration and a waste of time and resources. The business planning process discussed in Chapter 7 is one approach that can be used to examine the potential of implementing a new public health service. Using the business planning process does not guarantee that consumers will accept a new service, or that the service will meet organizational goals. However, business planning does help managers identify risks and assess the likelihood that a new service will be successful.

Many administrators require that their pharmacists develop written business plans to justify offering a new service. This helps administrators decide whether to allocate scarce resources (especially money, time, and personnel) to the development of any new service or idea. One important aspect to keep in mind about business planning is that administrators and

pharmacists are under no obligation to implement a plan. If the research done in the planning process indicates that a service will not meet consumer or organizational needs, that it would not be feasible to offer, or that the risks involved are greater than the organization cares to take, a decision can be made simply not to move forward with the plan. While it takes an investment of time to develop a business plan, not implementing a plan that is likely to fail consumes far less time, money, and other resources than developing a new service that does in fact fail.

Applying the business planning process to the development of public health pharmacist services is not that different from how the process is used to evaluate any other good, service, or idea. One of the first steps when starting the business planning process should be to identify the organization's strategic plan and mission statement. Since these documents represent the road map for what the organization wishes to become and how it plans to get there, it is important that the development of any new service bears these in mind. One question that almost all administrators will want to have answered is how the implementation of any new value-added service will help their organization achieve the goals set out in the strategic plan.

It is important to recognize that mission statements and strategic plans vary among types of organizations, especially within health care. The mission statement and strategic plan of a not-for-profit children's research hospital likely will be different from that of a for-profit pharmacy chain. The aspects of a professional service that will need to be emphasized in a business plan will vary as well. The not-for-profit children's research hospital may want to see how a new professional service will result in enhanced clinical outcomes or benefit the greatest number of children at the lowest possible cost. On the other hand, a for-profit pharmacy chain may want to see how the service will expand its market share or enhance its shareholders' value of owning the company.

The next step of the business planning process is to explore the prospects for various types of public health services. At this point, it is helpful to have several ideas for services that could be implemented. One of the best ways to do this is to speak with key stakeholders including administrators, staff pharmacists, support personnel such as technicians, patients, and potential collaborators in the community such as physicians. This is essential to learn more about their needs and can help business planners learn more about their environments (which will be important later in the process). In particular, it is important to work with administrators and organizations early in the business planning process, not only to keep them informed but also to learn what they desire from an administrative standpoint. Taking the views of administrative and organizational personnel into account throughout the process increases the likelihood that administrators will support and provide the resources necessary to implement value-added pharmacist services in the future. It also worthwhile for business planners to speak with others who have successfully implemented similar services. Many pharmacists who have already developed value-added services will gladly share what they have learned. Visiting a setting where value-added pharmacist services are already in place not only provides evidence of how these services actually work but also will answer many questions pharmacists may have later in the planning process. Payers (e.g., insurance companies, health maintenance organizations [HMOs], employers, and governments) may be willing to share ideas about value-added pharmacist services that may improve the health of their constituents while saving them money. These discussions have taken on added importance since the passage of the Affordable Care Act, the proliferation of accountable care organizations, and the creation of pay-for-performance measures.

It is also useful to identify existing expertise and skills that can be leveraged to develop a service (Kennedy & Biddle, 2014). In the scenario, Dr. Smith is building upon her training in public health and immunizations to develop a value-added service, in this case, immunization delivery. However, given the initial low uptake of the service it is not enough to focus on the clinical aspects, Dr. Smith now needs to think about the service from a business perspective.

Professional pharmacy and medical organizations (e.g., the American Pharmacists Association [APhA], the American Society of Health-System Pharmacists [ASHP], the National Community Pharmacists Association [NCPA], and the American Medical Association [AMA]) and health care organizations (e.g., the Advisory Committee on Immunization Practice [ACIP] and the American Diabetes Association [ADA]) also provide valuable information about many health conditions and value-added services. This information is important not only in the development of a service but also in justifying the need for a service with consumers and administrators. These organizations also provide treatment guidelines and additional resources that can be used when developing an operations plan for a service (see Chapter 8). Other sources for ideas about value-added public health services include evidence-based literature, clinical practice guidelines, colleagues, professional meetings and seminars, the Internet, consultants, books, and full-service wholesalers.

■ REVISITING THE SCENARIO

At Dr. Smith's annual performance review in April, her pharmacy manager let her know that she was disappointed that only 150 patients decided to get their flu shot at the pharmacy. They decided to have several meetings to plan for the upcoming flu season and to strategize ways to reach more patients to prevent the flu and improve the health of their patients. One solution proposed was to have the other three pharmacists obtain their immunization certification. Her pharmacy manager was in full support of this potential strategy. The pharmacy owner decided to pay for each of the pharmacist's training. This ensured that there was always an immunizing pharmacist working at the pharmacy.

Dr. Smith also proposed that they offer pneumonia vaccines to eligible patients when they received their flu shot to help increase vaccination rates and protection against pneumonia. They specifically decided to target high-risk groups such as older adults.

One additional strategy they considered was how to involve pharmacy students in their efforts to increase vaccination rates. Dr. Smith, along with her colleagues, was a pharmacy preceptor for pharmacy students on their introductory and advanced pharmacy practice experience rotations. They discussed opportunities to include students in both the development and delivery of the immunization services. She and her pharmacy manager decided to set up a meeting with the college of pharmacy's experiential education office to learn more and potentially expand their rotations. She also involved her pharmacy team in the design of patient brochures, posters, and outdoor signs that would advertise flu shot availability.

■ EVALUATING THE MARKET FOR PHARMACIST SERVICES

In evaluating potential pharmacist services, it is essential to consider the characteristics of the market where they will be offered. Since any service first must satisfy consumer needs before a pharmacist's personal, professional, or organizational goals can be met, evaluating potential consumers of a service should be the first aspect of the market that is considered.

When pharmacists think of potential consumers of their value-added services, the first (and often only) group they think about is patients. After all, pharmacists interact with patients on a daily basis. While patients are essential to the success of most value-added pharmacist services, pharmacists must remember that groups of consumers other than patients may benefit from pharmacist services as well.

When planning for value-added pharmacist services, pharmacists often classify consumers into one of the three Ps. These three groups are patients, physicians and other health care professionals, and payers (Table 29-1). Pharmacists should consider the characteristics and needs of each of these groups in the business planning process carefully.

It is not realistic to expect that all patients will benefit from a value-added service. Thus, it is important for pharmacists to identify subgroups of patients

Table 29-1.	Types of Consumers of Value-Added Pharmacist Services

Patients and caregivers
 Patients with particular disease states
 Patients who have multiple disease states
 Patients who are not well controlled on existing therapy
 Patients who have unmet preventive care needs (e.g., immunizations, health screenings)
 Patients who are impacted by public health emergencies or natural disasters
 Caregivers of children, older adults, and individuals with a disability

Physicians and other health care professionals
 Primary care physicians (e.g., family medicine, general medicine, internal medicine, and pediatricians)
 Specialists (e.g., cardiology and endocrinology)
 Physician assistants, nurse practitioners, and nurses
 Dentists, podiatrists, and veterinarians

Payers
 Private insurance companies HMOs
 PPOs
 Accountable care organizations
 Government programs (i.e., Medicare, Medicaid, and state and local assistance programs)
 Employers

who may benefit more directly from their services. For an immunization program, offering flu vaccinations is a good starting point because it is recommended by the CDC that generally all adults receive a flu shot annually (CDC, 2018), which means that many patients will be eligible for the service each year. However, flu shots occur seasonally, so Dr. Smith is thinking ahead to identify other patient groups who may benefit from other types of immunizations. In this case, she decides to focus on pneumococcal vaccinations in older adults since it is recommended that adults 65 years old or older get a pneumococcal vaccination (CDC, 2017) and her store has a large number of older adult patients. Likewise, a pharmacy that serves a high proportion of individuals living with diabetes might choose to focus on services to that could benefit those patients. Pharmacists who can convince their patients and caregivers, when applicable, that their services will address an important need and positively impact their health outcomes will be on their way to developing a successful service.

Pharmacists desiring to implement new services must develop relationships with other health care professionals such as physicians, nurses, therapists, and other specialists, which means building rapport and trust and being able to clearly articulate how the pharmacist service complements existing services and benefits health outcomes (Kennedy et al., 2014). For example, for a new anticoagulation monitoring service to be viable, a pharmacist needs patient referrals from cardiologists, internal medicine specialists, vascular surgeons, and other health professionals who prescribe anticoagulation therapy. The pharmacist will also need medical information about these patients and perhaps even support from the professionals in billing for their services. On the other hand, the health care professionals need information not only about their patients but also about drug therapy. Physicians are increasingly challenged in today's managed care environment and often need to see many patients per day to maintain their financial viability. This creates a potential opportunity for pharmacists to partner with physicians who may be seeking ways to extend their services while maintaining high-quality patient care. Chapter 30 describes ways in which pharmacists can develop and enhance relationships with other health care professionals.

One group of consumers whose needs are often overlooked by pharmacists is payers. Today, almost all pharmacy goods and services are paid for by someone other than the patient. These third-party payers include insurance companies, managed-care plans, employers, and local, state, and national government agencies. Most third-party payers have needs that pharmacists are in a unique position to satisfy. Payers generally want to obtain high-quality goods and services at the lowest possible costs. Payers also recognize that they may not always be getting optimal benefits from their expenditures, especially those related to drug therapy. Pharmacists, given their expertise in drug therapy and proximity to their enrollees, are in an ideal position to help payers improve the quality of care while controlling costs, especially through their value-added services. On the other hand, since payers are used to pharmacist services being tied to a product (i.e., medication), a good business plan that aligns with a payer's needs, such as decreasing expenditures on a high-cost condition like diabetes, is critical to approaching a payer with an idea for a new service. Pharmacists who can demonstrate the value of their services to payers often find that payers are willing to encourage their enrollees to use pharmacists for services beyond dispensing (APhA, 2016; Smith et al., 2014).

Another aspect of the market for any value-added pharmacist service that must be considered is the competition. When identifying competitors, it is important to acknowledge exactly what services the pharmacist will pursue. When identifying competitors for value-added services, pharmacists often limit their search to other pharmacies and pharmacists. While this may be appropriate for traditional pharmacy goods and services (e.g., dispensing medications), pharmacists considering new value-added services must cast a much broader net. Some value-added services offered by pharmacists are still at the introductory point of their product life cycles. Few, if any, other pharmacies may offer these services in a particular market. Other classes of competitors may be very well established. For example, while diabetes education services are currently not offered in many community pharmacies, physicians and certified diabetes educators (CDEs), who can be nurses, nurse practitioners, dieticians, and other health care professionals, have provided this service for a number of years (Zrebiec, 2014). In the scenario, Dr. Smith should consider competitors to be primary care clinics and hospitals where immunizations are traditionally delivered.

Recognizing and evaluating competitors is an important part of the business planning process (see Chapter 7). While competitors have an established clientele and represent a potential threat to the success of a new pharmacist service, much can be learned from observing how they provide their services. If a large number of competitors are present in a market, it may be daunting to think about how a new value-added pharmacist service can compete successfully for customers. Competitors represent a challenge, but with proper research and planning, many pharmacists find that these challenges can be overcome. One way is by positioning a value-added pharmacist service in the market such that consumers see it as different from the others. This is often referred to as *niche marketing* (Doucette & McDonough, 2002). A pharmacy that hopes to establish a smoking-cessation service may find that there are a number of established competitors in the market (e.g., physicians, psychologists, support groups, and OTC medications). However, if the pharmacist can provide its service in such a way that consumers recognize that it is more convenient or has higher quality or a lower price than competitors, the pharmacy and its smoking-cessation service still can be successful in the market. In Dr. Smith's case, the convenience of getting a vaccination in a pharmacy with no appointment and no cost of a clinic visit is one advantage for patients over the traditional primary care setting.

For any value-added pharmacist service to be viable, there must be a sufficiently large number of consumers in the market who may be willing to purchase the service. Investing too many resources into a service that benefits a small number of consumers ultimately will lead to the demise of any business venture. Several sources can be used to determine the size of a market for a professional service. The easiest place for a business planner to start is to review a pharmacy's patient profiles, purchasing and financial records, and other internal data. Knowing how many prescriptions are filled for different classes of medications will help the planner determine which conditions are the most prevalent among the pharmacy's

patients. The only downfall of this method is that the information is limited to the pharmacist's current clientele. Many pharmacies would like to provide value-added pharmacist services that attract new patients.

Reviewing the literature to learn the potential size of a market can be helpful, especially epidemiologic studies that describe the incidence and prevalence of a condition. Unfortunately, most of these studies are done on a state, national, or even international level and may not provide information about the prevalence of a condition in a specific geographic location of interest. This disadvantage can be offset in part by combining a literature review with interviews of other health care professionals in the pharmacy's market area. They may be able to provide specific information about the number of patients they and other professionals treat. For example, it is becoming more common for primary care clinics to have registries of patients with chronic conditions such as diabetes, hypertension, and/or asthma. Networking with other professionals to access these registries is a way to quickly estimate market size in an area. Another valuable resource can be the local health department website to give indications and prevalence of the area's major health burdens. Generally, these websites also have county level information, such as immunization rates, for some but not all counties.

Perhaps the most direct way to determine the size of a market for a value-added pharmacist service is to perform a market research study. Survey research methods can be used to gather information from potential customers. Not only can this information be used to determine the number of potential consumers in a specific area, but it can also provide additional information about consumers that can be useful in developing a value-added pharmacist service (e.g., if/ where they currently obtain this service, their level of satisfaction with the service, and their willingness to obtain the service from a pharmacist). Some of the drawbacks of market research include the specialized knowledge and skills needed to carry out a study properly, the amount of time involved, the relatively high cost of performing this type of research, and the potential biases that are inherent in any type of survey research. Several studies have been published that used market research to determine the size, characteristics, and willingness-to-pay of potential consumers of value-added pharmacist services (Feehan et al., 2017; Painter et al., 2018).

Even if there are a large number of consumers who might be interested in obtaining a value-added service from a pharmacist, the ultimate question that must be answered is whether these consumers are willing and able to make this purchase. Some consumers (especially patients) may be very interested in obtaining a health service from a pharmacist and actually may say on a survey that they would be willing to pay for this service. However, saying that one is willing to pay does not always result in an actual payment for the service. The consumer may not have the means to pay the price being charged by the pharmacist or may be able to obtain the service from another provider (e.g., a physician) for only a small insurance copayment. Similar to payers, consumers are also used to paying a copay for a medication and may need education about the value of pharmacist services not associated with a product.

Other groups of consumers may also be interested in obtaining a value-added pharmacist service and often have the financial resources to do so (e.g., other health care professionals, insurance companies, employers, and government agencies). However, pharmacists often find that these groups may not be willing to pay for these services until the pharmacist can demonstrate the value of the services (APhA, 2016). This has created a "chicken and egg" problem for many pharmacists. Pharmacists state that they cannot show the value of the service unless they are given the opportunity to provide it. At the same time, pharmacists state that they cannot afford to provide the service unless they are paid to do so. Numerous projects have been performed to show the value of professional services to various groups of consumers (Giberson et al., 2011; Matzke et al., 2018; Pellegrin et al., 2017). Medicare now provides opportunities for pharmacists to receive payment for MTM services through the Part D program and some Medicaid programs and private insurers will pay for pharmacist services, although it is not widespread (APhA, 2016). In Dr. Smith's case, immunizations are a billable service that pharmacists can receive payment from government (Medicare) and private insurers.

Several methods can be used to learn more about consumers' willingness and ability to pay for value-added pharmacist services. Getting to know consumers and observing their habits (e.g., what services they will pay for, how much they will pay, and what they expect to receive in return) can be done relatively quickly and easily in most practice settings. Market research and the pharmacy literature can also be used, but it is important to remember that what a consumer says he or she will pay for a value-added pharmacist service on a survey may not represent what he or she actually will pay when presented with the service in the pharmacy. The only way to truly determine what a consumer will pay for a value-added pharmacist service is to offer the service, charge a price, and observe whether the consumer actually makes the purchase. Unfortunately, this can occur only after the decision has been made to offer the service.

■ REVISITING THE SCENARIO

Dr. Smith was able to implement many of the strategies that she had discussed with her pharmacy manager and team. All of the pharmacists in her independent pharmacy attended a pharmacy-based immunization delivery certificate program during the summer. Before the start of this year's flu season, her independent pharmacy implemented a marketing plan (see Chapter 25) to inform their target markets that they would have flu and pneumonia shots available. They developed advertisement and put information on the pharmacy's web site which focused on the importance of vaccinations and how convenient it was to receive their flu and pneumonia vaccine at her pharmacy. She also worked with her pharmacy students and the local public health department to develop educational presentations for the community about the benefits of being vaccinated. Dr. Smith and her students then delivered the presentation at several independent living apartment buildings for older adults.

CAN A VALUE-BASED PHARMACIST SERVICE MEET THE NEEDS OF CONSUMERS?

Assuming that there is a consumer need and a market for a particular value-added pharmacist service, business planners must ask themselves a very serious question before moving forward. The question is whether they can actually meet the needs of consumers. The answer to this question is not always as easy as it might appear and requires a great deal of introspection on the part of the pharmacist and the organization.

One way that business planners can begin to answer this question is to perform a SWOT (i.e., *s*trengths, *w*eaknesses, *o*pportunities, and *t*hreats) analysis, as described in Chapters 6 and 7. SWOT analysis has applications in both strategic and business planning. In strategic planning, managers perform this analysis on a broad level, looking at the entire organization. In business planning, SWOT are evaluated only at the level of the service being considered. Strengths and weaknesses are considered to be internal to an organization and are the easiest to *initially* evaluate. They are also within the control of the organization, such that aspects that initially may be considered a weakness can be addressed and perhaps even become strengths of the organization in the future. Opportunities and threats generally exist external to an organization. Given that they are part of the external environment, they are often more difficult to control. At the same time, they can exert just as much influence over the success or failure of a value-added pharmacist service as internal strengths and weaknesses.

The first internal factor that an organization planning to offer a value-added pharmacist service should evaluate is the resources necessary to provide the service. This starts with the abilities and interests of the staff to provide the service. Many value-added pharmacist services require knowledge and skills beyond those used in traditional dispensing functions. Staff members may need to attend educational or training programs to gain the appropriate knowledge and skills. Some value-added services require that pharmacists become certified to demonstrate their knowledge and skills in an area before the service may be offered. States that allow pharmacists to administer immunizations often require that they become certified before providing this service (APhA, 2015). Medicare and many insurance companies require that pharmacists become CDEs before they will compensate them to provide diabetes education services. Becoming a CDE is time-intensive and involves completing a series of exercises, direct experience in providing diabetes education to patients, and passing an examination. This process generally takes about 2 years to complete (National Certification Board for Diabetes Educators [NCBDE], 2019).

It may go without saying that pharmacists should be interested in providing value-added services if they are to be successful. It is important to match the skills and interests of a pharmacy's personnel with the services the pharmacy intends to provide. If a pharmacist is not interested in providing a service, can he or she be provided with an incentive that may motivate him or her to do so? If not, can another pharmacist be hired who has the interest and skills needed to be successful?

Pharmacies need a number of physical resources to provide most value-added services. This usually begins with the layout of the pharmacy. Many value-added pharmacy services require at least some degree of privacy. Unfortunately, pharmacies that were designed to maximize the efficiency of the dispensing process often do not have a private office or classroom space necessary to provide patient care services. Other physical resources that may be needed to provide a professional service include computer hardware and software, testing devices, medical supplies, and office supplies. It is also important to consider how outcomes of a service will be documented. Are existing systems sufficient for documentation? Is new software required?

Pharmacies must be willing to commit financial resources to the development of a new value-added service. Working capital is needed to support the purchase of equipment, supplies, and marketing before the service can be offered. Since most services do not bring in enough income initially to cover their costs, money will also be needed to pay employees and continue to purchase needed resources. Business planners must consider how much working capital they will need to start a service and how long they are willing to support the service before it is expected to cover its costs and contribute to organizational profitability.

Another internal resource that cannot be overlooked is support from administrators within the organization. Administrators who "buy in" to the concept of providing value-added services are much more likely to support their development and provide the resources needed to get them off the ground. Pharmacists hoping to gain this support generally work to convince administrators how implementation of value-added services will help the organization reach its overall goals. In the scenario, the pharmacy manager showed buy-in by paying for the pharmacy remodel and for pharmacists to become immunization certified. The manager also gave feedback about the process, which allowed Dr. Smith to try different strategies when patient uptake was low.

Many external factors, such as patient demographic trends, can be viewed as both a threat and an opportunity for the development of a value-added service. The aging of the population, increasing chronic disease burden, and the increased reliance on drug therapy as a medical treatment have greatly increased the number of prescriptions filled in pharmacies (Kaiser Family Foundation, 2017). This can be seen as a threat in that pharmacy staff may not have as much time to provide other nondispensing services. On the other hand, these trends also present opportunities for pharmacists to implement new services that meet the increased patient needs for health information and drug therapy monitoring.

Other external factors that may influence the success or failure of a value-added service include laws and regulations affecting practice (both of pharmacists and of other health care professionals), reimbursement and compensation policies of third-party payers, competition from other pharmacies and health care providers, technology, and the ever-changing needs of health care consumers themselves. While these factors may be difficult for business planners to influence, they are manageable. Pharmacists willing to take a proactive stance regarding these issues (especially though involvement in professional organizations and other groups) are often able to have their voices heard and help to shape the policies that affect their futures.

■ REVISITING THE SCENARIO

At her next annual review, Dr. Smith's pharmacy manager reported that she was very pleased with the success of changes to the flu and pneumonia vaccine program. Not only was there an increase in the number of patients vaccinated at the pharmacy, many of the patients decided to transfer their prescriptions and were now regular pharmacy patients. This service was helping to increase the health of their patients and was also able to generate a revenue stream for the pharmacy. Going forward, Dr. Smith and her pharmacy manager strategized that offering vaccines off-site may be a viable option. Dr. Smith noticed that when she and her pharmacy students were providing the educational sessions to the residents of the independent living buildings that many of the residents would be interested in receiving their vaccines on site. This would allow them to reach the residents who had transportation difficulties to travel to the pharmacy. She also considered collaborating with local businesses to offer the vaccines to their employees during business hours. Her pharmacy manager was in complete support of this endeavor and they worked together to see what was needed for traveling offsite and for billing vaccine administrations outside of the pharmacy.

While the immunizations for influenza and pneumonia were highly successful, Dr. Smith realized that much of this service was occurring during September through December. She decided to meet again with her local public health department to see which additional immunizations would be of value to the public health of her community. She also decided to conduct a survey of patients who visited the pharmacy to gauge their interest level with other vaccines and other clinical services within the pharmacy. She worked with her pharmacy students to analyze the demographics of her patients to get a more complete picture of her patient population. Using all of these sources, Dr. Smith found that there was a need to provide herpes zoster (Shingles) vaccines as well as human papilloma virus (HPV) vaccines within the pharmacy to meet the community's need. In her discussions with the college of pharmacy, she noted that several students participated in international rotations. Across the university a number of students, faculty, and staff participated in international courses or mission trips each year. This opened her eyes to the potential for a partnership with the university to provide travel vaccines and medication to create a comprehensive pharmacist immunization program.

■ CONCLUSION

There are many opportunities for pharmacists to implement public health services. Value-added services cannot be developed with the hope that consumers will adopt them. Pharmacy managers can use business planning as a tool to evaluate consumer needs, the market, and their own resources before deciding whether to offer value-added services and which services would be most likely to succeed. While using business planning does not guarantee that a new value-added pharmacist public health venture will be successful, the process helps pharmacy managers manage the risks involved in this increasingly important area of their organizations.

■ QUESTIONS FOR FURTHER DISCUSSION

1. What are the dangers of only thinking about the clinical components of a new pharmacist service?
2. Compare and contrast the types of value-added public health pharmacist services that most likely would be accepted at not-for-profit, university-based medical center and a for-profit community pharmacy chain.
3. What obligations does a pharmacist have to provide services that benefit their community, in addition to those that benefit individual patients?
4. How would have developing a business plan before she implemented the immunization program helped Dr. Smith?
5. Given what you now know, what other professional services may also be viable for Dr. Smith to offer at her pharmacy?

REFERENCES

Accreditation Council for Pharmacy Education (ACPE). 2015. *Accreditation Standards and Key Elements for the Professional Program in Pharmacy Leading to the Doctor of Pharmacy Degree ("Standards 2016")*. Chicago, IL: ACPE.

American Association of Colleges of Pharmacy (AACP). 2005. *Council of Deans and Council of Faculties Joint Task Force. White Paper on the Role of Schools and Colleges of Pharmacy in Developing and Administering Combined/Dual Degree Programs*. Alexandria, VA: AACP.

American Pharmacists Association (APhA). 2015. Pharmacy-based immunization delivery certificate program. Available at http://www.pharmacist.com/pharmacy-based-immunization-delivery. Accessed January 14, 2019.

American Pharmacists Association (APhA). 2016. Pharmacists' patient care services digest. Building momentum. Increasing access. Available at http://media.pharmacist.com/documents/APhA_Digest.pdf. Accessed January 13, 2019.

American Pharmacists Association (APhA). 2017. Number of states authorizing pharmacists to administer influenza and number of pharmacists trained to administer vaccines. Available at https://www.pharmacist.com/sites/default/files/files/States_Authorizing_Pharmacists_vs_training_December_2017.pdf. Accessed January 13, 2019.

American Public Health Association (APHA). 2015. Policy statement: The role of the pharmacist in public health. Available at http://www.apha.org/policies-and-advocacy/public-health-policy-statements/policy-database/2014/07/07/13/05/the-role-of-the-pharmacist-in-public-health. Accessed January 12, 2019.

American Society of Health-System Pharmacists (ASHP). 2008. ASHP statement on the role of health-system pharmacists in public health. *Am J Health Syst Pharm* 65:462–467.

Athern KM, Linnebur SA, Fabisiak G. 2016. Proper disposal of unused household medications: The role of the pharmacist. *Consult Pharm* 31(5):261–266.

Bach AT, Goad JA. The role of community pharmacy-based vaccination in the USA: Current practice and future directions. *Integr Pharm Res Pract* 2015;4:67–77.

Centers for Disease Control and Prevention (CDC). 1994. The public health system and the 10 essential public health services. Available at https://www.cdc.gov/publichealthgateway/publichealthservices/essentialhealthservices.html. Accessed January 12, 2019.

Centers for Disease Control and Prevention (CDC). 2017. Pneumococcal vaccination. Available at https://www.cdc.gov/vaccines/vpd/pneumo/index.html. Accessed January 13, 2019.

Centers for Disease Control and Prevention (CDC). 2018. Vaccination: Who should do it, who should not and who should take precautions. Available at https://www.cdc.gov/flu/protect/whoshouldvax.htm. Accessed January 13, 2019.

Cochran G, Hruschak V, De Fosse B, Hohmeier KC. 2016. Prescription opioid abuse: Pharmacists' perspective and response. *Integr Pharm Res Pract* 5:65–73.

Darin KM, Scarsi KK, Klepser SA, et al. 2015. Consumer interest in community pharmacy HIV screening services. *J Am Pharm Assoc (2003)* 55:67–72.

Doucette WR, McDonough RP. 2002. Beyond the 4 P's: Using relationship marketing to build value and demand for pharmacy services. *J Am Pharm Assoc* 42:183–194; quiz 193–194.

Eades CE, Ferguson JS, O'Carroll RE. 2011. Public health in community pharmacy: A systematic review of pharmacist and consumer views. *BMC Public Health* 11:582.

Feehan M, Walsh M, Godin J, Sundwall D, Munger MA. 2017. Patient preferences for healthcare delivery through community pharmacy settings in the USA: A discrete choice study. *J Clin Pharm Ther* 42(6):738–749.

Fitzgerald TJ, Kang Y, Bridges CB, et al. 2016. Integrating pharmacies into public health program planning for pandemic influenza vaccine response. *Vaccine* 34(46):5643–5648.

Gerber BS, Cano AI, Caceres ML, et al. 2010. A pharmacist and health promoter team to improve medication adherence among Latinos with diabetes. *Ann Pharmacother* 44:70–79.

Giberson S, Yoder S, Lee MP. 2011. *Improving Patient and Health System Outcomes through Advanced Pharmacy Practice. A Report to the U.S. Surgeon General.* Office of the Chief Pharmacist. U.S. Public Health Service.

Gonzalvo JD, Lantaff WM. 2018. CDE pharmacists in the United States. *Diabetes Educ* 44(3):278–292.

Gortney JS, Seed S, Borja-Hart N, et al. 2013. The prevalence and characteristics of dual PharmD/MPH programs offered at US colleges and schools of pharmacy. *Am J Pharm Educ* 77(6):116.

Hannings AN, von Waldner T, McEwen DW, White CA. 2016. Assessment of emergency preparedness modules in introductory pharmacy practice experiences. *Am J Pharm Educ* 80(2):23.

Hill LG, Sanchez JP, Laguado SA, Lawson KA. 2018. Operation naloxone: Overdose prevention service learning for student pharmacists. *Curr Pharm Teach Learn* 10:1348–1353.

Institute of Medicine (IOM) of the National Academies, Committee on Assuring the Health of the Public in the 21st Century. 2003a. *The Future of the Public's Health in the 21st Century.* Washington, DC: National Academies Press.

Institute of Medicine (IOM) of the National Academies, Committee on Quality Health Care in America. 2003b. *Crossing the Quality Chasm: A New Health System for the 21st Century.* Washington, DC: National Academies Press.

Kaiser Family Foundation. 2017. State health facts: number of retail prescription drugs filled at pharmacies by payer. Available at https://www.kff.org/health-costs/state-indicator/total-retail-rx-drugs/?currentTimeframe=0&sortModel=%7B%22colId%22:%22Location%22,%22sort%22:%22asc%22%7D/. Accessed January 13, 2019.

Kennedy AG, Biddle MA. 2014. Practical strategies for pharmacist integration with primary care:

A workbook. Available at http://contentmanager.med.uvm.edu/docs/default-source/ahec-documents/practicalstrategiesforpharmacistintegrationwithprimarycare-workbook_000.pdf?sfvrsn=2. Accessed January 13, 2019.

Matzke GR, Moczygemba LR, Williams KJ, et al. 2018. Impact of a pharmacist-physician collaborative care model on patient outcomes and health services utilization. *Am J Health-System Pharm* 75(14):1039–1047.

Medina M, Plaza C, Stowe C, et al. 2013. Center for the Advancement of Pharmaceutical Education (CAPE) educational outcomes 2013. *Am J Pharm Educ* 77:162.

Melin K, Rodríguez-Díaz C. 2018. Community pharmacy response in the aftermath of natural disasters: Time-sensitive opportunity for research and evaluation. *J Prim Care & Com Health* 9(7):620-623.

National Association of Boards of Pharmacy (NABP). 2015. *Survey of Pharmacy Law*. Mount Prospect, IL: National Association of Boards of Pharmacy.

National Certification Board for Diabetes Educators (NCBDE). 2019. 2019 Certification examination for diabetes educators. Available at https://www.ncbde.org/certification_info/professional-practice-experience/. Accessed January 13, 2019.

Painter JT, Gressler L, Kathe N, Slabaugh L, Blumenschein K 2018. Consumer willingness to pay for pharmacy services: An updated review of the literature. *Res Soc Admin Pharm* 14(12):1091–1105.

Patel AR, Breck AB, Law MR. 2018. The impact of pharmacy-based immunization services on the likelihood of immunization in the United States. *J Am Pharm Assoc* 58:505–514.

Pellegrin KL, Krenk L, Oakes SJ, et al. 2017. Reductions in medication-related hospitalizations in older adults with medication management by hospital and community pharmacists: A quasi-experimental study. *J Am Geriatr Soc* 65:212–219.

Perry LA, Shinn BW, Stanovich J. 2014. Quantification of an ongoing community-based medication take-back program. *J Am Pharm Assoc* 54(3):275–279.

Queeno BV. 2017. Evaluation of inpatient influenza and pneumococcal vaccination acceptance rates with pharmacist education. *J Pharm Pract* 30(2):202–208.

Smith M, Cannon-Breland ML, Spiggle S. 2014. Consumer, physician and payer perspectives on primary care medication management services with a shared resource pharmacists network. *Res Soc Admin Pharm* 10:539–553.

Strand MA, Tellers J, Patterson A, Ross A, Palombi L. 2016. The achievement of public health services in pharmacy practice: A literature review. *Res Social Adm Pharm* 12:247–256.

Strand MA, Eukel H, Burck. 2018. Moving opioid misuse prevention upstream: A pilot study of community pharmacists screening for opioid risk. *Res Soc Adm Pharm* [Epub ahead of print].

Substance Abuse and Mental Health Services Administration (SAMHSA) Center for the Application of Prevention Technologies. 2018. Preventing the consequences of opioid overdose: Understanding naloxone access laws. Available at https://www.samhsa.gov/capt/sites/default/files/resources/naloxone-access-laws-tool.pdf. Accessed January 12, 2019.

Trinkley KE, Weed HG, Beatty SJ, Porter K, Nahata MC. 2017. Identification and characterization of adverse drug events in primary care. *Am J Med Qual* 32(5):518–525.

Truong H, Taylor C, DiPeitro N. 2012. The assessment, development, assurance pharmacist's tool (ADAPT) for ensuring quality implementation of health promotion programs. *Am J Pharm Ed* 76:1.

Vargas J, Dang C, Subramaniam V. 2011. Public health approaches in ethnically diverse populations. *Drug Top* 155:4.

Westrick SC. 2009. College/school of pharmacy affiliation and community pharmacies' involvement in public health activities. American Association of Colleges of Pharmacy Annual Meeting. 73:NIL.

Westrick SC, Patterson BJ, Kader MS, Rashid S, Buck PO, Rothholz MC. 2018. National survey of pharmacy-based immunization services. *Vaccine* 36:5657–5664.

Zrebiec J. 2014. A national study of the certified diabetes educator: Implications for future certification examinations. *Diabetes Educ* 40(4):470–475.

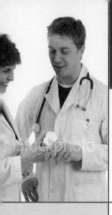

30

IMPLEMENTING VALUE-ADDED PHARMACIST SERVICES

Karl M. Hess

About the Author: Karl Hess earned his PharmD from the Massachusetts College of Pharmacy and Allied Health Sciences in Boston. He subsequently completed a PGY1 community pharmacy practice residency at the University of Southern California School of Pharmacy. Currently, Dr. Hess is an Associate Professor of Pharmacy Practice and the Director of Community Pharmacy Practice Innovations at Chapman University School of Pharmacy. Dr. Hess lectures on a variety of subjects on self-care therapeutics, immunizations, and travel health and medicine. In 2009, he received the Certificate in Travel Health from the International Society of Travel Medicine and in 2018, he received Associate Member status in the Faculty of Travel Medicine at the Royal College of Physicians and Surgeons in Glasgow, Scotland. Dr. Hess is also a past Speaker of the House for the California Pharmacists Association and received fellowship status from this association in 2011. Dr. Hess is interested in the implementation and practice of collaborative patient care services within the community pharmacy setting. His areas of academic and research interests include community pharmacy practice, travel health and medicine, vaccines, self-care therapeutics, and the safe and effective use of nonprescription medications and dietary supplements.

■ LEARNING OBJECTIVES

After completing this chapter, readers should be able to

1. Describe the types of value-added services that pharmacists have implemented in their practices.
2. Identify the components of a value-added service to consider before implementation, including key elements of a policy and procedures manual.
3. State how to manage the marketing mix during service implementation.
4. Describe the role that collaborative practice agreements (CPAs) have in value-added pharmacist services.
5. Describe strategies for pricing and obtaining payment for value-added pharmacist services.

■ SCENARIO

Amber Smith, the pharmacist-owner of Care-Rite Pharmacy, is interested in expanding her services. She has owned this pharmacy for several years and has built up an excellent reputation among her patients, with physicians, and the local community as her practice is recognized as patient friendly and service oriented. She would like to be able to leverage this by establishing a valued-added patient care service to help improve her patient's health and well-being while simultaneously adding to her pharmacy's bottom line as third-party prescription reimbursements continue to decline. Her pharmacy is located in a city with a population of approximately 100,000 people and she has not implemented any specific patient care service in the past. She has two full-time pharmacists and two part-time pharmacists who have been working at the pharmacy for a number of years (range 5–15 years). Recently, they completed a strategic plan, a strengths, weaknesses, opportunities, and threats (SWOT) analysis, and a survey of their patients. The results of the patient survey identified their key target market as women 50 years of age and older. Initially, they had wanted to implement a diabetes educational program, but their market research determined that a local hospital sponsored an American Diabetes Association (ADA)-recognized program. This hospital has a strong presence in their community and the hospital's diabetes educators were not interested in collaborating with local pharmacies. Amber's pharmacy also looked into developing a community based anticoagulation service, but after researching the reimbursement for this type of service, they realized that it would not be financially feasible. However, their market research did show that there was a need for a medication therapy management (MTM) program since they had noted that there was not a similar program elsewhere in their community. They already had a large percentage of patients who were taking multiple chronic medications and had several chronic medical conditions and were deemed to be high risk for medication-related problems. Many of these patients expressed a need for assistance with medication management issues. They also serve a large percentage of patients eligible for Medicaid and/or Medicare and they saw an opportunity to provide MTM services for those patients who may be eligible (have at least two chronic medical conditions, take between two to eight covered medications, and are likely to incur a predetermined minimum cost threshold for their medications) according to their prescription drug plan (Centers for Medicare and Medicaid, 2018).

■ CHAPTER QUESTIONS

1. What are the different types of value-added services that pharmacists have implemented in their practices? Describe the medication management process for each.
2. What are the components of a value-added service that pharmacists should consider and plan before implementation?
3. Why is a policy and procedures manual important to successful service implementation? What other resources should pharmacists have or develop to ensure success of the service?
4. How should pharmacists manage the marketing mix for value-added services?
5. How much do pharmacists typically charge for their value-added services? What strategies have been successful in obtaining reimbursement from patients? From third-party payers?
6. How can services, once implemented, be sustained over time?

■ INTRODUCTION

As discussed in previous chapters, implementing value-added pharmacist services requires a comprehensive strategic plan that should include a mission statement, SWOT analysis, goals and objectives that the service hopes to achieve, and strategies to achieve those objectives. Other areas that should be addressed when implementing a new service include setting financial goals and allocating financial resources to help ensure that the service is sustainable, understanding the service experience of the end user, managing pharmacy staff who will be helping to provide the service, and creating a dedicated space to provide the service (Feletto et al., 2010). This helps to provide further direction for the service, guides the allocation of resources and efforts, and helps ensure that the new service is successful. As the scenario above demonstrates, the planning process helped Amber, the pharmacy owner, identify a service that fits with her pharmacy's strategic plan, yet has a niche in the marketplace. Pharmacists can implement many types of services in their practices, but it is essential that they perform market research to determine the opportunities and threats in their specific marketplace to ensure the success of the new service and its sustainability overtime. A planning framework that takes into account pharmacist service characteristics (e.g., advantages of, complexity, costs) outer setting characteristics (e.g., patient needs and resources), inner setting characteristics (e.g., physical space available in the pharmacy, climate, and readiness for implementation), pharmacy staff characteristics (e.g., knowledge and skill set to provide the service), and process characteristics (e.g., planning, engaging, and executing the service) may aid in this process (Shoemaker et al., 2017). Pharmacist services that are more cost effective than usual care can help to create buy-in with providers and payers (Malet-Larrea et al., 2016). Ultimately, the success of any service depends both on market opportunities and the pharmacy's ability to provide the service.

■ TYPES OF VALUE-ADDED PHARMACIST SERVICES

Value-added pharmacist services can be thought to exist along a continuum (see Figure 30-1). On one end of the continuum, pharmacists are focused on medication therapy issues that arise during the dispensing process. On the other end of the continuum, pharmacists provide ongoing MTM services for select individuals who have multiple comorbidities requiring complex therapies (i.e., case management). Other types of services fall somewhere in-between these two ends (e.g., disease-state management programs such as anticoagulation or lipid clinics, and immunization services).

MTM can be focused or comprehensive and therefore can fall anywhere within the continuum. Focused MTM services can occur during the dispensing process when a medication therapy problem is identified and the pharmacist performs a targeted intervention. For example, it may be determined that the patient has an allergy to a specific medication. By focusing efforts on resolving this problem, information is collected pertaining to this allergy (allergic reaction, past history, etc.), an alternate medication is identified, the prescriber is called, the pharmacist's recommendation is made, and the medication is changed. An extension of the focused MTM service is a process called continuous medication monitoring (CMM). CMM is a proactive approach to medication management that incorporates a comprehensive review of the medication profile into the medication dispensing process for all patients as prescriptions are processed (McDonough, 2014). CMM, like other services, is possible in a busy community pharmacy, but

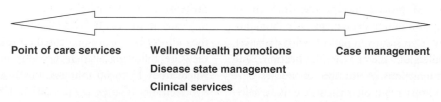

Figure 30-1. Value-added pharmacist services continuum.

it does require implementation of a technician-driven dispensing process, automation and technology, and the utilization of an electronic documentation system.

Comprehensive MTM services are at the other end of the continuum where the pharmacist provides a comprehensive medication review (CMR), identifies problems with the patient's medication therapy, develops a medication action plan (MAP) and a personalized medication record (PMR) in which they share with the patient, and finally the pharmacist sends the patient workup and recommendations to the physician or other health care provider. Medicare Part D recognizes pharmacists as MTM providers; therefore, pharmacists can get reimbursed for providing this service to Part D beneficiaries. Online platforms such as Outcomes MTM (https://www.outcomesmtm .com) and Mirixa (https://www.mirixa.com) are available for pharmacies to contract with which help to automate and streamline the comprehensive MTM process for Medicare beneficiaries.

The Appointment Based Model (ABM) can also be incorporated into MTM services. The ABM is a medication synchronization program that can help the patient with medication adherence. In this model, the pharmacist proactively reviews the patient's profile for medications that need to be refilled, contacts the prescriber for any new prescriptions needed, schedules a date for the patient to pick up all of their medications, and counsels the patient on their medications when they arrive at the pharmacy for their appointment. In addition to helping improve medication adherence, the ABM has also been shown to improve operational efficiency, increase patient enrollment in other pharmacist services, and increase refill volume (Patterson & Holdford, 2017).

Common therapy problems that may be found using any MTM process include identification of high-risk medications in older patients, need for additional therapy (e.g., statins in patients with diabetes), adherence, allergies, therapeutic duplication, and drug–drug interactions. A number of studies have examined the impact that pharmacists can have delivering MTM services. Pharmacist-provided patient care services have been found to improve laboratory

values such as A1C levels, systolic and diastolic blood pressure values as well as patient understanding of disease states and health-related quality of life (Caffiero et al., 2017; Murphy-Menezes, 2015; Okere et al., 2015; Pinto et al., 2014; Rodis et al., 2017; Schwartz et al., 2017; Shaya et al., 2015; Smalls et al., 2015).

Pharmacist monitoring/screening services and wellness/health-promotion programs are the next level of value-added services along the continuum. Examples of such services abound in the literature and include, but are not limited to, pharmacist-managed anticoagulation services (Bishop et al., 2015; Biszewski et al., 2015; Garwood et al., 2014; Hale et al., 2018; Lee et al., 2018; Manzoor et al., 2017; Philip et al., 2015; Singh et al., 2015) travel health (Durham et al., 2011; Hess et al., 2010; Seed et al., 2011), hormonal contraception prescribing (Manchikanti, 2017), naloxone dispensing and education (Puzantian & Gasper, 2018), lipid management services (Atanda et al., 2017; Bouwmeester & Chim, 2013), smoking cessation counseling (Smalls et al., 2015), osteoporosis screenings (Salvig et al., 2016), and lipid screenings with cardiovascular assessment (Smith et al., 2013). Health-promotion/screening programs utilizing point of care testing (POCT) for influenza, strep throat, and hepatitis C among others have been more recently adopted and implemented in community pharmacies (Isho et al., 2017; Klepser et al., 2016; Klepser et al., 2018).

The next types of services along the continuum are those which pertain to disease-state management. These services occur separately from the dispensing function over an extended period of time, but have an added feature of ongoing patient education and monitoring of medication therapy as it relates to attainment of the patient's therapeutic goals. A comprehensive patient chart is created and pharmacists may review the entire medication profile, although their efforts may be more focused on the disease state they are following. Patient sessions may last anywhere from 15 to 60 minutes. Pharmacist-managed hypertension (Carter et al., 2015; Khazan et al., 2017; Sisson et al., 2016), heart failure (Hale et al., 2017; Milfred-LaForest et al., 2017), diabetes (Halalau et al., 2018; Hansen et al., 2017; Kostoff et al., 2014; Maxwell et al., 2016; Schultz et al., 2018; Sease et al., 2013; Sullivan et al., 2016; Wang et al., 2016), and asthma (Pett & Nye, 2016) disease-state management programs have been cited frequently in the literature, and typically are associated with positive clinical outcomes which support their implementation.

The most comprehensive pharmacist service, and often the most challenging to implement, is that of case management. With this service, pharmacists are responsible for providing complete patient workups. A thorough patient history needs to be taken, a comprehensive review of all medications done with the patient, and the patient followed for an extended period of time. Pharmacists may also decide to perform physical assessment procedures (e.g., vital signs, review of systems, etc.) as part of this service in order to gain a better understanding of the effects of medications on the body. Case management typically involves patients with complex medical problems and multiple prescribers. Studies have investigated the impact of pharmacists' reviews in high-risk patients in the community setting and have found high levels of patient satisfaction of the service provided along with high rates of provider acceptance to pharmacist-made recommendations and care plans with resolution of most identified medication-related issues (Garcia-Cardenas et al., 2017; Smith MG, 2017).

Regardless of the specific service being offered, these types of services will require more patient data collection and often are delivered over an extended period to monitor for changes and attainment of therapeutic goals. Patient visits may also be prescheduled (as opposed to performed on a walk-in basis) and conducted in a face-to-face manner with the patient. Patient visits may also occur telephonically; however, the pharmacy will need to invest in secure communication technologies in order to facilitate this process and be compliant with the Health Insurance Portability and Accountability Act (HIPAA) and the Health Information Technology for Economic and Clinical Health Act (HITECH). Documentation is more comprehensive and focused on the assessment and plan being performed and developed, respectively.

However, the activities and process of medication management provided by pharmacists implementing a value-added service is relatively similar along the continuum and should follow the Pharmacists Patient Care Process (PPCP), which is a five step approach to patient care activities.

The first step of the PPCP is to collect the patient's medication history, medical history, laboratory data, physical assessment findings, as well as social history and lifestyle habits in order to gain a comprehensive overview of the patient. The second step is to evaluate and assess this information in order to make a decision regarding the appropriateness, effectiveness, and safety of the patient's current therapy. Additional items that could be assessed include the patient's adherence to medications, risk factors for disease, and need for immunizations. The third step is to develop an individualized patient-centered plan that addresses the patient's medication-related problems and sets goals for therapy. The fourth step is to implement that plan in collaboration with the patient's physician, nurses, and other health care providers as well as the patient's caregivers. The fifth and last step of the PPCP is monitoring the patient's progress toward therapeutic goals, evaluating whether they have attained these goals, and following up with the patient and the patients other providers as needed (Joint Commission of Pharmacy Practitioners, 2014). Appropriate documentation of these activities (either in a shared electronic documentation system or within the pharmacy management system [PMS]) is also an integral component and should occur at each step of the PPCP.

■ COMPONENTS OF A VALUE-ADDED PHARMACIST SERVICE

Once it is determined which service is to be implemented, it is important to put thought into the resources needed and processes and workflow for implementation. Use of the pharmacy's PMS or electronic medical record to help flag patients who are eligible for the service and shifting technical/non-discretionary tasks to technicians or other pharmacy staff to help free up the pharmacists in order to provide the service are two key interventions that may help the implementation and ultimate success of the service (MacKeigan et al., 2017). Below are important components to providing any pharmacist service which should be taken into account when planning and preparing for the service.

Data Collection

Patient data collection is a critical component of any value-added service. The information collected provides pharmacists with important baseline and monitoring parameters for patients. The amount and type of information needed from the patient or other health care providers may differ depending on the service, but nonetheless, this information is the foundation on which the other components of the service are built. Forms can be developed to help pharmacists collect this information (see Figures 30-2 to 30-4). In addition, consideration should be given to how this information will be stored, and the safety and security of that information (e.g., paper charts or an electronic patient database). The information that should be collected from the patient includes demographic information, medical history, family history, and medication history among others which can be obtained directly from a patient intake form. Some of this information may need to be collected from other providers and health care institutions, and an authorization to release medical information should be signed by the patient and kept as part of the chart (see Figure 30-5). Finally, pharmacists should ensure that their site is in compliance with HIPAA and HITECH and reinforce to their patients that the information they provide is confidential and secure at the pharmacy.

Pharmacy-Based Laboratory

Although pharmacists can receive objective patient data from outside laboratories or from physician offices, it may be decided that it is more convenient for the patient and pharmacist if a laboratory monitoring/screening service is performed as part of the service. Several types of monitors and equipment can be purchased by pharmacists and integrated into their practices. For example, pharmacists who implement wellness programs may purchase a body-fat analyzer, a weight scale, or a monitor that measures lipid and blood glucose levels. Alternatively, pharmacists who develop a diabetes program may wish to obtain a device that measures the glycosylated hemoglobin (A1C) of patients. Some pharmacists may decide to develop a women's health program and purchase a bone densitometer that measures bone mineral density to determine fracture risk owing to osteoporosis. In certain states, pharmacists may be able to order laboratory tests for medication therapy related problems themselves (American Pharmacists Association, 2019). Pharmacists should check with their State Board of Pharmacy to determine whether they can order laboratory tests in this manner and the process for doing so.

Pharmacies implementing monitoring/screening services must become familiar with the Clinical Laboratory Improvement Amendments of 1988 (CLIA) should they wish to utilize devices that measure patient specimens (e.g., blood or saliva samples). CLIA was enacted to ensure that all medical laboratories meet quality standards. These amendments are administered by the Centers for Medicare and Medicaid Services (CMS), which is responsible for laboratory registration, certificate generation, surveys, and surveyor guidelines for development and training. Tests typically performed by pharmacists in pharmacies (e.g., blood glucose, lipid panels, hemoglobin A1C, and international normalization ratio [INR] tests) are considered CLIA-waived tests. CLIA-waived tests are considered by the Centers for Disease Control and Prevention (CDC) and the Food and Drug Administration (FDA) to be simple to administer and have little risk of error. Pharmacists providing waived tests agree to follow good laboratory practices that include following the manufacturer's instructions on instrument operation and maintenance, performing quality-control procedures, appropriately documenting test data, and storing the monitoring equipment

Patient History Form

Name: _____   Phone: (H) _____   (W) _____

Address: _____   City: _____   State: _____

Date of Birth: _____   Height: _____   Weight: _____   Gender: _____

Marital Status: _____   Pregnancy Status: _____

Medical Alerts (examples; hearing aids, prosthesis, heart valves, eyeglasses, artificial hips): _____

_____

Allergies/reactions:

_____   _____

_____   _____

Smoking History: **Caffeine History:**

_____ Never Smoked   _____ Never Consumed

_____ Packs Per Day for_____Years   _____ Drinks Per Day

_____ Stopped_____ Years Ago   _____ Stopped _____ Years Ago

Alcohol History: **Dietary History:**

_____ Never Consumed   _____ Number of Meals Per Day

_____ Drinks Per Day   _____ Food Restrictions (explain)

_____ Stopped _____ Years Ago   Other: _____

Since health information may change periodically, I will notify the Pharmacist, to the best of my ability, of any new medications (prescription and non-prescription), any changes in directions of medicines, any new allergies, drug reactions or health condition changes. I authorize any releases of information and insurance benefit payments to the above pharmacy on my behalf.

_____   _____

Signature   Date

This information is requested by your Pharmacist as required by state regulations so that he/she can provide appropriate pharmacy services to you. This information will be kept confidential.

I do not wish to complete this form and WILL NOT HOLD THE PHARMACY RESPONSIBLE FOR ADVERSE SIDE EFFECTS I MAY INCUR.

_____   _____

Signature   Date

Figure 30-2. Patient history form.

Care-Rite Pharmacy
Patient Medical History Form

Medical History: Have you or any of your blood relatives had (mark all that apply)

Disease State	Self	Relative
High Blood Pressure		
Asthma		
Cancer		
Depression		
Lung Disease		
Diabetes		
Heart Disease		
Stroke		
Kidney disease		
Mental Illness		
Substance Abuse		
Other		

Medical Problems: Have you experienced or do you have any of the following?

Disease	Yes	No	Disease	Yes	No
Frequent urinary infections			Sores on legs or feet		
Difficulty with urination			Known blood clot problems		
Frequent urination at night			Leg pain or swelling		
Known liver problems			Unusual bleeding or bruising		
Trouble with certain foods			Anemia		
Nausea/Vomiting			Thyroid Problems		
Constipation/Diarrhea			Known hormone problems		
Bloody or black stools			Arthritis or joint problems		
Abdominal pain or cramps			Muscle cramps or weakness		
Frequent heartburn/cramps			Memory problems		
Stomach ulcers			Dizziness		
Shortness of breath			Hearing or visual problems		
Coughing up phlegm or blood			Frequent headaches		
Chest pain or tightness			Rash or hives		
Fainting spells or passing out			Change in appetite/taste		
Thumping or racing heart			Walking or balance problems		

Figure 30-3. Care-Rite Pharmacy patient medical history form.

Care-Rite Pharmacy
Medication History and Medical History

Collected by: _____ Date: _____

Patient Name: _____ Sex _____ Birth Date _____ Ht _____ Wt _____ LBW _____ Race _____

Prescribed Medications (Rx and OTC)					
Name/Strength	Dose/Sig	Duration	Indication	Dr	Comments

Past Medications Not Currently Taking (Rx and OTC)					
Name/Strength	Dose	Duration	Indication	Dr	Reason for Stopping

Figure 30-4. Care-Rite Pharmacy medication history and medical history.

AUTHORIZATION TO RELEASE MEDICAL INFORMATION

Date: _____   Date of Birth: _____

SSN: _____

Patient Name: _____

Address: _____

I, the undersigned, do hereby grant permission for the above named pharmacy to obtain from or
  release to:

_____

(Name of person or institution the information will be coming from)

_____

(Address of person or institution the information will be coming from)

The following information from the patient's clinical record:

_____

_____

_____

I understand that this information will be used for the purpose of:
❏ Providing information to allow pharmaceutical care to be provided to the patient
❏ Providing information to the physician regarding the care provided by the Pharmacist
❏ Supporting the payment of an insurance claim
❏ Other: _____

This authorization will be valid for the period of 12 months unless otherwise specified below.

I understand that I may revoke this consent at any time by sending a written notice to the above named pharmacy. I understand that any release which has been made prior to my revocation which was made in reliance upon this authorization shall not constitute a breach of my rights to confidentiality. I understand that I may review the disclosed information by contacting the above named pharmacy.

_____   _____
Signature of Patient or Patient's Authorized Representative/Date   Relationship of Authorized Representative

_____
Pharmacy Representative/Date

Specific authorization for release of information protected by state or federal law - I specifically authorize by writing my initials beside the category and signing below the release of data and information relating to:

❏ Substance abuse
❏ Mental Health
❏ AIDS/HIV

_____
Signature and date of Patient or Patient's Authorized Representative

❏   Release mailed or information sent _____
                          Signature/Date

Prohibition on Redisclosure
This form does not authorize redisclosure of medical information beyond the limits of this consent. Where information has been disclosed from records protected by federal law for alcohol/drug abuse, by state law for mental health records or HIV/AIDS related records, federal requirements (42 CFR Part 2) and state requirements (Iowa Code chs..228/141) prohibit further disclosure without the specific written consent of the patient, or as otherwise permitted by such law and/or regulation. A general authorization for the release of medical or other information is not sufficient for these purposes. Civil and/or criminal penalties may attach for unauthorized disclosure of alcohol/drug abuse, mental health or HIV/AIDS information.

Figure 30-5. Authorization to release medical information.

and its reagents properly. Approximately 100 tests have been approved for certificate of waiver (Centers for Medicare and Medicaid Services, 2014). If a pharmacy is interested in performing waived tests as part of its services, it must complete the appropriate forms. Instructions for how to obtain a certificate of waiver can be found at https://www.cms.gov/Regulations-and-Guidance/Legislation/CLIA. After receiving a CLIA number, the pharmacy may start providing the monitoring/screening service.

In addition to CLIA, pharmacists must be knowledgeable about the Occupational Safety and Health Act (OSHA) that regulates workplace safety. In particular, pharmacists who perform monitoring/screenings on patient specimens are at risk from exposure to blood-borne pathogens such as hepatitis B, hepatitis C, and HIV. Pharmacies that perform these tests must have a blood-borne pathogen exposure control plan that describes who should be trained about the hazards of blood-borne exposure, precautions that need to be taken to prevent exposure, and what to do should an exposure occur. Employers must also offer hepatitis B vaccination to their employees at risk of exposure. More information regarding OSHA can be found at the OSHA website: www.osha.gov.

Medication Management Protocols/ Collaborative Practice Agreements

The next component of a value-added pharmacist service is the medication management that pharmacists will provide once they have collected the patient's information (medication history, medical conditions, laboratory data, etc.). During this component of the service, pharmacists will assess patients, determine if they are reaching their goals of therapy, identify and resolve any medication therapy problems, and develop a care plan that helps to guide the pharmacists' follow-up and monitoring of the patients. For these services, protocols or collaborative practice agreements (CPAs) should be developed to help guide the pharmacists' therapeutic decisions. The requirements for a CPA or protocol are often spelled out in a state's pharmacy practice act, resulting in variations in requirements to

participate and the types of activities on which prescribers and pharmacists may collaborate. Protocols and CPAs are also used to formalize the relationship between pharmacists providing the service and physicians or other providers that they are working with. They spell out the responsibilities of each party and the acceptance of a mutually agreed-on process or steps for the service.

The components of a CPA typically include the information contained in the policies and procedures manual (discussed below), MTM protocols, and pharmacist/prescriber responsibilities. General decision pathways may also be incorporated into these documents to help guide pharmacists through the patient's clinical situation. The protocols/CPAs may be specific (e.g., adjustment of warfarin given a specific target INR) or more general without specific medication therapy recommendations regarding a patients' therapy. For example, in a comprehensive MTM service, a protocol/CPA may be developed to describe what activities the pharmacists will perform at each patient visit, the documents that will be created from the services provided, and the communication/documentation that the pharmacist provides to the physician or other prescriber to resolve identified medication therapy problems. Most importantly, any protocols, CPAs, and clinical decision pathways used as part of the service must be evidence-based and supported by national guidelines and the primary literature.

Pharmacists should seek input from prescribers regarding patient eligibility criteria and MTM protocols to help aid with their buy-in to the service. Once this information is agreed to, then physicians and pharmacists should sign an agreement form. A copy of the CPA or protocol should be kept at the pharmacy and at the physician practice.

The National Alliance of State Pharmacy Associations (NASPA) reports that pharmacists, depending upon the state in which they practice, may also be able to provide patient care services such as furnishing hormonal contraception, smoking cessation medications, travel medications, or naloxone to patients as well as administering Tuberculin Skin Tests though a state-wide protocol, standing-order, or CPA rather than through an individual one with a physician or other prescriber. In certain states, pharmacists may even be able to furnish (i.e., akin to prescribing by physicians) medications or products for identified medication therapy problems (K. Weaver, personal communication, November 26, 2018). Pharmacists should check with their State Board of Pharmacy to determine if there are any state-wide options available to them as this may be an opportunity to more easily create a value-added service. Additional information and resources about protocols and CPAs can be found at the NASPA website at https://naspa.us/resource/swp.

Patient Education

Patient education is a vital component of each type of value-added pharmacist service. The comprehensiveness of the education differs though, depending on the service being implemented. For example, pharmacists implementing lipid screenings may see patients for a limited time (during the screening) and provide them with baseline education to help them understand their cardiovascular risk factors, fasting lipid panel results, and lifestyle-modification strategies. However, pharmacists providing diabetes educational services may provide more comprehensive education by determining patients' educational needs, providing training for self-monitoring of blood glucose and insulin injection techniques, providing ongoing educational services to help them achieve their self-management goals, and assessing if patients are achieving their therapeutic endpoints. In this situation, there usually will be multiple educational sessions with patients, including comprehensive documentation. In both examples, patient education is a well-defined and integrated component of the service.

Pharmacists can create or identify existing patient educational resources (e.g., patient brochures, educational fliers, and flip charts) to reinforce important educational messages. These resources should be screened for accuracy and completeness. The patient's health literacy should also be assessed to make sure that difficult technical terms are replaced with more patient-friendly language (e.g., instead of blood glucose, use the term blood sugar). Another consideration is that some patients may not be able to read at all and some patients may speak English as a second language. Therefore, it is not appropriate to simply hand out educational materials without first assessing the patient's understanding and reading ability and making appropriate adjustments to educational material. Once educational resources are selected, it should be determined how they will be used as part of the service. Adequate copies should be ordered or created and these should be inventoried periodically to make sure that there are sufficient supplies to meet patients' demands.

■ OUTCOME MEASUREMENTS

Pharmacists should determine what outcomes they will be assessing to evaluate the effectiveness of their services. These measures will help pharmacists decide if certain aspects of the service need reviewing and altering if outcomes are not being achieved. A simple approach that pharmacists can use when developing services is to focus on the clinical (e.g., therapeutic targets and goals), humanistic (e.g., patient satisfaction), and/or economic (e.g., health care spending) outcomes of the service.

Clinical outcomes are the most readily apparent and easiest outcomes to assess. These outcomes include objective parameters such as blood pressure, lipid panels, blood glucose, A1C, and weight. Clinical outcomes usually are part of the patient chart and so are more easily accessed than other forms of data. More complex clinical outcomes may include hospital readmissions, emergency room visits, or physician visits. Humanistic outcomes (e.g., health-related quality of life and patient satisfaction) can be collected from surveys that become part of the service delivery. If such surveys do become a component of the service, then it should be determined how frequently patients should fill out the surveys and how the data will be stored and used. If economic outcomes are of interest, then a data-collection tool could be created that routinely requests these types of data. Pharmacists can partner with payers/insurers to see if claims data can be shared for mutual patients to determine the impact that pharmacists' clinical services have on total health spend or utilize the pharmacy's own PMS for this information. Patient knowledge also may be of interest to pharmacists who are providing comprehensive educational services. For this type of outcome, pre- and post-assessment surveys can be used.

It is important to note that while community pharmacies may use a variety of implementation strategies as the patient care service develops (e.g., educational materials and meetings to help engage patients and other providers, computer prompts to remind the staff of the service, financial incentives for patients and/or the pharmacy staff), their intended effect may be variable with only modest improvement observed. As a result, an attempt to target and personalize these components to their specific practice model, patient care service, and local community needs may be preferred (Watkins et al., 2015).

■ REVISITING THE SCENARIO: CARE-RITE PHARMACY AND SERVICE DEVELOPMENT

Data Collection

After performing a SWOT analysis and some market research, Amber and the other pharmacists at Care-Rite Pharmacy have decided to develop a MTM service. One of Amber's pharmacists volunteered to put together a prototype patient chart that will be used by the pharmacists to document their activities. The patient chart contains several forms, including a patient history form that requests some basic demographic information (see Figure 30-2), medical and medication histories forms (see Figures 30-3 and 30-4), and an authorization to release medical information that is signed and dated by the patient (see Figure 30-5). A communication form was also created to fax clinical information and pharmacists' recommendations to the prescriber (see Figure 30-6). Several copies of each individual form will be kept in separate folders in a file cabinet located in a secure area of the pharmacy. One of the staff will be responsible for

making sure that enough copies are always on hand. Completed charts will be kept in a filing cabinet that is arranged in alphabetical order by patient last name.

Pharmacy-Based Laboratory Testing

The pharmacists at Care-Rite Pharmacy decided to purchase a Cholestech LDX portable analyzer to measure the lipid profiles of their patients. They realized that many of their patients who they were targeting for the MTM service had cardiovascular disease. By purchasing the Cholestech LDX analyzer, they are able to assess lipid profiles and blood glucose levels for those patients who are willing to pay for this additional service. The system was chosen for its ease of use, quick results, and wide range of tests that it offers (e.g., lipid profile, glucose, and alanine aminotransferase [ALT]). The Cholestech LDX lipid profile is also considered a CLIA-waived test. The pharmacists sent in their completed application for a CLIA Certificate of Waiver, paid the biennial fee, and received their CLIA number. All the pharmacists were trained in use of the Cholestech LDX and how to perform quality-control procedures. The pharmacists were taught how to do finger sticks, appropriate procedures on how to minimize exposure to blood-borne pathogens, and proper disposal of used supplies. Each pharmacist was required to perform a test on another pharmacist to demonstrate his or her competency in using this analyzer. Finally, a cardiovascular risk assessment form was created. The results from the test are added to the form and reviewed with the patient during the 5-minute test.

Medication Management Protocols/Collaborative Practice Agreements

Owing to the complexities of the patients that the Care-Rite pharmacists were targeting for their MTM service, they determined that there was not one single type of protocol or CPA that they could use to assess and manage a patient. For patients who did have cardiovascular disease requiring lifestyle modifications and/or lipid-lowering therapy; however, a general CPA using a treatment algorithm from the AHA/ACC/AACVPR/AAPA/ABC/ACPM/ADA/AGS/APhA/ASPC/NLA/PCNA

Care Rite Pharmacy

Physician Communication Form

Physician: _____ Fax: _____ Telephone:_____

☐ Initial   ☐ Follow-up   ☐ New Problem   ☐ Preventative   ☐ Other

Patient Name: _____

Birth date: _____ Gender: _____

Pharmacist: _____   Date: _____

Subjective Findings:

Objective Findings:

Assessment:

Plan:

Recommended Pharmacist Follow-up Assessment: ☐ 4 weeks   ☐ 8 weeks   ☐ 6 months   ☐ Other

Pharmacist Signature: _____

Physician: _____   Date: _____

☐   I agree with the above recommendations:

☐   Proposed modified plan:

Pharmacist Follow-up   ☐ As recommended   ☐ Other: _____

Physician Signature: _____

Figure 30-6. Physician communication form.

Guideline on the Management of Blood Cholesterol was developed (see Figure 30-7). The protocol provided a clinical decision pathway to determine treatment strategies depending on the patients' atherosclerotic cardiovascular disease (ASCVD) risk. To help in their assessment of patients, the pharmacists used the ASCVD risk estimator from the American College of Cardiology and the American Heart Association (http://tools.acc.org/ASCVD-Risk-Estimator). The protocol, although providing direction for pharmacists, did not give specific recommendations regarding which medications to choose, but rather the intensity level of the statin needed to sufficiently lower LDL cholesterol (see Table 30-1). By using this

protocol, the pharmacists still had some discretion regarding medication options based on patient-specific factors.

Patient Education

The pharmacists of Care-Rite Pharmacy also developed patient educational tools to be used during the patient assessment and patient education components of the MTM service. Since many of the targeted patients have other medical conditions, education materials were developed for specific disease states, including hypertension, ischemic heart disease, diabetes, asthma, chronic obstructive pulmonary disease (COPD), and so on. Educational materials were also

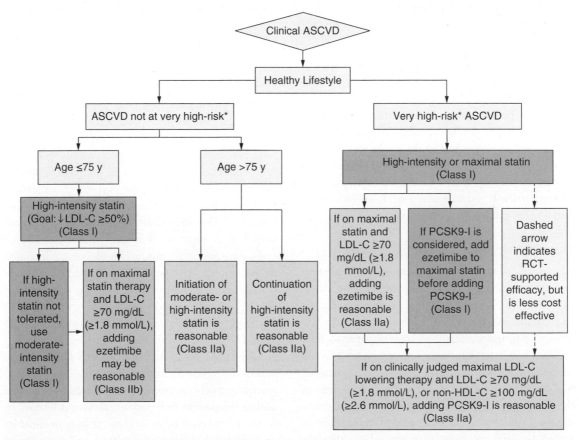

Figure 30-7. AHA/ACC/AACVPR/AAPA/ABC/ACPM/ADA/AGS/APhA/ASPC/NLA/PCNA 2018 Guideline on the Management of Blood Cholesterol.

Table 30-1.	Intensity Level of Statins		
LDL-C Lowering	**High Intensity** ≥50% Atorvastatin 40 mg Atorvastatin 80 mg Rosuvastatin 20 mg Rosuvastatin 40 mg	**Moderate Intensity** 30–49% Atorvastatin 10 mg Atorvastatin 20 mg Rosuvastatin 5 mg Rosuvastatin 10 mg Simvastatin 20–40 mg Pravastatin 40 mg Pravastatin 80 mg Lovastatin 40 mg Lovastatin 80 mg Fluvastatin XL 80 mg Fluvastatin 40 mg BID Pitavastatin 1–4 mg	**Low Intensity** <30% Simvastatin 10 mg Pravastatin 10–20 mg Lovastatin 20 mg Fluvastatin 20–40 mg

Reprinted from Grundy SM, Stone NJ, et al. 2018 AHA/ACC/AACVPR/AAPA/ABC/ACPM/ADA/AGS/APhA/ASPC/NLA/PCNA Guideline on the Management of Blood Cholesterol: A Report of the American College of Cardiology/American Heart Association Task Force on Clinical Practice Guidelines, Journal of the American College of Cardiology, Volume 73, Issue 24, 2019, Pages e285–e350.

developed for certain therapeutic classes of medications. The Care-Rite pharmacists also determined that many patients needed individualized education materials, so they implemented a drug information/educational service as part of the MTM service. With this service, patients can ask questions regarding their medical conditions and/or medication therapies. The pharmacists will research and provide an individualized written response for each patient.

Outcome Measures

The main patient outcome measures of interest to the pharmacists at Care-Rite Pharmacy were determined to be clinical outcomes, patient knowledge, and patient satisfaction. The pharmacists were also interested in monitoring prescriber response to their recommendations. The information collected would be kept in the patient chart. An electronic database was created to store and collate outcome data. One of the pharmacists is responsible for periodically entering data. The information garnered from these efforts would be used to identify areas needing improvement, to market the program to other providers, and to ensure payment from third-party payers.

Policies and Procedures

To help provide an organized approach to service delivery, a policies and procedures manual should be created to guide pharmacy staff during program implementation. The policies and procedures manual is a comprehensive road map to the service, providing information regarding the purpose of the service, patient eligibility, how patients will be evaluated, what happens during each clinic visit, and documentation workflow. A copy of all forms, patient educational tools, patient assessments, and protocols are included in the manual. The policies and procedures manual is a dynamic document that must be updated and changed as new information becomes known or as the program is modified. At a minimum, the manual should be reviewed annually.

The policies and procedures document should be kept at the pharmacy, used as a training tool for pharmacists and other personnel, and referred to as needed during the patient care process. It should be easy to access information in the manual. A table of contents should be included, sections tabbed, and an appendix created containing the forms that will be part of the program. National guidelines and key articles from the primary literature that support the service should also be included in the manual.

Revisiting the Scenario: Policies and Procedures for the Care-Rite Mtm Services

The Care-Rite pharmacists created a comprehensive policies and procedures document for their MTM service. They determined that the purpose of their program is to manage the medication therapy of high-risk patients. The criteria chosen to define the target population for the program were patients who used four or more chronic medications and had at least one chronic medical condition. As part of the service, pharmacists will:

- Assess patients using the PPCP process to identify medication therapy problems.
- Resolve medication therapy problems by working collaboratively with patients and their physicians and other prescribers.
- Provide comprehensive and ongoing education to patients and/or caregivers about common medication therapy problems, therapeutic goals, and the importance of becoming informed consumers of their own health care.

Next, they developed policies for the program. The policies contained information regarding the evaluation of patients. The initial evaluation will occur after the patient is enrolled into the MTM service either by a health plan, other health care provider, pharmacist staff member, or by patient self-referral. A patient chart will be created containing the patient's demographic information and medical and medication histories. The patients will sign an authorization to release medical information form and a contract that outlines the patient's responsibilities in the program. To be eligible for the program, patients must meet the eligibility criteria, be able to attend clinic appointments, and agree to come in for scheduled follow-up visits. Patients must also be willing to be active participants in their own health maintenance by attending all scheduled appointments with the pharmacist.

It was decided that there will be an initial visit and up to three follow-up visits within a 12-month period. All sessions will include a comprehensive review of medications, vital sign assessment and laboratory testing for CLIA-approved tests (as needed), patient education, and prescriber communication.

The initial session will last approximately 60 minutes, and the follow-up visits will last approximately 30 minutes. The follow-up visits will occur at 3 to 6 month intervals depending on the clinical situation. Pharmacists will assess the following information at each visit:

- Patient vital signs
- Dietary considerations
- Patient laboratory values
- Family history
- Medication history
- Vaccination history
- General activity
- Social history, including alcohol use, smoking status, and illicit drug use
- Health problems
- Adherence with current therapy
- Signs and symptoms of intolerance to a medication

Medication and/or dosage change recommendations will be made, if necessary, based on the pharmacists' assessment, and patients will be counseled on these proposed changes. The prescriber communication form will be used to communicate these recommendations, and when approved, the pharmacist will dispense the new medication(s). Where appropriate under the law, pharmacists will also independently furnish medications or products for any medication therapy-related problem. Patient education will be reinforced and documented. Patients will be instructed on when to return to the clinic, and referrals to physicians or other providers will occur as needed. The referrals may be based on patient complications of therapy or condition and need for ancillary services (e.g., eye examination, foot examination, etc.).

The documentation will occur via a patient chart. Subjective patient information and objective physical assessment and laboratory data will be stored in the chart. Assessments of patients during the clinic visit will be documented in pharmacist progress notes contained in the chart. Acceptance of pharmacist recommendations by prescribers will constitute an order change, and this will be documented in the patient record as well. Finally, patient outcomes (i.e., clinical, knowledge, and satisfaction) will be documented in the patient record.

The other components of the policies and procedures manual include the medication management protocol and detailed instructions on use of the Cholestech LDX analyzer. The appendix of the policies and procedure manual contains copies of the forms and patient educational tools used in the program.

■ PHARMACIST TRAINING

As with any successful implementation of a pharmacist service, education and training of pharmacy staff prior to the implementation of the service are essential for success. Pharmacists should achieve proficiency in providing the service before the start date of the service. The time needed to train pharmacy staff depends on the complexity of the service and the experience of the staff. Not only do the pharmacists need to be knowledgeable about the service, but they also must practice and become proficient in the skills required for the service (e.g., giving an influenza vaccine or completing a lipid panel). Therefore, there should be sufficient practice and a demonstration of competence before they work with actual patients. National pharmacy associations such as the American Pharmacists Association (APhA) or the American Society of Health-System Pharmacists (ASHP) offer structured and standardized certificate training and other programs to their members to help improve their knowledge and skill set.

■ REVISITING THE SCENARIO: PHARMACIST TRAINING FOR THE CARE-RITE MTM SERVICES

Care-Rite Pharmacy developed a comprehensive pharmacist educational/training program for its MTM service. This educational program had multiple components and activities that the pharmacists needed to demonstrate knowledge of or proficiency in before they were ready for service implementation. Initially, it was determined that a general knowledge of patient care, types and categories of drug therapy problems, and how to perform a patient assessment should be the foundation for the rest of their education. To help improve pharmacists' knowledge of this topic, the pharmacists were responsible for enrolling in certificate training programs to help them prepare for the service. It was determined that APhA's Delivering MTM Services and Pharmacy-Based Cardiovascular Disease Risk Management certificate training programs would be most appropriate. More information on these certificate programs can be found at https://www.pharmacist.com/apha-advanced-training-programs.

The pharmacists also watched a video provided by Cholestech that demonstrated how to perform a finger stick and a lipid panel. A component of the training included information regarding CLIA, the importance of good technique when performing a test, OSHA requirements, and discussions about the reduction of exposure to blood-borne pathogens. The pharmacists were given adequate time to practice using the Cholestech LDX analyzer. Once the practice was over, pharmacists were assessed on their competency to perform the test. A checklist with required activities that needed to be completed during a lipid panel was used as the grading criterion. Once the pharmacists were capable of providing the test, their proficiency with the Cholestech LDX analyzer was documented and stored in their personnel files.

■ MANAGING THE MARKETING MIX

Once the service is ready for implementation, recruiting patients into the program becomes the next activity. This requires a basic knowledge of marketing principles. Successful implementation of value-added pharmacist services requires that pharmacists manage each of the variables of the marketing mix.

■ REVISITING THE SCENARIO: MARKETING THE CARE-RITE MTM SERVICES

The product that Care-Rite Pharmacy is marketing is its MTM service. As discussed throughout this chapter, much attention has been given to developing each component of the service and planning for its implementation so that it is perceived as a quality service by patients and other providers. Pharmacists updated their knowledge regarding patient care and medication assessments and developed proficiency for testing patients' lipid panels. They hope to be perceived as knowledgeable and competent when providing the service. Finally, protocols, policies and procedures, and standardized forms were all created to ensure consistency in service delivery among the providers.

The next marketing-mix variables that need careful consideration are the place and physical facility. Care-Rite Pharmacy will be providing the MTM service on-site at the pharmacy. Therefore, pharmacy staff needs to consider the characteristics of their space to provide the service. In preparation for this service, Amber did some remodeling of her pharmacy. She created two semi-private patient areas using office partitions. One area was designated as the area where lipid testing would be performed. The Cholestech LDX analyzer and its supplies were stored in this area. Also, CLIA and OSHA guidelines were kept there as well. The second patient care area was created in case there were multiple appointments at the same time. Both areas had a small table, three chairs, and a computer terminal as standard equipment.

Price is the third marketing-mix variable. Amber and the pharmacy staff spent considerable time discussing the price of their service. They estimated the length of the time for each session, estimated the costs to provide the service, researched the price of office visits for other providers, and determined the profit level they needed to help them develop a pricing structure for their service. While no local pharmacies provided an MTM service, Amber decided to price the service to be competitive with similar services offered by physicians. The pricing structure for the service is as follows:

- Initial visit: $120
- Follow-up visits: $60 each
- Fasting lipid panel: $25

The pharmacists will monitor patient responses to these prices and their profitability before making any adjustments. The pharmacy will also determine whether or not any third-party payers will reimburse the pharmacists for providing the service.

The next marketing-mix component is promotion. Care-Rite has selected several promotional strategies to market their services. Amber has also created a marketing budget for the practice. The pharmacists will use press releases in local newspaper to announce the new service. Next, they decided to run an advertisement in the local newspaper twice per month promoting this service. They chose Sundays and Mondays as the days they would place the ads in the newspaper and on their website. Sunday was chosen because of the large readership of the newspaper, and Monday was chosen because the newspaper had a special health section on that day. They also purchased airtime on their local cable TV and radio to promote the service. They selected channels that attracted viewers and listeners whose demographics matched their target markets (e.g., women over age 50). They placed an ad for the program in a local magazine that was directed toward women, and they created a new ad for their pharmacy in the local telephone directory.

One of the pharmacists began to call on prescribers so that he could promote the services face-to-face. The pharmacist met with some of the local pharmaceutical company representatives to find out which prescribers should be identified as key targets for the promotional efforts. Amber contacted her wholesaler to find out if they had any programs that helped to identify key physicians in her area. They also created a physician newsletter entitled, "Progress Notes," that would be sent every other month to key physicians. The format of the newsletter includes sections on new drug updates, clinical pearls, and message updates about Care-Rite Pharmacy. The first newsletter was dedicated to the MTM service.

In-store signage and patient brochures were created to help market the program to current pharmacy patients. Pharmacists were instructed to market the program to patients they encountered who were receiving four or more chronic medications. A mailing list was created from the pharmacy's PMS based upon patients who were taking four or more chronic medications. A brochure describing the program was sent to each of those patients. The pharmacy updated their website and social media accounts to announce that they would be starting to offer MTM services. These announcements were designed in a manner to educate viewers as to what MTM services are and how they and those they care for could benefit. Finally, bag stuffers and monthly patient billing statements included information about the new program.

Process management, the next marketing-mix variable, refers to how Care-Rite Pharmacy incorporated the new MTM service into its existing practice. Workflow decisions were made regarding patient flow during the service. It was decided that the service would be by appointment only to minimize disruption of the other aspects of the practice. Schedules for pharmacists were created so that one pharmacist was responsible for clinic services while another covered the dispensing area.

The last marketing-mix variable that needs addressing is personnel. Care-Rite's pharmacists and staff were trained and assessed to ensure that they had adequate knowledge and skills regarding all aspects of pharmacotherapy management. Pharmacists need to take responsibility for the success or failure of the program. This means that they should continue to identify patient candidates for the lipid management program, use various promotional strategies to increase the community's awareness of the program, and ensure that they have the knowledge and skills to provide quality care to patients. Amber changed the format of her annual evaluations of pharmacists to include reviewing their impact on the MTM service. As a reward for their efforts, she has agreed to cover the costs for attendance at one national pharmacy meeting of their choice each year.

■ ONGOING MONITORING OF VALUE-ADDED PHARMACIST SERVICES

Sustainability can be thought of as another phase in the implementation process in which the service itself has become routine and institutionalized over time and has begun to attain expected service outcomes (Crespo-Gonzalez et al., 2017). Therefore, once the service has been implemented, several strategies should be in place to provide ongoing monitoring to ensure program quality and success. Scheduled staff meetings should occur regularly (e.g., biweekly to monthly), especially early during the implementation phase. These meetings could be used to discuss the number of patients who have enrolled, patient and prescriber acceptance of the service, feedback that has been received, and areas that need improvement. Staff can provide their own feedback on how they perceive the program's effectiveness and how it can be improved. These meetings can be used as educational offerings for the pharmacists to keep their therapeutic knowledge up to date. It is important to keep a time limit on these meetings to minimize disruption of the practice.

Another strategy to ensure program quality is to monitor the outcomes of the service of interest to the practice itself. One of the goals for service implementation is to create new business and generate additional revenue and profit for the pharmacy to ensure the service's success and future sustainability. The goals should be realistic to ensure economic viability for the practice. Both pharmacists and pharmacy staff should be held accountable for their efforts to help the practice reach its goals. Service outcomes that may be of interest to pharmacy staff are number of patients enrolled, revenue generated from the service, number of physician referrals, and profitability of the service (revenues minus expenses). If the service is not profitable, then it needs to be either altered (price increases or improved service delivery) or eliminated.

An additional continuous quality improvement strategy is to request feedback from patients who have completed the program and prescribers who have referred patients to the pharmacy. The feedback could be as simple as a 5-question survey about perceived value of the service or a one-page questionnaire asking open-ended questions to provide more qualitative comments about the service. The information that is gathered from these surveys and/or questionnaires can be used to improve patient and prescriber perception of the service. Furthermore, the request for feedback gives the impression that the practice is proactive toward meeting the needs of patients and other providers.

■ REVISITING THE SCENARIO: CARE-RITE PHARMACY'S CONTINUOUS QUALITY IMPROVEMENT STRATEGIES

Amber decided to schedule pharmacy staff meetings on the second Tuesday and fourth Thursday of each month. Those days were selected to ensure that all staff members had the opportunity to attend at least one meeting monthly. The meetings were scheduled at 11:00 A.M. because this usually is the least busy time for the pharmacy. The time limit for the meetings was 1 hour for pharmacists, and 30 minutes for the staff. The format of the meetings was as follows:

- Review of service outcomes (i.e., patient enrollment, revenue generation, and physician referrals): 5 minutes
- Discussion of program improvements: 15 minutes
- Review of feedback from patients and/or physicians: 5 minutes
- Miscellaneous issues: 5 minutes
- Therapeutic updates (for pharmacists): 30 minutes

Amber is tracking the service outcomes over time and documenting the staff's activities to ensure successful program implementation. She informed the staff about the change in their annual evaluations to include reviews of their impact on the program. She also developed a patient satisfaction survey that

patients are given after completing the program. A one-page prescriber questionnaire has been developed and is sent to prescribers who have had patients enrolled in the service.

Flexibility and Collaborative Working Relationships with Prescribers

Pharmacies have been described as being in one of four states of flexibility leading up to providing value-added patient services. Steady state is the first state of flexibility. In this state, the pharmacy provides traditional dispensing and other services such as home delivery, but has not changed their practice in any meaningful way to incorporate a patient care service. Pharmacies that exhibit steady state flexibility will often over-rely on external factors for their success (e.g., physicians sending prescriptions to the pharmacy, unsolicited patient referrals, etc.). Operational flexibility is the second state of flexibility. In this state, the pharmacy provides traditional products and services quickly and efficiently. Pharmacies that exhibit operational flexibility will extend their product and service offerings to help draw in additional customers, but do not yet provide value-added patient care services. Structural flexibility is the third state of flexibility. In this state, the pharmacy has expanded their offerings by developing one or more patient care services in key areas. Perhaps more importantly, pharmacies in this state have made the necessary internal changes to implement these services. Pharmacies that exhibit structural flexibility, while they may have implemented one or more services, often have not incorporated a business strategy for the longer-term success and sustainability of the service. Strategic flexibility is the fourth and last state of flexibility. In this state, the pharmacy proactively manages all aspects of the pharmacy and patient care services in order to achieve long-term success and sustainability. Pharmacies that exhibit strategic flexibility will utilize technicians and other pharmacy staff to help free the pharmacist from technical/non-discretionary duties in order to provide patient care services. Additionally, pharmacies in this state will focus on integrating its traditional products and services into the overall image of the pharmacy, often by incorporating internal processes to support the model (Feletto et al., 2010).

In concert with preparing the pharmacy to provide value-added patient care services is the need to develop collaborative working relationships (CWRs) with prescribers in order to develop and approve the pharmacy's protocols or CPA for the service. The development of CWRs between providers is a four-stage process, with the final stage usually representing the time when prescribers are most comfortable signing off on a CPA or protocol (McDonough & Doucette, 2001; Snyder et al., 2010).

Although physicians and pharmacists may be aware of one another in the community, they may not be collaborating, and they may communicate only during discrete episodes of care (Stage 0: professional awareness). Pharmacists who are interested in developing services that require the sharing of patient information and regular communication with physicians and other providers will need to increase their interaction with these other providers. For example, the owner of Care-Rite Pharmacy could meet with physicians in her community and discuss her desire to start an MTM service. During these meetings, she could provide the physicians with preliminary protocols and communication forms and request their feedback. By increasing her communication and face-to-face interactions, she moves into the next stage of the CWR (Stage 1: professional recognition).

In the professional recognition stage, physicians are not only aware that a pharmacy exists, but they also recognize that the pharmacy can offer services that go beyond dispensing medications. Since not all pharmacies are providing MTM services, Amber has set herself and her practice apart from other pharmacies in her community. Although attainment of Stage 1 is important early in the working relationship, there is still not much information being shared between providers. Therefore, pharmacists need to develop closer and stronger professional relationships with other providers. In Amber's situation, she requested and received feedback from one physician group regarding her protocol. The physicians in this practice, although initially sceptical of this new service, believed that some of their patients might benefit from the pharmacy's education regarding risk factors, medications, and lifestyle modifications. Therefore, it was agreed that they would refer one or two patients to Care-Rite's Pharmacy's MTM service (Stage 2: exploration and trial).

The exploration and trial stage is one in which physicians are ready to try the service. It is important that pharmacy staff is ready and able to perform at a high level because the physicians will be monitoring their patients' progress closely. Following along with the chapter's scenario, Amber's staff was fully prepared to provide high-quality services for the two patients that were referred to the program. They worked up the patients, performed the medication management services, provided the patient education, and communicated back to the physicians after each patient appointment. After the patients completed several appointments with the pharmacists, Amber met with the physicians to seek their input regarding the program. The feedback was positive, and the physicians' recommendations to improve the program and communication flow were integrated into the program. The physicians agreed to refer more patients to the MTM service (Stage 3: professional relationship expansion).

If physicians and other provides are satisfied with the quality and efficiency of a pharmacy service, they may be willing to increase their referrals. It is during this stage that communication between providers becomes more bilateral, and physicians and pharmacists are exchanging information more equally. Physicians may begin to develop expectations about the pharmacists and the service. It is important during this stage that pharmacists maintain or increase the quality of the service so that physicians see a benefit to referring patients (Stage 4: full CWR).

In the final stage, the CWR, pharmacists have proven their abilities, performed reliably and consistently, and gained the trust of physicians. Because of this trust, physicians may now be willing to sign a CPA or protocol. This is the case with Care-Rite Pharmacy. Amber and her pharmacists consistently helped the physicians' patients reach their goals of therapy. The patients became more compliant with lifestyle changes, and they spoke positively of their experience working with the pharmacists. At Amber's next meeting with the physicians, she discussed developing a CPA, and the physicians agreed to sign it and refer patients regularly to her practice. An example of a CPA for Care-Rite Pharmacy is shown in Figure 30-8.

■ RECEIVING PAYMENT FOR VALUE-ADDED SERVICES

Developing and implementing value-added pharmacist services can be challenging and time consuming. An equally challenging task is determining an adequate payment schedule to ensure that the service is economically viable and sustainable. Factors which must be considered when determining a payment schedule are the costs to provide the service, what competitors may charge for similar services (both other pharmacists and other health care professionals), and what third-party payers may be willing to pay pharmacists for the service.

The first component to pricing value-added services is to determine all the costs associated with providing the service. This can be especially challenging because all costs, fixed and variable, need to be considered. These costs include staff time, rent, overhead costs, equipment and technology, paperwork, and the costs associated with the process of care (e.g., chart generation, faxing, photocopying, etc.). It is important to closely review all aspects of the service to ensure that all costs have been included. The principles used to calculate the cost of dispensing a prescription can also be applied to estimate the costs of providing a value-added pharmacist service.

Once the costs are determined, then prices that will be charged for the services should be set. There are different pricing methodologies that have been used. Fee-for-service pricing is the traditional method of billing for health care. This is when a specific rate

Management by Care-Rite Pharmacists

1. Care-Rite pharmacists will complete lab orders and coordinate the finger stick to fit the patient's schedule.
2. Care-Rite pharmacists will assess the patients fasting lipid panel, atherosclerotic cardiovascular disease risk, medical and medication histories, and dietary and exercise habits.
3. Care-Rite pharmacists will follow the protocol mutually agreed to by the physician to manage the patient's lipid therapy according to the current guidelines on the management of blood cholesterol.
4. Care-Rite pharmacists will communicate their assessment and plan to the physician via fax.
5. The physician will communicate via fax with their response to the pharmacists' recommendations within 24 hours.
6. If the physician agrees to the recommendations, their signature will constitute a new order and the pharmacist will carry out their orders.
7. Care-Rite pharmacists will schedule patients for follow-up visits at the designated times discussed in the policy and procedures manual.
8. Ultimately, the physician is responsible for the care of the patient and at any time can discontinue the patient's involvement in the program.

_____   _____
Physician Signature   Date

_____   _____
Pharmacist Signature   Date

Figure 30-8. Collaborative practice agreement.

is charged for a service based on time or a specific intervention. This method has been criticized because of its inherent incentive to providers to provide more care (e.g., procedures, tests, follow-up appointments), even when it may not be warranted. In addition, since fee-for-service is focused on payment for actions of the provider, it may not fulfill patient needs for optimal health and quality of life. Another pricing method is the resource-based relative-value scale (RBRVS) in which payment is directly related to the level of service provided to the patient. This method uses International Classification of Diseases (ICD)-10 codes that identify the diagnosis of the patient and Current Procedural Terminology (CPT) codes that describe specific types of patient visits. Although CPT codes unique to pharmacists are not typically recognized by Medicare and other payers because pharmacists are not considered providers, pharmacists are recognized as MTM providers for Medicare Part D beneficiaries. Pharmacist-specific CPT codes that are used by some payers for MTM include:

99605: An initial encounter service performed face-to-face with a patient in a time increment of up to 15 minutes.

99606: For use for a subsequent or follow-up encounter with the same patient in a time increment of up to 15 minutes.

99607: An add-on code that may be used to bill for additional increments of 15 minutes of time to either of the above codes.

Other CPT codes that have been used by pharmacists include 99211, which is a code sometimes used by pharmacists who provide services as part of a patient's visit to their physician (commonly referred to as incident to services). Pharmacists may bill for lab tests performed in the pharmacy by using CPT codes 82465 for total cholesterol, 80061 for fasting lipid panel, 85610 for INR testing, 76977T for bone mineral density screening, 83036 for A1c, and G001 for a finger stick. Pharmacists who are trained and qualified to provide diabetes education may use G108 for individual patient training or G109 for group training. Pharmacists billing utilizing these codes normally use the CMS 1500 claim form. This form is used to bill medical services to an insurance program and is universally recognized and accepted for physician billing. Using the CMS 1500 form as the example, a proposed pharmacy superbill was created, using CPT codes recognized by CMS and other payers, to help pharmacists coordinate and bill for their non-dispensing services (Hogue et al., 2009).

CMS created a new CPT code 99490 for non-face-to-face care coordination services provided to Medicare beneficiaries with multiple chronic conditions also called chronic care management (CCM). Although, this is a newer code, CMS has acknowledged the services of pharmacists and they can potentially bill incident to the physician if the patient is referred to them. There are limitations to this code as only once practitioner can use it to bill monthly, but it does give potentially new opportunities for pharmacists and medication management is mentioned as part of the comprehensive care plan.

Finally, another pricing methodology is capitation. This is where a service is provided for a fixed fee, usually per patient per month, that is negotiated with a health plan. This payment methodology may be appealing to the payer because their costs are predetermined at a monthly rate. However, the provider is at risk because they need to keep their costs below the total monthly capitated amount if the services are to be profitable and sustainable.

Each pricing methodology can be used within a pharmacy practice depending on the service and needs and wants of the patient/payer. Regardless of methodology chosen, there are some basic considerations to setting a reasonable fee for a value-added pharmacist service. As discussed above, it is important to determine the cost of doing business, but it is also important to determine a reasonable profit. One general rule that has been used by some pharmacists is that the individual providing the service should generate two to three times their salary in revenue. Pharmacists may charge anywhere from $1.00 to $3.00 per minute per visit for a value-added pharmacy service (Zingone et al., 2007). However, the reality of the marketplace is that pharmacists will not be paid an unlimited amount based on their time spent with the patient, but rather most payers either have a fixed amount or a ceiling on the amount that they will pay. Since this is the most common scenario that pharmacists may face, it is essential that they become efficient with the service so that their costs (in particular their time) do not become excessive as to make the service unprofitable.

There are strategies that can be used to make value-added pharmacist services more profitable. First and foremost, the pharmacist has to be efficient. Therefore, patient interviews should be methodical and time efficient. Pharmacists should be current with their knowledge, be able to identify drug therapy problems from the information they collected from the patient, develop an action plan to resolve the problems, and communicate/document all this to the prescriber and patient. It is essential that pharmacists have a good working knowledge of therapeutics if they are to be successful.

Pharmacists should also empower their technicians (and other pharmacy staff) to provide clinical support for value-added services. Pharmacy technicians can be used to help enroll and schedule patients, prepare patient charts prior to their visit, document communications with other providers, bill patients and payers, and identify additional opportunities for services among other tasks (Hohmeier et al., 2018; Lengel et al., 2018). By utilizing staff in this manner, pharmacists are then freed up to spend their time working directly with patients to identify and resolve drug therapy problems and be able to practice at "the top of their license." In addition, some state boards of pharmacy have approved tech-check-tech (TCT) programs (National Association of Boards of Pharmacy, 2012). TCT programs have been implemented in health-systems and are expanding the community setting, particularly in medically underserved areas (Miller et al., 2018). Pharmacists should check with their state board to find out if TCT is possible in their state.

It is also important to realize that some services are more time intensive than others, making it more difficult to be profitable. For example, a routine immunization service may take a relatively short period of time to perform as the paperwork could be filled out by the patient; however, the pharmacist is usually reimbursed for an administration fee in addition to the vaccine fee. This makes immunizations particularly easy to implement and profitable. Services such as MTM tend to be more time intensive and require a lot of face-to-face time with the initial visit and possibly during subsequent visits. If the pharmacist does a comprehensive workup and has a thorough medical and medication history to draw from, follow-ups can be profitable. Unfortunately, the way the marketplace is paying for MTM services, it may only be once a year that a pharmacist can be reimbursed for a CMR, which makes it more challenging to be profitable. On the other hand, if the patient can be seen two to four times in a year, and the pharmacist reimbursed for follow-up visits, then there is a possibility of long-term service viability.

Pharmacists need to know all their costs, know how much they can be paid, and understand each payer's billing process. Once these factors are known, then pharmacists can determine the amount of time they can spend with a patient to ensure profitability. Costs need to be minimized as much as possible and efficiencies maximized. As more pharmacists begin to provide value-added services in their practice settings, alternative payment models that align with services such as MTM may become the norm over traditional fee-for-service models. These alternative payment models (e.g., fee-for-service tied to quality and value performance, CCM fees, etc.) could help to not only financially support the value-added service but also provide ongoing revenue to the pharmacy (Smith MA, 2017).

■ CONCLUSIONS

Pharmacists have implemented several types of value-added services in their practices from focused interventions to comprehensive case management. Regardless of the service, the care process remains relatively the same and should follow the PPCP. For pharmacists considering implementing new services, the essential components of the service (e.g., data collection, medication management, patient education, etc.) should be identified and a policy and procedure manual created to ensure standardization and consistency of the service. It is important that all pharmacists and pharmacy staff are trained to provide quality and efficient care. Pharmacists also need to manage the marketing mix and develop CWRs with other providers. Pharmacists can ensure their success with program implementation if they follow these steps. By pre-planning and preparing before service initiation, pharmacists can minimize the challenges with any new start-up program and ensure success, profitability, and sustainability over the long term.

■ **QUESTIONS FOR FURTHER DISCUSSION**

1. This chapter emphasized that the process of implementing value-added pharmacist services remains the same regardless of the service. What may be some differences in the forms used, protocols, and CPAs if the service were a diabetes educational program instead of a medication management service?

2. Discuss how the marketing mix may be similar/different from the scenario used in this chapter and a pharmacist implementing a heart failure clinic.

3. Think about a value-added service that you have an interest in implementing. What are the components of the service?

REFERENCES

American Pharmacists Association. Pharmacist Scope of Services. Available at https://www.pharmacist.com/sites/default/files/files/APhA%20-%20PAPCC%20Scope%20of%20Services.pdf. Accessed January 1, 2019.

Atanda A, Shapiro NL, Stubbings J, Groo V. 2017. Implementation of a new clinic-based, pharmacist-managed PCSK9 inhibitor consultation service. *J Manag Care Spec Pharm* 23(9):918–925.

Bishop L, Young S, Twells L, Dillon C, Hawboldt J. 2015. Patients' and physicians' satisfaction with a pharmacist managed anticoagulation program in a family medicine clinic. *BMC Res Notes* 9(8):233.

Biszewski M, Nitzki-George D, Zhou Y. 2015. Comparison of warfarin time in the therapeutic range at a pharmacist-run anticoagulation clinic and the RE-LY trial. *Am J Health Syst Pharm* 72(7):557–562.

Bouwmeester C, Chim C. 2013. Pharmacist-managed oral anticoagulation therapy in the community. *Consult Pharm* 28:280–294.

Caffiero N, Delate T, Ehizuelen MD, Vogel K. 2017. Effectiveness of a clinical pharmacist medication therapy management program in discontinuation of drugs to avoid in the elderly. *J Manag Care Spec Pharm* 23(5):525–531.

Carter BL, Vander Weg MW, Parker CP, Goedken CC, Richardson KK, Rosenthal GE. 2015. Sustained blood pressure control following discontinuation of a pharmacist intervention for veterans. *J Clin Hypertens* 17(9):701–708.

Centers for Medicare and Medicaid Services. 2018. Medicare Part D Medication Therapy Management (MTM) Programs. Available at https://www.cms.gov/Medicare/Prescription-Drug-Coverage/Prescription-DrugCovContra/Downloads/CY2018-MTM-Fact-Sheet.pdf. Accessed December 31, 2018.

Centers for Medicare and Medicaid Services. 2014. How to apply for a CLIA certificate, including international laboratories. Available at https://www.cms.gov/Regulations-and-Guidance/Legislation/CLIA/How_to_Apply_for_a_CLIA_Certificate_International_Laboratories.html. Accessed December 31, 2018.

Crespo-Gonzalez C, Garcia-Cardenas V, Benrimoj SI. 2017. The next phase in professional services research: From implementation to sustainability. *Res Social Adm Pharm* 13:896–901.

Durham MJ, Goad JA, Neinstien LS, Lou MA. 2011. A comparison of pharmacist travel-health specialists' versus primary care providers' recommendations for travel-related medications, vaccination, and patient compliance in a college health setting. *J Travel Med* 18:20–25.

Feletto E, Wilson LK, Roberts AS, Benrimoj SI. 2010. Building capacity to implement cognitive pharmaceutical services: Quantifying the needs of community pharmacies. *Res Social Adm Pharm* 6:163–173.

Feletto E, Wilson LK, Roberts AS, Benrimoj SI. 2010. Flexibility in community pharmacy: A qualitative study of business models and cognitive services. *Pharm World Sci* 32:130–138.

Garcia-Cardenas V, Benrimoj SI, Ocampo CC, Goyenechea E, Martinez-Martinez F, Gastelurrutia MA. 2017. Evaluation of the implementation process and outcomes of a professional pharmacy service in a community pharmacy setting. A case report. *Res Social Adm Pharm* 13:614–627.

Garwood CL, Curtis KD, Belanger GJ, et al. 2014. Preliminary data from a pharmacist-managed anticoagulation clinic embedded in a multidisciplinary patient-centered medical home: A coordinated quality, cost-savings model. *J Am Geriatr Soc* 62(3):536–540.

Halalau A, Shelden D, Keeney S, Hehar J. 2018. PharmMD; an open-label, randomized controlled, phase II study to evaluate the efficacy of a pharmacist-managed diabetes clinic in high-risk diabetes patients study protocol for a randomized controlled trial. *Trials* 19(1):458.

Hale A, Merlo G, Nissen L, Coombes I, Graves N. 2018. Cost-effectiveness analysis of doctor-pharmacist collaborative prescribing for venous thromboembolism in high risk surgical patients. *BMC Health Serv Res* 18(1):749.

Hale GM, Hassan SL, Hummel SL, Lewis C, Ratz D, Brenner M. 2017. Impact of a pharmacist-managed heart failure postdischarge (bridge) clinic for veterans. *Ann Pharmacother* 51(7):555–562.

Hansen F, Teeples H, Csati J, Gillespie SM. 2017. Pharmacy diabetes management of a veteran population in a long-term care setting: A program evaluation. *Consult Pharm* 32(11):676–681.

Hess KM, Dai CW, Garner B, Law AV. 2010. Measuring outcomes of a pharmacist-run travel health clinic located within an independent community pharmacy. *J Am Pharm Assoc* 50:174–180.

Hogue M, McDonough R, Bennett MA, et al. 2009. Development of a medication management superbill for ambulatory care/community pharmacy practice. *J Am Pharm Assoc* 49:232–236.

Hohmeier KC, McDonough SLK, Rein LJ, Gibson ML, Powers MF. 2018. Exploring the expanded role of the pharmacy technician in medication therapy management service implementation in the community pharmacy. *J Am Pharm Assoc* 59:187–194.

Isho NY, Kachlic MD, Marcelo JC, Martin MT. 2017. Pharmacist-initiated hepatitis C virus screening in a community pharmacy to increase awareness and link to care at the medical center. *J Am Pharm Assoc* 57(3S):S259–S264.

Joint Commission of Pharmacy Practitioners. 2014. The Pharmacists Patient Care Process. Available at https://jcpp.net/patient-care-process. Accessed December 31, 2018.

Khazan E, Anastasia E, Hough A, Parra D. 2017. Pharmacist-managed ambulatory blood pressure monitoring service. *Am J Health Syst Pharm* 74(4):190–195.

Klepser DG, Klepser ME, Smith JK, Dering-Anderson AM, Nelson M, Pohren LE. 2018. Utilization of influenza and streptococcal pharyngitis point-of-care testing in the community pharmacy practice setting. *Res Social Adm Pharm* 14(4):356–359.

Klepser DG, Klepser ME, Dering-Anderson AM, Morse JA, Smith JK, Klepser SA. 2016. Community pharmacist-physician collaborative streptococcal pharyngitis management program. *J Am Pharm Assoc* 56(3):323–329.e1.

Kostoff MD, Boros ML, Moorman JM, Frazee LA. 2014. Evaluation of factors associated with achieving glycemic control in a pharmacist-managed diabetes clinic. *Am J Ther* 21(4):234–239.

Lee JC, Horner KE, Krummel ML, McDanel DL. 2018. Clinical and financial outcomes evaluation of multimodal pharmacist warfarin management of a statewide urban and rural population. *J Pharm Pract* 31(2):150–156.

Lengel M, Kuhn CH, Worley M, Wehr AM, McAuley JW. 2018. Pharmacy technician involvement in community pharmacy medication therapy management. *J Am Pharm Assoc* 58:179–185.

MacKeigan LD, Ijaz N, Bojarski EA, Dolovich L. 2017. Implementation of a reimbursed medication review program: Corporate and pharmacy level strategies. *Res Social Adm Pharm* 13:947–958.

Malet-Larrea A, Garcia-Cardenas V, Saez-Benito L, Benrimoj SI, Calvo B, Goyenechea E. 2016. Cost-effectiveness of professional pharmacy services in community pharmacy: A systematic review. *Expert Rev Pharmacoecon Outcomes Res* 16(6);747–758.

Manchikanti Gomez A. 2017. Availability of pharmacist-prescribed contraception in California, 2017. *J Am Med Assoc* 318(22):2253–2254.

Manzoor BS, Cheng WH, Lee JC, Uppuluri EM, Nutescu EA. 2017. Quality of pharmacist-managed anticoagulation therapy in long-term ambulatory settings: A systematic review. *Ann Pharmacother* 51(12):1122–1137.

Maxwell LG, McFarland MS, Baker JW, Cassidy RF. 2016. Evaluation of the impact of a pharmacist-led telehealth clinic on diabetes-related goals of therapy in a veteran population. *Pharmacotherapy* 36(3):348–356.

McDonough RP. 2014. A paradigm change in community pharmacy practice. *Pharmacy Today* 20(12):34.

McDonough RP, Doucette WR. 2001. Developing collaborative working relationships between pharmacists and physicians. *J Am Pharm Assoc* 41:682–692.

Milfred-LaForest SK, Gee JA, Pugacz AM, et al. 2017. Heart failure transitions of care: A pharmacist-led post-discharge pilot experience. *Prog Cardiovasc Dis* 60(2):249–258.

Miller RF, Cesarz J, Rough S. 2018. Evaluation of community pharmacy tech-check-tech as a strategy for practice advancement. *J Am Pharm Assoc* 58:652–658.

Murphy-Menezes M. 2015. Role of the pharmacist in medication therapy management services in patients with osteoporosis. *Clin Ther* 37(7):1573–1586.

National Association of Boards of Pharmacy. 2012. *Survey of pharmacy law*. Mount Prospect, IL: National Association of Boards of Pharmacy.

Okere AN, Renier CM, Tomsche JJ. 2015. Evaluation of the influence of a pharmacist-led patient-centered medication therapy management and reconciliation service in collaboration with emergency department physicians. *J Manag Care Spec Pharm* 21(4):298–306.

Patterson J, Holdford D. 2017. Understanding the dissemination of appointment-based synchronization models using the CFIR framework. *Res Social Adm Pharm* 13:914–921.

Pett RG, Nye S. 2016. Evaluation of a pharmacist-managed asthma clinic in an Indian Health Service clinic. *J Am Pharm Assoc* 56(3):237–241.

Philip A, Green M, Hoffman T, et al. 2015. Expansion of clinical pharmacy through increased use of outpatient pharmacists for anticoagulation services. *Am J Health Syst Pharm* 72(7):568–572.

Pinto SL, Kumar J, Partha G, Bechtol RA. 2014. Pharmacist-provided medication therapy management (MTM) program impacts outcomes for employees with diabetes. *Popul Health Manag* 17(1):21–27.

Puzantian T, Gasper JJ. 2018. Provision of naloxone without a prescription by California pharmacists 2 years after legislation implementation. *J Am Med Assoc* 320(18):1933–1934.

Rodis JL, Sevin A, Awad MH, et al. 2017. Improving chronic disease outcomes through medication therapy management in federally qualified health centers. *J Prim Care Community Health* 8(4):324–331.

Salvig BE, Gulum AH, Walters SA, et al. 2016. Pharmacist screening for risk of osteoporosis in elderly veterans. *Consult Pharm* 31(8):440–449.

Schultz JL, Horner KE, McDanel DL, et al. 2018. Comparing clinical outcomes of a pharmacist-managed diabetes clinic to usual physician-based care. *J Pharm Pract* 31(3):268–271.

Schwartz EJ, Turgeon J, Patel J, et al. 2017. Implementation of a standardized medication therapy management plus approach within primary care. *J Am Board Fam Med* 30(6):701–714.

Sease JM, Franklin MA, Gerrald KR. 2013. Pharmacist management of patients with diabetes mellitus enrolled in a rural free clinic. *Am J Health Syst Pharm* 70:43–47.

Seed SM, Spooner LM, O'Connor K, Abraham GM. 2011. A multidisciplinary approach in travel medicine: The pharmacist perspective. *J Travel Med* 18:352–354.

Shaya FT, Chirikov VV, Rochester C, Zaghab RW, Kucharski KC. 2015. Impact of a comprehensive pharmacist medication-therapy management service. *J Med Econ* 18(10):828–837.

Shoemaker SJ, Curran GM, Swan H, Teeter BS, Thomas J. 2017. Application of the consolidated framework for implementation research to community pharmacy: A framework for implementation research on pharmacy services. *Res Social Adm Pharm* 13:905–913.

Singh LG, Accursi M, Korch Black K. 2015. Implementation and outcomes of a pharmacist-managed clinical video telehealth anticoagulation clinic. *Am J Health Syst Pharm* 72(1):70–73.

Sisson EM, Dixon DL, Kildow DC, et al. 2016. Effectiveness of a pharmacist-physician team-based collaboration to improve long-term blood pressure control at an inner-city safety-net clinic. *Pharmacotherapy* 36(3):342–347.

Smalls TD, Broughton AD, Hylick EV, Woodard TJ. 2015. Providing medication therapy management for smoking cessation patients. *J Pharm Pract* 28(1):21–25.

Smith MA. 2017. Implementing primary care pharmacist services: Go upstream in the world of value-based payment models. *Res Social Adm Pharm* 13:892–895.

Smith MG, Ferreri SP, Brown P, Wines K, Shea CM, Pfeiffenberger TM. 2017. Implementing an integrated care management program in community pharmacies: A focus on medication management services. *J Am Pharm Assoc* 57:229–235.

Smith MC, Boldt AS, Waston CM, Zillich AJ. 2013. Effectiveness of a pharmacy care management program for veterans with dyslipidemia. *Pharmacotherapy* 33:736–743.

Snyder ME, Zillich AJ, Primack BA, et al. 2010. Exploring successful community pharmacist-physician collaborative working relationships using mixed methods. *Res Social Adm Pharm* 6(4):307–323.

Sullivan J, Jett BP, Cradick M, Zuber J. 2016. Effect of clinical pharmacist intervention on hemoglobin A1C reduction in veteran patients with type 2 diabetes in a rural setting. *Ann Pharmacother* 50(12):1023–1027.

Wang Y, Yeo QQ, Ko Y. 2016. Economic evaluations of pharmacist-managed services in people with diabetes mellitus: A systematic review. *Diabet Med* 33(4):421–427.

Watkins K, Wood H, Schneider CR, Clifford R. 2015. Effectiveness of implementation strategies for clinical guidelines to community pharmacy: A systematic review. *Implementation Science* 10:151.

Zingone MM, Malcolm KE, McCormick SW, Bledsoe KR. 2007. Analysis of pharmacist charges for medication therapy management services in an outpatient setting. *Am J Health-Syst Pharm* 64:1827–1831.

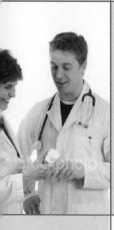

SECTION VII

MANAGEMENT APPLICATIONS IN SPECIFIC PHARMACY PRACTICE SETTINGS

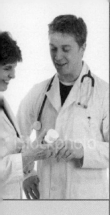

31

ENTREPRENEURSHIP AND INNOVATION

Leticia R. Moczygemba and Shane P. Desselle

About the Authors: Dr. Moczygemba is an associate professor and associate director of the Texas Center for Health Outcomes Research and Education at The University of Texas College of Pharmacy. Her research program focuses on working with communities and health systems to mitigate health disparities by developing patient-centered interventions to optimize medication-related health outcomes. She has worked to advance the health care of homeless individuals, older adults, and those living in rural areas through the development, implementation, and evaluation of care models that integrate pharmacists with health care teams. She teaches in the health care systems course in the PharmD program and is engaged in interprofessional education initiatives with a focus on quality improvement and patient safety.

Dr. Desselle is professor of Social, Behavioral, and Administrative Pharmacy at Touro University California College of Pharmacy. His research program focuses on optimizing roles for pharmacy technicians, development of mentorship programs, and in promoting health organizational cultures and citizenship behaviors in professional settings. He is a Fulbright Specialist Scholar having completed a project to develop a Center of Assessment for the University of Pristina in Kosovo. Dr. Desselle is Founding Editor-in-Chief of the international peer-reviewed journal, Research in Social and Administrative Pharmacy, with graduate students and collaborations worldwide on various projects such as medication safety and medication adherence issues with informal caregivers. Dr. Desselle also is a primary author for the Pharmacy Management Tips of the Week on AccessPharmacy that accompany this textbook.

The authors acknowledge Brad Tice for his contributions to this chapter in the fourth edition of the book.

■ LEARNING OBJECTIVES

After completing this chapter, readers should be able to

1. Define entrepreneurship.
2. Discuss characteristics and types of entrepreneurs.

3. Discuss the applicability of entrepreneurship principles in the profession of pharmacy.

4. Given an "opportunity concept," apply the process of entrepreneurship to evaluate, pursue, execute, and harvest the venture.

■ CHAPTER QUESTIONS

1. What are the three common characteristics of entrepreneurs?

2. What are the four types of entrepreneur personalities, which one do you most identify with, and what leads you to identify yourself with this characterization?

3. Why is the understanding and use of the "process" of entrepreneurship an important component in the establishment of entrepreneurship as its own body of knowledge?

4. Why is it important for an entrepreneur to be able to clearly and succinctly communicate the business concept?

■ SCENARIO

Pharmacist John Adams works for a chain pharmacy in a large city with a population of over 1 million. He has been out of school for several years and has worked as a staff pharmacist and as a pharmacy manager. In the last year, he has begun focusing his work on patients living with diabetes. He has incorporated a comprehensive diabetes program into his practice that includes classes on a general overview of diabetes, blood glucose monitoring, insulin administration, meal planning, and healthy eating for patients with diabetes. He also offers one-on-one counseling sessions, which can be tailored to individuals' needs. During the course of delivering these sessions, John has discovered that a recurring problem patients have is not getting enough blood for a measurement when they stick their fingers to check their blood sugar. Additionally, patients often find this painful and do not do this as often as they should. One day, John develops a device that is very effective at getting the necessary blood sample from patients and is nearly pain-free. The device is very popular among his patients, and he begins to get referrals for the device.

While the high salary as a pharmacist was attractive to John at first, he is now beginning to feel more confident in his abilities and would like a new challenge and opportunity. He wonders if this lancet device he has developed could be worth something. He did not take any business classes in pharmacy school; however, when he was growing up, his father ran the hardware store in their small town, so he has some exposure to running a business. He thought that his father might be interested in helping him out. John has developed a number of relationships with businesspeople through his involvement in the community and thinks that he might solicit their advice, too.

Some questions running through his mind are:

• Should he pursue developing this idea into a product?

• If he does, should he do this through the company that he is currently with or on his own?

• If he chooses to do this on his own, would he need to completely quit what he is currently doing?

• How much money will he need, and is he really ready to commit his money to this?

■ BACKGROUND

Entrepreneurship has been a long-standing component of the profession of pharmacy, going back to the earliest days of the corner drugstore. Coca-Cola (Coca-Cola Company, 2012) and Dr. Pepper (Dr. Pepper Museum, n.d.) are two examples of products that arose from some of the earliest days of that practice setting. In an era when industrialized medicinal products did not exist, pharmacists were in the position of creating new recipes and formulations to meet physicians' orders and treat patients. As the industry evolved and more standardized and large-scale methods were developed, the profession of pharmacy evolved with it. Traditionally, independently owned pharmacies were started and run usually with one pharmacist opening up the store as an owner-operator. Some pharmacists saw opportunities beyond single-store ownership and pursued and developed multiple stores. This led to the development of what is now referred to as *chain store pharmacies*. These pharmacies are often thought of as not being a place for individual pharmacists' entrepreneurship to thrive; however, chain pharmacy itself is an example of entrepreneurship, and as will be discussed later, there are opportunities for entrepreneurship within large companies. Within the hospital setting, clinical pharmacy was developed in the 1960s and eventually made its way into the community pharmacy practice setting. In the last 30 years, the concept of *pharmaceutical care* was established and transitioned into medication therapy management (MTM), which has led to many entrepreneurial activities and endeavors in disease management, immunization delivery, and other new businesses.

Entrepreneurial endeavors within the profession have been undertaken largely without formal training in entrepreneurship within the pharmacy curriculum. However, it is likely that formal training in entrepreneurship can increase the success rate of these entrepreneurial endeavors. This has been recognized in formal pharmacy education and training with the most recent Accreditation Council for Pharmacy Education (ACPE) Standards for Doctor of Pharmacy Programs including Innovation and Entrepreneurship as a key element of Standard 4, Personal and Professional Development [Accreditation Council for Pharmacy Education (ACPE), 2015]. Beyond the content focused on entrepreneurism that is required for all pharmacy students, some schools have begun to offer additional training in entrepreneurism in the form of electives, certificate programs, or tracks (Mattingly et al., 2018; Shealy & McCaslan, 2018). Additionally, many pharmacy programs now offer the opportunity

to earn a Master of Business Administration (MBA) or Master of Science degree in pharmacy administration while concurrently completing the PharmD degree.

■ WHAT IS ENTREPRENEURSHIP?

The word *entrepreneurship* has come to have many definitions. One commonly used definition is "the process by which individuals pursue opportunities without regard to resources they currently control." One of the key aspects of this definition is that entrepreneurship is a process. This has several implications. First of all, a process is something that can be taught and is something that is repeatable. It also implies characteristics of passion and perseverance. In pursuing opportunities without regard to resources currently controlled, the entrepreneur must believe in and have a passion to succeed that will carry them through difficult times and brave the risks that come with entrepreneurial endeavors (Brazeau, 2013). The end goal is achieving the vision. The ACPE Standards indicate that pharmacy graduates must be able to "engage in innovative activities by using creative thinking to envision better ways of accomplishing professional goals" (ACPE, 2015). As health care moves toward value-based payment and more patient-centered care, pharmacists, with their accessibility to the public, are ideally positioned to contribute to the development of novel approaches to patient care that may be viable business opportunities. As mentioned in Chapter 1, effective business management and patient care are not mutually exclusive goals; they often go hand-in-hand. In fact, entrepreneurship has been observed to be one of the main drivers in pharmacy practice change (Doucette et al., 2012; Kaae et al., 2011).

■ WHO IS AN ENTREPRENEUR?

There are often misperceptions about *who* an entrepreneur is (Kuratko & Hodgetts, 2004). Some common stereotypes are that an entrepreneur is someone who is lucky, highly charismatic, greedy, and often that they are just "born" this way. The definition given earlier helps to debunk these misperceptions. The process orientation and ability to teach the process shows that entrepreneurship is not something a person is just born with or that just depends on luck.

Likely because of these misperceptions, the area of identifying who is an entrepreneur is one of the most heavily researched areas in the field. Some of the common characteristics of entrepreneurs include a high level of achievement motivation, an internal locus of control, and a tolerance for ambiguity. Those with an entrepreneurial spirit have been described as unique, creative, risk-taking, adaptive, and savvy in business (Brazeau, 2013; Dawkins, 2007). John Miner, in his book, *The Four Routes to Entrepreneurial Success* (Miner, 1996), identifies four types of entrepreneurs (Table 31-1). Each of these types has unique characteristics that can help to break through the stereotypes. For instance, the "super sales person" is the more charismatic individual typical of some stereotypes, but the other three types help to identify where less charismatic people fit as entrepreneurs. Additionally, "real managers" identifies the type of entrepreneur that can fit into corporate entrepreneurship. One characteristic that is not present in the descriptions of entrepreneurs is "high-risk gamblers." Entrepreneurs have been found to have a tolerance for ambiguity but not to be inclined to take unnecessary risks and even have been found to be more risk averse than people who are not entrepreneurs (Xu & Ruef, 2004).

An important aspect of entrepreneurs to recognize is that they are not necessarily experts in all areas of business (e.g., finance, accounting, marketing, operations, etc.). It is not possible for one person to be an expert in every area necessary to start, grow, and run a business. Entrepreneurs are typically very good at establishing networks of people who can help them in areas that are not their strengths. An example of this is Henry Ford (Hill, 1960). During World War I, a Chicago newspaper called Mr. Ford an "ignorant pacifist." Mr. Ford did not like this and took the paper to court. When Mr. Ford was on the witness stand, the attorney drilled him with questions to test his knowledge with the intent of showing that Mr. Ford was unable to answer the questions and was indeed "ignorant." After getting frustrated with the line of questioning, Mr. Ford stated that if he really wanted to know the answer to any question, he had a row of electronic buttons on his desk. By pushing the right buttons, he could summon to his aid someone who could answer any question he could think to ask, and then asked why he should clutter up his mind with this knowledge. The attorney was stumped, and Mr. Ford showed that he was not an "ignorant" man. Knowing how to get access to the people and information needed and not being afraid to ask are important characteristics of entrepreneurs.

Another important characteristic of entrepreneurs is *passion*. Passion is important because the entrepreneurial road is seldom easy. There are peaks and valleys the entrepreneur must navigate to bring

Table 31-1. Types of Entrepreneurs	
Personal Achievers	**Super Sales People**
Need for feedback	Capacity to understand others, empathize
Need for achievement	Belief that social processes are important
Strong commitment	Good at external relationship building
Internal locus of control	Belief in sales force
Expert Idea Generators	**Real Managers**
Build venture around new products	Desire to take charge, compete, be decisive, stand out
Involved with high-tech companies	Desire to be corporate leader, desire for power
Desire to innovate	Positive attitude toward authority
Intelligence as source of competitive advantage	

the business idea to fruition. There likely will be times of challenges in cash flow, challenges in bringing the product or service to market, and challenges with hiring, to name a few. Passion for the business concept is required to provide the perseverance to make it through challenging times. Investors and key hires also look for this trait. Investors want to know the person they are investing their money with has the fortitude to make it through challenging times. Key hires also want to know they are going to be with someone who is steadfast in their commitment to help pull them through demanding circumstances. Specific to pharmacy, the profession needs passionate professionals who are motivated to improve the profession without regard to resources they feel are under their control (Brazeau, 2013).

■ THE ENTREPRENEURIAL PROCESS

Understanding the process of entrepreneurship and its application is one of the most important aspects of "learning" entrepreneurship because it provides a structured approach that can be repeated, analyzed, and improved upon. For these reasons, integrating the process of entrepreneurship into pharmacy practice is likely to provide a methodology that can increase the success of entrepreneurial activities and ultimately advance the profession.

Identifying an Opportunity

Ideas can come in many different forms and from many different places. Table 31-2 lists categories where ideas can come from. While this table was not created specifically to address pharmacy, there are many opportunities in each category on the list that exist within pharmacy. Once trained to look at life through the lens of an entrepreneur, an individual will likely generate many ideas (e.g., the "expert idea generator" type) and see opportunity where others do not. McGrath and MacMillan (2000), in their book, *The Entrepreneurial Mindset*, indicate that entrepreneurs often generate and maintain an *opportunity*

register. This is an ongoing list of ideas for opportunities. The entrepreneur then chooses which one to pursue and maintains the list to go back to when he or she is ready to move to the next opportunity. It is impossible and imprudent to pursue every idea. The entrepreneur must be disciplined in the selection of opportunities to pursue because resources likely will be limited and pursuit of an opportunity requires focus, perseverance, and dedication.

Developing the Concept

As the opportunities are identified, the next step is to develop the concept further and determine where the best market opportunity lies. Most ideas have multiple ways that they can be implemented. Table 31-2 lists some of the possible options. Determining which idea to pursue and how to execute the opportunity are key decisions for the entrepreneur to make. To guide these decisions, the entrepreneur will often perform a *feasibility analysis* (Berry, 2017).

In the feasibility analysis, extensive research is performed on the product/service, industry, market, organizational feasibility, and financial feasibility of the opportunity. This is an extremely important component of the decision to pursue or not pursue opportunities and speaks to the risk-averse nature of entrepreneurs. Much of this research will go into the building of a business plan (see Chapter 7).

When pursuing opportunities within a corporation, the feasibility analysis can be used to weigh opportunities, or projects, against each other. This type of entrepreneurship is called *corporate entrepreneurship or intrapreneurship* (Bouchard & Fayolle, 2017).

One might argue that pharmacist John in the scenario has demonstrated perhaps as much intrapreneurship as entrepreneurship. The device he developed might be shared with management and corporate executives, and they might be able to help determine how this device might better position the company, or how John might leverage this innovation to the best possible benefit to both him and to patients/society. Intrapreneurship, like entrepreneurship, has its potential pitfalls, including potential envy among coworkers, potential piracy of ideas,

Table 31-2.   The Entrepreneurial Process

Identify an Opportunity	Changing demographics Emergence of new 　market segments Process needs New technologies Incongruities Regulatory change Social change	**Acquire the Necessary Resources**	Debt Equity Leveraging Outsourcing Leasing Contract labor Temporary staff Supplier financing
Develop the Concept	New products New services New processes New markets New organizational 　structure/forms New technologies New sales or distribution 　channels		Joint ventures Partnerships Barter Gifts
		Implement and Manage	Implementation of concept Monitoring of performance Payback of resource 　providers Reinvestment Expansion
Determine the Required Resources	Skilled employees General management 　expertise Marketing and sales 　expertise Technical expertise Financing Distribution channels Sources of supply Production facilities Licenses, patents, and 　legal protection	**Harvest the Venture**	Achievement of perfor- 　mance goals Absorption of new con- 　cept into mainstream 　operations Licensing of rights Family succession Sell venture Go public Shut down the venture

Reproduced with permission from Morris MH, Kuratko DF, Schindehutte M. 2001. Towards integration: Understanding entrepreneurship through frameworks. *International Journal of Entrepreneurship and Innovation* 2(1):35–49.

and having the corporation take ownership of the concept. However, an intrapreneurial spirit is one of the more sought-after qualities in organizations, and often positions someone to ascend high and quickly up the organizational chart. Intrapreneurism is actually a necessary component of an ever-changing health care environment, and from a management perspective, should be encouraged among employees without fear of retaliation or other repercussions. Innovative ideas that propel an organization forward are often born from innovative pursuits of intrapreneurs. From the employee perspective, being an intrapreneur can provide significant advantages to you and the organization while providing a safety net of steady employment. A culture of intrapreneurism allows someone to unlock their creative juices, thus increasing their own work satisfaction, before they might eventually decide to go off into a more "nontraditional" path, such as starting up their own company and becoming more *entrepreneurial*.

Determining the Required Resources

As the definition at the beginning of the chapter describes, entrepreneurs typically will not have all the resources needed to pursue the identified opportunity. This step in the process, which can be a part of the feasibility analysis, will help to identify what resources are needed and help to determine if the entrepreneur can obtain those needed resources. The list in Table 31-2 identifies at least some of the areas to be included in the analysis. This is an especially important point for pharmacists to evaluate because pharmacists have a specialized body of knowledge and are often not diverse in their training in business, management, marketing, finance, and other areas important to pursuing an entrepreneurial venture. It is important to realize that this does not have to be a limiting factor but rather a factor that can and needs to be managed.

This step in the process will also help to identify the extent to which financial resources need to be acquired and at what stage in the business development timeline they are needed. In general, when outside financial resources are needed, they are not all acquired at the same time. To maintain an equity position for those starting the business, rounds of funding are established that enable the business to develop, having enough capital to operate but not an overabundant amount of money as to be wasteful. Acquiring capital from investors results in awarding those investors with shares of the business. The investors who are in at the earliest time are subject to the most risk and, therefore, get more shares for less money. Conversely, this early money is costing the business owner more equity for the dollars he or she is getting. Acquiring the money in stages, often called tranches, lets the owner maintain a larger equity position in the business. It should be noted that one of the biggest mistakes entrepreneurs make is not being willing to give up equity to fund their venture. While it can be important to be smart about how and when to give up equity, one analogy in entrepreneurship compares equity to manure (yes, manure). The more manure is piled up, the more it smells, but the more it is spread around (on a field), the more it helps things to grow.

Acquiring the Necessary Resources

Once the entrepreneurial idea and venture have been well defined and researched through the feasibility analysis, resources are acquired to pursue the idea. Table 31-2 lists some of the ways to acquire resources. Usually, to help get others to invest, the entrepreneur will have to put some of their own money into the development. This is referred to as having "skin in the game," and having skin in the game usually means that this person will care that much more and take responsibility for business outcomes. Entrepreneurs can get very creative in how to get their businesses started. Grants and small business loans are often used, but grants can take longer to acquire than other methods. The benefit of not having to pay back the financing or to give up equity in the company can be very attractive. A lot of "sweat equity" (time put into developing the business without receiving payment for the time put in) is also usually required, and this typically does not translate into actual dollar equity. If the entrepreneur cannot identify enough resources himself or herself, identifying an *angel investor* may be the next best alternative. An angel investor is someone who can supply the money himself or herself. This person also often helps to mentor the entrepreneur to ensure success. Crowdfunding, seeking money from an online community (e.g., Kickstarter or Indiegogo), is a growing method of raising capital for new business ventures (Merriam-Webster, n.d.). However, a recent article found that out of 40 pharmacy- and medication-related products, such as medication adherence tools, on the Kickstarter and Indiegogo platforms, only 13 achieved funding goals (Holmes et al., 2019).

It can also be beneficial to go after *strategic money*. Once someone provides capital to the business, he or she is likely to have a vested interest in seeing the business succeed. Money from individuals who can help make connections to potential customers and other stakeholders can be an important part of getting the business established. Joint ventures and partnering can also help to speed up the adoption process and get buy-in to the business.

Financial resources are not the only types of resources that will need to be acquired. One of the most important resources to be acquired is a management team. Finding key people who can drive the business idea forward is an essential component of the success of the business. As implied earlier in the example of Henry Ford, having a strong network is an extremely powerful characteristic of an entrepreneur. Entrepreneurs who are able to identify key individuals and make connections through the people they know can get the right people to work for them, obtain funding, and get work done (e.g., marketing and business development/client recruitment) without having to spend as much money on regular outsourcing.

Implement and Manage

Implementation and management of the startup, growth, and ongoing operations are also critical components of the entrepreneurial process. The skills needed for this level of the process can be self-taught or learned in more formal training. Entire business degrees focus on the different areas where expertise is needed to run a business. Still, there are many successful business owners who do not have a formal degree in business. Decision-making abilities and experience are two of the most important attributes for success in this process. While some people may seem "born" with natural abilities in these areas, both decision-making ability and experience are often learned over time and can be learned within the profession of pharmacy after licensure. Pharmacists are put in many decision-making positions in professional practice (see Chapter 4). This experience, along with others that can be gained in managing a pharmacy, growing a practice, or working in a business unit of a large company, can serve as training and provide confidence to pharmacists to decide later in their career to pursue an opportunity. These same attributes can be acquired outside the profession and earlier as well.

Any exposure to running a business or decision-making positions can help to provide training that is beneficial to developing entrepreneurial abilities. The 5 + 5 + 5 Bernelli Entrepreneurial Learning (BEL) method (Table 31-3) was developed by a pharmacist, Cynthia Ianerelli, now President of Bernelli University, who left the profession to help with the family business. In pursuing more formal training to run the business, she realized that many of the decisions in business school were easier for her than for others. She attributes this to her growing up around the family business and the subtle experiences she had in doing so. Her research has focused in this area and developed this method of teaching entrepreneurship that focuses on experiential learning, even starting as early as preschool, to train for entrepreneurship. As seen in Table 31-3, the BEL method identifies five stages of development and provides initially for exposure and hands-on experience. Once the individual has this, they can grow into broader experiences. It is not until after the person has these earlier experiences that they build into formal entry and leadership stages. Research and reports (Hnatek, 2015) also support the value of experience in developing entrepreneurial thinking.

For any business, the key to implementing and managing the opportunity will center on cash flow. First, acquiring capital to get the business started, as discussed earlier, and then, once the business is started,

Table 31-3. The 5 + 5 + 5 Bernelli Entrepreneurial Learning Method		
Five Stages of Development	**Five Skills to Teach at Each Stage**	**Five Steps to Transmit the Information Effectively**
Exposure	Self-starting skills	Continuity
Hands-on	People skills	Problem solution
Broadening experience	Marketing skills	Meet and greet
Formal entry	Money skills	Create networks
Leadership	Leadership skills	Recap

balancing the expenditure of money with the need to obtain more to keep the business going. Businesses often fail because they do not have enough cash when they start. It is recommended that a business have enough cash to support it for 3 years when it is started. However, this is often difficult to obtain. Additionally, in opportunities where the business is obtaining funding through investors and venture capital and is giving up equity, it is typical for the business to pursue rounds of funding. This means that funds need to be raised in incremental steps as a product is developed. A funding round often begins with a concept or idea (i.e., pre-seed) and then moves to a seed round where funds are raised to begin product development and market testing. Next, are series rounds (A, B, C, etc.) where each step requires proof of concept and more data to demonstrate success (Cremades, 2018). The reason for this is that investors at the earlier stages get more equity for the money they put in because it is a riskier stage of the business. As the business develops and can demonstrate success, funding is not as risky and requires less equity to be given up.

Balancing the use of cash to operate the business with the need for funds to grow the business is delicate. Typically, the business is using funds to acquire supplies and resources to support the product. If the business is not paid expediently when sales are made, it can be difficult to replenish the supplies and resources for the next round of sales, and this can cause difficulty for the business in paying its bills on time.

Harvest the Venture

Harvesting the venture refers to how the entrepreneur will reap the rewards of the endeavor. There are many ways that an entrepreneur can "exit" the business. Some of these include selling the business to someone else, passing the business on to someone in the family, licensing the rights of the intellectual property developed in the business, going public with the business, or simply shutting the business down. To maximize the reward of the opportunity, it is important to develop the *exit strategy* (see Chapter 7) or list of potential exit strategies early on in the concept-development process. Often, the best time to cash in on a venture will be when the venture is blossoming. This can be a difficult time to part with the venture unless a strategy is mapped out in advance. Having the exit strategy(ies) mapped out in advance can help in business planning and execution and in identifying opportunities to maximize rewards.

■ MENTORSHIP FOR INTRAPRENEURS/ ENTREPRENEURS

Mentorship is important for breaking down barriers to entrepreneurship. As noted above in the BEL method, having the opportunity for exposure to entrepreneurship is an important key to developing entrepreneurial abilities. Having a mentor provides someone with experience to troubleshoot ideas, provide guidance on important decisions, and to shepherd the less experienced entrepreneur through the journey. There will be many decisions to make and many opportunities for missteps that a mentor can help steer through. Junior entrepreneurs and pharmacists should pay close attention to the types of persons they choose to work with early in their careers, as this can shape and mold them for future opportunities and career growth (Eesley & Wang, 2017). Mentorship is critical to success in many ways, and many pharmacy organizations, community programs, and Fortune 500 programs have initiated mentorship programs that focus on the mentee's quality of work life and whole-life actualization, while having the mentor hone the mentee's skills to navigate political minefields and become more savvy about communicating their ideas of innovation for greater acceptance by important stakeholders.

■ APPLICATION WITHIN PHARMACY

Work has been done to understand the characteristics of entrepreneurship within the pharmacy profession. Research examining practice change that considers both the environment and characteristics of individuals and practices related to implementing patient-care services has been performed. This research reinforces the work previously mentioned specific to the field of entrepreneurship. Doucette and Jambulingham (1999) described a PHARMacist Entrepreneurial Orientation (PHARMEO), which is a multidimensional model for measuring market entry to practice change and "refers to the processes, practices, and decision-making activities that lead to market entry." In this model, six dimensions are identified that can indicate a pharmacy's entrepreneurial orientation. These include proactiveness, innovativeness, risk-taking, autonomy, competitive aggressiveness, and work ethic. Four antecedents, or factors leading to a pharmacist's entrepreneurial orientation, were identified. These include dynamism (the degree to which new products and services are being introduced in the market), environmental munificence (the extent to which an organization can support sustained growth), pharmacy type (being an independently owned pharmacy or small chain), and organicity of the pharmacy structure (the degree to which the policies and structure are less rigid), lending to more of an entrepreneurial orientation.

Willink and Isetts (2005) also examined the characteristics of pharmacists implementing advanced patient-care activities. They identified essential components, including profession-related aspects such as philosophy of practice and clinical knowledge, in addition to patient-care processes, and environmental aspects of the practice. A group of highly successful, entrepreneurial pharmacists all reported on being empathic toward patients, giving back to the community, emphasizing relationship building, and fostering climates of innovation in their pharmacies. Holland and Nimmo (1999) identified a "three-ring circus" of required elements to achieve practice change to include having the appropriate practice environment, having appropriate training, and the presence of appropriate motivational strategies.

Mapping the work done in the pharmacy literature to the previously discussed process of entrepreneurship provides insights into pharmacy entrepreneurship. Most of what has been identified focuses on characteristics of identifying new opportunities and developing the concept to be introduced to the market. Referring back to the definition introduced earlier in this chapter of an entrepreneur pursuing opportunities without regard to resources currently controlled, these models mostly suggest that the environment has to be appropriate for entrepreneurship in pharmacy to occur. Opportunities for further inquiry would be to identify if entrepreneurs self-select into environments where they can see their ideas being more easily implemented, or if the environmental factors help to prompt the entrepreneurial spirit.

The opportunities for intrapreneurism and entrepreneurism in pharmacy are virtually endless. Many pharmacists have developed alternative dosage forms or repackaged prefabricated products in a way that meets a consumer demand; developed software that helps clinical pharmacists document and bill for MTM services; used their expertise in compounding to create new products sold at the local or national level; begun to niche into the handling and storage of specialty pharmaceuticals; identified opportunities for particular target markets, such as veterinary pharmacy; and began consulting firms to provide insight on more effective buying of pharmaceutical goods and/or developing care management plans, just to name a few.

■ INTELLECTUAL PROPERTY

One of the most important aspects of entrepreneurship is protecting the idea, referred to as *intellectual property*. Intellectual property can take many forms, from logos, to products, to business processes, as some examples. Types of protection include copyrights, trademarks, and patents (Allen, 2003).

Copyright protection is the easiest and least costly to acquire. However, it also generally provides the least amount of protection. This protection does not protect the ideas, processes, or methods of the intellectual property. It only protects the form, or original work, which is the end result of the ideas, processes, or methods. For example, if your pharmacy developed an innovative diabetes management service called PhA1c, a copyright might protect the name and graphic used in its distribution material or signage, but not the processes used in its execution. Copyrights can be obtained officially through the U.S. Copyright Office for $35 to $85.

Trademarks are used to protect names, brands, logos, and other marketing devices that are distinctive. Trademarks are somewhat more expensive. They generally can be filed for $750. It is possible to conduct a trademark search on the Internet through the U.S. Patent and Trademark Office website (www .uspto.gov). It is also possible to pay attorneys to do the search for you.

Patents offer the highest level of protection. They take the most time and money to acquire, usually taking at least 2 years and several to many thousands of dollars to file. It is generally necessary to hire intellectual property attorneys to assist with the filing and defense of the patent. Patents protect the idea, method, and design of products and businesses. (For a full description of patents and the filing process, go to www.uspto.gov.) It is important to research the timelines for filing—generally within 1 year of use—and to decide if you need only a patent in the United States or a patent filed in other countries as well (and there are specific timelines on when this needs to be done).

■ INCUBATORS

A useful concept for entrepreneurs that may be especially applicable to pharmacist entrepreneurs is the *incubator*. This term describes an entity that exists to help get new businesses started. As stated earlier, entrepreneurs cannot be experts in every area required of entrepreneurship. Incubators bring all or many of the necessary areas together (e.g., accounting, business plan development, legal, capital acquisition, etc.) to help entrepreneurs bring their ideas to market. As discussed previously, investment early in the idea development process costs the most. Incubators usually take

significant equity of the business to get started. The entrepreneur must assess how much is really needed and how much the incubator is really going to contribute before signing on. Incubators are often found connected to academic institutions, especially those with entrepreneurship programs. They can also exist within an area's business community and can serve as a method for local investors to formalize or outsource their investment process. For example, a person wishing to invest in new opportunities can use the incubator to screen opportunities and provide structure to the opportunities to lessen the risk of the investment. Locating an incubator can also be done by searching on the Internet.

■ TIMING AND COMPETITION

One of the most important aspects of bringing an idea to market is timing. No matter how good the idea is, if the market is not prepared for it, it will not reach its full potential. First-movers, the first person to bring a concept to market, can have what is called *first-mover advantage,* allowing them to gain the rewards of early entry into a market. At other times, the second person into the market can gain the advantage because the first-mover has had to go to all the effort to train and educate the market about the concept and also work out "kinks" that inevitably arise in the early stages. Deciding exactly when an opportunity is ripe is one of the most important decisions an entrepreneur must make. Research, focus groups, forecasting, and competitive analysis can go a long way toward identifying when the timing is right. However, many companies spend enormous resources to identify when the timing is right and exactly what the product should be only to see their product fall flat or short of expectations. As described by Zaltman (2002), people cannot tell in advance of a product offering what their true reaction to the product will be. Zaltman's research showed that 95% of people's thinking occurs in their subconscious mind, so their true reaction can be seen only with exposure to the product and all the parallel decisions accompanying it. For example, many patients and even health care professionals have the traditional image of a pharmacist behind the counter dispensing medications in mind when they think about pharmacist services. Therefore, regardless of how good a disease management or MTM service may be in addressing a particular need, it may be difficult for a patient or physician to move beyond the traditional pharmacist services to more direct patient-care activities until they actually participate in it. One often counterintuitive factor that can help to identify a product's success is whether or not a similar product offering exists. Competition, in general, can be a positive sign that the market is ready for the concept and can serve to bring down the costs of bringing the product to market. The competition's presence and marketing can serve to validate the need for the product, increase awareness of the need for the product, and help tear down walls of resistance to the new product.

■ SELLING THE CONCEPT

To sell the opportunity effectively, the entrepreneur must be able to quickly communicate the value proposition associated with the product, service, or business. In entrepreneurship circles, this is referred to as the *elevator pitch*. The elevator pitch refers to the ability to pitch the concept to a potential investor in the amount of time it takes to get on an elevator and then get off. The idea behind this is for the entrepreneur to be ready to pitch the concept clearly and concisely at any time. This skill actually fits in well for pharmacists because it is similar to how pharmacists often must counsel patients and make drug therapy recommendations to prescribers. One method of getting additional training in doing this effectively is explained in the book, *How to Get Your Point Across in 30 Seconds or Less* (Frank, 1986). Three key questions that may be helpful to address are the following:

1. What is the benefit?
2. How is the opportunity new and different?
3. What is the reason to believe?

A common mistake made by inexperienced entrepreneurs and pharmacists in "selling" their product or service is to focus on its *features*. They describe these features or aspects of the product or service but do not relate to the customer or how the features provide benefit or value. Benefits relate directly to how the product or service will make buyers' lives better (see Chapter 5). Investors are looking for an obvious value proposition and preferably one that is recurring or leads to multiple selling opportunities.

■ ADDITIONAL RESOURCES

There are many resources for entrepreneurs. Searching the Internet can easily identify a number of resources.

Networking in the community with business owners can also identify mentors who can be a vital resource as well. Some recommended resources include the following:

- *The DELTA Rx* Institute (http://www.drake.edu/deltarx/). The DELTA Rx Institute is based at the Drake University College of Pharmacy & Health Sciences. DELTA stands for "Drake Entrepreneurial Leadership Tools for Advancement." The website provides resources on entrepreneurship, profiles pharmacy entrepreneurial leaders, and provides tools and courses that can help to get pharmacists started on the path to entrepreneurship.
- *The Stanford Technology Ventures Program* (http://stvp.stanford.edu/). This is a website through the Stanford University School of Engineering that is "dedicated to accelerating high-technology entrepreneurship research and education to engineers and scientists." The website has many resources and podcasts from entrepreneurs, including many from successful entrepreneurs in Silicon Valley that can provide great insights.
- *The Entrepreneurship and Emerging Enterprises Program at Syracuse University* (http://http://whitman.syr.edu/programs-and-academics/academics/eee/index.aspx). This website also has many resources that can assist in growing entrepreneurial capabilities and links to other sites targeted to entrepreneurship.

■ REVISITING THE SCENARIO

John Adams decides that the time is right to pursue this opportunity. He decides that to really give this opportunity the chance for success that it needs, he will focus his attention by fully researching the opportunity, identifying a mentor, and setting everything in place. Once that is accomplished (under a planned timeline), he will turn to this as a full-time opportunity, leaving his current employment. John is wisely pursuing his intrapreneurial goal and keeping the shelter of his current employment until a greater amount of time must be dedicated to his venture and becoming an entrepreneur. John is also willing to take some risks, given that in the event his venture does not reach the goals he had hoped for, he can always return to his position as a full-time staff pharmacist, with some valuable experience under his belt that can propel him forward in any setting/organization for which he might come back to work.

■ CONCLUSION

Entrepreneurship has strong roots in the pharmacy profession. The specialized knowledge, skills, and practice of pharmacy provide a solid foundation for identifying and pursuing entrepreneurial endeavors. While stereotypes often portray entrepreneurs as charismatic, high-risk gamblers, evidence suggests that people can be successful entrepreneurs with a variety of personal characteristics. Passion for the profession and business concept are important aspects of building the opportunity. Relationship building, empathy, understanding internal/external forces, and performing hard work and due diligence are also paramount. Importantly, identifying that entrepreneurship is a formal process that can be repeated and taught shows that it is not simply a trait individuals are "born with." Applying the described process of entrepreneurship can provide a framework for success and for quality improvement through refinement of the process. Financing the entrepreneurial endeavor requires a skillful balance of managing cash flow and equity to bring the opportunity to market successfully.

Throughout pharmacy's history, entrepreneurship has been a strong component of the profession that has helped it to adapt and strengthen itself over the years. With the explosive growth of entrepreneurship education and the rapid change in today's world, there is no doubt that it will be just as vital in moving the profession forward. Pharmacists should look for a mentor early in their career and choose who they work with carefully, as this can both shape them and provide opportunities to build their career.

■ QUESTIONS FOR FURTHER DISCUSSION

1. Describe the importance of networking for entrepreneurs, and identify methods of networking in the profession, community, and business world.
2. What, in your opinion, is the most difficult step in the process of entrepreneurship? Describe and explain why.
3. Describe an approach to financing an entrepreneurial venture. Include a discussion of the pros and cons of debt acquisition, using personal and "friends and family" funds, and venture capital.
4. After identifying an opportunity, develop a 30-second elevator pitch that clearly communicates the value of the concept.
5. Which category from Table 31-1 do you most readily identify with, and how would you see this leading toward your own individual entrepreneurship?

REFERENCES

Accreditation Council for Pharmacy Education. 2015. Accreditation Standards and Key Elements for the Professional Program in Pharmacy Leading to the Doctor of Pharmacy Degree. Available at https://www.acpe-accredit.org/pdf/Standards2016FINAL.pdf. Accessed May 2, 2019.

Allen KR. 2003. *Launching New Ventures: An Entrepreneurial Approach*, 3rd ed. Boston, MA: Houghton Mifflin.

Berry GR. 2017. Feasibility analysis for the new venture nonprofit enterprise. *New Engl J Entrepreneurship* 20:52–70.

Bouchard V, Fayolle A. 2017. *Corporate Entrepreneurship*. London: Taylor & Francis Group; Available at https://doi.org/10.4324/9781315747989. Accessed July 21, 2019.

Brazeau G. 2013. Entrepreuneurial spirit in pharmacy. *Am J Pharm Educ* 77(5):Article 88.

Coca-Cola Company. 2012. *The Chronicle of Coca-Cola: Birth of a Refreshing Idea*. Available at https://www.coca-colacompany.com/stories/the-chronicle-of-coca-cola-birth-of-a-refreshing-idea. Accessed April 14, 2019.

Cremades A. 2018. How funding rounds work for startups. Forbes. Available at https://www.forbes.com/sites/alejandrocremades/2018/12/26/how-funding-rounds-work-for-startups/#699a50947386. Accessed May 5, 2019.

Dawkins J. 2007. How to define entrepreneurial spirit. Available at https://ezinearticles.com/?How-To-Define-Entrepreneurial-Spirit&id=738736. Accessed May 3, 2019.

Doucette WR, Jambulingham T. 1999. Pharmacy entrepreneurial orientation: antecedents and its effect on the provision of innovative pharmacy's services. *J Soc Adm Pharm* 16:26–37.

Doucette WR, Nevins JC, Gaither C, et al. 2012. Organizational factors influencing practice change. *Res Social Adm Pharm.* 8:274–284.

Dr. Pepper Museum. n.d. *History of Dr. Pepper*. Available at https://drpeppermuseum.com/history/. Accessed April 14, 2019.

Eesley C, Wang Y. 2017. Social influence in choice: Evidence from a randomized field experiment on entrepreneurial mentorship. *Res Policy.* 46:636–650.

Frank MO. 1986. *How to Get Your Point Across in 30 Seconds or Less*. New York, NY: Pocket Books.

Hill N. 1960. *Think and Grow Rich*. New York, NY: Ballantine Publishing Group.

Hnatek M. 2015. Entrepreneurial thinking as a key factor of family business success. *Procedia—Social Behav Sciences.* 181:342–348.

Holland RW, Nimmo CM. 1999. Transitions in pharmacy practice, part 3: effecting change—the three-ring circus. *Am J Health Sys Pharm* 56:2235–2241.

Holmes TM, Aungst TD, Smith CC, Metcalf MD. 2019. Crowdfunding pharmacy- and medication-related products: How successful is it? *J Am Pharm Assoc* 59(2):S57–S62.

Kuratko DF, Hodgetts RM. 2004. *Entrepreneurship: Theory, Process, Practice*, 6th ed. Mason, OH: Thomson Learning.

Kaae S, Sondergaard B, Haugbolle LS, Traulsen JM. 2011. The relationship between leadership style and provision of the first Danish publicly reimbursed cognitive pharmaceutical service—A qualitative multicase study. *Res Social Adm Pharm* 7:113–121.

Mattingly TJ, Mullins CD, Melendez DR, Boyden K, Edington ND. 2018. Entrepreneurship in pharmacy practice and education: A systematic review. *Am J Pharm Educ.* 2019;83(3):7233.

McGrath RG, MacMillan I. 2000. *The Entrepreneurial Mind-set*. Boston, MO: Harvard Business School Press.

Merriam-Webster. n.d., Crowdfunding. Available at https://www.merriam-webster.com/dictionary/crowdfunding. Accessed May 4, 2019.

Miner JB. 1996. *The Four Routes to Entrepreneurial Success*. San Francisco: Berrett-Koehler.

Morris MH, Kuratko DF, Schindehutte M. 2001. Towards integration: Understanding entrepreneurship through frameworks. *International Journal of Entrepreneurship and Innovation.* 2(1):35–49.

Shealy KM, McCaslan M. 2018. Incorporating an entrepreneurial certificate into the pharmacy curriculum. *Am J Pharm Educ* 82(8):Article 6701.

Willink DP, Isetts BJ. 2005. Becoming 'indispensable': Developing innovative community pharmacy practices. *J Am Pharm Assoc* 45:376–386.

Xu H, Ruef M. 2004. The myth of the risk-tolerant entrepreneur. *Strategic Organization.* 2:331–355.

Zaltman G. 2002. *How Customers Think: Essential Insights into the Mind of the Market*. Boston, MO: Harvard Business School Press.

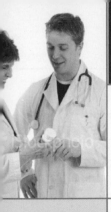

32

APPLICATIONS IN INDEPENDENT COMMUNITY PHARMACY

Thad Schumacher

About the Author: Dr. Schumacher is a pharmacist and owner of Fitchburg Family Pharmacy located in Fitchburg, Wisconsin. He received his Doctor of Pharmacy (PharmD) degree from Creighton University. He began his career working in community settings throughout four different states. For the past decade he has lived in Wisconsin and practiced in independent pharmacy settings, and now owns his own pharmacy. Dr. Schumacher has served for 6 years as the Chair of the Pharmacy Examining Board for the State of Wisconsin. He was awarded the Bowl of Hygiea in 2017 for his community service, including serving on the Board of Directors for the Boys and Girls Clubs of Dane County, and hosting a cycling group that raises money for charities. He is a member of the Pharmacy Society of Wisconsin and his pharmacy is accredited by the Wisconsin Pharmacy Quality Collaborative (WPQC) and the Community Pharmacy Enhanced Services Network—Wisconsin affiliate (CPESN-WI). He has a love for cycling and it has led him to delivery prescriptions via bicycle. This has branded him the cycling pharmacist, by his friends, patients, and colleagues.

■ LEARNING OBJECTIVES

After completing this chapter, readers should be able to

1. Identify evolutionary changes leading to current independent community pharmacy practice.
2. Identify the characteristics of entrepreneurship and describe the opportunities that exist within independent community pharmacy practice.
3. Compare and contrast starting up a new independent community pharmacy versus purchasing an established pharmacy.
4. List and describe the steps necessary for starting an independent community pharmacy.
5. Identify methods of purchasing an established pharmacy.
6. List and discuss various issues facing independent community pharmacy practice.

■ SCENARIO 1

As Sue Franklin was completing her last Advanced Pharmacy Practice Experience (APPE) rotation during her final year of pharmacy school, she began to think about where she wanted to work after graduation. As part of her required and elective APPE rotations, Sue gained experience in a number of practice settings. She really enjoyed the critical care rotation at University Medical Center. However, she knew that a residency probably would be required to land a clinical position there. Sue had completed a rotation with the Indian Health Service and had thoroughly enjoyed her experience caring for a Native American population in New Mexico. She also had gained experience working at a chain pharmacy and then a supermarket pharmacy during holidays and vacations throughout pharmacy school. "What am I going to do?" thought Sue. She had so many great experiences and in some ways too many employment options. She had already received job offers from the chain and supermarket pharmacies, each paying a very good salary. She also received an offer from Professional Pharmacy, a local independent community pharmacy in which she completed two rotations, community and administrative. Sue was surprised by the offer, because she had spent only 10 weeks in the pharmacy. Prior to her rotations, Sue had never considered working in an independent community pharmacy. One of her favorite APPE projects was the development of an immunization program for Professional Pharmacy. Sue loved the ability to create new programs and offer specialty services to patients in need. Darrel Burke, the owner of Professional Pharmacy, was very enthusiastic about the ideas Sue had shared with him regarding the development of other patient care specialty services. As Sue thought back about her experience, she was also impressed with Mr. Burke's management style. She remembered that the workflow was very organized and that the employees enjoyed taking care of patients and took pride in their jobs. Mr. Burke took great care of the entire staff. He was the only manager that Sue had worked with to hold brief staff meetings every couple of weeks to find out how things were going and to take action on issues raised during the meetings. Sue was also amazed at how much the patients cared for Mr. Burke and the staff, and vice versa. She could not remember receiving cookies from a patient whom she had helped on any other rotation. While the salary offered by Professional Pharmacy was slightly lower than those offered by other prospective employers, Sue realized how unique Professional Pharmacy is and began to see the value of working in a place that accepted and even encouraged its employees to seek creative strategies for enhancing customer service.

■ CHAPTER QUESTIONS

1. What is independent community pharmacy—from a practitioner's perspective and from a patient's perspective?
2. What are the benefits that are unique to independent pharmacy practice? What are the unique benefits of owning a pharmacy practice?
3. How can an independent community pharmacy owner of 15 years keep the entrepreneurial spirit alive in the pharmacy?
4. What are the advantages and disadvantages of starting a new pharmacy versus purchasing an existing one?

■ INTRODUCTION

As stated in Chapter 1, "The managerial sciences of accounting, finance, economics, human resources management, marketing, and operations management are indispensable tools for today's practitioner." Each of the tools referred to is critical to all pharmacy practitioners in varying degrees. This statement could not be more accurate when discussing independent community pharmacists. An independent community pharmacist works in an environment that demands a unique level of understanding of the proper use of each tool in providing patient care, in addition to running a respected business in a community. While a discussion of managing an independent community pharmacy practice could incorporate most of the concepts from this book, the goal here is to provide an overview of independent pharmacy and discuss the application of management tools critical to this environment.

WHAT IS INDEPENDENT COMMUNITY PHARMACY?

For almost as long as medications have been used to treat disease, those with expertise in preparing and using these medications have sought ways to sell their products. The first "pharmacies" were operated in the Middle East as early as the 8th century (Higby, 2003). Shops selling "materia medica" operated in Europe through the Middle Ages and Renaissance, almost always being owned and operated by the person whose expertise was in obtaining and preparing these products in a manner where they could be used, the precursor to today's pharmacist. In the United States, long before there were chain pharmacies, discount stores, or grocery stores with pharmacy departments, there were privately owned pharmacies, operated by a pharmacist, that not only filled prescriptions but also took care of patients and their families. This type of pharmacy has been described in many ways: a "mom and pop" shop, a drugstore, a chemist's shop, an apothecary, a prescription shop, or hundreds of brand names ranging from Abe's Drug to Zimmerman's Pharmacy. Today, we have come to describe this type of practice as an independent community pharmacy. While the latter half of the 20th century saw rapid growth in other types of pharmacies, there are still thousands of independent community pharmacies throughout the United States, with new pharmacies opening to develop new ways to serve patients.

A stereotypic description of an independent community pharmacy might include the existence of a small business with a prescription counter operated by the pharmacist/owner and located in the back of the store. The front of the store might contain a wide variety of offerings that could range from a small section of over-the-counter (OTC) medications, vitamins, and other health-related products to an expanded OTC area with additional offerings, such as greeting cards, candy, gifts, and health and beauty products. In general, one might find a relatively small but very helpful and friendly staff that know their customers by name and provide great service.

Historical Perspective

Pharmacy practice in the United States was founded on the shoulders of independent community pharmacy owners. Beginning with the earliest apothecary shops in colonial America, independent practices manufactured most medications that were provided to customers. In the early 1800s, apothecaries and drugstores became more prominent in cities and towns (Higby, 2003). Reasons surrounding this growth include the evolution of medicine and pharmacy into separate professions and the growing need for medications as the country and its population continued to expand. The drugstore became recognized as the place to purchase medicine. These practices diversified and began to offer additional products and services to their respective communities.

In the late 1800s, the pharmacy began to stock and sell more products that were being created by pharmaceutical manufacturers. With this change, pharmacies needed less space for compounding products. The prescription department moved to the back of the store, with the front opening up for salable goods and creation of the soda fountain. Since the pharmacist had a background in chemistry and experience with mixing and flavoring, the soda fountain was a perfect fit for the pharmacy. While the soda fountain attracted customers, events such as the prohibition movement greatly increased its popularity. A unique combination of prescription department, general store, and soda fountain established the drugstore as a cultural icon (Higby, 2003).

Independent community pharmacy practice evolved with the rest of the profession through the education reform of the early 1900s, increased competition from the development of chain and mass-merchandiser pharmacies, and the decreased need for practitioners compounding coinciding with the increased availability of mass-produced medications.

The 1950s ushered in the "count and pour" era of pharmacy practice: a momentous surge in antibiotics and other medications coming to market, increases in the number of prescriptions dispensed, limited roles of pharmacists in patient care, and boom times for pharmacy businesses (Higby, 2003).

The 1960s witnessed a new era that dramatically changed the face of independent community pharmacy practice. Legislation created the Medicare and Medicaid programs and, with that, the birth of public pharmaceutical benefit programs (Williams, 1998). These events drastically changed the economics of independent pharmacy practice by introducing greater influence from government and private payers. Also during this time, the profession was beginning to embrace the concept of clinical pharmacy. Eugene White, an independent pharmacist, was advocating patient-oriented professional pharmacy practices, by example, with the development of a patient drug profile and an office-based practice (Ukens, 1994). The public, which had been viewed only as customers, was now recognized as patients (Higby, 2003).

Through the 1980s, community pharmacists began carving out their own niche in health care as drug information experts by expanding their scope of practice into patient care areas such as consulting, home health care, and long-term care. Independent community pharmacists began to accept this expanded role and fostered the pharmacist–patient relationship by continuing to provide high-quality, personalized service to all patients.

The dawn of clinical pharmacy provided the groundwork for the shift to the pharmaceutical care era. With significant changes in the areas of law (e.g., the Omnibus Budget Reconciliation Act of 1990 and the Health Insurance Portability and Accountability Act of 1996), health care reimbursement (e.g., the rise of managed care), and scope of practice (e.g., disease-state management programs, wellness programs, and collaborative practice agreements between pharmacists and physicians), independent practice has had to diversify and change to meet the needs of the various players in this environment. In addition, the independent community pharmacist has had to become a better manager in order to survive in such a competitive marketplace.

The 2000s brought major changes to health care and pharmacy in particular. In 2003, the Medicare Prescription Drug, Improvement and Modernization Act was passed that provided prescription drug coverage through Medicare Part D. With its implementation at the beginning of 2006, the nation's community pharmacies bore the burden of this new program by experiencing increased prescription volume and major delays in reimbursements (Kostick, 2006). In 2010, health care reform took center stage as a major national issue, providing a venue for President Obama to sign into law the first health care reform legislation in decades (American Pharmacists Association [APhA], 2019a). The two laws that make up the Affordable Care Act—the Patient Protection and Affordable Care Act and Health Care and Education Reconciliation Act of 2010—include pharmacy-related provisions regarding medication therapy management (MTM), recognizing the pharmacist's role in medication use, and improving patient access to medications and service (APhA, 2019a). Independent community pharmacists continue to be very active participants in these areas to improve the care of their patients (Hoey, 2011).

The most recent advocacy efforts of the profession have been focused on provider status: pharmacists being recognized as health care providers by federal law (APhA, 2019b). Pharmacists and pharmacists' patient care services are not included in key sections of the Social Security Act, particularly in Medicare Part B (APhA, 2013). By enabling Medicare Part B beneficiaries access to pharmacist-provided services, this legislation would finally recognize pharmacists as providers (NCPA, 2015). The profession has come together in a united front to support this critical pharmacy issue, demonstrated by the formation of the Patient Access to Pharmacists' Care Coalition (PAPCC). The PAPCC is a coalition comprised of organizations representing patients, pharmacists, and pharmacies (PAPCC, 2019). While as of 2019 pharmacists have yet to garner provider status at the federal level, they have been successful in gaining this status in a number of states, including California (Gabay, 2014) and Ohio (Balick, 2019). This has enabled pharmacists, and in particular pharmacists at independent pharmacies, the ability to implement and bill insurance companies for a variety of clinical services related to medications and their use.

Today's Independent Community Pharmacy

According to various agencies, a strict definition of *independent community pharmacy* means that no more than three pharmacies are owned and operated by one person (Smith, 1986). Even with this established definition, other organizations have expanded the number of pharmacies that can be owned to as many as 11. A better sense of what independent community pharmacy is can be gained from the views of various stakeholders.

What do patients think? Beginning in 1976, Gallup has conducted a survey of Americans to rate the honesty and ethical standards of a variety of professions (Brenan, 2018). Since 1981, pharmacists have consistently been rated one of the most trusted and respected professions identified in the Gallup survey. In recent years, *Consumer Reports* has been conducting a survey of their readers and asking them to rate drugstores. In 2018, a Consumer Reports study of over 78,000 respondents found that independent pharmacies consistently rated better than chain pharmacies on measures such as pharmacists' knowledge and expertise, accuracy, courtesy, helpfulness, and even the speed of filling prescriptions and making purchases at the checkout (Gill, 2018). In the annual U.S. Pharmacy Study conducted by J.D. Power and Associates, independent community pharmacies received the highest rankings of all pharmacy practice settings for customer satisfaction (J.D. Power and Associates, 2018).

While these examples provide a look at patient perceptions, it is important to get a sense of what independent community practitioners think. One of the principal advantages of this type of practice frequently pertains to personal control. Referred to in various ways, such as "being my own boss," "wanting to do

things my way," and "besides my patients, I answer to no one but myself," the issue of personal control is a driving force for individuals to become owners. This ability to control their time and their practice enables independent pharmacists many opportunities to "practice at the top of their license," with their imagination, and not the mandate of an employer, serving as the only limit as to what services they can provide for their patients. Many independent pharmacists feel that they are able to care for their patients' needs because they, the pharmacist, has the ultimate control over what they will and will not do. Other factors, such as involvement and recognition in the community and personal motivations, are also considered to be advantages of this practice setting (Smith, 1986). One of the predominant disadvantages of independent community pharmacy relates to the increased responsibilities assumed by the owner: financial, legal, and professional. Because the pharmacy is a business, in some sense everyone (e.g., customers, employees, payers, and regulators) is the "boss" of the independent (Smith, 1986). The independent pharmacist is the public face of their pharmacy, which means that it's very difficult for owners to separate their professional life from their personal time. Independent pharmacy owners are responsible for all aspects of their pharmacy's operations, and in particularly their cash flow and finances. An additional disadvantage that also might be included are the long hours typically put in by the owner, especially during the business's formative years (Smith, 1986).

■ THE ENVIRONMENTS OF INDEPENDENT COMMUNITY PHARMACY

Overall Health Care Environment

Pharmacy continues to assume a large portion of the health care dollar. Spending for prescription drugs in retail outlets such as community pharmacies was $333 billion in 2017, accounting for almost 10% of all health care spending in the United States (Centers for Medicare and Medicaid Services [CMS], 2018).

When combined with spending on durable medical equipment, OTC medications, and other health goods commonly sold in community pharmacies, there is evidence that there continues to be ample and growing consumer demand for health goods and services in community pharmacies.

Community pharmacies must navigate a complicated and ever-changing landscape with regard to reimbursement for their goods and services. Gone are the days when pharmacies purchased drugs directly from a manufacturer, covered their costs of doing business by charging a 50% mark-up on the cost of the drug, and then dispensed the prescription to a patient who paid cash for their medication at the time they picked it up at the pharmacy. Today almost 90% of prescriptions dispensed in an independent community pharmacy are paid for by a government program (Medicaid, Medicare Part D) or another third-party payer, such as the health insurance one receives through their employer (NCPA, 2018).

As the payer mix for prescription drugs has changed, so have the challenges to pharmacists and pharmacies for obtaining reimbursement for their goods and services. While third-party payers, and particularly government programs like Medicaid and Medicare Part D, have enabled many patients who were previously unable to afford prescription medications to now obtain them, pharmacies are no longer able to set the prices they will charge for their goods and services. Instead, these are determined by the contracts established by the third-party payer (See Chapter 23). Third-party reimbursement has created unique challenges for independent pharmacists and pharmacies. Unlike chain pharmacies, who can leverage their size and scope when negotiating reimbursement terms with third party payers, independent pharmacies are limited in their ability to negotiate with payers on reimbursement terms. This is not only time consuming for the pharmacy owner, but also increases the risk that they will not have access to networks which their patients use to obtain coverage and pay for their services. Recently, independent pharmacies have banded together to form Community Pharmacy Enhanced Services Networks (CPESNs)

(CPESN, 2019). A CPESN is an integrated health improvement network, which lays the groundwork for individual pharmacies to meet and discuss providing clinical services for regional and national health insurance providers separate from the drug benefit (which still must be negotiated by each individual entity). This helps independent pharmacies develop and receive reimbursement for clinical services without the risk of violating anti-trust laws.

Internal Pharmacy Environment

The *NCPA Digest,* sponsored by Cardinal Health, is an annual survey that compiles and summarizes financial data from independent pharmacies nationwide (NCPA, 2018). Data from the *NCPA Digest* are used as a benchmark to describe the typical independent community pharmacy, as shown in Table 32-1. In general, the typical independent community pharmacy has a total sales volume of just over $3.5 million. Over 59,000 prescriptions are filled annually, with 89% of those prescriptions being paid for by a third party: 17% by Medicaid, 36% by Medicare Part D, and 36% by other third-party payers.

Independent community pharmacies have incorporated various elements of technology into the practice setting, including specialized software that

Table 32-1.	Characteristics of a Typical Independent Community Pharmacy	
		2017[a]
Prescription volume (annually)		59,137 Rxs
Third-party prescription coverage		89%
Medicare Part D		36%
Medicaid		17%
Other third-party programs		36%
Total sales		$3,540,013
Cost of goods sold		78.2%
Gross profit		21.8%
Cost of dispensing		$10.79

[a]Based on 2018 NCPA Digest.

checks for medication errors, fills and labels each prescription, and even processes the sales transaction. Additional uses have grown to include automated dispensing machines, specialized compounding and intravenous mixing equipment, and customized software that can be used in the management of patients with particular disease states such as diabetes. Emerging trends in technologies now include the expanded use of social media for pharmacies (NCPA, 2018).

A typical *NCPA Digest* pharmacy offers patients a number of specialized services including, but not limited to, delivery, compounding, health screenings, hospice, durable medical goods, and providing specialty medications, which require an intensive level of service from the pharmacist and their staff (NCPA, 2018). The trend to offer clinically oriented specialty services in independent community pharmacies continues to increase. According to the 2018 NCPA Digest, almost 90% of independent community pharmacies offer medication adherence services to their patients, with services ranging from medication synchronization and automated refill reminders to dispensing medications in customized packaging designed to enhance medication adherence (NCPA, 2018). Disease management service offerings continue to increase in frequency. The most frequently offered programs are immunizations, diabetes training, and blood pressure monitoring. Pharmacies who offer and bill for clinical services are now forming networks to enhance payer knowledge of their services, and provide financial benefits to payers who contract with the network (CPESN, 2019). As of 2019 over 2,000 pharmacies were members of a CPESN network (NCPA, 2018).

In addition to patient care services, another area that has been expanded by Medicare Part D has been MTM services and programs. MTM programs are designed to improve medication use, enhance patient safety, and increase patient adherence to medication regimens (NCPA, 2007). The 2007 *NCPA-Pfizer Digest* reported that over 46% of independent community pharmacies offered MTM services, with an average charge of $40, and that 48% of the pharmacies are receiving reimbursement under Medicare

Part D. The most recent *Digest* reported an increase in pharmacies offering MTM services to 79%, with a corresponding increase in point of care testing, such as cholesterol screening and A1C and international normalized ratio testing (NCPA, 2018).

■ CHARACTERISTICS OF THE INDEPENDENT COMMUNITY PHARMACIST

Independent community pharmacy provides a unique venue for an individual pharmacist. Opportunities exist to be an owner and run the pharmacy, a part-time employee interested in staying in touch with community pharmacy practice, an entrepreneur with ideas for creating new service offerings for patients, or an employee working for the owner/manager. In this venue, the individual is limited only by his or her imagination. Thus, with this in mind, who chooses a career path in independent community pharmacy?

Whether one is interested in ownership or not, one of the key characteristics for a pharmacist in this practice setting is the importance of interacting with people. The independent community pharmacy provides pharmacists with a great opportunity to help patients. Problem-solving skills are critical as a pharmacist, and this setting provides constant challenges that require those skills. Other characteristics that are fostered by the independent setting are the ability to embrace change, deal with risk, and adapt to an ever-changing environment.

It is important that stereotypes sharing a negative connotation of independent community pharmacists be addressed. In some cases, pharmacists who are business-oriented have been viewed in a negative light. In addition, many individuals interested in independent community pharmacy practice have been falsely accused of generalities such as "They are only going into business for the money," "They are not very clinical," and "They have a lack of professionalism."

Based on the descriptions of independent community pharmacy practice and the characteristics of the individuals who pursue this career path, several points must be made. First, independent pharmacists are placed in a difficult situation because of their need to possess expertise in pharmacy practice and business. All pharmacy organizations must stay in business so that they may provide goods, services, and care to patients. Second, independent community pharmacy practice represents one of the most accessible health care venues for patients. Because of this, there exist numerous clinical opportunities for pharmacists in the provision of quality patient care and positive patient outcomes. Third, independent community pharmacists contribute to the overall health of any community not only in the care provided but also in contributions to the economic and civic health of the community. As a health care provider, the pharmacy adds a stable business to any town's economic structure. In addition, through involvement of the owner and other staff members in civic organizations, these individuals serve as volunteer leaders in activities ranging from school and hospital boards to elected offices.

Today's Independent

In visiting one of nearly 22,000 independent community pharmacies across the country, one might find the following two different types of pharmacists. The first type of pharmacist is the younger of the two. This pharmacist received a PharmD degree in the past 15 years. There is a chance that this individual completed an MBA in conjunction with the pharmacy degree or at least had the chance to take some business courses. During his or her professional education, this pharmacist took the required courses that introduced issues such as management, marketing, and economics into pharmacy practice. If available at the university where they attended pharmacy school, any electives focusing on subjects ranging from pharmacy management and economics to entrepreneurship and ownership also would have been taken. This pharmacist had opportunities to be active in pharmacy school organizations, such as student chapters of the American Pharmacists Association (APhA-ASP) or the National Community Pharmacists Association (NCPA). After graduation, this pharmacist may have gained work experience at various practice settings

or may have completed a community pharmacy residency. They have gained a variety of experiences from practice settings that range from a single independent pharmacy to experiences in hospital, chain, and other specialty practice areas, such as long-term care, home infusion therapy, or compounding pharmacy. This pharmacist is in the process or has already established a specialty patient care service, such as an immunization program or disease-specific monitoring program in diabetes or asthma, and has received national certification in these various specialty areas.

The second type of pharmacist has been an owner for over 30 years. This pharmacist received a Bachelor of Science degree, having graduated from pharmacy school prior to the transition to the PharmD as the sole first-professional degree in the early 2000s. While this pharmacist may have some business courses in pharmacy school, the vast majority of their knowledge stems from their experience, often focused in community practice. This pharmacist may have spent time working in a chain, a hospital clinic, or even another independent before pursuing ownership of his or her own practice. This pharmacist manages personnel that includes other pharmacists, technicians, clerks, delivery personnel, and individuals such as bookkeepers, accountants, part-time help, and contract employees. The pharmacist has been a preceptor and has provided a recognized rotation site for several schools of pharmacy since opening the store. This pharmacist has always felt that students provide the pharmacy with as much as the pharmacy gives to them. This pharmacist may also have additional training experiences available, such as an administrative rotation or a community residency program. In addition, this pharmacist is an active member of several civic groups in the community, such as Rotary and the Chamber of Commerce. They are politically active, knowing the state and federal senators and representatives and voicing concerns to them regarding issues related to independent pharmacy practice. They support various activities of the local schools, such as speaking at career days and sponsoring various programs. The pharmacy may sponsor a little league team in the summer and a basketball team in the winter. This pharmacist knows his or her patients and is now taking care of several generations of families. He or she continues to participate in various certificate training programs and has implemented a variety of specialty services.

It is clear that both types of pharmacists enjoy their jobs from a professional, clinical, and personal perspective. They value the freedom to care for their patients through the variety of services they provide. Their career choices provide them with a salary that can support them individually and their families, if appropriate. They are constantly learning and growing as practitioners, managers, and businesspeople. For both types of pharmacists, management plays an important role in their lives. The application of management tools is critical to the success of these individuals, as well as to the success of the independent community pharmacy.

■ SCENARIO 2

Sue has been on staff at Professional Pharmacy for 6 months. She is beginning to feel comfortable with the employees, customers, and flow of the business. The immunization program that she helped institute while as a student has continued to grow, now offering vaccinations year-round for influenza, diphtheria, and tetanus, in addition to miscellaneous travel and childhood vaccinations.

Sue began to realize that a large portion of Professional Pharmacy's patient population was diabetic. As she learned more by participating in diabetes-related continuing education programs, Sue started to see opportunities for enhanced patient services that could be provided to this specific population of patients. In one of the continuing education programs that she attended, Sue learned how to create a business plan (see Chapter 7) for the development of a diabetes care center. Sue created a business plan for a service that would help patients identify whether they were diabetic, as well as to help educate and train those with diabetes to care for themselves and enhance their quality of life.

■ ENTREPRENEURSHIP/ INTRAPRENEURSHIP

In Scenario 2, Sue has formulated an idea, developed the idea through education and analysis, and created a business plan to test the strength of the idea. The process that Sue progressed through and the steps she took to develop her idea implicate her as a potential entrepreneur (see Chapter 31).

It is easy to see why most small business owners, including independent community pharmacy owners, are categorized as entrepreneurs. Yet there is more to being an entrepreneur than just setting up a business. Entrepreneurs typically demonstrate the effective application of a number of enterprising attributes such as creativity, initiative, risk-taking, problem-solving ability, and autonomy and often will risk their own capital to set up a business (Bloomsbury Publishing, 2002).

Prior to a more descriptive discussion regarding the characteristics of an entrepreneur, Scenario 2 must be re-examined. Although it was suggested that Sue may be a potential entrepreneur, she is not really starting a business. She is an employee of Professional Pharmacy, and Sue's idea will provide a new business opportunity for the pharmacy and Mr. Burke, the owner. A more accurate definition of Sue in this scenario is as an intrapreneur. An *intrapreneur* is an employee who uses the approach of an entrepreneur within an organization (Bloomsbury Publishing, 2002). As a business ages and grows, the original entrepreneurial spirit can diminish. Intrapreneurs are critical to any established business in that they question the establishment and provide the internal spark to pursue innovation and new opportunities.

Characteristics of Entrepreneurs

Entrepreneurship is a growing area of research. A major area of interest is in identifying the combination of characteristics that makes a successful entrepreneur. Over 40 traits believed to be associated with entrepreneurship have been identified. Five of the more frequently identified characteristics include the following (Daft, 2015; Gartner, 1985):

- *Internal locus of control.* A belief by individuals that they are in control of their future and that other external forces will have little or no influence.
- *Need to achieve.* A human quality in which people are motivated to excel, so they pick situations in which they will be challenged but where success is likely.
- *Tolerance for ambiguity.* The psychological characteristic that allows a person to be untroubled by disorder and uncertainty.
- *Risk-taking propensity.* The likelihood of being a risk taker no matter the circumstance.
- *Demographics factors.* These factors focus on a number of characteristics, including past work experience (experience in independent settings supports entrepreneurial tendencies), entrepreneurial parents (more likely to be entrepreneurial when parents have been as well), and age (most businesses are launched between the ages of 25 and 40).

ENTREPRENEURIAL OPPORTUNITIES IN INDEPENDENT COMMUNITY PHARMACY

The history of independent community pharmacy provides a wealth of examples of entrepreneurship. Independent pharmacists were some of the first to provide and use (Gumbhir, 1996)

- Complete patient medication profiles
- Total parenteral nutrition
- Delivery of products and care to prisons and long-term care facilities
- Home infusion services
- Veterinary pharmacy
- Specialty compounding services
- Point of care testing

In today's marketplace, entrepreneurial opportunities are everywhere. Individuals are limited only by their imagination in developing new services or other innovations. The biggest concern for any business is the ability to keep the entrepreneurial spirit alive. To continue that spirit, the owner/manager must create a climate that will support and foster the entrepreneurs and intrapreneurs in the pharmacy. Some rules that can be used in creating that climate in the pharmacy include (1) encourage action, (2) tolerate failure and use as a learning example, (3) be persistent in getting an idea to market, (4) use informal meetings to provide opportunities to share ideas, (5) provide challenges with the staff to help problem-solve given situations, and (6) reward and/or promote innovative personnel (Daft, 2015).

SCENARIO 3

Sue loves her job. In the 3 years that she has been at Professional Pharmacy, she has developed patient care services in areas such as immunizations and osteoporosis, created a disease management program in diabetes, and successfully marketed the pharmacy's services to other health care providers in town. She has a great relationship with Mr. Burke, the owner, and thoroughly enjoys the people she works with and the patients she cares for in the community. While she is pleased with her accomplishments, she is beginning to detect the emergence of several obstacles. Mr. Burke has been very supportive of her ideas, and even when he has disagreed, he has carefully explained his position against an idea. Over the past year, Sue has become more involved in the area of specialty compounding. A new dermatologist recently moved to the area, and during one of Sue's "detailing" visits to the Midtown Physicians Group, she struck up a conversation that has evolved into a steady stream of prescriptions for his "special" ointments and creams. Mr. Burke, although appreciative of the new business, is not interested in any expansion of the pharmacy to incorporate additional technology for use in compounding specialty items. Sue has been thinking so much about the potential for such a service that she sketched out a rough business plan one night when she could not sleep. Sue believes that this is a major local market that is going untapped; however, she knows that Mr. Burke wants no part in this venture.

If she were her own boss, she could direct the business in the direction she saw fit. "Hmmm," she thought, "should the idea be shelved for a while, or is it time to look at the potential for owning her own business?"

■ INDEPENDENT COMMUNITY PHARMACY OWNERSHIP

While working for an independent owner can be a very fulfilling experience for many, one of the most attractive aspects of the independent setting is the opportunity to own a pharmacy. Interest in ownership has peaked and waned over the past 30 years. A significant decline in the number of independent community pharmacies occurred between 1990 and 1997 (National Association of Chain Drug Stores [NACDS], 2003). From the late 1990s to 2006, the number of independent practices hovered around 24,000 sites (NCPA, 2007). As of December 2017 there were 21,909 independent community pharmacies in the United States. Together, they make up over 35% of all community pharmacies (including chains, supermarkets, and mass merchants with pharmacy departments) and a $77.6 billion share of the health services market (NCPA, 2018).

Some of the top reasons for wanting to go into business include self-management, creative freedom, and financial independence. Other reasons include (1) not having to answer to others regarding the focus of the pharmacy, (2) being recognized and playing an important role in the business, (3) optimizing the health of their patients, while addressing the health care needs of their community, (4) achieving a level of self-fulfillment and pride, and (5) continuing the legacy of pharmacy ownership established by family and/or mentors (Smith, 1986, 1996). Each individual who pursues ownership is driven by his or her own reasons. Once the decision of pharmacy ownership is made, the prospective owner must do the following: identify available pharmacies for sale or suitable locations for a new pharmacy, determine a satisfactory purchase price, evaluate and determine capital needs,

and investigate and select the best source of capital (Gagnon, 1996). He or she must determine whether to start a new independent practice or purchase an established pharmacy.

Option 1: Starting from Scratch

Sue is determined to pursue her idea of creating a compounding specialty service. After her discussions with Mr. Burke confirmed his lack of interest, she realized that she has two options: find another pharmacy that would be interested in pursuing this specialty service or start her own business. Sue decides that despite how well things have been for her at Professional Pharmacy, the time is right to start her own business.

The act of starting a new independent community pharmacy practice follows a long and rich history. As mentioned previously, a new pharmacy appears for various reasons, ranging from support of unmet health care needs for a particular patient population to taking advantage of a potentially lucrative business opportunity. Starting a new pharmacy, as with any business, requires considerable planning.

A number of distinct advantages are available to an owner opening a new independent community pharmacy. The opportunity to select and purchase each item of this new venture, such as fixtures, equipment, and inventory, is a great advantage. Also, hiring your own personnel, finding a great location, creating sound policies and procedures, and avoiding paying for intangible assets are additional advantages.

One of the intangible assets that requires further attention is goodwill. By definition, goodwill is an intangible asset of a company that includes factors such as reputation, continued patronage, and expertise, for which a buyer of the company may have to pay a premium (Bloomsbury Publishing, 2002). For an independent community pharmacy, specific factors that contribute to goodwill include the prescription files and accounts receivable (Smith, 1996). Since goodwill is related to the profitability of the pharmacy, the most frequently used method to estimate goodwill is some multiple of the annual net profit. The most recent year's net profit is generally considered the minimum price for goodwill, whereas a common value for goodwill is estimated at 1 to 2 years of net profit (Jackson, 2002; Smith, 1996).

If the venture is not planned carefully, the advantages of opening a new pharmacy can turn into disadvantages. There is a greater amount of risk that must be assumed by the owner and an increased chance of experiencing unforeseen events. For one, the lag time between start-up and profit tends to be longer. Moreover, the challenge to secure capital is a formidable one.

How to Get Started

An individual interested in starting a new business can find a great number of books on the topic. While there are few books that specifically relate to the opening of a pharmacy, the general topics covered in the new business development literature are pertinent to any business type. The National Community Pharmacists Association (NCPA) also offers a pharmacy ownership workshop to help prospective owners consider the steps of the business planning process (NCPA, 2019). This section offers a list of steps that can be followed on the path toward independent community pharmacy ownership:

1. Decide on the type of pharmacy.
2. Assess the potential market.
3. Develop a detailed business plan.
4. Determine the organization's structure.
5. Identify financing options.
6. Select a location.
7. Obtain licenses, permits, and insurance.
8. Develop a marketing and promotion plan.
9. Establish the management philosophy of the business.

Decide on the Type of Pharmacy

This question can only be answered by the potential owner. While it seems like a very simple question, the answer requires considerable contemplation. As in Sue's case, most individuals have a general idea of what type of business they want to start. For Sue, a compounding specialty pharmacy is her wish. Now Sue must begin to evaluate her idea thoroughly by resolving such questions as follows:

- What products and services will I sell?
- From what base will I derive my customers?
- What skills do I bring to this business?
- Where should I be located?
- Will I have any competition?

Assess the Potential Market

Based on her evaluation of the type of pharmacy she would like to open, Sue has decided that she will start a compounding prescription business in the community where she currently lives. She has had a great deal of specialized training in this area and believes that there is a need for this type of pharmacy in the community. Now she must assess the potential market.

As described in Chapter 25, Sue must undertake a complete market assessment of the area in which she plans to locate. Some of the questions to resolve include the following:

- What is the potential customer base?
- How many physicians are in the community? Specialists?
- What is the competition? Other pharmacies? Other businesses?

Develop a Detailed Business Plan

It is important that the plan is well thought out and that due diligence is paid to eliminate as much uncertainty as possible when starting a new pharmacy (see Chapter 7).

Determine the Business Structure of the Pharmacy

A decision regarding the legal structure of the pharmacy must be made fairly early in the business development phase. Deciding on the legal structure of the pharmacy is critical to the overall success of the business. Each business venture is unique, and there is no one single ownership structure that suits every situation. The prospective owner should consult with an accountant and an attorney to help select the ownership structure that will best meet her needs.

In general, three legal structures are available to pharmacy owners: sole proprietorship, partnership,

Table 32-2.   Comparisons Between Business Structures

	Sole Proprietor	Partnership	S Corp	C Corp	LLC
Number of owners	One	Two or more	No more than 75 shareholders	Unlimited	No maximum, 1 person LLC permitted in most states
Level of liability	Unlimited, personal liability	Unlimited, all partners jointly liable for actions of other partners	Limits personal liability to the amount invested to the limit of assets of the company	Limits personal liability to the amount invested to the limit of assets of the company	Limits personal liability to the amount invested
Tax issues	Owner pays tax on personal returns	Profits divided among partners; individuals must pay taxes	Profits flow to shareholders; individual pays taxes	Corporation pays tax on profit; shareholders pay on dividends	Flexibility, profits flow to members; individual pays taxes
Can deduct losses on personal tax returns?	Yes	Yes	Yes	No	Yes
Ability to transfer ownership	Totally transferable	May need consent of other parties	May be limited in order to preserve S status	Totally transferable	Generally need consent of all owners

Data from SBA, 2019a; Spadaccini, 2009; Tootelian, 1993.

and corporation. Table 32-2 identifies some of the unique characteristics of each legal structure (SBA, 2019a; Spadaccini, 2009; Tootelian & Gaedeke, 1993).

SOLE PROPRIETORSHIP This is the simplest ownership form because the business is owned by one individual. The sole proprietor owns all the assets, receives all profits, and is responsible for all aspects of the business. While the owner receives all the profits generated from the business, there is also no legal distinction between the business and the owner, making the owner completely responsible for any liabilities

and debts. This form of ownership is ideal for starting a business (Spadaccini, 2009). However, as a business grows, there are other ownership forms that provide more security to the owner and the business.

PARTNERSHIP By definition under the Uniform Partnership Act, a partnership is an association of two or more persons to carry on as co-owners of a business for profit (Tootelian & Gaedeke, 1993). While seemingly straightforward, partnerships have the potential to be complex. Because of this, it is strongly recommended that a written legal agreement between the partners be executed. The agreement, also referred to as *articles of partnership,* should outline issues including, but not limited to, profit-sharing, business decisions, resolving disputes, adding additional partners, and dissolving the partnership.

There are two types of partnership for consideration: general and limited. A *general partnership* entails all partners to divide the responsibility for management and liability, as well as profit or loss (Tootelian & Gaedeke, 1993). In addition, partners are jointly and individually liable for the actions of one another. While this is usually considered the least favorable form of ownership, a partnership can be less complicated than a corporation. For example, a payroll is not required for the partners in this relationship, and this provides for less paperwork and similar tax benefits to a sole proprietor (Spadaccini, 2009). A *limited partnership* consists of at least one general partner and one or more "limited" partners (Tootelian & Gaedeke, 1993). *Limited partners* are individuals who provide capital to the business but are held liable only for the amount of their investment. These same individuals are not involved in any of the management decisions or operational issues of the business.

CORPORATION A *corporation* is a business that is chartered by the state and legally operates as a separate entity from its owners. The Supreme Court defined the corporation in 1819 as "an artificial being, invisible, intangible, and existing only in contemplation of the laws" (Tootelian & Gaedeke, 1993). This means that a corporation can be sued, taxed, own property, and enter into contractual agreements, whereas the owners of the corporation, the stockholders, are protected from liability. The stockholders elect a board of directors to oversee the entity and adopt bylaws to govern the corporation during its existence.

While incorporating a business seems like a good move with regard to the limited personal liability experienced by the owners, there are challenges to consider. The complexity of corporations requires a great deal of time and money for the setup and running of such an organization. Based on this structure, operating in accordance with local, state, and federal governments may result in higher taxation and require additional resources.

There are three forms of corporations that most businesses use: the S corporation, the C corporation, and the limited-liability corporation (LLC) (Table 32-3). Over 96% of all independent community pharmacies were organized as corporations in 2017, with the majority (60%) being organized as a S corporation, followed by 25% as LLCs and 11% as C corporations (NCPA, 2018).

Identify Financing Options

Once the business plan has been outlined and the organizational structure has been selected, the next step for the soon-to-be owner is financing the pharmacy. Some questions that must be resolved include the following:

- What are the financial needs for this venture?
- What type of financing will be best for the given situation?
- Where does one go to obtain capital for such a venture?

FINANCIAL NEEDS Every business has financial needs. These needs vary with the type and individualistic nature of each business. For example, the financing needs of a new compounding pharmacy requiring specialized equipment, expensive inventory, and complicated reimbursement may be quite different than the financing needs of a more traditional community pharmacy offering prescriptions, OTC medications, and durable medical equipment. The buyer must understand the needs of the business venture. These financial needs refer to capital. *Capital* is wealth, in the form of cash, equipment, property, or a combination of these factors, that can be used in the production or creation of income (Kelly, 1996).

There are three areas of capital need: set-up capital, start-up capital, and operating capital (Tootelian & Gaedeke, 1993). Each area represents a period of time in the life of a business during which particular activities that require capital are conducted.

Establishing a pharmacy, whether starting new or making changes to an existing business, often requires a considerable amount of capital. The activities that represent the largest initial capital expenditure focus

Table 32-3.   Summary of Corporation Types

Type of Corporation	Advantages	Disadvantages
S corporation	Limited personal liability	Shareholder restrictions
	Corporate losses can pass through to shareholders	Employee benefit expenses are included in gross income
	No corporate taxes	All shareholders must agree to the election of S corporation status
	Shareholders and employees do not pay Medicare or FICA on profits/dividends	
C corporation	Deduct 100% of health insurance paid for employees	If corporation loses money, owners cannot deduct on personal income tax
	Deduct fringe benefits such as qualified education costs, portion of life insurance, and employer-provided transportation for work	Corporate taxes on profit
		If profits distributed to shareholders, they must pay personal income tax on dividends
	Profits up to $50,000 annually are taxed at lower rate if left in corporation rather than pay higher personal income tax rate	More complicated and requires close monitoring
LLC	Owners are protected from personal liability as with corporation	Owners experience same self-employment tax treatment as partners and sole proprietors
	As with partnership, income or losses are reported on member's individual tax return	States may differ in tax treatment
	In general, fewer restrictions and more flexibility	Newer corporation form—less precedents

Data from SBA, 2019a; Spadaccini, 2009.

on the physical aspects of the business. The remodeling and renovation of the pharmacy, purchasing of fixtures and equipment, finalizing the building's lease deposit if it is not owned directly, and purchasing the beginning inventory, prescription and non-prescription merchandise, are the major sources of capital expenditure. Most of the other activities in the area of start-up relate more to paperwork and attention to detail. Such activities include prepaying insurance and utilities, obtaining the appropriate licenses and permits, and covering the professional fees of hired advisors (e.g., attorneys and accountants).

TYPES OF FINANCING Having identified a number of financial needs that come with the purchase of a pharmacy, the next step is to identify the type of funding available. Three main types of financing will be discussed: personal, debt, and equity.

Personal financing is just what it sounds like, the use of personal funds to finance the purchase of the pharmacy. It is no different from saving money for that first bicycle, car, or even one's retirement; personal savings is an important type of funding. This type of funding provides the buyer with the best possible funding source because there is no cost or payback terms, the amount can be unlimited, and it is relatively easy to use, whereas the only detractor is that there is a risk of loss (SBA, 2019b). However, in most cases, the buyer will need additional funds for the purchase, set-up, start-up, or operation of the pharmacy.

A common type of funding for a pharmacy is debt financing. *Debt financing* can be defined as something of value such as money that is borrowed at interest for a specified period of time (Kelly, 1996). Debt financing provides a buyer with an advantage by allowing him or her to borrow the needed capital without having to share any of the profits with the lender and to keep control of the management of the pharmacy. The disadvantages of debt financing highlight the fact that if something is borrowed, it must be returned. Loans must be repaid, with some measure of interest, over a defined period of time. In addition, the amount of debt incurred is limited by the value of assets and earning record of the borrower (Tootelian & Gaedeke, 1993). Debt financing can consist of either/or a combination of short- and long-term strategies (see Chapter 21).

Used less frequently, *equity financing* results in the buyer sharing ownership with investors who contribute funds. This level of investor ownership brings with it varying degrees of involvement in management of the business. Depending on the structure of the pharmacy, investors could be recognized as anything from a partner to a stockholder in the business. An advantage to equity financing is the chance to reduce the debt that must be repaid on a particular scale. Depending on the fiscal health of the business, partners or stockholders may or may not receive paid dividends. A significant disadvantage is that ownership of the pharmacy is spread among a larger group of individuals, thus reducing the owner's decision-making abilities (Tootelian & Gaedeke, 1993). Most small businesses, such as a pharmacy, are unable to attract much funding in this manner owing to the risk of small business survivals.

SOURCES OF FINANCING Banks are not the only source for obtaining capital. In fact, establishing an entirely new independent community pharmacy may not be appealing to a bank. Banks view the purchase of an established pharmacy as less risky, generally because these pharmacies have established collateral in the form of accounts receivable, inventory, and a track record of patients and prescription volume. But even with this knowledge of an existing pharmacy, there is no guarantee of obtaining a loan.

The choice of a funding source is critical to the future of a business venture and should be made carefully. The buyer must thoroughly weigh the options regarding the types of financing and the specific requirements provided for by each funding source. Table 32-4 provides a brief list of potential lenders (Kelly, 1996; SBA, 2019b; Tootelian & Gaedeke, 1993).

Select a Location

The familiar mantra Sue hears consists of three words: Location! Location! Location! The selection of the trade area, as well as the actual physical site of the pharmacy, is a primary factor in determining the success of the business. Sue has already incorporated the idea of location into her planning process by deciding on the type of pharmacy she wants to start and in conducting a market analysis.

Sue must evaluate the location of her pharmacy thoroughly with regard to population, potential customers, competition, physician availability, and community trends ranging from general health to economic issues (Kelly, 1996). To help Sue in accomplishing this task, a number of information resources are available to help analyze her pharmacy's location, including, but not limited to, public libraries; realty companies; utility companies; local, state, and federal documents and websites; state and national small business administration (SBA) offices; and individually conducted or contracted surveys, interviews, or traffic counts. Sue is also reminded continuously that this is a process that will be time-consuming and take hard work. She should not depend solely on what the computer provides in the way of information. By putting in the work on the front end, the next steps will be smoother.

Obtain Licenses, Permits, and Insurance

As the owner of this new pharmacy, Sue will need to obtain specific licenses and permits to operate. While local zoning laws, building permits, and standards set by health, fire, and police are requirements that must be met by all businesses in a given community, Sue

Table 32-4.   Potential Capital Sources for Financing a New or Established Pharmacy Business

Source	Type	Positive	Negative
Personal savings	Personal	Easy, inexpensive	Risk of loss
Family	Personal, debt, or equity	Flexible	Can cause problems
Friends	Personal, debt, or equity	Flexible, usually good rate	Can cause problems
Granting agencies	Personal	Cash awarded	Few, competitive, restricted regarding use
Credit cards	Debt	Easy to qualify, no collateral	Small amounts, high interest
Banks/savings and loans	Debt	Most common debt source	Hardest to qualify for
Commercial finance companies	Debt	More flexible alternative to banks	More expensive, collateral more important
Consumer finance companies	Debt	Personal loan, not loan to business; no restrictions on use of funds	High interest, personal collateral, not business
Wholesalers/suppliers	Debt	Line of credit, sometimes loans	Terms and conditions, requirements for use as wholesaler/supplier
Small business administration	Debt	Longest payback time	Complex and competitive process
Venture capitalists	Equity	Can be large amounts	Hard to find, share ownership

Data from SBA, 2019b; Kelly, 1996; Tootelian, 1993.

also must ensure compliance with a variety of state and federal regulations that pertain specifically to pharmacy (National Association of Boards of Pharmacy [NABP], 2018; Tootelian & Gaedeke, 1993). Insurance is of critical importance to a pharmacy. Sue will need to find an insurance agent to help with creating a comprehensive insurance plan that covers events ranging from natural disasters and physical accidents to employee health and workers' compensation. In addition, Sue must examine and acquire professional liability insurance for herself, professional staff members, and the business. Chapter 11 provides more detailed information on risk management strategies available to pharmacy owners.

Develop a Marketing and Promotion Plan

How will Sue inform the community of her new pharmacy and the innovative services that she will be offering? Using the techniques and tools provided in Chapter 25, Sue will be able to develop a specific marketing plan to educate the community. Through the use of the local newspapers, radio, television, websites and social media, Sue will be able to execute a specific promotion plan for the new pharmacy. Sue should not focus all her marketing and promotional efforts on potential customers. A critical area for her specialty pharmacy will be the community of health care professionals, ranging from physicians and nurse practitioners to specialty practices such as dermatologists and veterinarians.

Establish the Management Philosophy of the Business

The owner of an independent community pharmacy sets the tone for the business. The owner has been involved in virtually every aspect of the business, from conceptualization and planning to development and completion. As the new owner, Sue will be involved in all aspects of the business. In addition to the potential tools available in print, the experience that she has gained from working in an independent community pharmacy will be even more valuable to the dissemination of her management philosophy.

Option 2: "Why Reinvent the Wheel?"— Purchasing an Established Pharmacy

Sue has worked for Professional Pharmacy for 3 years. As she was closing up the pharmacy one night, Mr. Burke, the owner, brings up the idea that he is starting to think about retirement. He and his wife Helen eventually would like to move into a beachfront property. There they could take out their boat and have a place for their kids and grandchildren to visit. Sue is shocked by this sudden revelation. Mr. Burke reassures her that retirement is still a ways off, but he wants to chat about her future career goals and whether those goals might include pharmacy ownership.

For a potential buyer, looking for the right pharmacy may seem like a daunting task. There are a number of places to begin a search. In many cases, the potential buyer already may have identified several businesses either through research or as a result of his or her current job. Professional brokers who deal on the business side of the real estate market can be contacted and hired. There also exist specialty services provided by local, state and national pharmacy organizations. One example of this is the Independent Pharmacy Matching Service (IPMS), found on www.PharmacyMatching.com that is coordinated by the National Community Pharmacists Association (NCPA) (Pharmacy Matching, 2019). The IPMS helps match prospective buyers and sellers on various criteria, including geographic location.

Once a potential pharmacy is identified, an important question to ask is, "Why is this pharmacy for sale?" (Cotton, 1984). Is the owner retiring? Has the neighborhood changed due to increased competition or economic changes to "sour" the location? Is the pharmacy on the verge of bankruptcy? These are just a few of the many questions that should be asked

regarding the pharmacy. These questions reinforce the importance of researching the business and obtaining advice from various sources.

Purchasing an established pharmacy can provide an excellent opportunity to a potential buyer. Identifying the advantages and disadvantages of this ownership alternative will provide valuable insight into an individual's decision-making process regarding ownership (Smith, 1986, 1996; Tootelian & Gaedeke, 1993).

Advantages and Disadvantages

According to many in the pharmacy and business literature, there are a number of advantages to purchasing an established pharmacy (Table 32-5). An established pharmacy already has eliminated a number of the unknowns that the start-up of a new pharmacy faces. There is a lower level of risk on the

Table 32-5.   Advantages and Disadvantages of Purchasing an Established Pharmacy

Advantages

Lower level of risk for the buyer

No additional competition added to the current marketplace

Reduced start-up costs/less risk

Less time required to show a profit

Buyer receives established goodwill

Business has an established clientele

Business provides buyer with trained employees, inventory, physical facilities, and established relationships area health care providers

Disadvantages

Inadequate facilities

Old/outdated fixtures and equipment

Inventory that is too large and/or unsalable

Established policies and procedures do not match with new ownership's philosophy

Inflated sale price

Problems with the location

Undesirable established leases

buyer's part because the pharmacy has an established history. Pending thorough research and assessment, the buyer should have fewer uncertainties regarding the pharmacy, ranging from the physical facility, inventory, and equipment to the personnel and patient base of the pharmacy. Based on this transfer of ownership, the pharmacy obtains new management while not adding another business to a competitive marketplace. Another advantage is that an established pharmacy provides the buyer with great potential for reducing start-up costs and decreasing the length of time between start-up and profitability. In addition, the buyer receives the goodwill and reputation of the pharmacy.

The advantages related to this method of ownership can just as easily become disadvantages. The established assets, such as facilities and equipment, may be outdated or inadequate to meet the needs of the interested parties. The inventory of the business in question could consist of a large amount of out-of-date and unsalable items or even be too large for the pharmacy to support. The previously established policies and procedures could be in direct conflict with what the potential owner has in mind, thus creating potential human resources management problems. In addition, the pharmacy's location may not be optimal, and the purchase price may be overinflated by goodwill.

During the negotiation of such a transfer of ownership, the careful review of all leases is a critical factor that is often overlooked. A *lease* refers to a long-term agreement to use or rent a fixture, a piece of equipment, the physical structure in which the pharmacy is located, or the land the business occupies (Gagnon, 1996).

Value Assessment and Price Determination

Once the decision has been made to purchase an established pharmacy and a specific property has been identified, the next step is to determine the value of the business. Prior to a value assessment, the future owner should conduct a thorough review of the external environment of the business; that is, the community in which the business is located.

The predominant method of determining the value of a business is through financial analysis. Chapter 21 discussed the basic principles of financial analysis. In determining the fiscal health of the business, its financial records (income statements and balance sheets) from at least the past 3 to 5 years should be reviewed. From these data, the various facets of financial analysis—solvency, liquidity, efficiency, and profitability—can be determined for the business, and trends can be projected based on the time frame analyzed. A number of financial formulas are used to provide a range of values that serve as a guide for either the buyer or seller to begin the negotiation process (Jackson, 2002). It is important to note that while there is no single formula that must be used, each formula determines the value of the business from various perspectives, providing a range of values that can be used to determine an initial buying or selling price.

Based on the preceding discussion, it should be obvious that determining the value of a business is not an exact science. While a number of established techniques may be used, each business is unique. In fact, the value of a business is ultimately determined through negotiation between the buyer and the seller (Jackson, 2002). The agreed-on price will usually lie somewhere between the initial price of the seller and the initial offer of the buyer. The valuation of a business is based on the assessment of facts about the business, informed judgment, and some common sense (Jackson, 2002).

Purchasing Methods

The next step for the prospective owner is to finance the cost of purchasing the pharmacy.

FINANCING As was done during the preceding discussion regarding the financing of a new pharmacy, similar questions regarding the needs of the business, the type of financing, and the sources of capital must be addressed for the purchase of an established pharmacy. Whether purchasing an established pharmacy or starting one from scratch, a significant amount of capital will be needed to cover the cost of the venture. In this case, the buyer has a significant advantage over someone starting a new business because the established pharmacy will have lower start-up costs and should take less time to begin making a profit.

From a buyer's perspective, various types of financing are available for purchase of a pharmacy. While personal, debt, and equity financing are examples available to the buyer, the main question that must be determined is will the pharmacy be bought outright, or will there need to be some financial arrangement made for purchasing over a period of time. In most cases, an individual buyer would have great difficulty in securing financing to buy a pharmacy outright. With this in mind, the following discussion illustrates a transfer of ownership that provides a win-win scenario for both the buyer and the seller.

JUNIOR PARTNERSHIP A junior partnership provides an opportunity for a buyer to purchase a pharmacy with little or no initial capital and a seller to ease out of ownership and keep the legacy of the independent pharmacy alive in the community (Jackson, 2002). Instead of trying to figure out a way to sell the pharmacy when the owner is ready for retirement, this option allows the current owner to transfer ownership to a buyer, continue to have an income, and prepare for retirement.

The advantages of a junior partnership range from less risk and less initial capital needed by the potential buyer to the continued presence of an independent pharmacy to the economic and health care needs of the community. A junior partnership has disadvantages that are similar to those of any partnership arrangement. However, in this situation, because of the established relationship, the chance for both parties to determine compatibility, and the detailed nature of the agreement, a junior partnership proves beneficial.

■ SCENARIO 4

It has been 4 years since Sue entered into a junior partnership with Mr. Burke, and at the end of next year, she will be majority owner of Professional Pharmacy. While the time has just flown by, Sue marvels at all she has learned about pharmacy practice from both the business and professional sides. Sue came to this realization shortly after her first scheduled meeting with this year's community pharmacy resident, Cindy Ryan. After laughingly explaining to Cindy that there is no such thing as a typical day when you are in the business of caring for patients, Sue offered the following description:

> As the owner, I am responsible for the 40-member staff that makes up Professional Pharmacy, Incorporated. This includes the main pharmacy, Professional Pharmacy West, and the compounding/home infusion pharmacy, Professional Pharmacy East. My day usually begins at East, where I check in with Jerry, the manager, to review the workload for the day and take care of any problems, usually human resources issues. I am usually at East for most of the morning, taking care of e-mail, mail, and so on. I usually spend the afternoons at West. There I meet with Lois, the store manager, to go over things for the day and take care of problems. In each facility, on a weekly basis, an all-staff meeting is conducted to update staff regarding procedure changes and new third-party coverage, address employee concerns, and check in with everyone. The meeting can last up to 20 minutes. As the owner, I have had to spend more time managing the business and less time working with the compounding center and the diabetes care program that we established several years ago. While I miss the time with patients, I have come to realize that becoming the best manager I can be of help to ensure that the patients we serve receive the best possible care.

■ CURRENT ISSUES/ OPPORTUNITIES FACING INDEPENDENT PHARMACY PRACTICE

The life of an independent community pharmacy owner provides numerous challenges and can be highly rewarding. As Sue pointed out, most of her responsibilities have evolved into a management role.

As a manager, the success or failure of the business is that individual's responsibility, and that success is dictated by the decisions made and actions taken.

The owner must balance a number of issues and ideas related to the pharmacy. Today's owner must be able to evaluate the issues, determine the feasibility of ideas, and take action. The following is a list of four issues that require a great deal of attention by an owner of an independent community pharmacy: competition, third parties, patient care service development, and niche development.

Competition

Independent community pharmacy practices operate in one of the most dynamic and competitive marketplaces. Most competition is readily apparent, such as traditional chain drugstores, supermarket pharmacies, and mass-merchandisers. Independent community pharmacies also have experienced competition from other less obvious entities. This additional group of competitors consists of mail-order pharmacies, managed-care pharmacies, hospital ambulatory clinics and pharmacies, and even Internet pharmacies. While the total number of community pharmacies has remained relatively steady, the community pharmacy market continues to change. Independents have experienced a small decline in total numbers in the past 20 years. Pharmacy chains and other community pharmacies are not immune from these trends, with larger pharmacies consolidating smaller pharmacies, and even some chains choosing to discontinue their pharmacies altogether (Gibson, 2019). Pharmacies compete not only on the basis of the price of the goods and services which they sell but also on their location, accessibility, willingness to participate in insurance programs, and the mix of goods and services which they offer.

Third-Party Issues

For an independent community pharmacy, addressing third-party issues is critical not only to the success of the business but also to its very survival. Addressed previously in this chapter, the average *NCPA Digest* pharmacy reported that 89% of prescriptions filled were paid for by a third party (NCPA, 2018). This relationship identifies the importance of understanding third-party issues for owners and managers.

Third-party issues are wide ranging. One of the most prominent issues from this arena focuses on the reimbursement rates for prescription medications that are received by independent community pharmacies from third parties (see Chapter 23). It is a constant struggle between third parties, who want to lower costs by lowering reimbursement rates to pharmacies, and independent practitioners, who must monitor the rates constantly to ensure that the pharmacy will be able to cover costs and have some profit margin. Independent pharmacies can affiliate with a Pharmacy Services Administration Organization (PSAO), who contract with many insurance companies, pharmacy benefits managers (PBMs) and other third-party payers and in turn, allow their member pharmacies access to their networks. While PSAOs offer independent pharmacies some levels of efficiency and access, there are costs to joining these groups, and the individual pharmacy is not able to negotiate with each of the third-party payers. The must "take or leave" the medication and service reimbursement payment terms that they are offered.

Patient Care Service Development

Independent community pharmacies have a rich tradition of service to patients. This tradition has evolved into a number of identifiable patient care services that are offered in many pharmacies. Patient care services can range from home delivery and patient charge accounts to specialized patient care such as disease-state management programs focusing on diabetes or asthma. The development of such services is usually based on the fact that patients needed to be cared for and the pharmacist began stocking the product and creating the service to help their patients. In areas such as herbal medicine, homeopathy, and nutrition, patients not only obtain specific products but also receive valuable information and learn that the pharmacist is a valuable information resource. As a complement to this continued development of patient care services comes the MTM programs and services (NCPA, 2018). All of pharmacy is striving to develop quality and cost-effective services that will continue to provide their patients with exceptional customer service while also helping to further secure the means to receive compensation directly for such services. New outcome measures and payment models are being developed which may provide additional incentives for independent pharmacists to provide adherence management, MTM and other patient care services (Urick et al., 2018). Continued political and professional pressure will be needed for pharmacists to bill for patient care services, as well as the ever-shrinking compensation for the medication itself.

Niche Development

The nature of independent community pharmacies and pharmacists is to develop and offer patient care services. In specific cases, certain services may be developed to fill a niche in the community. In Scenario 4, Sue identified and developed a niche with the creation of her compounding specialty business. The specialty service was created and succeeded because there was an unmet need for compounding services in the community. As was discussed in the entrepreneurship section of this chapter, independent community pharmacies provide a wealth of opportunities to develop specialty services based on an idea, such as administering immunizations and other medications, blood pressure monitoring, and offering patient education services such as smoking cessation and diabetes education. The development of niches provides the pharmacy and its staff with new challenges and opportunities for additional business success through the introduction of potential revenue streams.

■ CONCLUSION

Independent community pharmacy practice provides a vast array of opportunities for professional development and personal satisfaction. This venue accommodates all types of practitioners, ranging from allowing entrepreneurs and intrapreneurs the freedom to develop their ideas into actual goods or services to offering individuals interested in "being their own

boss" the chance to start their own pharmacy and pursue unique practice niches. The independent community pharmacy continues to evolve from its earliest appearance in the United States to the technologically advanced patient care service entities of the 21st century. Independent pharmacists will continue to deal with unique issues facing their practices, and yet they will continue to innovate and provide quality patient care.

■ QUESTIONS FOR FURTHER DISCUSSION

1. Do you consider yourself to be entrepreneurial? Intrapreneurial? Why or why not? Can you identify another individual as being entrepreneurial and/or intrapreneurial? Explain why you selected that person.
2. After reading this chapter, what interests (or what does not interest) you about a career in independent community pharmacy practice?
3. Imagine that you are the owner of a new independent community pharmacy. If money were no object, where would you be located? What patient care services would you offer? Would you have a general or specialized practice?
4. What is the most difficult management responsibility for the owner of an independent community pharmacy?
5. In your opinion, what is the future of independent community pharmacy? What are the largest challenges facing independent practice this year? In 5 years? In 10 years?

REFERENCES

American Pharmacists Association (APhA). 2019a. *Health Care Reform—The Affordable Care Act*. Available at https://www.pharmacist.com/health-care-reform-affordable-care-act. Accessed February 5, 2019.

American Pharmacists Association (APhA). 2019b. *Pharmacists Provide Care.* Available at http://www.pharmacistsprovidecare.com. Accessed January 31, 2019.

American Pharmacists Association (APhA). 2013. *The Pursuit of Provider Status: What Pharmacists Need to Know.* Washington, DC: American Pharmacists Association.

Balick R. 2019. *Ohio Hits Provider Status Milestone with New Law.* Available at https://www.pharmacist.com/article/ohio-hits-provider-status-milestone-new-law?is_sso_called=1. Accessed February 4, 2019.

Bloomsbury Publishing (ed.). 2002. *Business: The Ultimate Resource.* Cambridge, MA: Perseus Publishing.

Brenan M. 2018. *Nurses Again Outpace Other Professions for Honesty, Ethics.* Available at https://news.gallup.com/poll/245597/nurses-again-outpace-professions-honesty-ethics.aspx. Accessed January 31, 2019.

Centers for Medicare and Medicaid Services (CMS). 2018. *National Health Expenditure Accounts: Methodology Paper, 2017; Definitions, Sources and Methods.* Available at https://www.cms.gov/Research-Statistics-Data-and-Systems/Statistics-Trends-and-Reports/NationalHealthExpendData/downloads/dsm-17.pdf. Accessed January 31, 2019.

Cotton HA. 1984. Pharmacy for sale: How to arrive at a fair price. *Curr Concepts Retail Pharm Manag* 2:2.

CPESN. 2019. *CPESN.com: Re-imagine Healthcare Delivery in America.* Available at https://cpesn.com. Accessed February 4, 2019.

Daft RL. 2015. *Management,* 12th ed. Boston, MA: Cengage Learning.

Gabay M. 2014. A Step Forward: Review of the New California Provider Status Law. *Hosp Pharm* 49(5):435–436.

Gagnon JP. 1996. Establishing and financing a community pharmacy. In Huffman DC Jr (ed.) *Effective Pharmacy Management.* Alexandria, VA: National Association of Retail Druggists, p. 87.

Gartner WB. 1985. A conceptual framework for describing the phenomenon of new venture creation. *Acad Manage Rev* 10:696.

Gibson K. 2019. *Shopko Stores Files for Bankruptcy, Plans 100 Store Closings.* Available at https://www.cbsnews.com/news/shopko-filing-for-bankruptcy-green-bay-wisconsin-based-retail-chain-closing-more-than-100-stores/. Accessed February 4, 2019.

Gill LL. 2018. *Consumers Still Prefer Independent Pharmacies. CR's Ratings Show.* Available at https://www.consumerreports.org/pharmacies/consumers-still-prefer-independent-pharmacies-consumer-reports-ratings-show/. Accessed January 31, 2019.

Gumbhir AK. 1996. Entrepreneurship. In Huffman DC Jr (ed.) *Effective Pharmacy Management.* Alexandria, VA: National Association of Retail Druggists.

Higby GJ. 2003. From compounding to caring: An abridged history of American pharmacy. In Knowlton CH, Penna RP (eds.) *Pharmaceutical Care.* Bethesda, MD: American Society of Health-System Pharmacists.

Hoey BD. 2011. *Community Pharmacists Can Help Improve Health Outcomes. The Hill's Congress Blog.* Available at http://thehill.com/blogs/congress-blog/healthcare/162603-community-pharmacists-can-help-improve-health-outcomes. Accessed February 5, 2019.

Jackson RA. 2002. Maintaining our independents. *America's Pharmacist* 124:54.

J.D. Power and Associates Reports. 2018. US Pharmacies Raise Bar for Customer Satisfaction, Setting Stage for Fierce Competition in Digital/Mail-Order Market. Westlake Village, CA: J.D. Power and Associates. Available at https://www.jdpower.com/business/press-releases/2018-us-pharmacy-study. Accessed February 5, 2019.

Kelly ET 3rd. 1996. Location analysis and lease evaluation. In Huffman DC Jr (ed.) *Effective Pharmacy Management.* Alexandria, VA: National Association of Retail Druggists.

Kostick JH. 2006. *Medicare Part D: A Financial Drain for Pharmacies? Mediscape Pharmacists.* Available at http://www.medscape.com/viewarticle/537279. Accessed February 5, 2019.

National Association of Boards of Pharmacy (NABP). 2018. *Survey of Pharmacy Law.* Mount Prospect, IL: National Association of Boards of Pharmacy.

National Association of Chain Drug Stores (NACDS). 2003. Industry Statistics. Arlington, VA: National Association of Chain Drug Stores.

National Community Pharmacists Association (NCPA). 2007. *NCPA-Pfizer Digest.* Alexandria, VA: National Community Pharmacists Association.

National Community Pharmacists Association (NCPA). 2015. *NCPA Digest.* Alexandria, VA: National Community Pharmacists Association.

National Community Pharmacists Association (NCPA). 2018. *NCPA Digest.* Alexandria, VA: National Community Pharmacists Association.

National Community Pharmacists Association (NCPA). 2019. *Pharmacy Ownership Workshop.* Available at https://www.ncpanet.org/meetings/ownership-workshop. Accessed February 4, 2019.

Patient Access to Pharmacists' Care Coalition (PAPCC). 2019. Available at http://pharmacistscare.org/. Accessed February 5, 2019.

Pharmacy Matching. 2019. *Pharmacy Matching: Buying and Selling a Pharmacy*. Available at http://pharmacy-matching.com/wp/. Accessed January 31, 2019.

Small Business Administration (SBA). 2019a. *Business Guide, Launch Your Business, Choose a Business Structure*. Available at https://www.sba.gov/business-guide/launch-your-business/choose-business-structure. Accessed February 5, 2019.

Small Business Administration (SBA). 2019b. *Business Guide, Plan Your Business, Fund Your Business*. Available at https://www.sba.gov/business-guide/plan-your-business/fund-your-business. Accessed February 5, 2019.

Smith HA. 1986. *Principles and Methods of Pharmacy Management*. Philadelphia, PA: Lea & Febiger.

Smith HA. 1996. Purchasing an established pharmacy. In Huffman DC Jr (ed.) *Effective Pharmacy Management*. Alexandria, VA: National Association of Retail Druggists, p. 57.

Spadaccini M. 2009. *The Basics of Business Structrure. Entrepreneur*. Available at http://www.entrepreneur. com/startingabusiness/startupbasics/article200516.html. Accessed May 12, 2011.

Tootelian DH, Gaedeke RM. 1993. *Essentials of Pharmacy Management*. St. Louis, MO: Mosby Year Book.

Ukens C. 1994. Whatever happened to pharmaceutical care? *Drug Top* 138:38.

Urick BY, Ferreri SP, Shasky C, Pfeiffenberger T, Trygstad T, Farley JF. 2018. Lessions learned from using global outcome measures to assess community pharmacy performance. *J Manag Care Spec Pharm* 24(12):1278–1283.

Williams CF. 1998. *A Century of Service and Beyond*. Alexandria, VA: National Community Pharmacists Association.

INDEX

Note: Page numbers followed by *f* and *t* indicate figures and tables.

AAC. *See* Actual acquisition cost
AACP. *See* American Association of Colleges of Pharmacy
ABB. *See* Activity-based budgeting
Abbreviations, medication errors from, 212–213, 213*f*
ABC. *See* Activity-based costing
ABM. *See* Appointment Based Model
Absolute systems, for performance appraisals, 397–401, 398*t*
ACA. *See* Patient Protection and Affordable Care Act
Accent discrimination, 350
Accepting assignment clause, in third-party payer contracts, 474
Accommodator negotiators, 285
Accountability
    leadership and, 49
    for medication errors, 222–224
Accounting, 15, 16*t*, 418, 419–420
Accounting equation, 419
ACCP. *See* American College of Pharmacy
Accreditation Commission for Health Care, 115
Accreditation Council for Pharmacy Education (ACPE), 659
Acid test, 423*t*, 425
ACPE. *See* Accreditation Council for Pharmacy Education; American Council for Pharmacy Education
Acquisition cost, 460–461, 464, 564, 566
Action plans
    in business planning, 118–119, 119*f*
    in operations management, 133–135, 134*t*
    strategic planning and, 102*t*
Active end medication errors, 208

Activity-based budgeting (ABB), 446–448, 446*f*, 447*t*
Activity-based costing (ABC), 445–446, 445*f*, 446*f*
Actual acquisition cost (AAC), 460, 460*t*
Ad hock performance reviews, 341
ADA. *See* American Diabetes Association; Americans with Disabilities Act of 1990
Adaptive leadership, 40–41
ADCs. *See* Automated dispensing cabinets
ADEA. *See* Age Discrimination in Employment Act of 1967
Adequate service level, 497
ADEs. *See* Adverse drug events
Adherence, 164
    medication errors from, 222
    MTM and, 9, 82
    pharmacy technicians for, 376
Adhocracy, 304
Administration Industrielle et Generale (Fayol), 24
Adverse drug events (ADEs), 207
Advertising, 525–526, 529*f*
Affordable Care Act. *See* Patient Protection and Affordable Care Act
Age Discrimination in Employment Act of 1967 (ADEA), 328, 328*t*, 348, 353
Agency for Healthcare Research and Quality (AHRQ), 229
Agreeableness, 314
AHRQ. *See* Agency for Healthcare Research and Quality
AICPA. *See* American Institute of Certified Public Accountants
Alcohol abuse, 12, 356–357
Alcoholic beverage sales, 589
Allen, F., 419
All-products clause, in third-party payer contracts, 475
Alston, Greg L., 3, 75, 127, 187

Alternation ranking, for performance appraisals, 398*t*, 402
AMA. *See* American Marketing Association; American Medical Association
Ambiguous order medication errors, 213–215, 214*f*
American Association of Colleges of Pharmacy (AACP), 6–7
American College of Pharmacy (ACCP), 7, 112
American Council for Pharmacy Education (ACPE), 11
American Diabetes Association (ADA), 614
American Institute of Certified Public Accountants (AICPA), 418
American Marketing Association (AMA), 486
American Medical Association (AMA), 614
American Pharmaceutical Association (APhA), 112, 642
    Code of Ethics of, 7, 57, 63, 235
    independent community pharmacies and, 678
    pharmacist technicians and, 370
    on value-added services, 614
American Pharmacists Association (ASP), 678
American Society of Health-Systems Pharmacists (ASHP), 173
    on drug shortages, 663
    PAI of, 92
    on pharmacist technicians, 370, 373–374
    on pharmacist training, 642
    on value-added services, 614
American Society of Hospital Pharmacists, 8
Americans with Disabilities Act of 1990 (ADA), 328*t*, 329, 354–356, 592
AMP. *See* Average manufacturer price
"Analysis but no action," 105
Analytic negotiators, 285
Analytic time managers, 261, 262*t*
Angel investors, 663
Anticipatory stock, 570
AOG. *See* Arrival of goods
APhA. *See* American Pharmaceutical Association
Appointment Based Model (ABM), 628
APT. *See* Association of Pharmacy Technicians
Arbinger Institute, 44
Arrival of goods (AOG), 572

Articles of partnership, 684
ASHP. *See* American Society of Health-Systems Pharmacists
ASP. *See* American Pharmacists Association
Asplund, J., 138
Assertive negotiators, 285
Assets, 419
Association of Pharmacy Technicians (APT), 370
Assurance, 498, 539*t*. *See also* Quality assurance
Autocratic leaders, 314
Automated compounding equipment, 221
Automated dispensing cabinets (ADCs), 216–218
Automation
    barcodes, 198–199
    human tradeoffs with, 199
    for QI, 166
Auxiliary label medication errors, 219
Average actual acquisition cost (AvAC), 460*t*, 461, 464
Average collection period, 426
Average manufacturer price (AMP), 462
Average net profit comparison, 465–469, 468*t*–469*t*
Average wholesaler price (AWP), 460–462, 460*t*

Backorder programs, 574
Bailey, D. E., 305
Bailey, K., 551
Balance sheet, 420–421, 420*t*, 421*t*, 429*t*
Barcodes, 198–199
Barker, K. N., 226
BARS. *See* Behavior-anchored rating scale
BATNA. *See* Best alternative to a negotiated agreement
Behavior-anchored rating scale (BARS), 398*t*, 400, 401*t*
Behavioral theories, of leadership, 314
BEL. *See* 5 + 5 + 5 Bernelli Entrepreneurial Learning
Benau, E. M., 270–271
5 + 5 + 5 Bernelli Entrepreneurial Learning (BEL), 664, 664*t*
Best alternative to a negotiated agreement (BATNA), 282–283
BFOQ. *See* Bona fide occupational qualifications

Bledstein, B. J., 235
Blunt end medication errors, 208
Bodie, Z., 419
Bolman, L. G., 50
Bona fide occupational qualification
    (BFOQ), 395
Bonds, 435
Boone, Steve, 187
Borkowski, N., 306
Boundaryless organization, 304–305
Brealy, R., 419
Broadcast media advertising, 526
Brodie, D. C., 8
Budget, 437–452
    ABC and, 445–446, 445f, 446f
    administration of, 448–449
    behavioral effects of, 450–452
    communication for, 439–440
    master, 441–448, 442f, 447t
    for not-for-profit organizations, 444–445
    for operations, 440, 443–444
    participative, 451–452
    for product lifecycle costs, 449–450
    purchasing and, 570–571
    purposes of, 439–440
    resource allocation in, 440
    types of, 440–441
Budget padding, 451
Budgeted financial statements, 441, 445
Buffer stock, 570
Bulatao, Peter T., 75
Bundled pricing, 524
Bureau of Labor Statistics, 25, 361
Burglary, 359
Burnout, 12, 310–311
Business concept, 111–113
Business management, 9, 10t
Business owner's insurance, 193
Business planning, 94t, 109–124
    action plan in, 118–119, 119f
    communication in, 121–123, 122n3, 122t
    competitor analysis in, 114
    exit plan in, 119–121
    financial projections in, 117–118, 118t

market research for, 113–114
marketing strategy in, 116–117
for operations, 115–116, 116f
regulations in, 114–115
steps of, 113–121
strategic planning and, 96
SWOT in, 119, 120t, 121t
target market in, 114
for value-added services, 613–614
Business-function attack, 198
Bynum, Leigh Ann, 347

Caldas, Lauren M., 325
Campbell, Patrick J., 161
CAPE. See Center for the Advancement of Pharmacy
    Education
Capital budget, 441
Career planning, 396
    self-management for, 257–258
Carpal tunnel syndrome, 200
Case management, 629
Case mix index (CMI), 434t, 436
Cash budget, 444
Cash disbursement budget, 444
Cash discounts, 571–572
Cash patients, 467
Cash receipts budget, 444
CBO. See Congressional Budget Office
CDC. See Centers for Disease Control and
    Prevention
CE. See Continuing education
Center for Pharmacy Practice Accreditation (CPPA),
    173
Center for the Advancement of Pharmacy Education
    (CAPE), 67–68
Centers for Disease Control and Prevention (CDC),
    630
Centers for Medicare and Medicaid Services (CMS),
    173, 630
    receivable turnover ratio and, 426
Central tendency, for performance appraisals, 399,
    399t
Centralization, 300, 302–303
CEO. See Chief Executive Officer

Certified pharmacy technician (CPhT), 248
CFO. *See* Chief Financial Officer
Chain store pharmacies, 659
Charters, W. W., 6–7
Checklists
    medication errors and, 225
    for performance appraisals, 397, 398*t*
Chief Executive Officer (CEO), 95, 95*n*2, 111, 113,
    130, 300
Chief Financial Officer (CFO), 92, 92*n*1, 111, 113,
    130
Chief Operating Officer (COO), 130, 301
Cho, B. H., 439
Christensen, D. B., 492
Chronic diseases
    adherence in, 82
    leadership for, 50
Chui, M. A., 379
Civil law, 244–245
Civil money penalties (CMPs), 243
Civil Rights Act of 1964, 328, 328*t*, 329, 348,
    349–353
Civil Services Reform Act, 394
Clawbacks, 475
Cleveland Clinic, 97
Clinical Laboratory Improvement Amendments
    (CLIA), 362–363, 630, 635, 642
Cloud computing, 449
CMI. *See* Case mix index
CMM. *See* Comprehensive medication management;
    Continuous medication monitoring
CMPs. *See* Civil money penalties
CMR. *See* Comprehensive medication review
CMS. *See* Centers for Medicare and Medicaid
    Services
Coaching, 337–338
COD. *See* Collect on delivery; Cost of dispensing
Code of Ethics, of American Pharmaceutical
    Association (APhA), 7, 57, 63, 235
COGS. *See* Cost of goods sold
Cohen, S. G., 305
Coinsurance, 192
Collaborative practice agreements (CPAs), 635–636,
    645–647, 647*f*

Collaborative prescribing, 246
Collect on delivery (COD), 572
Collins, Jim, 39–40
Color discrimination, 349–350
Columbia Tragedy, 327–328
Command intent, 131–133
Communication
    as barrier to planning, 105
    for budget, 439–440
    in business planning, 121–123, 122*n*3, 122*t*
    with employees, 30
    influence and, 72
    in leadership, 40
    medication errors and, 207
    of organizational teams, 306
    of performance appraisals, 395
    in principled negotiation, 281
Community Pharmacy Enhanced Services Networks
    (CPESNs), 676
Company slogan, 98
Compassion, 59–60
Competing values framework, 298–299, 298*f*
Competition
    of entrepreneurship, 667–668
    of independent community pharmacies, 691
    for value-added services, 616–617
Competitor analysis, in business planning, 114
Complementary and alternative medicine, 14–15
Compounded sterile preparations (CSPs), 220
Comprehensive medication management (CMM),
    10
Comprehensive medication review (CMR), 628
Computerized prescriber order entry (CPOE), 209
Conchie, B., 40
Confidentiality, 57
Confirmation bias, 218
Conflict
    leadership and, 49
    in organizational teams, 306
    role, 395
Congressional Budget Office (CBO), 76
Consumer price index (CPI), 117
Contingency approach, to organizational behavior,
    304

Contingency planning, 94*t*

Continual quality improvement (CQI), 167–171, 167*f,* 171*t*
    for medication errors, 223

Continuing education (CE), 384

Continuous budget, 441

Continuous medication monitoring (CMM), 11, 627–628

Contribution margin, 469

Controlled Substance Ordering System (CSOS), 568–569

Controlled substances
    e-procurement of, 568–569
    PDMPs for, 244
    robbery of, 358
    shrinkage of, 566

Controlled Substances Act of 1970, 247

COO. *See* Chief Operating Officer

Cooperative gaming theory, 278

Copyrights, 666–667

Corporate entrepreneurship, 661

Corporate model, for organizational behavior, 307

Corporations, 683*t,* 684, 685*t*

Cost center, 435

Cost of dispensing (COD), 458, 464–465, 466*t*

Cost of goods sold (COGS), 424, 425–426, 443, 560, 572
    average net profit comparison and, 465–469
    ITOR and, 564–565

Counterfeiting, 440

Courtney, Robert, 235

Coverage, of insurance, 192

Covey, Stephen, 25, 38, 46–47, 47*t,* 72, 262–263

CPAs. *See* Collaborative practice agreements

CPESNs. *See* Community Pharmacy Enhanced Services Networks

CPhT. *See* Certified pharmacy technician

CPI. *See* Consumer price index

CPOE. *See* Computerized prescriber order entry

CPPA. *See* Center for Pharmacy Practice Accreditation

CQI. *See* Continual quality improvement

Critical-incident performance appraisals, 397, 398*t*

Cross-merchandising, 598

Cross-selling, 595

Cross-training, 337

CSOS. *See* Controlled Substance Ordering System

CSPs. *See* Compounded sterile preparations

Cultural competence, 14

Culture
    for HRM, 339–340
    for organizational behavior, 296–299, 298*f*

Cumulative quantity discounts, 571

Current ratio, 423*t,* 425, 436

Customer concept, 491

Customer satisfaction, 498–499

Customer service, 135, 535–552
    for difficult patients, 550–551
    of employees, 548–550, 548*t*
    feedback on, 547–548
    with MTM, 540
    prevention of conflict and complaints in, 551–552
    principles for, 538, 538*t*
    satisfaction surveys for, 547–548
    service failure of, 540–541
    service recovery of, 541–547, 542*f*
    standards for, 538–540, 539*t*
    word-of-mouth on, 546–547

Cybersecurity, 199

Cycle stock, 570

Daft, R. L., 23

Daily Plan Payment report, 427, 427*t*

DARN CAT. *See* Desire, Ability, Reasoning and Need/Commitment, Activation and Taking steps

Data collection
    for marketing, 501–502
    pharmacy technicians for, 378
    for value-added services, 630, 631*f*–634*f*

Dating, 572

Days inventory on hand, 423*t,* 426

De Quervain tenosynovitis, 200

DEA. *See* Drug Enforcement Administration

Deal, T. E., 50

Debt financing, 686

Deductible, 192

Deer hunt, 278
Deferred discounts, 571
Define, measure, analyze, improve, control (DMAIC), 136
Delayed dating, 572
Delegation, 69–71
Demand planning, 561–564
Demands, 488–489
Democratic leaders, 314
Department of Health and Human Services, U.S. (DHHS), 196, 200, 229, 242, 370
Departmentalization, 300, 304
Desire, Ability, Reasoning and Need/Commitment, Activation and Taking steps (DARN CAT), 287–289
Desired service level, 497
Desk audits, 474
Desselle, Shane P., 3, 367, 391
Developmental organizational culture, 299
DF. See Dispensing fee
DHHS. See Department of Health and Human Services, U.S.
Dichter report, 7
Differential analysis, 469–470, 470t
Differentiation
    of organizational behavior, 299–302, 301f
    for QI, 166
Difficult patients, 550–551
Digital veil, 199
Direct costs, 465
Direct marketing, 14
Direct observation, for medication errors, 226
Director of Pharmacy (DOP), 92, 99, 113
Disabilities. See Americans with Disabilities Act of 1990
Disability insurance, 192, 194
Disconfirmation of expectations, 540, 546
Discounts, 571–572
Discrimination. See Civil Rights Act of 1964
Disease and medication therapy management, 10t
Disease-state management, 628–629
Dispensing fee (DF), 456, 459–461
Dividends, 419, 435
Division of labor, 300, 303, 308

Divisional structure, for organization behavior, 304
DMAIC. See Define, measure, analyze, improve, control
Donnelly, Andrew J., 91, 109
DOP. See Director of Pharmacy
Doucette, W. R., 502, 666
Douglass, D. N., 262–263
Douglass, M. E., 262–263
Draper, R., 64
Drive-through windows, 600–601, 602f
Drucker, Peter F., 25, 29, 41, 135
Drug abuse, 12, 377. See also Controlled substances
Drug Enforcement Administration (DEA), 357, 568–569
Drug Importation Act of 1848, 236
Drug shortages, 85
    product mix and, 563
Drug Supply Chain Security Act (DSCSA), 558, 580–581
Drug testing, 356–357
Drug utilization review (DUR), 165, 166, 195, 215, 372, 374
Drug-allergy interactions, 239
Drug-drug reactions, 239
Drug-Free Workplace Act, 356
DSCSA. See Drug Supply Chain Security Act
DUR. See Drug utilization review
Durham, Carl, 237
Durham–Humphrey amendment, 7, 237

e-Budgeting, 448–449
e-prescribing. See Electronic prescribing
e-procurement, 568–569
EAC. See Estimated acquisition cost
EAPs. See Employee assistance programs
Earnings, 422
ECHO model, 164
Economic Order Quantity (EOQ), 567, 570
Economics, 15, 16t
Economies of scale, 469, 469n1
Economy, P., 29
EDM models, 58–64
    integration of, 63–64

of Markula Center for Applied Ethics, 58–59, 59f
moderating factors in, 65
PLUS EDM, 60–61
rationalist model for, 61–62, 61f
sensemaking, 64–67
EEOC. See Equal Employment Opportunity
    Commission
EFT. See Electronic funds transfer
EHR. See Electronic health records
EI. See Emotional intelligence
Electronic funds transfer (EFT), 568, 572
Electronic health records (EHR), 200–201
Electronic medication administration records
    (eMARs), 214
Electronic prescribing (e-prescribing), 200–201
    medication errors in, 209–210, 209f, 210f, 225
Electronic Quality Improvement Platform for Plans
    and Pharmacies (EQuIPP), 464
Electronic word of mouth (eWOM), 499
Elevator pitch, 668
Elixir Sulfanilamide, 236–237
eMARs. See Electronic medication administration
    records
Embezzlement, 360
Emergency planning, 94t
Emotional intelligence (EI), 44–45, 313
    leadership and, 318
Emotional labor, 313
Emotional stability, 314
Emotions, organizational behavior and,
    312–313
Empathy, 313, 498, 539t
Employee assistance programs (EAPs), 363–364
Employee engagement, in Human Sigma, 139
Employees. See also Human resources management;
    Job; Organizational behavior
    communication with, 30
    customer service of, 548–550, 548t
    delegation to, 69–71
    empowerment of, 29–30, 69–71
    labor demand decline for, 76
    laws for, 347–365
    management of, 27
    marketing dat from, 502

    performance appraisals for, 391–411
    regulation of, 347–365
    support for, 30
    theft by, 360–361
    training of, under HIPAA, 241
    violence and, 361–362
Employers of choice, 332–333
End caps, 595, 596f
Engagement
    of employees, 139
    well-being and, 312
English-only rules, 350
Enright, Sharon Murphy, 50
Entertainer time managers, 262
The Entrepreneurial Mindset (McGrath and
    MacMillan), 661
Entrepreneurship, 657–669
    competition of, 667–668
    defined, 659
    incubators for, 667
    in independent community pharmacies,
    679–680
    intellectual property and, 666–667
    mentorship for, 665
    process of, 661–665, 662t
    resources for, 668
    types of, 659–661, 660t
EOB. See Explanation of Benefits
EOQ. See Economic Order Quantity
EPA. See Equal Pay Act
Equal Employment Opportunity Commission
    (EEOC), 330, 334, 349, 351, 352, 355
Equal Pay Act (EPA), 329, 348, 353–354
Equilibrium, in negotiation, 278
EQuIPP. See Electronic Quality Improvement
    Platform for Plans and Pharmacies
Equity financing, 686
Essay method, for performance appraisals,
    397, 398t
Essential Medicines List (WHO), 384
Essentialism: The Disciplined Pursuit of Less
    (McKeown), 39
Estimated acquisition cost (EAC), 460–461, 460t
Ethical dilemmas, problem-solving with, 57–58

Ethics, 55–73
  APhA Code of Ethics, 7, 57, 63, 235
  EDM models for, 58–64, 59*f*, 61*f*
  leadership and, 56–57, 67–68
  in organizational behavior, 308
  pharmacist standards from, 235
  of pharmacy technicians, 383
  vision and mission and, 68–69
eWOM. *See* Electronic word of mouth
Exchange, in marketing, 487–488
Exit plan, 119–121
Expectations
  disconfirmation of, 540, 546
  in marketing, 497–498
Expense report, 431, 432*t*–433*t*
Explanation of Benefits (EOB), 427
External fraud, 198–199
Extroversion, 314

Facing, of product, 597–598
Fail-safes, for medication errors, 224
Failure mode and effects analysis (FMEA), 168,
  169*t*, 219
Fair Labor Standards Act of 1938
  (FLSA), 329
Family and Medical Leave Act of 1993 (FMLA),
  328*t*, 329, 330
FASB. *See* Financial Accounting Standards Board
Fayol, Henri, 24–25, 29
FDA. *See* Food and Drug Administration
FDAAA. *See* Food and Drug Administration
  Amendments Act
Fee-for-service (FFS), 37, 440
Feedback
  on customer service, 547–548
  in HRM, 340–342
  with performance appraisals, 395–396, 398*t*,
    400–401, 409–410
Field audits, 474
Fifth-tier stakeholders, 85
Finance and financing, 15, 16*t*, 419
  for entrepreneurship, 663–664
  for independent community pharmacies,
    684–686, 687*t*

performance appraisals and, 396–397
  in preplanning phase of strategic planning, 99
Financial Accounting Standards Board (FASB), 420,
  423
Financial budget, 441, 444
Financial Management for Health-System Pharmacists
  (Wilson), 428
Financial planning models, 448
Financial projections, 117–118, 118*t*
Financial ratios, 423–426, 423*t*
Financial reports, 417–436
Financial statements, 420–423, 420*t*, 432*t*
Find, organize, clarify, understand, select, plan, do,
  check, and act (FOCUS-PDCA), 167
First-tier stakeholders, 83
The Five Dysfunctions of a Team (Lencioni), 46
Fleming, J. H., 138
Flexner reports, 6, 7
Flowcharts, for QI, 169
FLSA. *See* Fair Labor Standards Act of 1938
FMEA. *See* Failure mode and effects analysis
FMLA. *See* Family and Medical Leave Act of 1993
Focus groups, 502
FOCUS-PDCA. *See* Find, organize, clarify,
  understand, select, plan, do, check, and act
Food, Drug, and Cosmetic Act of 1938, 7,
  236–237
Food and Drug Administration (FDA), 85, 199,
  362, 580, 630
  on drug shortages, 663
  NDA to, 237
  REMS of, 115, 576–577
Food and Drug Administration Amendments Act
  (FDAAA), 576–577
Forced distribution, for performance appraisals,
  398*t*, 402
Forced-choice rating, for performance appraisals,
  398*t*, 401, 401*t*
Forcing functions, for medication errors, 225
Ford, Henry, 660, 664
Forecasting
  of sales, 441–443
  sensemaking and, 67
Forgery, 360

Formal feedback, 341

Formalization, 300, 302, 307

Formularies
  inventory management of, 567
  product mix and, 562

Four P's, of marketing, 491–497, 521–525

The Four Routes to Entrepreneurial Success (Miner), 660

Fourth-tier stakeholders, 84

Frame-of-reference training, 405

Frank, M. O., 668

Frankl, V. E., 308

Fraud, 198–199

Free-flow layout, 594

Fridy, K., 474

Front end medication errors, 208

Full-time equivalents (FTEs), 115, 115*n*2, 431, 434*t*

Function, 95

Functional discount, 524

Functional quality, 498

Future dating, 572

GAAP. *See* Generally accepted accounting principles

Gaedeke, R. M., 23, 594

Gag clauses, 475

Gaither, Caroline A., 293

Gantt chart, 119, 119*f*

Ganz, Marshal, 45

GDUR. *See* Generic drug utilization rate

General partnership, 684

Generally accepted accounting principles (GAAP), 418

Generic drug utilization rate (GDUR), 456, 460*t*, 462, 463

Generic drugs, 562–563, 566, 571

Generic effective rate (GER), 462

Goals. *See also* Strengths, weaknesses, opportunities, threats
  of CQI, 170
  leadership and, 317
  in operations management, 132–133, 133*t*
  of organizational teams, 306

in performance appraisals, 395–396
  strategic planning and, 100*f*, 102, 102*t*
  for time management, 262–264

Golden Rule, 30, 62

Goleman, Daniel, 44

Good to Great (Collins), 39–40

Gordon, J., 306

GPO. *See* Group Purchasing Organization

Graphic rating, for performance appraisals, 397–400, 398*t*, 399*t*

Grid layouts, 594–595

Gross profit margin, 423*t*, 424, 436, 458

Group organizational culture, 299

Group Purchasing Organization (GPO), 575

Gummesson, E., 503–504

Halo effect, 400

Harassment, 349, 352–353

Harrison, D. L., 103

Hartley, Dan, 361

Harvesting the venture, 665

HDA Research Foundation, 578

Health Care and Education Reconciliation Act of 2010, 674

Health care stakeholders, 83–85, 84*f*, 309–310

Health Insurance Portability and Accountability Act of 1996 (HIPAA), 62, 188, 196, 240–243, 249, 592–593, 593*f*, 674

Health literacy, 221–222

Health Maintenance Act of 1973, 7

Health maintenance organizations (HMOs), 7

Health Plan Employer Data and Information Set (HEDIS), 172

Health-related quality of life (HRQoL), 164–165, 166

Healthy Living Champions, 384

HEDIS. *See* Health Plan Employer Data and Information Set

Heifetz, R. A., 40

Heizer, J., 130

Hepler, C. D., 485

Hersey, P., 315

Hersh, R. H., 61

Hierarchical organization culture, 299

High-reliability organizations (HROs), 223
Hill-Burton (Hospital Survey and Construction) Act of 1946, 7
Hilts, Philip J., 236–239
HIPAA. *See* Health Insurance Portability and Accountability Act of 1996
HMOs. *See* Health maintenance organizations
Hohmeier, Kenneth C., 367
Holistic marketing, 491
Holmes, Erin, 347
Horizontal differentiation, 300
Hospital Survey and Construction (Hill-Burton) Act of 1946, 7
Hostile workplace, 353
How to Get Your Point Across in 30 Seconds or Less (Frank), 668
HRM. *See* Human resources management
HROs. *See* High-reliability organizations
HRQoL. *See* Health-related quality of life
Human factors principles, 165
Human resources management (HRM), 15, 16*t*, 325–344
    coaching in, 337–338
    culture for, 339–340
    development in, 337–338
    interviews in, 334–337, 336*t*, 337*t*
    performance appraisals in, 391–411
    performance feedback in, 340–342
    pharmacy practice and, 327–328
    placement in, 331–337, 332*f*
    in preplanning phase of strategic planning, 99
    recruitment in, 331–333, 332*f*
    regulation of, 328–330, 329*t*
    terminations in, 342–343
Human Sigma, 135–138
Humphrey, Hubert, 237
Hunt, S. D., 486, 487
Hunter, J. C., 50

Illegible handwriting medication errors, 210–211, 249
Immigration Reform and Control Act of 1986 (IRCA), 329, 350
Immunizations, 374, 377, 612

Income statement, 420*t*, 421, 422*t*, 430*t*
Incubators, for entrepreneurship, 667
Indemnity insurance, 457
Independent community pharmacies, 671–692
    characteristics of, 677–679
    competition of, 691
    entrepreneurship in, 679–680
    environments of, 675–677, 676*t*
    finance for, 684–686, 687*t*
    history of, 673—675
    insurance for, 686–687
    intrapreneurship in, 679–680
    licenses for, 686–687
    marketing for, 687
    ownership of, 681–690, 683*t*, 685*t*
    patient care services of, 691–692
    permits for, 686–687
    purchasing established pharmacy, 688–690, 688*t*
    third-party payers for, 676, 691
Independent pharmacy insurance, 194–195
Independent Pharmacy Matching Service (IPMS), 688
Indirect costs, 465
Individual professional liability insurance, 194
Influencer marketing, 499
Informal feedback, 340, 409–410
Information attack, 198
Information technology-related risk (ITRR), 196
Informational organizational structure, 306–307
Injectables, medication errors with, 219–221
Institute of Medicine (IOM), 163, 165, 207, 227–228, 610
Institute of Safe Medication Practice (ISMP), 85
    on ADCs, 218
    on medication errors, 208–210, 212–213, 226, 228*t*, 229
    Sterile Preparation Compounding Safety Summit of, 220
Insurance, 14
    HIPAA and, 62, 188, 196, 240–243, 249, 592–593, 593*f*, 674
    for independent community pharmacies, 686–687
    for liability, 192, 193

receivable turnover ratio and, 426
risk in, 190
risk management and, 192–195
Intellectual property, 666–667
Internal fraud, 198
Internal Revenue Service (IRS), 420
Internet marketing, 528–530
Interpersonal management, 28
Interviews
  in HRM, 334–337, 336t, 337t
  for performance appraisals, 406–407
Intranet, 198
Intrapreneurship, 661, 679–680
Inventory management, 564–569
Inventory turnover ratio (ITOR), 436, 564–566, 565t
IOM. *See* Institute of Medicine
IPMS. *See* Independent Pharmacy Matching Service
IRCA. *See* Immigration Reform and Control Act of 1986
IRS. *See* Internal Revenue Service
Isetts, B. J., 666
ISMP. *See* Institute of Safe Medication Practice
Item-movement report, 568
ITOR. *See* Inventory turnover ratio
ITRR. *See* Information technology-related risk

Jambulingham, T., 666
Jap, S. D., 503
JIT. *See* Just-in-time deliveries
Job description, 333–334, 335t
Job rotation, 337
Job satisfaction, 12, 309–310
Job training, 337
Job turnover, 311–312, 396
The Jungle (Sinclair), 236
Just-in-time deliveries (JIT), 565

Kefauver–Harris Amendments, 237
Keller, K. L., 486, 491, 492, 498
Kelsey, Frances, 237
Kenna, G., 356
Kennedy, John F., 277

Kenton, W., 446
Keresztes, Jan M., 367
Key person insurance, 194
Kilmann, R. H., 50
Kohlberg, L., 61–62, 61f
Kotler, P., 486, 489, 490, 491, 492, 498
Kotter, John, 38, 40–41
Kouzes, J. M., 43, 50

Label similarity medication errors, 218, 218f
Laboratories, 630–631
Laissez-faire leaders, 314
Larson, L. N., 502
Latent end medication errors, 208
Leader-member exchange (LMX), 316, 385–386, 385f
Leader-participation model, 316–317
Leadership, 48t
  accountability and, 49
  adaptive, 40–41
  behavioral theories of, 314
  for chronic diseases, 50
  communication in, 40
  conflict and, 49
  defined, 39
  delegation and, 69–71
  empowerment and, 69–71
  ethics and, 56–57, 67–68
  inertia and, 41
  influence in, 71–72
  inspiration from, 71–72
  management and, 23, 38–39, 38t
  by management teams, 45–49
  mission and, 68–69
  non-positional, 39
  organizational behavior and, 313–318
  passion in, 39–40
  in pharmacy practice, 35–51
  positional, 39
  relationships and, 44–45
  results and, 48–49
  self-awareness in, 41
  self-management and, 45
  sensemaking in, 67

Leadership (*Cont.*):
    short-term wins in, 41
    situational theories of, 315–316
    strategic vision in, 40
    strengths-based approach to, 41–44, 42*t*
    time management for, 261
    trait theories of, 314
    transactional, 317–318
    transformational, 317–319
    trust of, 46–48, 47*t*
    values and, 43
    vision and, 68–69
The Leadership Challenge (Kouzes and Posner), 43, 50
Leading Change (Kotter), 40–41
Leading/directing, in management, 26
Leaner organizations, 305
Leapfrog Group, 173
Learned intermediary doctrine, 195
Leland, K., 551
Lencioni, Patrick, 46
Lenz, T. L., 440
Levitt, Theodore, 493
Liabilities, 419
Liability
    for illegible handwriting, 249
    insurance for, 192, 193
    risk management for, 244–245
Licenses, for independent community pharmacies,
    686–687
Limited partnership, 684
Liquidity ratios, 423*t*, 425
List price, 461
LMX. *See* Leader-member exchange
Long-range budgets, 441–442
Long-term planning, 96
Look-alike drug name medication errors, 211, 211*f*
Lovelock, C., 502, 503
Loyalty, 500
Loyalty programs, 505, 506*t*

MAC. *See* Maximum allowable cost
Machine bureaucracy, 304
MacKeigan, L. D., 502
MacMillan, I., 661
Macroenvironment, 516, 516*f*

Management. *See also specific types*
    activities of, 26–27, 27*f*
    classical and modern views of, 23–25, 24*t*,
        29–30
    control/evaluation in, 26–27
    defined, 22–23
    of employees, 27
    leadership and, 23, 38–39, 38*t*
    leading/directing in, 26
    levels of, 28–29
    mission and, 68–69
    of money, 27
    organizational behavior and, 313
    organizing in, 26
    planning in, 25–26, 93–95
    process of, 25–29, 26*f*
    resources of, 27–28
    study reasons for, 30–31, 32*f*–33*f*
    of value, 75–86
    vision and, 68–69
Management by crisis, 105
Management by objective (MBO), 403–404
Management functions, 21–31
Management teams, 45–49, 305
Managerial sciences, 15–17, 16*t*
Manolakis, Michael L., 55
Market research
    for business planning, 113–114
    for independent community pharmacies, 682
    for value-added services, 615–618
Marketing, 15–16, 16*t*, 485*n*1
    applications, 513–533
    in business planning, 116–117
    company orientations to, 489–491
    data collection for, 501–502
    definitions and concepts, 486–487
    for employee recruitment, 331–333, 332*f*
    exchange in, 487–488
    expectations in, 497–498
    four P's of, 491–497, 521–525
    fundamentals of, 483–508
    for independent community pharmacies, 687
    on Internet, 528–530
    for MTM, 485, 494
    to needs, wants, and demands, 488–489

PDMA on, 243
by pharmacy technicians, 384
in preplanning phase of strategic planning, 99
quality in, 498–499
relationship, 503–507, 505t, 506t
satisfaction in, 498–499
science of, 487
of services, 9, 10t, 494n8
situation analysis for, 516–517
steps of, 515, 515f
strategic planning for, 515
value in, 499–500, 500f
of value-added services, 643–644
Marketing concept, 490
Marketing control, 531
Marketing efficiency, 505
Marketing mix, 491–497, 521–525, 642
Marketing myopia, 493–494
Markula Center for Applied Ethics, EDM model of,
    58–59, 59f
Marshall, L. L., 271–272
Master budget, 441–445, 442f, 446–448,
    447t
Master list, for time management, 264–265
Maximum allowable cost (MAC), 456, 460t
MBO. See Management by objective
MBWA. See Practice
    management-by-walking-around
McCarthy, E. J., 492
McConnell, W. E., 226
McDonough, R. P., 489, 502
McGrath, R. G., 661
McKeown, Greg, 39
Medicaid
    HIPPA and, 243
    receivable turnover ratio and, 426
    as third-party payer, 457
    340B Drug Pricing Program and, 579
Medicare
    EHR for, 200
    HIPPA and, 243
    Part D of, 76, 104, 173, 457–458, 674
    PDPs for, 426
    prospective payment system for, 7
    as third-party payer, 457–458

Medicare Improvements for Patients and Providers
    Act (MIPPA), 200
Medicare Prescription Drug, Improvement and
    Modernization Act (MMA), 9, 104, 674
Medication adherence. See Adherence
Medication Error Reporting Program (MERP), 228f,
    229
Medication errors, 12
    from abbreviations, 212–213, 213f
    accountability for, 222–224
    from adherence, 222
    from ambiguous orders, 213–215, 214f
    auxiliary labels and, 219
    communication and, 207
    in e-prescribing, 209–210, 209f, 210f, 225
    fail-safes for, 224
    forcing functions for, 225
    HRM and, 327
    from illegible handwriting, 210–211, 249
    in independent community pharmacies, 676
    with injectables, 219–221
    from label similarities, 218, 218f
    from look-alike drug names, 211, 211f
    from packaging similarities, 216, 217f
    patient counseling and education and,
        221–229
    prevention and management of, 205–230
    redundant checks for, 215–219
    reporting of, 226–229, 228f
    risk identification methods for, 226–229
    risk-reduction strategies for, 224–226, 224t
    from sound-alike drug names, 211–212
Medication therapy management (MTM), 9–11, 76,
    104
    adherence and, 9, 82
    budget for, 443
    clinical purists in, 12
    CPAs for, 635
    customer service with, 540
    with good management practice, 13–15, 14t
    independent community pharmacies and, 674
    marketing for, 485, 494
    by pharmacy technicians, 373
    pharmacy technicians for, 374, 378–379
    QI and, 163–164, 166

Medication therapy management (MTM) (*Cont.*):
  third-party payers and, 478
  value-added services and, 627–628
Medwatch, 580
Mentorship, 665
Merchandising, 585–604
  collaborations for, 587–588, 588*f*
  pharmacy design for, 589–593, 590*f,*
    592*f,* 593*f*
  pharmacy layout for, 593–595, 594*f*
  of prescription department, 599–601, 600*f,* 601*f*
  technology in, 601–603
  trends in, 588–589
MERP. *See* Medication Error Reporting Program
Merrill, R. R., 46–47, 47*t*
Meyer, Urban, 339
MI. *See* Motivational interviewing
Microenvironment, 516, 516*f*
Milanovic, Randy, 258
Millis Commission, 8, 370
Miner, John, 660
Minimum wage, 329
Mintzberg, H., 304
MIPPA. *See* Medicare Improvements for Patients and
    Providers Act
Mirror to Hospital Pharmacy, by American Society of
    Hospital Pharmacists, 8
Mission
  leadership and, 68–69
  product mix and, 562
  strategic planning and, 97–98, 100*f,* 102*t*
  for time management, 262–264
MMA. *See* Medicare Prescription Drug,
    Improvement and Modernization Act
Moczygemba, Leticia R., 3, 391
Moderating factors, in EDM models, 65
Modular organizations, 304–305
Modularity, 198
Moments of truth, 504
Monaghan, M. S., 440
Money management, 27
Monitoring
  CMM, 11, 627–628
  PDMP, 239, 244–245

of performance appraisals, 407–408
of strategic plan, 103
of value-added service, 644–645
Moral reasoning, 61–62, 61*f*
Morgenstern, J., 263–264, 268
Mosavin, Rashid, 417
Most favored nation clause, in third-party payer
    contracts, 475
Motivational interviewing (MI), 287–289
MTM. *See* Medication therapy management
Multi-rater assessment, for performance appraisals,
    398*t,* 400–401
Multisource drugs, 462
Myers, S., 419
Mystery shopping, 502

NABP. *See* National Association of Boards of
    Pharmacy
Narver, J. C., 489
NASA. *See* National Aeronautics and Space
    Administration
Nash, John, 278–279
NASPA. *See* National Alliance of State Pharmacy
    Associations
National Academies of Medicine, 312
National Aeronautics and Space Administration
    (NASA), 327–328
National Alliance of State Pharmacy Associations
    (NASPA), 635–636
National Association of Boards of Pharmacy
    (NABP), 173
National Committee for QA (NCQA), 172
National Community Pharmacy Association
    (NCPA), 424, 614, 678, 682, 688
National Coordination Council for Medication
    Error Reporting, 166
National Council for Prescription Drug Programs,
    244
National Institute for Occupational Safety and
    Health (NIOSH), 361
National Institute on Drug Abuse (NIDA),
    243–244, 377
National origin discrimination, 350
National Pharmacist Workforce Survey, 305

NCPA. *See* National Community Pharmacy
  Association
NCPA Digest, 676–677
NCQA. *See* National Committee for QA
NDA. *See* New drug application
Needs, 488–489
  value-added services and, 619–620
Negative goods, 489
Negligence
  in insurance, 192
  liability of, 244
  OBRA 90 and, 195
Negotiation, 275–292
  BATNA, 282–283
  dirty tricks in, 285–286
  equilibrium in, 278
  MI for, 287–289
  options in, 282
  phrases to use in, 284–285, 284*t*
  positional, 279–282, 279*t*, 289–290
  principled, 279–282, 279*t*, 283*t*,
    290–291
  recommendations for, 282
  standards for, 281
  traditional styles of, 277–279
  types of, 285
Nelson, B., 29
Nelson, Mel L., 161
Net income, 422
Net profit, 422
Net profit margin, 423*t*, 424, 436
Net-profit-to-average-inventory ratio, 566
Networked organizations, 304–305
Never Split the Difference (Voss and Raz), 283
New drug application (NDA), 237
NIDA. *See* National Institute on Drug Abuse
NIOSH. *See* National Institute for Occupational
  Safety and Health
Noncumulative quantity discounts, 571
Non-positional leadership, 39
Nonrationalist model, in moral reasoning,
  61–62, 61*f*
Nonresponse bias, 548
Normative marketing, 487

Obesity, 355
Objective price, 494
Objective quality, 498
OBRA 90. *See* Omnibus Budget Reconciliation Act
  of 1990
Occupational Safety and Health Act of 1970
  (OSHA), 330–331, 362, 635, 642
Odd pricing, 523
Office of Inspector General (OIG), 243
Office of Pharmacy Affairs (OPA), 579–580
Office of Technology Assessment, U.S. (OTA),
  162–163
OHIO. *See* Only Handle It Once
OIG. *See* Office of Inspector General
Oliver, R. L., 501
Omnibus Budget Reconciliation Act of 1990
  (OBRA 90), 165, 195, 239–240, 674
Only Handle It Once (OHIO), 264
OPA. *See* Office of Pharmacy Affairs
Open-to-buy budget, 570–571
Openness to experience, 314
Operational planning, 94*t*, 102–103
Operational risk, 198–200, 201*t*
Operationalization, of strategic plan, 102
Operations
  budget for, 440, 443–444
  business planning for, 115–116, 116*f*
  strategic planning in, 91–106
Operations management, 16, 16*t*, 127–140
  action plan in, 133–135, 134*t*
  command intent in, 131–133
  goals in, 132–133, 133*t*
  Human Sigma and, 135–138
  role of, 130–131, 131*t*
Opioid crisis, 104, 244–245, 357
Opportunity costs, 197
Organizational behavior, 293–318
  centralization of, 300, 302–303
  culture for, 296–299, 298*f*
  defined, 294–296
  departmentalization in, 300, 304
  differentiation of, 299–302, 301*f*
  division of labor in, 300, 303, 308
  emotions and, 312–313

Organizational behavior (*Cont.*):
  ethics in, 308
  formalization for, 300, 302, 307
  informal, 306–307
  leadership and, 313–318
  management and, 313
  principles of, 296–307, 297*f*
  professional model for, 307–309
  span of control in, 300, 303–304
  stress and, 310–311
  structure for, 299–302, 301*f*
  unity of command in, 300, 303
Organizational commitment, 310
Organizational Culture Profile, 299
Organizational identification, 311–312
Organizational management, 28–29
Organizational planning, 94*t*
Organizational rewards, 408–409
Organizational teams, 305–306
Ortmeier, B. G., 103
OSHA. *See* Occupational Safety and Health Act of
  1970
OTA. *See* Office of Technology Assessment, U.S.
OTC. *See* Over-the-counter drugs
Outcome-oriented systems, for performance
  appraisals, 403–404, 403*t*
Over-the-counter drugs (OTC)
  ITOR for, 564
  marketing of, 485
  medication errors with, 207
  pharmacy layout for, 594
  pharmacy technicians and, 373, 374
  pro-DUR for, 239
  regulation of, 237
  right quantity of, 569
Overall evaluation surveys, 502
Overtime wages, 329
Ovretveit, J., 163
Owner's equity, 419
Ownership programs, 574

Packaging similarity medication errors, 216, 217*f*
PAI. *See* Practice Alignment Initiative
Paid family leave, 330

Paired comparisons, for performance appraisals,
  398*t*, 402
Palmatier, R. W., 503
PAPCC. *See* Patient Access to Pharmacists' Care
  Coalition
Parallel teams, 305
Parenteral nutrition (PN), 219
Participative budget, 451–452
Partnerships, 683–684, 683*t*
Passion
  of entrepreneurs, 660–661
  in leadership, 39–40
Patents, 667
  expiration of, 562–563
Patient Access to Pharmacists' Care Coalition
  (PAPCC), 674–675
Patient care services
  budget for, 443–444
  of independent community pharmacies, 691–692
Patient counseling and education
  medication errors and, 221–229
  OBRA 90 and, 239
  as value-added service, 612, 636
Patient days, 434*t*, 436
Patient Protection and Affordable Care Act (ACA),
  76, 82
  independent community pharmacies and, 674
  Medicare and, 9
  third-party payers and, 457–458
  340B Drug Pricing Program and, 579
  value-added services and, 614
Patient Safety and Quality Improvement Act of
  2005, 229
Patient Safety and Quality Improvement final rule,
  by U.S. Department of Health and Human
  Services, (DHHS), 229
Patient Safety Organizations (PSOs), 229
Patient-centered care delivery, 10*t*
Patient-centered medical home model (PCMH), 82
Patton, George S., 132
Pay equity laws, 329–330
Pay for performance. *See* Value-based reimbursement
PBM. *See* Pharmacy benefit manager
PCMH. *See* Patient-centered medical home model

PDA. *See* Pregnancy Discrimination Act of 1978

PDAPs. *See* Prescription drug assistance programs

PDMA. *See* Prescription Drug Marketing Act of 1987

PDMP. *See* Prescription drug monitoring program

PDPs. *See* Prescription Drug Plans

People, in four P's of marketing, 496

Perceived price, 494

Perceived quality, 498

Perceived value (PV), 77, 79–82

Perfectionism, 260

Performance, in four P's of marketing, 496–497

Performance appraisals
    absolute systems for, 397–401, 398*t*
    BARS for, 398*t*, 400, 401*t*
    budget and, 440
    communication of, 395
    defined, 393
    for employees, 391–411
    feedback for, 395–396, 398*t*, 400–401, 409–410
    finance and, 396–397
    forced-choice rating for, 398*t*, 401, 401*t*
    goals in, 395–396
    graphic rating for, 397–400, 398*t*, 399*t*
    informal feedback and, 409–410
    interviews for, 406–407
    monitoring of, 407–408
    motivation and, 409–410
    organizational rewards and, 408–409
    outcome-oriented systems for, 403–404, 403*t*
    QI and, 405–406
    rationale for, 393–396, 394*t*
    relative systems for, 398*t*, 401–403
    reliability of, 407–408
    rewards and, 396
    rewards differentiation in, 405
    special considerations for, 404–405
    types of, 397–404, 398*t*
    validity of, 407–408

Performance risk, 197–198, 201*t*

Peril, in insurance, 193

Periodic method, for inventory management, 567

Permits, for independent community pharmacies, 686–687

Perpetual method, for inventory management, 567

Personal financing, 686

Personal selling, 530–531

Personalized medication record (PMR), 628

Pharmaceutical care, 8–11
    domains of, 9, 10*t*

PHARMacist Entrepreneurial Orientation (PHARMEO), 666

Pharmacist-in-Charge (PIC), 238–239

Pharmacists
    as prescribers, 246
    standards for, 235–236

Pharmacists for the Future: The Report of the Study Commission on Pharmacy (Millis), 8

Pharmacists Mutual, 357

Pharmacists' Patient Care Process (PPCP), 246, 629

Pharmacists training, for value-added services, 642

Pharmacy benefit manager (PBM), 427
    customer service and, 540
    third-party payers and, 457

Pharmacy networks, of third-party payers, 458–459

Pharmacy practice
    as career path, 129–130
    history of, 6–8
    HRM and, 327–328
    labor demand decline for, 76
    leadership in, 35–51
    myths on, 11–12
    profit margins in, 14–15
    QI in, 162–175
    risk management in, 187–202
    technology in, 15
    time management in, 268–270
    trust in, 14

Pharmacy Practice Accreditation, 115

Pharmacy Quality Alliance (PQA), 173, 245, 464

Pharmacy Reconciliation Report (PRR), 427–428

Pharmacy services administrative organizations (PSAOs), 459

Pharmacy Technician Certification Board (PTCB), 371, 372

Pharmacy Technician Education Council (PTEC), 371

Pharmacy technicians, 367–387
  for adherence, 376
  certification of, 371
  current landscape for, 379–384, 380*t*–383*t*
  for DUR, 372, 374
  education and training of, 373
  ethics of, 383
  history of, 369–370
  international perspectives on, 383–384
  for MTM, 373, 374, 378–379
  OTC products and, 373, 374
  performance appraisals for, 404
  for public health initiatives, 376–377
  QA and, 374
  regulation of, 248
  roles of, 375–379
  supervision of, 384–386, 385*f*
  for transitions of care, 375–376
Pharmacy-buying groups, 575–576
PharmD degree, 8, 12
  public health in, 612
  stress of, 271
PHARMEO. *See* PHARMacist Entrepreneurial
  Orientation
PHI. *See* Protected health information
Piaget, Jean, 61
PIC. *See* Pharmacist-in-Charge
PillPack, 8
Place, in four P's of marketing, 494–495, 524–525
Placement, in HRM, 331–337, 332*f*
Plan-o-grams, 597–598, 597*f*
Planning. *See also* Business planning; Strategic
  planning
  barriers to, 104–105, 105*t*
  budget for, 439
  limitations to, 105–106
  in management, 25–26, 93–95
  steps in, 95*t*
  types of, 94*t*
PLUS EDM Model, 60–61
PMR. *See* Personalized medication record
PN. *See* Parenteral nutrition
Point-of-care testing, 377
Point-of-purchase materials, 598–599

Point-of-sale (POS), 567
Poison Prevention Packaging Act, 247–248
POS. *See* Point-of-sale
Positional leadership, 39
Positional negotiation, 279–282, 279*t*, 289–290
Positioning, in four P's of marketing, 495–496
Positive affect, 313
Positive marketing, 487
Posner, B. Z., 43, 50
Post-conventional stage, in moral reasoning, 62
Post-transaction surveys, 502
Postplanning phase, of strategic planning, 101–102
PPCP. *See* Pharmacists' Patient Care Process
PQA. *See* Pharmacy Quality Alliance
Practice Alignment Initiative (PAI), 92
Practice management-by-walking-around (MBWA),
  340
Preconventional stage, in moral reasoning, 62
Predicted service level, 497
Pregnancy Discrimination Act of 1978 (PDA),
  328–329, 328*t*, 348, 352
Preplanning phase, of strategic planning, 98–99
Prescription department, merchandising of,
  599–601, 600*f*, 601*f*
Prescription drug assistance programs (PDAPs), 376
Prescription Drug Marketing Act of 1987 (PDMA),
  243
Prescription drug monitoring program (PDMP),
  239, 244–245
Prescription Drug Plans (PDPs), 426
Preventing Medication Errors (IOM), 207
Price
  in four P's of marketing, 494, 523–524
  in RVT, 78–79
Principled negotiation, 279–282, 279*t*, 283*t*,
  290–291
Principles of Corporate Finance (Brealy, Myers and
  Allen), 419
The Principles of Scientific Management (Taylor), 24
Print media advertising, 526–528, 529*f*
Prisoner's dilemma, 278–279
Privacy, 57
  drug testing and, 356
  HIPAA on, 240, 241

Private-label products, 574, 599

Pro forma analysis, 470–471, 472*t*–473*t*

Pro forma financial statements, 441

Pro-DUR. *See* Prospective drug use review

Problem-solving
delegation for, 69–71
empowerment for, 69–71
with ethical dilemmas, 57–58

Processes, in four P's of marketing, 496

Procurement, 569–576

Procurement costs, 564

Product
facing of, 597–598
in four P's of marketing, 492–494, 522–523

Product concept, 490

Product lifecycle costs, budget for, 449–450

Product mix, in supply chain management, 561–563

Production budget, 441, 443

Production concept, 489–490

Productivity ratios, 434, 434*t*

Professional model, for organizational behavior,
307–309

Profit margins
gross, 423*t*, 424, 436, 458
net, 423*t*, 424, 436
PV and, 81
shrinking of, 14–15

Profitability ratios, 423*t*, 424

Profits
accounting for, 419–420
average net profit comparison, 465–469,
468*t*–469*t*
budget for, 440
net, 422

Programs, in four P's of marketing, 496

Progressive discipline, 341

Project teams, 305

Promotion
in four P's of marketing, 495, 525
of independent community pharmacies, 687

Property insurance, 193

Prospective drug use review (Pro-DUR), 195, 239,
240

Prospective payment system, for Medicare, 7

Protected health information (PHI), 196, 200,
240–241

PRR. *See* Pharmacy Reconciliation Report

PSAOs. *See* Pharmacy services administrative
organizations

PSOs. *See* Patient Safety Organizations

Psychological pricing, 523

Psychosocial risk, 200, 201*t*

PTCB. *See* Pharmacy Technician Certification Board

PTEC. *See* Pharmacy Technician Education
Council

Public health
immunizations for, 612
value-added services and, 609–621

Publicity, 531

Purchase-trend report, 568

Purchasing, 569–576
of established pharmacy, 688–690, 688*t*

Pure Food and Drug Act of 1906, 236

Pure risk, 90

PV. *See* Perceived value

QA. *See* Quality assurance

QC. *See* Quality control

QI. *See* Quality improvement

Quality
in marketing, 498–499
service, 498–499

Quality assurance (QA), 167
for automated compounding equipment, 221
pharmacy technicians and, 374

Quality control (QC), 166

Quality improvement (QI), 162–175
accreditation for, 171–173
defined, 162–163
measurement of, 163–165
methods for, 166–167
in other industries, 165–166
performance appraisals and, 405–406
for value-added services, 645–647

Quality of life
HRQoL, 164–165, 166
time management for, 259

Quality of performance standards, 407–408

Quantity discounts, 571
Quick ratio, 423*t*, 425, 436
Quid pro quo sexual harassment, 353
Quinn, R. E., 298–299, 298*f*

Race discrimination, 349
Radial tunnel syndrome, 200
Radiofrequency identification (RFID), 199, 440, 569
Rath, T., 40
Rational organizational culture, 299
Rationalist model, in moral reasoning, 61–62, 61*f*
Raz, T., 283, 284, 285
RCA. *See* Root cause analysis
Reasonable accommodation, 355–356
Receipt of goods (ROG), 572
Receivables turnover ratio, 423*t*, 425–426, 436
Recruitment, 331–333, 332*f*
Reframing Leadership (Bolman and Deal), 50
Regulation and regulators
   in business planning, 114–115
   case examples of, 247–249
   compliance with, 233–249
   effect of, 245
   of employees, 347–365
   as fourth-tier stakeholders, 84
   future of, 245–246
   of HRM, 328–330, 329*t*
   necessity of, 236–237
   of OTC, 237
   PIC and, 238–239
   by states, 237–238
Reichheld, F. F., 501
Relationship marketing, 503–507, 505*t*, 506*t*
Relationships
   in Human Sigma, 138
   leadership and, 44–45
   in situational leadership, 315
Relative systems, for performance appraisals, 398*t*, 401–403
Relative value (RV), 77
Relative value theorem (RVT), 79*f*
   price in, 78–79

PV in, 77, 79–82
   service in, 79
Relator time managers, 261–262
Reliability
   of customer service, 539*t*
   HROs, 223
   of performance appraisals, 407–408
   of service quality, 498
Religious discrimination, 350–351
Reminders, medication errors and, 225
REMS. *See* Risk Evaluation and Mitigation Strategies
Render, B., 130
Reorder point, 570
Repackaging services, 574
Repetitive-motion injuries, 200
Resource allocation
   in budget, 440
   for entrepreneurship, 663–664
Resource planning, 94*t*
Responsiveness
   of customer service, 539*t*
   of service quality, 498
Rest, James, 6, 61
Restocking errors, 216
Retail class of trade, 462
Return on assets (ROA), 424, 436
Return on equity (ROE), 424
Returned-goods policies, 566
Revolving budget, 441
Rewards
   organizational, 408–409
   in performance appraisals, 396, 405
RFID. *See* Radiofrequency identification
Rider, on insurance policy, 193
Right price, in purchasing, 571–572
Right quantity, in purchasing, 569–571
Right time, in purchasing, 569–571
Risk
   defined, 189–190
   in insurance coverage, 190
   ITRR, 196
   operational, 198–200, 201*t*
   paradigm, 201, 201*t*
   performance, 197–198, 201*t*

psychosocial, 200, 201*t*

quantitative and qualitative approach to, 201

strategic, 196–197, 201*t*

Risk Evaluation and Mitigation Strategies (REMS), 115, 576–577

Risk management, 9, 10*t*

insurance coverage and, 192–195

for liability, 244–245

in pharmacy practice, 187–202

process of, 190–191

strategy for, 190

techniques for, 191–192

ROA. *See* Return on assets

Robbery, 357–358, 358*t*, 360*t*

Robinson, Evan T., 55

ROE. *See* Return on equity

ROG. *See* Receipt of goods

Rohrbaugh, J., 298–299, 298*f*

Role ambiguity, 395

Role conflict, 395

Role stress, 395

Rolling budgets, 441

Root cause analysis (RCA), 168–169, 169*t*, 219

Rosenthal, M. M., 440

Rough, S., 434

RV. *See* Relative value

RVT. *See* Relative value theorem

SAAS. *See* Software-as-a-service

SAC. *See* Statistical Analysis Center

Safety stock, 570

Sales forecasting, in master budget, 441–443

Sales promotions, 531

Sales revenue budget, 441

Satisfaction

job, 12, 309–310

in marketing, 498–499

from service recovery, 545

surveys, for customer service, 547–548

SBIRT. *See* Screening, Brief Intervention, and Referral to Treatment

Schumock, Glen T., 91, 109

Schwartz, M. S., 63–64

Scope of practice laws, 246

Screening, Brief Intervention, and Referral to Treatment (SBIRT), 377

Seasonal discount, 524

SEC. *See* Securities and Exchange Commission

Second-tier stakeholders, 83–84

Securities and Exchange Commission (SEC), 420

SEIPS. *See* Systems engineering initiative for patient safety

Self-assessments, for medication errors, 226

Self-awareness

delegation and, 71

in leadership, 41

leadership and, 318

sensemaking and, 66

Self-management, 28, 255–272

for career planning, 257–258

leadership and, 45

stress and, 270–272, 271*t*

time management in, 258–272, 260*f*, 261*t*, 267*t*, 269*t*

Self-reflection, sensemaking and, 66–67

Self-service kiosks, 601–602

Selling concept, 490

Semi-variable costs, 464–465

Sensemaking, in ethics, 64–67

Serial discounts, 572, 572*t*

The Servant Leader (Hunter), 50

Service benefit plans, 457

Service blueprint, 493

Service criticality, 541

Service failure, 540–541

Service quality, 498–499

Service recovery, 541–547, 542*f*

Service recovery paradox, 547

Services. *See also* Customer service; Value-added services

marketing of, 9, 10*t*, 494*n8*

in RVT, 79

SERVQUAL, 498

The 7 Habits of Highly Effective People (Covey), 38

Sex discrimination, 352–353

Sexual harassment, 352–353

Sheth, J. N., 503
Shoplifting, 359–360, 361t
Short-range budgets, 441
Short-term wins, in leadership, 41
Shrinkage, 566
Sick leave, 360
Signature Themes of talent, 41
Sinclair, Upton, 236
Sinek, Simon, 36
Single-payer reimbursement, 14
Situation analysis, 99
    for marketing, 516–517
Situational theories, of leadership, 315–316
Six Sigma, 136
SMART. *See* Specific, measurable, achievable,
    realistic, and timed
Social Security Act, 243, 249
Societal marketing concept, 491
Society for Human Resource Management, 364
Software-as-a-service (SAAS), 449
Sole proprietorship, 683, 683t
Sorensen, Todd D., 35
Sound-alike drug names medication errors, 211–212
Sourcing, 572–573
Span of control, 300, 303–304
Spatial differentiation, 302
Specialty distributors, 559, 573–575, 575f
Specialty drugs, 577–579, 578t
    strategic planning for, 104
Specific, measurable, achievable, realistic, and timed
    (SMART), 100–101, 100t, 263
Speculative risk, 189–190
Speculative stock, 570
Speed of Trust (Covey and Merrill), 46–47, 47t
Standardization
    medication errors and, 225
    for organizational behavior, 307
    of pharmacy technician education, 373
    for QI, 165–166
Standards
    for customer service, 538–540, 539t
    for negotiation, 281
    for pharmacists, 235–236
Start with Why (Sinek), 36

State boards of pharmacy, 237–238
State of Pharmacy Compounding Survey, 219
State pharmacy practice acts, 237–238
Statement of cash flows, 420t, 422–423, 422t
Statement of retained earnings, 422, 422t
Statistical Analysis Center (SAC), 361
Sterile Preparation Compounding Safety Summit, of
    ISMP, 220
Stock depth, 570
Strand, L. M., 485
Strategic money, 663
Strategic planning, 94t, 95–104, 103t
    defined, 96
    examples of, 102t, 103–104
    for marketing, 515
    mission and, 97–98
    in operations, 91–106
    time horizon for, 96–97
    vision and, 97–98
Strategic risk, 196–197, 201t
Strategic vision, in leadership, 40
Strengths, weaknesses, opportunities, threats
    (SWOT), 101, 101f, 119, 120t, 121t, 514,
    516–519, 518t
Strengths-based approach, to leadership,
    41–44, 42t
Strengths-Based Leadership (Rath and Conchie), 40
StrengthsFinder, 41
Stress
    organizational behavior and, 310–311
    self-management and, 270–272, 271t
    time management and, 270–272, 271t
Supply chain management, 557–582, 560f
    demand planning and, 561–564
    functions of, 560–561, 561t
    inventory management and, 564–569
    procurement in, 569–576
    product mix in, 561–563
Suspensions, 342
SWOT. *See* Strengths, weaknesses, opportunities,
    threats
System failures, 199–100
Systems engineering initiative for patient safety
    (SEIPS), 164, 379

Tactics, 102
Target market, 520–521, 521*t*
   in business planning, 114
Taylor, F. W., 24–25, 29
Teas, R. K., 499
Tech-check-tech, 374, 377–378, 404
Technical quality, 498
Technology
   for inventory management, 568–569
   ITRR, 196
   in merchandising, 601–603
   in pharmacy practice, 15
Terminations, in HRM, 342–343
Terms of sale, 571
Thalidomide, 236, 237
The Joint Commission (TJC), 115, 171–172, 226
Theft, 359–361
   pharmacy layout and, 595
Therapeutic duplication, 239, 628
Thiel, C. E., 65
Third-party assistance services, 575–576
Third-party payers, 14, 455–478, 459–462, 460*t*
   contract terminology of, 474–475
   direct and indirect remuneration by, 462
   financial impact of, 464–471
   future of, 477–478
   for independent community pharmacies,
      676, 691
   pharmacy networks of, 458–459
   receivable turnover ratio and, 426
   response to reimbursement response for, 475–476
   for value-added services, 616, 647–649
Third-tier stakeholders, 84
Thomas, K. W., 50
Thomas–Kilmann Conflict Mode (Thomas and
      Kilmann), 50
340B Drug Pricing Program, 579–580, 579*t*
360-degree feedback, for performance appraisals,
      398*t*, 400–401
Thurman, Howard, 39
Time journal, 261
Time management, 258–272, 261*t*, 267*t*, 269*t*
   goals for, 262–264
   for leadership, 261

master list for, 264–265
mission for, 262–264
myths and pitfalls of, 259–260, 260*f*
in pharmacy practice, 268–270
prioritization of tasks in, 265–266
review, revise, and modify in, 268
schedule of tasks in, 266
stress and, 270–272, 271*t*
systems for, 266–267
Tipton, D. J., 544
Title VII, 328*t*, 329, 348, 349–353, 394
TJC. *See* The Joint Commission
To Err Is Human (IOM), 207, 227–228
Tobacco cessation, 376–377
Tootelian, D. H., 23, 594
Total parenteral nutrition (TPN), 219–221
"The Toxic Pharmacist" (Draper), 64
TPN. *See* Total parenteral nutrition
Trademarks, 667
Traditional distributors, 559, 573
Trait theories, of leadership, 314
Transactional leadership, 317–318
Transactions, 488
Transfers, 488
Transformational leadership, 317–318
Transitions of care, pharmacy technicians for,
      375–376
Triple Aim, 37
Trust
   delegation and, 71
   of leadership, 46–48, 47*t*
   in pharmacy practice, 14
   from service recovery, 547
Turner, Kyle M., 35
Turnover ratios, 423*t*, 425–426

U&C. *See* Usual and customary pharmacy price
Umbrella liability, 193
Unclaimed prescriptions, 566
Underwater MACs, 462
Undue hardship, 351, 355
Uniform Guidelines on Employee Selection
      Procedures of 1978, 334
Unity of command, 300, 303

Use of performance appraisal results, 408
Usual and customary pharmacy price (U&C), 460
Utilitarianism, 59
Utilization Review Accreditation Commission, 115

Validity, of performance appraisals, 407–408
Value
   creation, 16–17, 16*t*
   examples of, 84
   for health care stakeholders, 83–85, 84*f*
   management of, 75–86
   in marketing, 499–500, 500*f*
   RVT, 77–82, 79*f*
Value-added services, 627*f*
   business planning for, 613–614
   competition for, 616–617
   components of, 629–636
   data collection for, 630, 631*f*–634*f*
   immunizations, 612
   implementation of, 625–650
   market research for, 615–618
   marketing mix for, 642
   marketing of, 643–644
   monitoring of, 644–645
   MTM and, 627–628
   needs and, 619–620
   outcome measurements of, 636–637
   patient counseling and education as, 612, 636
   pharmacists training for, 642
   public health and, 609–621
   QI for, 645–647
   third-party payers for, 616, 647–649
   types of, 615*t*, 627–629
Value-based reimbursement, 37, 463–464
Values, leadership and, 43
Vendors, 573–576, 573*t*, 574*f*, 575*f*
Verbal warning, 341
Vertical differentiation, 300–301
Veterans Administration, 8, 85
Virtual organizations, 304–305

Vision
   leadership and, 68–69
   strategic planning and, 97–98, 100*f*, 102*t*
Visual method, for inventory management, 567
Von Bertalanffy, L., 165
Voss, C., 283, 284, 285
Votta, R. J., 270–271

WAC. *See* Wholesaler acquisition cost
Wants, 488–489
Warholak, Terri L., 161
Weick, Karl, 64–65
Weitz, B. A., 503
Well-being, 312
   marketing for, 491
WHO. *See* World Health Organization
Wholesaler acquisition cost (WAC),
   460–461, 460*t*
Wholesalers, as fifth-tier stakeholders, 85
Wick, J. Y., 271
Willink, D. P., 666
Wilson, Andrew, 428
Wood, M., 356
Woodhull, A. V., 261, 262
Word-of-mouth
   on customer service, 546–547
   eWOM, 499
Work standards approach, to performance appraisals,
   398*t*, 404
Work teams, 305
Worker's compensation, 193, 194
Workgroups, 305
World Health Organization (WHO), 384
Wright, L., 502, 503
Written warning, 341–342
Wynn, William, 127

Zanni, G. R., 271
Zgarrick, David P., 3, 21
Zone of tolerance, 497, 546